WM 224 H

KINGSWAY HOSPITAL MEDICAL LIBRARY

Early-Onset Dementia:
a multidisciplinary approach

Early-Onset Dementia:
a multidisciplinary approach

Edited by
John R. Hodges

MRC Cognition and Brain Sciences Unit
Cambridge
and
Department of Neurology
University of Cambridge
Addenbrooke's Hospital

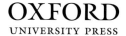

OXFORD

UNIVERSITY PRESS

Great Clarendon Street, Oxford OX2 6DP

Oxford University Press is a department of the University of Oxford.
It furthers the University's objective of excellence in research, scholarship,
and education by worldwide in

Oxford   New York

Athens Auckland Bangkok Bogotá Buenos Aires Cape Town
Chenai Dar es Salaam Delhi Florence Hong Kong Istanbul
Karachi Kolkata Kuala Lumpur Madrid Melbourne Mexico City Mumbai
Nairobi Paris São Paulo Shanghai Singapore Taipei Tokyo Toronto Warsaw

and associated companies in Berlin   Ibadan

Oxford is a registered trade mark of Oxford University Press
in the UK and in certain other countries

Published in the United States
by Oxford University Press Inc., New York

A catalogue record for this title is available from the British Library.

Library of Congress Cataloging in Publication Data

Early-onset dementia : a multidisciplinary approach / edited by John R. Hodges.
Includes bibliographical references and index.
1. Presenile dementia   2. Dementia   I. Hodges, John R.
RC522 . E37 2001   616.8′3–dc21   2001021614

ISBN 0 19 263034 2 (Hbk)

10   9   8   7   6   5   4   3   2   1

Typeset by EXPO Holdings, Malaysia
Printed in Great Britain
on acid-free paper by
Biddles Ltd.,
Guildford & King's Lynn

Preface

The idea of putting together this book arose in 1997 at the same time as we decided to start a multidisciplinary clinic in Cambridge for patients with presenile dementia. Although uncommon in comparison to dementia in the elderly, each case represents a tragedy for the patient and their family, which often includes both children and parents. There are also different medical issues to confront with in young patients with dementia: diseases that are rare in the elderly are represented to a much greater extent, and some (such as frontotemporal dementia and the inborn errors of metabolism) occur only under the age of 65 necessitating a thorough search for the rarer and occasionally reversible causes of dementia; genetic factors are also considerably more important in this age group.

Colleagues visiting the new clinic and those who referred patients began to ask where they could read up about clinical issues related to presenile dementia and the latest advances in the field. Although there existed many fine texts dealing with dementia in general and detailed monographs on specific disorders there were no books dedicated to the special problems of early onset dementia. After initial soundings from local friends I decided to edit a book which would encompass the topics of special interest to me — notably the clinical and neuropsychological features of the dementias — and also include reviews of the advances in the relevant neurosciences and the important issue patient management. This plan was greeted with enthusiasm by Richard Marley from Oxford University Press who had steered the book through its sometimes stormy gestation. After some discussion we decided on the title of early onset, rather than presenile, dementia which avoids any strict age cut-off and is less pejorative.

I was extremely fortunate that such an eminent and conscientious group of colleagues from around the world agreed to contribute and accepted graciously my editorial suggestions. Each author was asked to critically evaluate the state of current knowledge for the non-expert and to provide as many visual aids in the forms of tables and figures as possible, and most importantly a summary of key 'take-away' points. All have done an excellent job.

The structure of the book is fairly conventional. After an introductory chapter on epidemiology, the first section contains chapters dealing with the clinical, neuropsychiatric, and neuropsychological evaluation, and psychiatric conditions mimicking dementia. The enormous growth in imaging techniques is mirrored by the inclusion of separate chapters on structural and functional brain imaging. There follows appropriately substantial chapters on the advances in molecular pathology, neurochemistry, and neuropathology.

The next section of the book is dedicated to the main players in the causation of dementia; Alzheimer's disease, frontotemporal dementia, dementia with Lewy bodies, vascular dementia, Huntington's disease, prion diseases, and inflammatory disorders. The chapter on dementia in young adults is rather different: as well as covering the rarer inherited metabolic disorders it also deals with the general approach to investigating exceptionally young patients with dementia.

The final section contains chapters on drug interventions, both specific disease- and general behaviour-modifying treatments, and the practical non-pharmacological management.

I owe enormous debt to colleagues in Cambridge particularly Karalyn Patterson at the Medical Research Council Cognition and Brain Sciences Unit (MRC CBU) and our numerous research assistants, students, and fellows who have worked on dementia related topics over the past decade; Barbara Sahakian and Trevor Robbins who have continued to be a source of inspiration throughout our long-term collaborative relationship; German Berrios and the late Kristin Breen who co-founded with me the Memory Disorders Clinic at Addenbrooke's Hospital; Diana Caine my clinical neuropsychology colleague in the Neurology Department; Carol Gregory and Sinclair Lough who helped establish the Early Onset Dementia Clinic; Neil Scolding, Alistair Compston, Jerry Brown, and the other neurologists at Addenbrooke's who have tolerated and even encouraged my interest in neuropsychology; Angela O'Sullivan, John Xuereb, and the staff of the Cambridge Brain Bank Laboratory; Nagui Antoun, John Pickard, Adrian Carpenter, Martin Graves and the staff of the MRIS and WBIC imaging centres; and especially my secretaries at the MRC CBU Judith Pride and Marion Wilkinson without whom this project, and many others, would not have been completed.

This book is dedicated to Nelson Butters, the man who first started me off on this trail during my year as an MRC travelling fellow at the Alzheimer Disease Research Centre at the University of California San Diego in 1988. Nelson was a giant among men who died at a tragically young age. It is a great pleasure that his heir and my friend David Salmon was able to contribute to the book.

John R. Hodges
Cambridge 2001

List of Contributors

Gene E. Alexander   Laboratory of Neurosciences, National Institute on Aging, National Institutes of Health, Bethesda, MD, USA.

G. E. Berrios   Department of Psychiatry, University of Cambridge, Addenbrooke's Hospital (Box 189), Hills Road, Cambridge CB2 2QQ, UK.

Konrad Beyreuther   Center for Molecular Biology, The University of Heidelberg, D-69120 Heidelberg, Federal Republic of Germany.

Paul Brown   Laboratory of Central Nervous System Studies, National Institute of Neurological Disorders and Stroke, National Institutes of Health, Bethesda, MD, USA

Nigel J. Cairns   Department of Neuropathology, Institute of Psychiatry, King's College, De Crespigny Park, London SE5 8AF, UK.

Julia A. Chung   Department of Neurology, UCLA School of Medicine, Los Angeles, California. CA 90095-1769 USA.

Jeffrey L. Cummings   Department of Neurology and Psychiatry and Behavioural Sciences, UCLA School of Medicine, Los Angeles, California. CA 90095-1769 USA.

Nick C. Fox   Dementia Research Group, Institute of Neurology, Queen Square, London WCIN 3BG, UK.

Douglas Galasko   Department of Neurosciences, University of California, San Diego, 9500 Gilman Drive, La Jolla, CA 92093-0948, USA.

Rose Goodchild   MRC Building Centre Development in Clinical Brain Ageing, Newcastle General Hospital, Newcastle upon Tyre, NE 4 6BE, UK.

Naida L. Graham   MRC Cognition and Brain Science Unit, Cambridge. CB 22EF, UK.

Carol A. Gregory   University Department of Psychiatry, University of Cambridge School of Clinical Medicine, Addenbrooke's Hospital, Hills Road, Cambridge CB2 2QQ, UK.

Lawrence A. Hansen   Department of Pathology and Neurosciences, University of California, San Diego, La Jolla, CA, USA.

Richard J. Harvey   Dementia Research Group, Institute of Neurology, University College London & Division of Neurosciences, Imperial College London, The National Hospital for Neurology and Neurosurgery, Queen Square, London WC1N 3BG, UK.

John R. Hodges   MRC Cognition and Brain Sciences Unit, 15 Chaucer Road, Cambridge CB2 2EF, UK. Department of Neurology, University of Cambridge, Addenbrooke's Hospital, Hills Road, Cambridge CB2 2QQ, UK.

A. M. Kennedy   West London Neurosciences Centre, Charing Cross Hospital, Fulham Palace Road, London W6 8RF, UK.

Peter L. Lantos   Department of Neuropathology, Institute of Psychiatry, King's College, De Crespigny Park, London SE5 8AF, UK.

Sinclair Lough   Psychiatric Services for the Elderly, Fulbourn Hospital, Addenbrooke's NHS Trust, Cambridge, UK.

I. S. Marková   Department of Psychiatry, Coniston House, East Riding Campus, University of Hull, Willerby HU10 6NS, UK.

Colin L. Masters   Department of Pathology, The University of Melbourne, Victoria, 3010, Australia.

Catriona A. McLean   Department of Pathology, The University of Melbourne, Victoria, 3010, Australia.

Bruce Miller   UCSF/Mt. Zion Hospital, 1600 Divisadero Street, Box 1691, San Francisco, California 94115, USA.

Peter Nestor   University of Cambridge Neurology Unit, Box 165, Addenbrooke's Hospital, Cambridge CB2 2QQ, UK.

P. K. Panegyres   Department of Neuropathology, Royal Perth Hospital, Perth, Western Australia.

Jane S. Paulsen   The University of Iowa Department of Psychiatry, Iowa City, IA 52242-1000, USA.

Elaine Perry   MRC Building Centre Development in Clinical Brain Ageing, Newcastle General Hospital, Newcastle upon Tyre, NE 4 6BE, UK.

Pietro Pietrini   Department of Human and Environmental Sciences, University of Pisa, Pisa, Italy.

Margaret Piggott   MRC Building Centre Development in Clinical Brain Ageing, Newcastle General Hospital, Newcastle upon Tyre, NE 4 6BE, UK.

Shibley Rahman   University Department of Psychiatry, University of Cambridge School of Clinical Medicine, Addenbrooke's Hospital, Hills Road, Cambridge CB2 2QQ, UK.

Robert G. Robinson   The University of Iowa Department of Psychiatry, Iowa City, IA 52242-1000, USA.

M. N. Rossor   Dementia Research Group, The National Hospital for Neurology and Neurosurgery, Queen Square, London WC1N 3BG, UK.

Barbara J. Sahakian   University Department of Psychiatry, University of Cambridge School of Clinical Medicine, Addenbrooke's Hospital, Hills Road, Cambridge CB2 2QQ, UK.

David P. Salmon   Department of Neurosciences (0948), University of California, San Diego, 9500 Gilman Drive, La Jolla, CA 92093-0948, USA.

Neil Scolding   MRC Cambridge Centre for Brain Repair, University Forvie Site, Robinson Way, Cambridge CB2 2SR, UK.

John M. Stevens   Department of Neuroradiology, The National Hospital for Neurology and Neurosurgery, Queen Square, London WCI 3BG, UK.

Heather C. Wilson   University of Cambridge Neurology unit, Addenbrooke's Hospital, Hills Road, Cambridge CB2 2QQ, UK.

Contents

Abbreviations

ACE	Addenbrooke's Cognitive Examination
AChE	acetylcholinesterase
AD	Alzheimer's disease
ADL	activities of daily living
ALD	adrenoleukodystrophy
AMN	adrenomyeloneuropathy
ApoE	apolipoprotein E
APP	amyloid precursor protein
ATP	adenosine 5′ triphosphate
BSE	bovine spongiform encephalopathy
CADASIL	cerebral autosomal dominant arteriopathy with subcortical infarcts and leukoencephalopathy
CAMDEX	Cambridge Mental Disorders of the Elderly Examination
CBD	corticobasal degeneration
CDR	Clinical Dementia Rating Scale
ChAT	choline acetyltransferase
CJD	Creutzfeldt-Jakob disease
CN	caudate nucleus
CSF	cerebrospinal fluid
CT	computed tomography
CVLT	California Verbal Learning Test
DFT	dementia of frontal type
DLB	dementia with Lewy bodies
DPD	depressive pseudo-dementia
DRPLA	dentatorubral-pallidoluysian atrophy
DRS	Dementia Rating Scale
DSM-IV	Diagnostic and Statistical Manual of Mental Disorders, revision IV
EDTA	ethylenediaminetetraacetic acid
EEG	electroencephalogram
FFI	fatal familial insomnia
FLD	frontal lobe degeneration
FTD	frontotemporal dementia
GDS	Global Deterioration Scale
GOM	granular osmiophilic material
GSS	Gerstmann-Sträussler-Scheinker disease
HD	Huntington's disease
HDRS	Hamilton Depression Rating Scale
HIAA	hospital inpatient activity analysis
5-HT	serotonin
IMC	Information Memory Concentration test
MCB	membranous cytoplasmic bodies
MELAS	mitochondrial myopathy, encephalopathy, lactic acidosis and stroke-like episodes
MERRF	myoclonic epilepsy with ragged red fibres
MHA	mental health enquiry

MID	multi-infarct dementia
MLD	metachromatic leukodystrophy
MMSE	Mini-Mental State Examination
MRI	magnetic resonance imaging
MS	multiple sclerosis
NADH	nicotinamide adenine dinucleotide, reduced form
NE	noradrenergic
NFT	neurofibrillary tangle
NIT	Number Information Test
NP	neuritic plaques
NPH	normal pressure hydrocephalus
NPI	Neuropsychiatric Inventory
PD	Parkinson's disease
PET	positron emission tomography
PPA	primary progressive aphasia
PRNP	prion protein gene
PrP	prion protein
PS	presenilin
PSP	progressive supranuclear palsy
SCA	spinocerebellar ataxia
SLE	systemic lupus erythematosus
α-SN	α-synuclein
SPECT	single photon emission computed tomography
SSPE	subacute sclerosing panencephalitis
TFC	Total Functional Capacity scale
TME	transmissible mink encephalopathy
TSE	transmissible spongiform encephalopathies
VaD	vascular dementia
vCJD	variant Creutzfeldt-Jakob disease
VLCFA	very long chain fatty acids
WBC	white blood cells

1 Epidemiology of presenile dementia

Richard J. Harvey

1 Introduction

Epidemiology is the study of disease in relation to populations. In the field of dementia epidemiological research is concerned with estimating the frequency of disease, its severity, and with identifying potential risk factors. Accurate epidemiological data on dementia is needed in many areas of science and health care. Within basic scientific research, estimates of frequency place findings in context of the importance of the disease, and guide funding priorities and decisions. Moreover, data on risk factors generate hypotheses relating to causes and mechanisms prompting new research questions.

For health service planners and public health specialists, the availability of accurate estimates of frequency encourages the development of needs lead and cost-effective services. The identification of significant risk factors, such as the possible link between BSE (bovine spongiform encephalopathy) and human variant CJD (Creutzfeldt–Jakob disease), can promote environmental or public health measures aimed at disease prevention.

For the clinician, placing the patient in the consulting room within the context of a population is part of the diagnostic process, while investigation of potential risk factors, such as in vascular dementia, may have the potential to alter the course of the disease.

Finally, patients themselves, and their carers are consumers of epidemiological information about their disease. Moreover, evidence of frequency of disease promotes awareness and hopefully better assessment, while specific diagnosis is often the route to better support.

Early onset dementia is an excellent example of how epidemiological data has lead to better knowledge and understanding of the disease, improved support though dedicated services, and National public health initiatives.

The aims of this chapter are first to summarize the major epidemiological methods, and then to review published studies of the epidemiology of early onset dementia.

2 Epidemiological methods

Other than clinical trials, which are outside the scope of this chapter, all epidemiology is essentially observational, using techniques that may be divided into descriptive methods, and analytical methods. Two of the most important factors that determine the quality of epidemiological studies are those of case definition and sampling methods.

2.1 Case definition

For many diseases outside of the fields of neurology and psychiatry, diagnoses are defined by signs and symptoms backed up with specific diagnostic laboratory tests. Unfortunately in the study of dementia there are virtually no perfect diagnostic tests, and even where these are available, such as through genetic testing, they are of limited applicability and unsuitable for use in population studies. Therefore, although dementia is a neuropathological disease, the diagnosis in life is made using clinical skills, usually supported by standardized assessment procedures and the application of clinical diagnostic criteria. The need to make a clinical diagnosis of dementia presents significant challenges to the epidemiologist.

2.1.1 Case definition in clinical populations

Most epidemiological studies of early onset dementia have been based on clinical populations of patients. The main issue in interpreting these data are understanding the case definition used to identify subjects for the study. Because early onset dementia is rare, a broad 'net' needs to be cast to identify individuals with cognitive impairment or dementia before more detailed diagnostic assessments are made. Considering the problem in a hierarchical way can help to make the issues clearer.

At the broadest level, cognitive impairment alone could be the case definition; this is reasonably easy to demonstrate using a simple cognitive screening test such as the Mini-Mental State Examination (MMSE) (Folstein *et al.* 1975). In this case, individuals in the population scoring below a critical cut-off are defined as subjects. Although this will identify a population of cognitively impaired subjects, they may have a range of causes far wider than dementia for their symptoms. For example, brain injuries and learning disability will both be included, while patients with mild dementia, or unusual diseases for which the MMSE is insensitive, such as frontotemporal dementia, may not be identified.

The next level of the hierarchy would be identification of patients with organic brain disease, the case definition here might now define exclusion criteria such as learning disability or traumatic brain injury. However, this definition would still ultimately be including subjects with diseases other than primary progressive dementia.

The next level in the hierarchy would be to more precisely define dementia. The issue then becomes one of definition, and how this definition can be operationalized and applied to subjects being sampled or surveyed in the population under investigation. The DSM-IV (Diagnostic and Statistical Manual of Mental Disorders, Revision IV) (American Psychiatric Association 1994) provides a helpful and concise definition of dementia which is summarized below:

A. Development of multiple cognitive deficits that include memory impairment and at least one of:
    1. Aphasia
    2. Apraxia
    3. Agnosia
    4. Disturbance of executive function
B. The cognitive deficits must be sufficiently severe to cause impairment in occupational or social functioning and must represent a decline from a previously higher level of functioning.
C. A diagnosis of dementia should not be made if the cognitive deficits occur exclusively during the course of a delirium.
D. Dementia may be etiologically related to a general medical condition, to the persisting effects of substance use (including toxin exposure), or to a combination of these factors.

It is relatively simple to operationalize this definition so that it can be used either in community surveys, reviews of case notes, or searching of computerized case registers.

The penultimate grading covers differential diagnosis, where diagnostic criteria are available. This would include Alzheimer's disease (McKhann *et al.* 1984), vascular dementia (VaD) (Roman *et al.* 1993), dementia with Lewy bodies (DLB) (McKeith *et al.* 1996), frontotemporal dementia (FTD) (Brun *et al.* 1994), and alcohol related dementia (American Psychiatric Association 1994). The accuracy of these clinical criteria vary according to the pathological criteria against which they are judged and the experience of those applying them. In general 80–98% specificity is possible, although there is often a trade-off with sensitivity, and for criteria such as those for vascular dementia there may be relatively low sensitivity (Erkinjuntti *et al.* 1997).

Beyond these major, clinically well defined, causes of dementia there are a large number of diseases that result in cerebral degeneration and dementia. In a study of rare diseases such as the early onset dementias it is important not to exclude any specific diseases that result in syndromes fulfilling the criteria for dementia. For diseases that do not have well validated formal diagnostic criteria clinical judgement based upon research findings and reports of case series form the basis of the clinical diagnosis. Diseases in this group include HIV/AIDS related dementia (Lipton 1997), Huntington's disease (Jones *et al.* 1997), multiple sclerosis (Rao *et al.* 1991), corticobasal degeneration (Schneider *et al.* 1997), progressive supranuclear palsy (PSP) (Rossor and Brown 1995), and the prion diseases (Collinge *et al.* 1993), including variant Creutzfeldt–Jakob disease (vCJD) (Will *et al.* 1996).

The most significant sources of bias or error in the case definition of early onset dementia is likely to occur at the top level of this hierarchy. If the top level is too narrow a proportion of cases of interest may be excluded at an early stage, leading to a biased underestimate of specific diseases further down. Other biases may occur depending on the definition of the disease, such as whether early onset disease is defined by the age at onset of symptoms, or age at diagnosis. This is a particular issue with those developing the disease close to the age of 65.

2.1.2 Neuropathological case definition

The dementias are diseases ultimately defined by their neuropathology, which forms the 'gold standard' against which clinical diagnostic criteria are judged. The seminal papers that helped to define the causes of senile dementia were carried out on large post-mortem case series (Blessed *et al.* 1968; Tomlinson *et al.* 1968). To date, few of the epidemiological studies of early onset dementia have included follow-up to autopsy. Within our own study in West London (Harvey *et al.* 1998) we have sought consent for brain donation from all subjects, however, as this is neither compulsory, nor an inclusion criteria, the sample of subjects who eventually undergo an autopsy may not be representative of the cohort as a whole. There is also some anecdotal evidence that subjects with atypical or more unusual dementias may be more likely to come to autopsy. Nevertheless it is good practice and methodologically sound to include neuropathological follow-up in epidemiological studies. This inevitably involves very long-term follow-up, although once a good proportion of cases have been given a pathological diagnosis a reappraisal of the accuracy of the clinical diagnosis can be made, with revision of prevalence estimates as appropriate.

Patients with early onset dementia are more likely to undergo a cerebral biopsy (Hulette *et al.* 1992) on clinical grounds, and the results of such an investigation should be sought whenever it is available.

Obtaining death certificates for subjects who are part of a cohort can provide some information on mortality rates and cause of death. Robust mechanisms to ensure the completeness of these data are available through flagging of the NHS Central Register (*www.statistics.gov.uk*). However, up to 35% of cases of confirmed early onset dementia, the presence of dementia is not mentioned on the death certificate (Newens *et al.* 1993*a*). Alzheimer's disease is the most likely diagnosis to be mentioned (75% of cases), while vascular dementia (52%) and other causes of dementia (33%) were much less likely to appear. The use of death certificates alone would therefore lead to a significantly biased underestimate of the prevalence of early onset dementia.

2.2 Sampling methods

Having established a case definition, the next methodological issue is the sampling method to be used to identify potential cases. The classical epidemiological methods are cross-sectional, cohort, and case-control studies. Each of these are applicable to early onset dementia, while more recent techniques such as capture-recapture may offer distinct advantages in the study of rare neuropsychiatric disorders.

2.2.1 Population surveys, prevalence studies, and cohort studies

In general, pure cross-sectional studies or *population surveys* are impractical for rare diseases. They are based upon the assumption that the frequency of a condition within the total population can be estimated from its frequency in a sample of the population. To obtain an unbiased estimate of frequency for a rare disease would require impractical and uneconomic sample sizes. Even multi-stage sampling, used in studies of dementia in older people, where a large sample is screened using a simple test such as the MMSE, and those scoring below a defined cut-off are then examined in detail, are also impractical when the initial sample size needs to be several hundred thousand.

Most studies of early onset dementia, for practical reasons, have used a *prevalence study* methodology. This bases case ascertainment on affected individuals who have come to medical attention. Inherent in this strategy is the potential for generating an underestimate of the rate due to either undiagnosed cases in the community, or a failure to identify all of those who have received a diagnosis.

The first potential source of bias, undiagnosed cases, is likely to be of minor importance in early onset dementia. The diseases, although rare, have profound effects on the sufferer and their family, and are unlikely to be ignored or fail to receive medical attention. This is unlike dementia in the elderly where mild dementia in very elderly people might be dismissed as part of normal ageing.

The most important potential source of bias is therefore failure to identify prevalent cases that have received medical attention. Once again, good experimental design and careful attention to methodology can minimize this problem. The key to maximizing case identification is to make no assumptions about the professionals who are likely to be seeing cases, and to be all-inclusive in identification methods. In terms of the UK health service, these methods are supported by using catchment areas that follow local administrative boundaries such as health regions, local health authorities, or social services boundaries. Once the catchment area is defined there need to be a thorough process to identify all possible professionals who might see cases, together with other sources of information for case finding. In different areas, the success of case finding may vary dramatically, for example in our study we used two local authority boroughs. Table 1.1 summarizes the sources from which cases were identified and the marked discrepancies between the two areas.

Table 1.1 Primary sources of identification for 227 subjects with dementia in a London UK based epidemiological study of early onset dementia

Source of case identification	Study area[a]		
	Area 1 n (%)	Area 2 n (%)	Total n (%)
Psychologist	47 (46.1%)	0	47 (20.7%)
Hospital IT systems	9 (8.8%)	37 (29.6%)	46 (20.3%)
Neurologist	17 (16.7%)	22 (17.6%)	39 (17.2%)
Psychiatrist	5 (4.9%)	27 (21.6%)	32 (14.1%)
Social worker	0	21 (16.8%)	21 (9.3%)
General practitioner	8 (7.8%)	6 (4.8%)	14 (6.2%)
Physician (non-neurologist)	12 (11.8%)	2 (1.6%)	14 (6.2%)
Community nurse	0	9 (7.2%)	9 (4.0%)
Other	4 (3.9%)	1 (0.8%)	5 (2.2%)
Total	**102**	**125**	**227**

[a] Area 1 was the London Borough of Hillingdon, area 2 was defined by the Health Authority Boundaries for Kensington, Chelsea, and Westminster.

The major sources of identification are computerized information systems and direct contact with clinicians or other professionals. Computerized information systems are becoming increasingly widespread within the health service and a thorough search for all possible systems should be made at the start of any study. Historically, hospital and health authority level data has been obtainable, dating back a number of years, from the Hospital Inpatient Activity Analysis (HIAA), Mental Health Enquiry (MHA), and Körner inpatient data systems. More recently, many Hospital Trusts have purchased their own more detailed systems, and each Trust within a catchment area should be contacted with a request to search their databases. Unfortunately, diagnostic coding is poor on many of these systems, with previous studies suggesting that 17% of early onset dementia patients may not be identified, and up to 23% wrongly classified (McGonigal *et al.* 1992). Individual clinicians and departments may also maintain their own databases, which may provide a more accurate source of diagnosis. Social services departments are also now extensively computerized, although they rarely hold medical diagnostic information in a structured way, and may be difficult to search effectively. In every case, involving a senior IT analyst in developing the search strategy is critical for success. While GPs are also increasingly computerized, the prevalence of early onset dementia in any individual practice is low, and therefore unless large consortia of GPs maintain centralized data, searching multiple GP systems may not yield many extra cases. In our own study only 14 cases (6%) were primarily identified from GPs, while in another study only one additional case was identified from contact with 47 practices (Newens *et al.* 1993*b*).

Contact with clinicians is the second most useful source of cases, and should cover the specialities of neurology, adult psychiatry, old age psychiatry, general medicine, and elderly medicine. In addition to personal or departmental databases, manual searching of discharge summaries, clinic letters, and domicilliary visit reports are the best means of identifying cases. Personal contact also needs to be made with psychology, radiology, occupational therapy, and social services departments both within hospitals and in community. Social services may have a combination of hospital-based, community-based, and special needs departments all of whom may hold cases. In our own study, social services was particularly helpful for identifying and tracking cases, diagnosed several years before, who had since entered residential or nursing home care.

Having identified subjects through a prevalence study, it is then possible to follow these individuals longitudinally as a cohort. This can vary from intensive follow-up where subjects are reassessed at regular intervals, to simple mortality rate follow-up by flagging of the NHS central register. Identifying known cases of early onset dementia retrospectively over long periods of time can allow estimates of incidence to be made, without the need to recruit and follow large at-risk cohorts prospectively.

2.2.2 Case-control studies

While prevalence and cohort studies can provide frequency data such as prevalence, incidence, mortality, etc., assessing risk factors requires a control group and a case-control methodology. The objective of a case-control study is to identify a population of subjects with the index disease, and match them to a control population who differ only in not having the disease. Matching is usually based on age and sex as beyond this it can be difficult to identify the control group, and the sample becomes increasingly biased. The choice and source of the control group is the most difficult part of designing a case-control study.

These types of studies are, however, relative cheap, quick to perform, can assess a wide variety of risk factors, and are useful in rare diseases. However, they are also prone to bias in the selection of cases and controls, and to observer and responder bias where an association with a risk factor is either reported more frequently by affected individuals, or searched from more aggressively in the case population.

2.2.3 Capture-recapture techniques

Capture-recapture is a common technique in biology that is now being adapted for use in neuro-epidemiology (Martyn 1998; Hook and Regal 1998). The basis of the method is that cases with an index condition are identified in the target population using the methods discussed in Section 2.2.1. Those cases identified are then 'flagged' using a case register. A second survey is then carried out in the same area, the proportion of 'flagged' cases to new cases identified being used to provide a more accurate estimate of the true prevalence of the disease.

2.2.4 Sampling bias

I have briefly discussed potential sources of bias in all of the above methods. Identifying and minimizing potential sources of bias in epidemiological studies is most important when accurate estimates are required. Inevitably, in rare disease neuroepidemiology, complete removal of bias is never going to be possible. Major sources of bias can be addressed by careful case definition, together with broad and comprehensive case ascertainment followed by detailed diagnostic evaluation. Having identified possible confounding factors it may also be possible to correct for the effect of these in the final analysis.

2.3 Statistical methods

Before reviewing data from epidemiological studies of early onset dementia is useful to briefly consider the statistical methods that will have been used to analyse these data. Broadly, observational epidemiological studies can generate frequencies (rates) of disease and outcome, survival data, and associations with risk factors.

2.3.1 Frequency

The most common frequency measure reported by studies of early onset dementia is *prevalence rate*. This is more correctly a ratio of the number of cases of disease present to the total population at a defined point in time. It is usual to express this as the number of cases per unit of population at risk, e.g. 6/100 000 (6 cases per 100 000 people at risk).

The second most useful frequency measure is *incidence*, defined as the number of new cases of disease that develop in the population at-risk during a defined time period. However, following large cohorts of at-risk individuals prospectively and ascertaining new cases for early onset dementia has so far been impractical, and the incidence estimates available have mostly been estimated from retrospective cross-sectional data collected from large time frames.

Unlike incidence, the *mortality rate* or frequency of death in a defined time period for a population of cases can be relatively easily estimated in the UK through flagging of the NHS Central register for notification of death.

Having derived crude frequencies for these measures, it is then possible to derive age- and gender-specific rates, which can describe the diseases in much more detail. Similarly, a prevalence rate for dementia can be subdivided into individual prevalence rates for each of the underlying causes of dementia.

2.3.2 Survival

While mortality is a crude cross-sectional measure of survival, it provides little information about the course of the illness. More detailed survival analysis provide a way of presenting and analysing data that describe the outcome for a population from a particular *time origin* to a well-defined outcome (Collett 1994). The outcome may be mortality, institutionalization, or progression to a particular definable disease state. Data are presented as probabilities of survival to a particular time point and give much more detail about the course of the disease.

2.3.3 Risk factors

The results of case-control studies are presented as *odds of exposure* or risk in each group, and the *odds ratio* or relative risk to compare the case and control group as follows:

The odds of exposure in the cases group is a/c, while in the control group it is b/d. The odds ratio *OR* for the risk factor is therefore (a/c) / (b/d). An OR less than 1 suggests that the exposure

Table 1.2 A 2 × 2 contingency table for a case-control study

	Cases	Controls
Number exposed	a	b
Number not exposed	c	d

is having a protective effect, while an OR greater than 1 suggests that the exposure is a potential risk factor. The 95% confidence interval for the OR provides valuable information about significance; if the confidence interval includes 1.0, then this suggests that the effect seen is not statistically significant in the size of the sample studied.

2.3.4 Meta-analysis

Meta-analysis is a statistical technique that takes published data from multiple independent studies and combines them to provide more accurate estimates of the outcome of interest. The technique has used particularly effectively for studies of dementia in older people (Jorm *et al.* 1987; Jorm and Jolley 1998). Similarly, raw data from multiple comparable studies can be combined and re-analysed to provide more robust results, a good example of which are the EURODEM studies (Hofman *et al.* 1991; van Duijn and Hofman 1992). This type of analysis would seem to be attractive for studying early onset dementia, although to date there have been no published meta-analyses.

3 Frequency of early onset dementia

The rest of this chapter is devoted to a review of the available data on the epidemiology of the early onset dementias. The types of published studies divide into the handful of papers that are devoted to early onset dementia, and those studies of older people with dementia where the lower age cut-off is below 65 years. Table 1.3 summarizes the major studies from which frequency data for early onset dementia can be derived.

3.1 Prevalence rates

3.1.1 Dementia

Prevalence data on the broad diagnosis of dementia in people under the age of 65 years are summarized in Table 1.4, and represented graphically in Figure 1.1.

It is immediately clear from studies such as those performed in Lundby, that the crude estimates are related to having too small numbers of subjects screened for a disease of low prevalence. It is notable from Figure 1.1 that those larger studies who have used a similar methodology derive consistent prevalence figures.

3.1.2 Alzheimer's disease

Prevalence data for Alzheimer's disease diagnosed using acceptable clinical criteria are summarized in Table 1.5 and Figure 1.2.

As with the data for broad dementia, those studies using a similar methodology based on case finding show good consistency in the estimated prevalence of AD. This seems to show that AD is very rare before the age of 45 years, doubling in frequency every five years up to the age of 65 years. Beyond 65 the upward trend of doubling frequency every five years is now well documented (Rocca *et al.* 1991).

3.1.3 Vascular dementia

Identification of early onset VaD (multi-infarct) patients is included in only three studies, although once again, the two UK studies that follow similar methodology derive consistent estimates of age specific prevalence.

Table 1.3 Major studies reporting the prevalence and incidence of early onset dementia

Study	Reference	Size of under 65 years at-risk population included	Method of case ascertainment	Diagnoses included	Case definition
Finland (1)	Molsa et al. 1982	Incidence study	Population survey	Alzheimer's disease, vascular dementia	Clinical diagnosis
Finland (2)	Sulkava et al. 1985	6117	Two stage screen with review by a neurologist.	Severe dementia (excludes mild dementia)	DSM-III
Rochester, USA	Schoenberg et al. 1985	4422 aged 40–59 years 2277 aged 60–69 years	Two stage screen with review by a neurologist.	Severe dementia	Clinical diagnosis
Lundby, SE	Rorsman et al. 1986	1162	Follow-up of earlier cohort with two phase survey and review by a psychiatrist.	Dementia	Own criteria which are similar to DSM-III-R
Israel	Treves et al. 1986	Incidence study based on the population of Israel, denominator not stated	Israeli National Neurologic Disease Registry.	Alzheimer's disease (excludes other causes of dementia)	Criteria equivalent to DSM-III-R
Framingham, USA	Bachman et al. 1992	285	Longitudinal cohort study. Two stage screening using MMSE.	Dementia and all subtypes	Clinical assessment of all subjects and DSM-III-R
Northern Region, UK	Newens et al. 1993b	655 800	Hospital information systems and supplementary sources, followed by case note review.	Alzheimer's disease (excludes other causes of dementia)	ICD-9
Scotland, UK	McGonigal et al. 1993	Population of Scotland, denominator not stated	Government diagnostic register followed by case note review.	Alzheimer's disease, vascular dementia	ICD-9
Manchester, UK	Baldwin 1994	120 000	Call for referrals.	Dementia	Clinical diagnosis based on structured assessment
West London, UK	Harvey et al. 1998	193 493	Information systems and case note searching.	Dementia and all subtypes	DSM-IV and other specific diagnostic criteria
Rotterdam	Ott et al. 1998	4448 person-years at risk (incidence study only)	Three stage screening and assessment.	Dementia	CAMDEX, NINCDS/ADRDA, and DSM-III

Table 1.4 Age specific prevalence of dementia (per 100 000 population) in the under 65s

	Age group (years)							
Study	25–29	30–34	35–39	40–44	45–49	50–54	55–59	60–64
Finland (2)					260 (16/6120)[a]			
Rochester	–	–			45			351[b]
Lundby				0 (0/467)[b]				100 (1/100)
Framingham		0			77	40	86	249
Manchester[c]	20			17		23		83
West London		13	8	16	33	62	152	166

[a] Where study was population cohort based, the actual number of cases identified and subjects screened is shown in brackets.
[b] Age group 60–69.
[c] Prevalence estimated from raw data for age bands and population figures for the catchment area.

3.1.4 Prion disease

The prion diseases represent a special case amongst the early onset dementias, particularly in the UK. The potential association between prion disease in cattle and a new variant of CJD affecting young adults (Will *et al.* 1996) has lead to intense epidemiological surveillance co-ordinated by the UK CJD Surveillance Unit. Regularly updated figures for the number of confirmed cases of

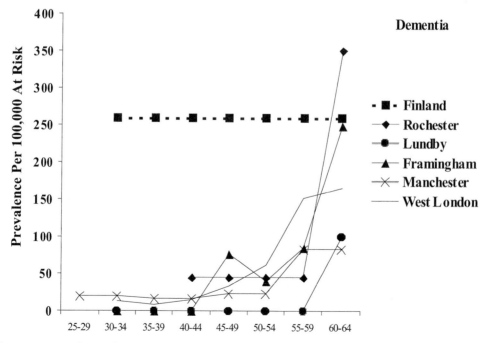

Figure 1.1 Prevalence of dementia.

Table 1.5 Age specific prevalence of Alzheimer's disease (per 100 000 population)

Study	Age group (years)						
	30–34	35–39	40–44	45–49	50–54	55–59	60–64
Finland (2)				30 (2/6120)			
Lundby				0			27ᵃ
Framingham				0		86	50
Northern Region	–	–	–	2.4	11.8	35.6	87.3
Scotland	–	–	1.4ᵇ (3.1)	8.1 (11.9)	27.6 (42.8)	39.7 (69.1)	37.8 (80.4)
West London	0	0	2.6	6.0	16.4	50.7	77.3

ᵃ Age group 60–69.
ᵇ Figures are for NINCDS probable AD (and broad AD).

CJD are published by the UK Government, and a detailed longitudinal epidemiological study of CJD in UK has recently been published (Cousens *et al.* 1997).

3.1.5 Other causes of dementia

Alzheimer's disease, vascular dementia, and prion disease are the main causes of early onset dementia for which there are more than one detailed epidemiological study reporting prevalence

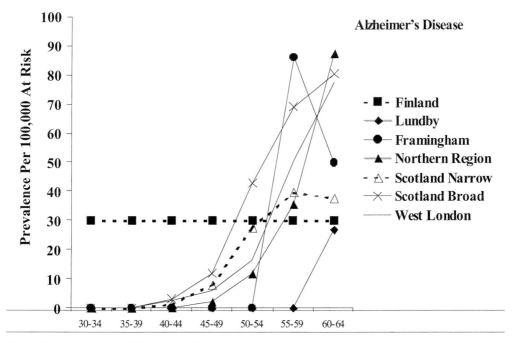

Figure 1.2 Prevalence of Alzheimer's disease.

Table 1.6 Age specific prevalence of vascular dementia (per 100 000 population)

Study	Age group (years)						
	30–34	35–39	40–44	45–49	50–54	55–59	60–64
Finland (2)				80 (5/6120)			
Scotland	–	–	3.5	5.3	12.9	27.0	52.2
West London	0	0	0	0	6.6	32.6	38.7

rates. Very little data is available for early onset dementia with Lewy bodies, the frontotemporal dementias, alcohol related dementia, or other rarer diseases. Table 1.7 and Figure 1.4 reports age specific prevalence rates for some of the other causes of dementia from our West London study.

The available data on prevalence are derived from studies of differing methodology and consider only the most common dementias as found in the elderly. Only one study considers frontotemporal dementia, a disorder known to occur relatively commonly in clinic based samples of younger people with dementia (Neary 1990; Ferran *et al.* 1996; Harvey *et al.* 1996). These data suggest that it is the third commonest cause of dementia in people under 65 years, with a rate approximately half that for AD, and similar to the rate for VaD, suggesting that one in seven cases of dementia in people under the age of 65 years is likely to be due to FTD. Patients diagnosed with FTD according to the Manchester/Lund criteria are a mixed population of cases of Pick's disease, frontal lobe degeneration (FLD), and FLD with motor neuron disease. Epidemiological studies of older patients appears to fail to identify FTD as a significant

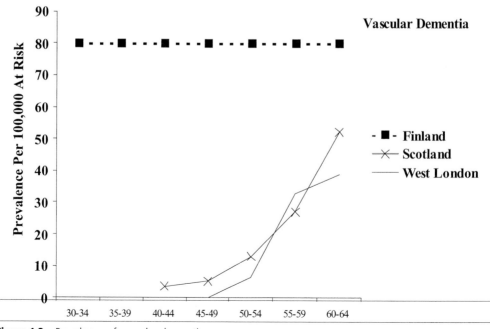

Figure 1.3 Prevalence of vascular dementia.

Table 1.7 Age specific prevalence (per 100 000 population) of other causes of dementia from West London study

	Age group (years)						
	30–34	35–39	40–44	45–49	50–54	55–59	60–64
Frontotemporal dementia	0	0	0	12	3	25	23
Alcohol related dementia	0	0	0	6	20	18	12
Dementia with Lewy bodies	0	0	0	2	3	7	4

cause of dementia; supporting our previous hypothesis that FTD is a more prevalent disease amongst younger people (Harvey *et al.* 1996).

By comparison, dementia with Lewy bodies appears to be proportionally rarer in the population of younger dementia patients, although again this is based only on a single study. It has been suggested that DLB accounts for up to 20% of dementia in older people (Byrne *et al.* 1989; Perry *et al.* 1989); the epidemiological evidence to date suggests it is an unusual cause of dementia in younger people.

There is a discrepancy of approximately 20% between the prevalence figures for broad dementia, and the total of all of the subtypes. Of these cases, at least a quarter are below the age of 35 years, the very young age group, where the more common forms of dementia are extremely rare. The most common cause of dementia in this very young group is Huntington's disease with a prevalence rates in Europe of 0.5–8/100 000 and in the US of 5–7/100 000 (Chiu 1994). Other

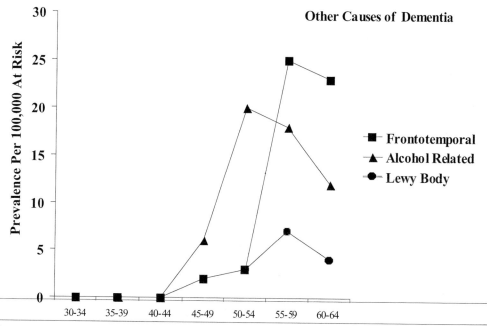

Figure 1.4 Prevalence of other causes of dementia.

causes include dementia in multiple sclerosis (4/100 000) (Rao *et al.* 1991), corticobasal degeneration (< 1/100 000), and dementia in Parkinson's disease (< 1/100 000).

Dementia associated with Down's syndrome is a further important group which can be grouped with the early onset dementia. A recent detailed study has estimated prevalence rates of 3.4% in the 30–39 age group, 10.3% in the 40–49 age group, and 40% in those aged 50–59 years (Holland *et al.* 1998).

The main points that can be concluded from this review of prevalence studies of early onset dementia area that firstly Alzheimer's disease accounts for less than one-third of cases of dementia in people under the age of 65 years. Taking this into account, we should be diagnosing AD in younger patients much less frequently than in older people. VaD appears to be proportionally as common among younger as older patients, while one in seven cases of early onset dementia may be due to FTD. While awareness of this disease is increasing we should be vigilant for the diagnosis when presented with a younger person with dementia.

3.2 Incidence rates

Studies reporting the incidence of dementia are less common for both elderly and early onset populations, however useful data is available which is summarized in Table 1.8. Figure 1.5 graphically displays incidence data for early onset Alzheimer's disease, while Figure 1.6 shows similar data for broad dementia diagnosis and vascular dementia.

Figure 1.5 suggests that there is considerable variability between studies on the estimates of incidence of AD. This probably reflects differences in methodology, some based on population studies, while others are based on prevalence studies, the use of diagnostic criteria, and whether age at symptom onset or age at diagnosis is used. The trends in all of the studies show an increase in incidence with age, which is consistent with increasing prevalence with age.

Table 1.8 Incidence rates for dementia, Alzheimer's disease, and vascular dementia (rate per 100 000 population at risk per year)

	Age group (years)				
	40–44	**45–49**	**50–54**	**55–59**	**60–64**
Finland (1) (AD)	–	——6.3——		——16.5——	
Israel (AD — Jews of	0	10	40	90	95
European–American origin) Israel (AD — Jews of	9	10	20	40	50
African–Asian origin) Rotterdam (dementia)	0	0	0	0	120
Scotland (probable AD)	1.4	8.1	27.6	39.7	37.8
Scotland (broad AD)	3.1	11.9	42.8	69.1	80.4
Scotland (VaD — men)	5.0	7.2	17.2	34.0	70.8
Scotland (VaD — women)	2.0	3.4	8.7	20.5	33.6
Northern Region (AD)	0	0.9	4.9	8.1	14.5

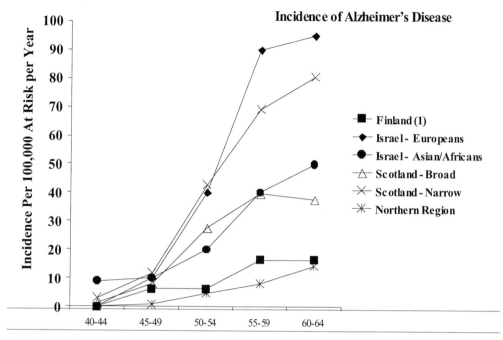

Figure 1.5 Incidence of Alzheimer's disease.

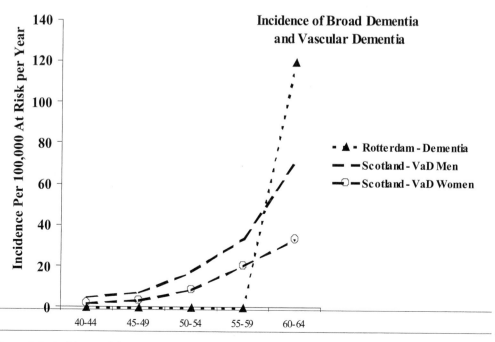

Figure 1.6 Incidence of dementia and vascular dementia.

4 Prognosis

Having generated frequency data for the number of cases of early onset dementia, and the numbers of new cases likely to develop each year, the next challenge for epidemiologists is to inform the course of the disease and prognosis. These type of data can be obtained both from both prevalence studies and population surveys. The simplest cross-sectional analyses provide information on levels of disability and dependency, while longitudinal follow-up can examine survival and outcomes for a population.

4.1 Severity

Disease severity is an important measure in dementia, being directly related to dependency, cost-of-illness, and need for institutional care. Understanding the likely distribution of severity in a population of patients with dementia can assist health care planning. There are a number of methods available to assess dementia severity, varying from comprehensive assessment scales such as the Clinical Dementia Rating (CDR) (Hughes *et al.* 1982) or Global Deterioration Scale (GDS) (Reisberg *et al.* 1988), though Activities of Daily Living (ADL) scales to simpler cognitive based severity assessments such as the Mini-Mental State Examination (Folstein *et al.* 1975).

Most of these assessments require direct contact with the patient and/or caregiver, and hence, unlike case note based prevalence studies subjects need to be traced, contacted, and to agree to participate in the study. Consequently data will be based upon a sample of cases that may not be representative of the whole population.

Two main studies report data on severity of epidemiological based samples of patients with early onset dementia (Newens *et al.* 1995; Harvey *et al.* 1998). In the study from the Northern Region 109 cases identified from their original epidemiological study, who were still living in the community, underwent a detailed interview. Only patients with AD were included, and it is interesting to note that more than 10% of cases that had previously been recorded as cases of AD for the prevalence survey, were subsequently thought to have other diagnosis following direct clinical assessment. The results of the study indicated that the need for assistance in basic ADLs (dressing, bathing, toileting, transferring, feeding, and continence) increase progressively with time. Five years after diagnosis 57% of patients were still able to live in the community, but 20% require assistance in all areas of ADL.

In our own study in West London, dementia severity was rated using the CDR scale. Figure 1.7 shows the cross-sectional distribution of dementia severity in the population, which includes both those resident in the community and those in institutional care. The data suggest a skewed distribution of severity in the population with more patients in the mild to moderate band than in the more severe categories.

4.2 Clinical course and mortality

The course and rate of progression of dementia varies dramatically between different diseases. Older patients with Alzheimer's disease may live for up to 20 years after diagnosis, while patients with CJD may be dead within six months, or less, of the first symptom. Several epidemiological studies report survival data for their cohorts (Treves *et al.* 1986; Newens *et al.* 1993*b*; Samson *et al.* 1996; Thomas *et al.* 1997).

Table 1.9 and Figure 1.8 summarize the survival probabilities for patients with early onset AD in three of these studies:

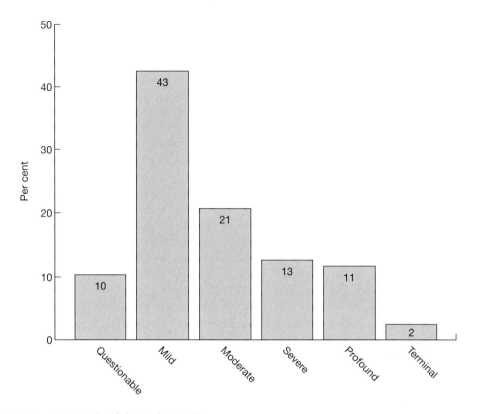

Figure 1.7 Cross-sectional dementia severity.

Table 1.9 Survival probabilities in early onset AD

	Years from diagnosis/presentation									
	1	**2**	**3**	**4**	**5**	**6**	**7**	**8**	**9**	**10**
Israel[a] (Treves *et al.* 1986)	96	93	88	83	71	67	58	50	27	14
Northern Region — incident cases[a]	92	78	63	54	40					
Northern Region — prevalent cases[a] (Newens *et al.* 1993)	96	95	85	77	65	56				
Scotland — AD — male[b] (Thomas *et al.* 1997)	83	75	61	44	32	21	14	8	5	3
Scotland — AD — female[b]	95	85	73	62	43	34	25	15	8	7
Scotland — VaD — male[b]	76	62	44	30	22	15	11	8	6	4
Scotland — VaD — female[b]	85	67	59	50	36	29	21	16	11	8

[a] By life table/actuarial analysis.
[b] By Kaplan-Meier analysis.

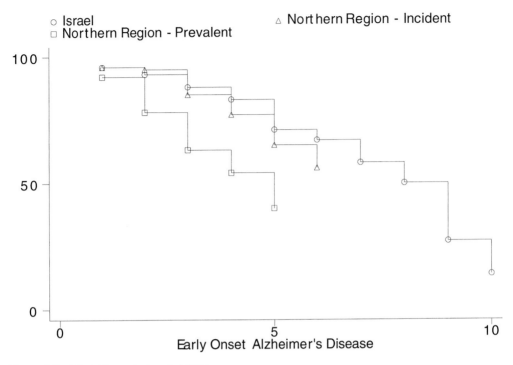

Figure 1.8 Life table survival probabilities.

Figure 1.8 displays the life table based survival probabilities for early onset AD, while Figure 1.9 displays Kaplan-Meier based survival estimates from the Scottish study. By either method, these data suggest that approaching 30–50% of patients with early onset AD will have died within five years.

All three of these studies were based on prevalence studies. Cohorts of patients from case-control studies can also be followed longitudinally to examine the association of particular risk factors with clinical course and mortality. Only one study has used this methodology (Samson *et al.* 1996) however they were able to show that the presence of tremor, rigidity, or myoclonus were all associated with significantly reduced survival at 5 years after diagnosis. For example patients with tremor survived for a median of only 2.5 years from diagnosis, while those without tremor had a median survival of 6.1 years.

5 Risk factors

Studies of risk factors in early onset dementia have focused on two main areas, genetics and environment. In terms of genetics, the majority of the autosomal dominant genes result in early onset disease (Harvey and Rossor 1998). While inherited forms of dementia are rare, there have been few studies that have attempted to measure the prevalence of pathogenic genetic mutations in populations of patients with dementia. The most extensive survey to date on an epidemiological series of 101 familial and sporadic cases of early onset AD showed an overall prevalence of 6% for presenilin 1 (PS1) mutations and 1% for presenilin 2 (Cruts *et al.* 1998). All of these patients were negative for amyloid precursor protein (APP) mutations. However, when only those cases with a clear family

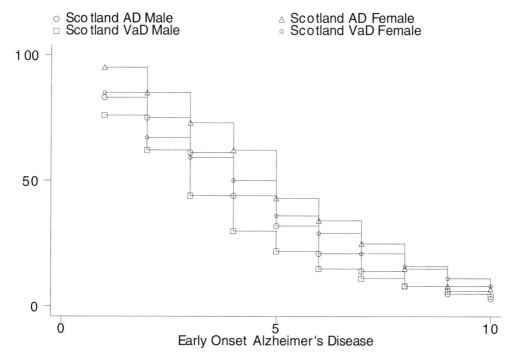

○ Sco tland AD Male
□ Sco tland VaD Male
△ Sco tland AD Female
○ Sco tland VaD Female

Figure 1.9 Kaplan-Meier survival probabilities.

history were included, the prevalence of PS1 mutations rose to 18%. These data suggest that APP and presenilin are rare causes of AD in the general population, and moreover, they account for less than one-fifth of strongly familial cases.

The risk factors for CJD have also been subjected to a large case-control study. Van Duijn *et al.* (1998) studied 405 patients with definite or probable CJD collected from across Europe, with controls matched for age and sex. There was evidence of significant familial aggregation of the disease (relative risk: 2.26) (95% CI: 1.31–3.90), but there was no association with surgery, blood transfusion, or consumption of beef veal, lamb, cheese, or milk. There was however a significantly increased risk associated with eating raw meat (RR: 1.63) and brain (RR: 1.68), and to extensive exposure to leather or fertilizer containing hoof and horn. This was however, a retrospective case-control study which methodologically introduces significant potential for both recall bias and observer bias. There were also considerable regional variations which suggest that these data needs to be interpreted cautiously.

Case-control studies on environmental risk factors for the common causes of early onset dementia have been carried out on both the Northern Region (Forster *et al.* 1995). The major risk factor identified in both cohorts was a family history of dementia, accounting for a odds ratio of 2.5 (1.05–6.56) in the Northern Region and 2.35 in the Scotland. These data again highlight the importance of genetic factors in early onset dementia.

Data from the Scottish cohort on more than 800 cases showed associations between socio-economic deprivation and early onset vascular dementia, and between parental age and early onset AD. Occupation was unrelated to risk, although having a father who was a coal miner was associated with increased risk for both AD and VaD. Non-random geographical distribution of cases was concluded to be related to genetics factors rather than environment (Whalley and Holloway 1985; Whalley *et al.* 1994, 1995; Starr *et al.* 1997 *a, b*).

Within the cohort from the Northern Region, which included 109 cases, there were no significant associations with environmental risk factors such as cigarette smoking, maternal age, medical history, or exposure to aluminium.

Overall, these are relatively small studies, which are all based on retrospective data. A clear conclusion is the association with familial clustering and genetic risk factors. Genetics may be the strongest factor influencing the development of dementia in younger people, and once these are better understood future research may be able to control for these in the analysis and so show more subtle interacting effects with environmental factors.

6 Conclusions

Epidemiological studies of dementia in younger people need to be based upon very large populations at risk, and for practical purposes usually have to follow a prevalence study methodology. The three major UK based studies identified cases from multiple sources, which minimizes the risk of missing cases. In the Scottish study, the completeness of their data was tested by examining case registers which confirmed that the majority of cases of presenile dementia in Scotland were admitted as inpatients at some time during their illness (McGonigal *et al.* 1992). Putting data from all of the available studies together provides a clearer overview of prevalence, incidence, and survival in early onset dementia. As future studies are published there may be opportunities to go further than this using the techniques of meta-analysis.

An important issue for future investigators will be the need to justify, test, and confirm the completeness of their data, particularly for retrospective studies. In the UK, the NHS reforms that have been occurring during the late 1980s and 1990s are likely to make prevalence studies based on case note research more difficult. The closure of large mental hospitals and the introduction of community care has resulted in the establishment of many smaller Community Mental Health Trusts, each usually having its own case notes, and computerized patient databases. In parallel with this, the number of acute hospital beds has been declining, and increasingly, medical investigation is carried out on an outpatient basis. In the new NHS, it may be less likely that every younger patient with dementia will have an inpatient admission for diagnosis. Moreover, the Community Care Act (1990) has changed the organization of social services, one effect of which has been that rather than being placed in state run residential or nursing homes in their local area, patients may be more likely to be placed in contracted private care outside of their home area. Careful review and consideration of all of these factors is needed when assessing the methodological quality of early onset dementia epidemiological studies.

The epidemiological data summarized here will hopefully be used by researchers, clinicians, and planners to estimate the number, and differential diagnoses of patients who may use their services, or participate in their research. Following the publication of the ADS strategy document on young onset dementia (Alzheimer's Disease Society 1996), some Health Authorities and Trusts have begun to consider the needs of this group of patients in their area. The data presented here can be easily applied to census figures for a particular population to estimate, with some accuracy, the number of patients and the range of diseases that are likely to be present.

7 Key points

1   Epidemiological studies of early onset dementia require a different methodology to studies of dementia in older people. Methods developed for studying rare diseases are the most appropriate and can derive consistent estimates of prevalence, incidence, survival, and risk factors.

2   Prevalence studies show that Alzheimer's disease (AD) accounts for less than one-third of all cases of early onset dementia. Prevalence and incidence of AD approximately double every five years from the age of 40 years onwards.

3   Dementia is very rare before the age of 45 years, most cases are caused by rare and unusual diseases.

4   Frontotemporal dementia may account for one in seven cases of early onset dementia, although it appears to remain relatively under-recognized in clinical practice.

5   Up to 50% of patients with early onset dementia may die within five years of diagnosis. Features such as tremor, myoclonus, and rigidity predict a more rapid course.

6   The strongest risk factor for early onset dementia is a family history, few other environmental risk factors have been shown to be strongly or consistently associated.

References

Alzheimer's Disease Society. (1996). Younger people with dementia: a review and strategy. London: Alzheimer's Disease Society.

American Psychiatric Association. (1994). *Diagnostic and statistical manual of mental disorders* (4th edn) (DSM-IV). APA, Washington, DC.

Bachman, D. L., Wolf, P. A., Linn, R., Knoefel, J. E., Cobb, J., Belanger, A., *et al.* (1992). Prevalence of dementia and probable senile dementia of the Alzheimer type in the Framingham Study. *Neurology*, **42**, 115–19.

Baldwin, R. C. (1994). Acquired cognitive impairment in the presenium. *Psychiatric Bulletin*, **18**, 463–5.

Blessed, G., Tomlinson, B., and Roth, M. (1968). The association between quantitative measures of dementia and of senile change in the cerebral grey matter of elderly subjects. *British Journal of Psychiatry*, **114**, 797–811.

Brun, A., Englund, B., Gustafson, L., Passant, U., Mann, D. M. A., Neary, D., *et al.* (1994). Clinical and neuropathological criteria for frontotemporal dementia. *Journal of Neurology, Neurosurgery and Psychiatry*, **57**, 416–18.

Byrne, E. J., Lennox, G., Lowe, J., and Godwinausten, R. B. (1989). Diffuse Lewy body disease — clinical-features in 15 cases. *Journal of Neurology, Neurosurgery and Psychiatry*, **52**, 709–17.

Chiu, E. (1994). Huntington's disease. In *Dementia* (ed. A. Burns and R. Levy), pp. 753–62. Chapman and Hall, London.

Collett, D. (1994). *Modelling survival data in medical research*. Chapman and Hall, London.

Collinge, J., Palmer, M. S., Rossor, M. N., Janota, I., and Lantos, P. L. (1993). Prion dementia. *Lancet*, **341**, 627.

Cousens, S. N., Zeidler, M., Esmonde, T. F., De, S. R., Wilesmith, J. W., Smith, P. G., *et al.* (1997). Sporadic Creutzfeldt–Jakob disease in the United Kingdom: analysis of epidemiological surveillance data for 1970–96. *British Medical Journal*, **315**, 389–95.

Cruts, M., Vanduijn, C. M., Backhovens, H., VandenBroeck, M., Wehnert, A., Serneels, S., *et al.* (1998). Estimation of the genetic contribution of presenilin-1 and -2 mutations in a population based study of presenile Alzheimer disease. *Human Molecular Genetics*, **7**, 43–51.

Erkinjuntti, T., Ostbye, T., Steenhuis, R., and Hachinski, V. (1997). The effect of different diagnostic criteria on the prevalence of dementia. *New England Journal of Medicine*, **337**, 1667–74.

Ferran, J., Wilson, K., Doran, M., Dhadiali, E., Johnson, F., Cooper, P., *et al.* (1996). The early onset dementias: A study of clinical characteristics and service use. *International Journal of Geriatric Psychiatry*, **11**, 863–9.

Folstein, M., Folstein, S., and McHughs, P. (1975). The 'Mini Mental State': a practical method for grading the cognitive state of patients for the clinician. *Journal of Psychiatric Research*, **12**, 189–98.

Forster, D. P., Newens, A. J., Kay, D. W. K., and Edwardson, J. A. (1995). Risk factors in clinically diagnosed presenile dementia of the Alzheimer type: A case-control study in northern England. *Journal of Epidemiology and Community Health*, **49**, 253–8.

Harvey, R. J., Roques, P., Fox, N. C., and Rossor, M. N. (1996). Non-Alzheimer dementias in young-patients. *British Journal of Psychiatry*, **168**, 384–5.

Harvey, R. J. and Rossor, M. N. (1998). Elucidating the genetic factors of Alzheimer's disease. *Progress in Neurology and Psychiatry*, **2**, 35–8.

Harvey, R. J., Rossor, M. N., Skelton-Robinson, M., and Garralda, M. E. (1998). Young onset dementia: Epidemiology, clinical symptoms, family burden, support and outcome. http://dementia.ion.ucl.ac.uk/, London: Dementia Research Group.

Hofman, A., Rocca, W. A., Brayne, C., Breteler, M. M. B., Clarke, M., Cooper, B., *et al.* (1991). The prevalence of dementia in Europe — a collaborative study of 1980–1990 findings. *International Journal of Epidemiology*, **20**, 736–48.

Holland, A. J., Hon, J., Huppert, F. A., Stevens, F., and Watson, P. (1998). Population-based study of the prevalence and presentation of dementia in adults with Down's syndrome. *British Journal of Psychiatry*, **172**, 493–8.

Hook, E. B. and Regal, R. R. (1998). Capture-recapture methods in epidemiology: Methods and limitations. *American Journal of Epidemiology*, **148**, 1219.

Hughes, C. P., Berg, L., Danziger, W. L., Coben, L. A., and Martin, R. L. (1982). A new clinical scale for the staging of dementia. *British Journal of Psychiatry*, **140**, 566–72.

Hulette, C. M., Earl, N. L., and Crain, B. J. (1992). Evaluation of cerebral biopsies for the diagnosis of dementia. *Archives of Neurology*, **49**, 28–31.

Jones, A. L., Wood, J. D., and Harper, P. S. (1997). Huntington disease: advances in molecular and cell biology. *Journal of Inherited Metabolic Disease*, **20**, 125–38.

Jorm, A. F. and Jolley, D. (1998). The incidence of dementia — A meta-analysis. *Neurology*, **51**, 728–33.

Jorm, A. F., Korten, A. E., and Henderson, A. S. (1987). The prevalence of dementia: a quantitative integration of the literature. *Acta Psychiatrica Scandinavica*, **76**, 465–79.

Lipton, S. A. (1997). Neuropathogenesis of acquired immunodeficiency syndrome dementia. *Current Opinion in Neurology*, **10**, 247–53.

Martyn, C. N. (1998). Capture-recapture methods in surveys of diseases of the nervous system. *Journal of Neurology, Neurosurgery and Psychiatry*, **64**, 2–3.

McGonigal, G., McQuade, C., and Thomas, B. (1992). Accuracy and completeness of Scottish mental hospital in-patient data. *Health Bulletin*, **50**, 309–14.

McGonigal, G., Thomas, B., McQuade, C., Starr, J. M., MacLennan, W. J., and Whalley, L. J. (1993). Epidemiology of Alzheimer's presenile dementia in Scotland, 1974–88. *British Medical Journal*, **306**, 680–3.

McKeith, I. G., Galasko, D., Kosaka, K., Perry, E. K., Dickson, D. W., Hansen, L. A., *et al.* (1996). Consensus guidelines for the clinical and pathologic diagnosis of dementia with Lewy bodies (DLB): Report of the consortium on DLB international workshop. *Neurology*, **47**, 1113–24.

McKhann, G., Drachman, D., Folstein, M., Katzman, R., Price, D., and Stadlan, E. M. (1984). Clinical diagnosis of Alzheimer's disease: Report of the NINCDS–ADRDA work group under the auspices of Department of Health and Human Services Task Force on Alzheimer's disease. *Neurology*, **34**, 939–44.

Molsa, P. K., Marttila, R. J., and Rinne, U. K. (1982). Epidemiology of dementia in a Finnish population. *Acta Neurologica Scandinavica*, **65**, 541–52.

Neary, D. (1990). Non Alzheimer's disease forms of cerebral atrophy. *Journal of Neurology, Neurosurgery and Psychiatry*, **53**, 929–31.

Newens, A. J., Forster, D. P., and Kay, D. W. (1993a). Death certification after a diagnosis of presenile dementia. *Journal of Epidemiology and Community Health*, **47**, 293–7.

Newens, A. J., Forster, D. P., Kay, D. W., Kirkup, W., Bates, D., and Edwardson, J. (1993b). Clinically diagnosed presenile dementia of the Alzheimer type in the Northern Health Region: ascertainment, prevalence, incidence and survival. *Psychological Medicine*, **23**, 631–44.

Ott, A., Breteler, M. B., vanHarskamp, F., Stijnen, T., and Hofman, A. (1998). Incidence and risk of dementia — The Rotterdam Study. *American Journal of Epidemiology*, **147**, 574–80.

Perry, R., Irving, D., Blessed, G., Fairbairn, A., and Perry, E. (1989). Senile dementia of the Lewy body type. A clinically and neuropsychologically distinct form of Lewy body dementia in the elderly. *Journal of the Neurological Sciences, 95*, 119–39.

Rao, S. M., Leo, G. J., Bernardin, L., and Unverzagt, F. (1991). Cognitive dysfunction in multiple-sclerosis. 1. Frequency, patterns, and prediction. *Neurology, 41*, 685–91.

Reisberg, B., Ferris, S. H., de Leon, M. J., and Crook, T. (1988). Global deterioration scale (GDS). *Psychopharmacology Bulletin, 24*, 661–3.

Rocca, W. A., Hofman, A., Brayne, C., Breteler, M. M. B., Clarke, M., Copeland, J. R. M., *et al.* (1991). Frequency and distribution of Alzheimer's disease in Europe — a collaborative study of 1980–1990 prevalence findings. *Annals of Neurology, 30*, 381–90.

Roman, G. C., Tatemichi, T. K., Erkinjuntti, T., Cummings, J. L., Masdeu, J. C., Garcia, J. H., *et al.* (1993). Vascular dementia: Diagnostic criteria for research studies. Report of the NINDS–AIREN International Workshop. *Neurology, 43*, 250–60.

Rorsman, B., Hagnell, O., and Lanke, J. (1986). Prevalence and incidence of senile and multi-infarct dementia in the Lundby study: a comparison between the time periods 1947–1957 and 1957–1972. *Neuropsychobiology, 15*, 122–9.

Rossor, M. N. and Brown, J. (1995). Progressive supranuclear palsy — neuropathologically based diagnostic clinical-criteria. *Journal of Neurology, Neurosurgery and Psychiatry, 59*, 343.

Samson, N. W., Vanduijn, C. M., Hop, W. C. J., and Hofman, A. (1996). Clinical-features and mortality in patients with early-onset Alzheimers disease. *European Neurology, 36*, 103–6.

Schneider, J. A., Watts, R. L., Gearing, M., Brewer, R. P., and Mirra, S. S. (1997). Corticobasal degeneration: neuropathologic and clinical heterogeneity. *Neurology, 48*, 959–69.

Schoenberg, B. S., Anderson, D. W., and Haerer, A. F. (1985). Severe dementia prevalence and clinical features in a biracial US population. *Archives of Neurology, 42*, 740–3.

Starr, J. M., Thomas, B. M., and Whalley, L. J. (1997*a*). Familial or sporadic clusters of presenile Alzheimer's disease in Scotland: II. Case kinship. *Psychiatric Genetics, 7*, 147–52.

Starr, J. M., Thomas, B. M., and Whalley, L. J. (1997*b*). Familial or sporadic clusters of presenile dementia in Scotland: I. Parental causes of death in Alzheimer and vascular presenile dementias. *Psychiatric Genetics, 7*, 141–6.

Sulkava, R., Wikstrom, J., Aromaa, A., Raitasalo, R., Lehtinen, V., Lahtela, K., *et al.* (1985). Prevalence of severe dementia in Finland. *Neurology, 35*, 1025–9.

Thomas, B. M., McGonigal, G., McQuade, C. A., Starr, J. M., and Whalley, L. J. (1997). Survival in early onset dementia: Effects of urbanization and socio- economic deprivation. *Neuroepidemiology, 16*, 134–40.

Tomlinson, B. E., Blessed, G., and Roth, M. (1968). Observations on the brains of demented old people. *Journal of Neurological Science, 7*, 331–56.

Treves, T., Korczyn, A. D., and Zilber, N. (1986). Presenile dementia in Israel. *Archives of Neurology, 43*, 26–9.

van Duijn, C. M., Delasnerie Laupretre, N., Masullo, C., Zerr, I., deSilva, R., Wientjens, D. M., *et al.* (1998). Case-control study of risk factors of Creutzfeldt–Jakob disease in Europe during 1993–95. *Lancet, 351*, 1081–5.

van Duijn, C. M. and Hofman, A. (1992). Risk factors for Alzheimer's disease: the EURODEM collaborative re-analysis of case-control studies. *Neuroepidemiology, 11* (Suppl 1), 106–13.

Whalley, L. J. and Holloway, S. (1985). Non-random geographical distribution of Alzheimer's presenile dementia in Edinburgh 1953–76. *Lancet*, 578.

Whalley, L. J., Thomas, B. M., and Starr, J. M. (1995). Epidemiology of presenile Alzheimer's disease in Scotland (1974–88). 2. Exposures to possible risk factors. *British Journal of Psychiatry, 167*, 732–8.

Whalley, L. J., Thomas, B. M., Starr, J. M., McGonigal, G., McQuade, C., and Black, R. (1994). Migration and risk-factors for Alzheimers presenile dementia in Scotland. *Neurobiology of Aging, 15*, S75 (Abstract).

Will, R. G., Ironside, J. W., Zeidler, M., Cousens, S. N., Estibeiro, K., Alperovitch, A., *et al.* (1996). A new variant of Creutzfeldt–Jakob disease in the UK. *Lancet, 347*, 921–5.

2 The clinical approach to assessing patients with early onset dementia

Peter Nestor and John R. Hodges

1 Introduction

The clinical assessment of patients with suspected dementia should, ideally, be multidisciplinary. Neurology, neuropsychology, and psychiatry each have an important role to play in the diagnostic process. Whether one chooses to offer these in a joint assessment clinic or as series of separate consultations will probably depend more on practical than clinical expediencies. Each has its own advantages and disadvantages; our approach, which we have found particularly rewarding, is the joint assessment clinic in which complex referrals are seen by all three arms of the team on the same day (the Cambridge Memory Clinic is described in detail elsewhere: see Berrios and Hodges 2000). This offers the opportunity for a multidisciplinary case-conference at the end of the individual assessments and is convenient where patients have travelled long distances to be seen. The principle disadvantages are that some patients find such an intensive approach quite tiring and there are also occasions when with hindsight a single medical consultation would have been adequate, for example where a patient is clearly in the moderate to severe stages of Alzheimer's disease.

No matter how one chooses to set up the clinic, it is of paramount importance to adopt a methodical approach to sorting out the various possibilities This is best achieved by first considering the diagnostic categories one is likely to encounter in a memory clinic setting as summarized in Figure 2.1. Patients will fall into four broad groups: the worried-well, the psychiatrically ill (particularly depression), those with a degenerative dementia, and a miscellaneous group (delirium, focal brain pathologies, metabolic disorders, inflammatory diseases, Korsakoff's, etc.).

The first aim is the separation of the worried-well: often made complicated because the worry is generated by a positive family history. For a significant number, follow-up over time will be the only way of making absolutely sure that subtle complaints do not herald the onset of an organic syndrome. Next is the detection and management of treatable psychiatric illness. It is important to note, however, that a significant number of those with organic brain disorders will exhibit concurrent psychiatric symptomatology, particularly features of depression (see Chapter 5). As these groups are not mutually exclusive, it is not uncommon to instigate a trial of anti-depressant therapy in parallel with investigations for organic causes of cognitive complaints. Follow-up is again the key to separating depression with cognitive symptoms from dementia with prominent affective symptoms.

For those who show evidence of organic impairment of cognition, the aim is to reach a specific diagnosis. Clinical features of delirium will necessitate extensive general medical

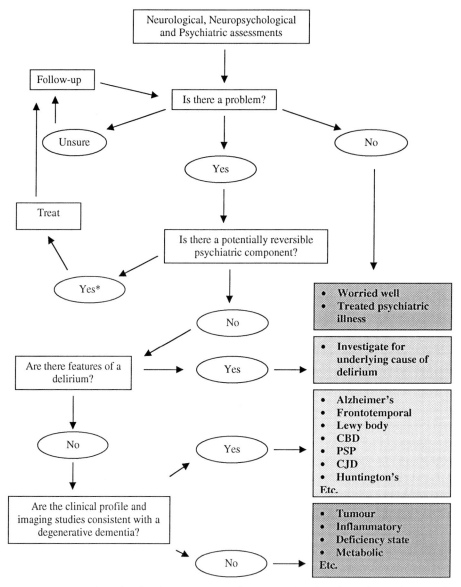

Figure 2.1 Diagnostic algorithm for the assessment of cognitive disorders. (*Psychiatric features do not exclude the possibility of organic pathology and it may be appropriate to investigate further whilst a trial of therapy is in progress). PSP = progressive supranuclear palsy; CJD = Creutzfeldt–Jacob disease; CBD = corticobasal degeneration.

investigation often including EEG and cerebrospinal fluid examinations. The features of delirium are summarized in Table 2.1. The proportion of cases with a potentially reversible acute brain syndrome will vary according to local referral patterns; in our memory clinic, the vast majority of patients with an organic disease will have a degenerative dementia. A final useful subclassification is into those with a relatively pure cognitive syndrome and those with associated neurological signs; the clinical patterns for the major degenerative dementias are summarized in Table 2.2.

Table 2.1 The features of delirium

Onset	Usually acute/subacute
Course	Fluctuating, nocturnal exacerbations
Conscious state	May be impaired, derangement of normal sleep/wake cycle
Cognitive profile	Disoriented in time and place
	Severe impairment of attention (with knock-on effects to other cognitive domains, i.e. due to poor registration etc.)
Psychiatric features	Incoherent and perseverative
	Mood disorders: agitation, apathy
	Visual illusions and hallucinations
	Paranoid ideas common
Physical signs	Asterixis
	May be evidence of general medical illness (pyrexia, signs of hepatic failure etc.)

2 History

Unlike other specialist medical consultations, patients referred to a clinic for assessment of cognitive function may not possess a clear understanding of why they are attending. The clinician, therefore, needs to be somewhat circumspect in their initial contact with the patient. After introductions, it is worthwhile to inquire into the patient's understanding of the purpose of the visit. If it transpires that they do not understand the reasons for their referral, one should introduce the topic with care: otherwise the patient is liable to find the experience a traumatic one and this will also impede the diagnostic process. It is best to err on the side understatement in this circumstance (e.g. '*well, your doctor was concerned that your memory is not as good as it was a few years ago and asked us to check things out ... have you noticed anything along those lines?*').

Otherwise history taking in dementias follows the same principles as those of any medical consultation though there are two other notable exceptions. First, the necessity to obtain a corroborative history from an informant and, second, the history, as told by the patient, will also form part of the cognitive examination.

2.1 Informant

There are a number of reasons why it is mandatory to obtain a history from an informant. Most obviously, a patient with memory or language impairment may simply be unable to give an adequate account of their problems. Another issue, in more subtle cases, is that of insight; while patients with Alzheimer's disease typically have some degree of insight, they tend to underestimate the extent of their problems. Frontal dementias (such as the frontal variant of frontotemporal dementia) are characteristically associated with lack of insight; this is frequently so extreme that the patient cannot even comprehend the reason for the clinic appointment. Given that such patients' problems manifest initially with qualitative changes in personality, lack of informant testimony makes it virtually impossible to distinguish early frontal dementia from, for instance, a life-long eccentric personality.

Table 2.2 Typical clinical profiles of the major categories of degenerative dementia

	Memory	Language	Visuospatial	Attention	Frontal behavioural symptoms	Neurological signs
Alzheimer's disease	++++	++	++	++	±	–
Alzheimer's: biparietal variant	+/++	+	++++	++	±	–
Dementia with Lewy bodies	++	+	+++	+++	±	++
Frontotemporal dementia:						– (unless associated with MND)[a]
Semantic dementia	+	++++	±	+	++	
Frontal variant	+	+	±	++	++++	
Progressive non-fluent aphasia	±	++++	±	+	+	
Corticobasal degeneration	+	+	+++	++	++	+++
Progressive supranuclear palsy	+	+	+	+++	++	+++
Huntington's disease	+	+	+	+++	++	+++

[a] MND = motor neuron disease.

An informant history is also important in helping identify the 'worried-well' and those with non-organic memory complaints: in such cases there is usually a marked contrast between their subjective complaints and the informants account of normal everyday functioning.

An informant should, wherever possible, be someone who lives with the patient or at the very least someone who has been acquainted with the patient for an extended period (i.e. have knowledge of their premorbid state). Information obtained from such sources gives far more first-hand insight into the impact the presenting problem has on the patients ability to carry on with activities of daily living.

One should always interview the informant in the patient's absence. This will allow a far franker discussion which is particularly important as, for instance a spouse, may find many of the behavioural aspects of dementias (e.g. sexual disinhibition) awkward to brooch in front of the patient. Separate interview of the informant is also kinder to the patient: for instance, a patient with mild Alzheimer's can become very distressed if forced to listen to an account of the extent of their cognitive impairment. Whilst it may seem that excluding the patient from this part of the consultation may create suspicion or mistrust, provided the clinician prefaces the need for the informants interview with a thoughtful explanation there is seldom a problem (e.g. *'Mr Smith, because you feel there is possibly a problem with your memory, I would now like to go over the details of your story with your wife, separately, in case there are any important details you have forgotten'*). An outline of the useful areas of inquiry is given in Table 2.3.

Table 2.3 Checklist of points to cover from informant's history

General features	Duration of problem(s)
	Initial symptoms
	Course (gradual, stepwise, static, etc.)
Cognitive symptoms	Memory
	Working (attention slips, poor concentration)
	Episodic (recall of specific events)
	Semantic (general knowledge, vocabulary)
	Language and speech (coherence of expression, comprehension)
	Visuospatial/perceptual (topographical and face recognition problems)
	Calculation (bills and money)
	Executive function (planning and organization)
Neuropsychiatric symptoms	Personality and behavioural change
	Disinhibition
	Loss of empathy/interest for family
	Apathy
	Stereotyped/ritualistic habits
	Impulsivity or challenging behaviours
	Mood (depression, euphoria)
	Psychotic phenomena (especially hallucinations)
	Eating habits (stereotyped, or especially, craving of sweet foods)
	Sleep pattern
	Sexual behaviour
Activities of daily living	Grooming
	Housework
	Shopping
	Hobbies
	Driving
	Work
	Social events

Based on our experience running a memory and early onset dementia clinic over the past decade we have developed a questionnaire (the Cambridge Behavioural Inventory) which carers complete prior to attending the clinic. This incorporates most of the sections in Table 2.3 and serves as a useful screening instrument. It derives largely from the Neuropsychiatric Inventory (Cummings *et al.* 1994) described in more detail in Chapter 4.

2.2 The history as a part of the examination

The other fundamental way in which the clinical assessment of suspected dementia differs from other medical conditions is that the mental faculties used by the patient to construct a narrative description of their presenting problem are also the areas under scrutiny as potentially defective. The clinician can supplement details missing from the patient's account, because of impaired cognition, from the informants history (see Section 2.1) but it is extremely important not to disregard the patient's account of themselves: even if it provides little objective information, their version of the history should be examined for what it can reveal of the underlying problem. This is especially true in the domains of language and memory.

2.2.1 Spontaneous language

Although formal examination of language is discussed below (Sections 2.3.2 and 4.2), much information can be gained from a patient's spontaneous conversation. In particular, the examiner should note language fluency: does conversation flow freely with reasonable sentence and phrase lengths, or does it appear effortful, non-fluent, and punctuated by frequent pauses or phonological errors (e.g. 'bobble' for 'bottle'). The latter may suggest a non-fluent aphasia as part of a frontotemporal dementia.

If spontaneous language is fluent, then one should assess whether it conveys meaningful information or, alternatively, whether it is vacuous and circumlocutive (e.g. *'Oh you know, the thing you put the stuff in when your going somewhere and …'*) as is seen in the fluent aphasia of semantic dementia or in the fluent anomia which typically accompanies the middle stages of Alzheimer's disease. These groups also, characteristically, make semantic paraphasic errors (substitution of a word related in meaning: instead of 'zebra', 'horse' or a broad superordinate response like 'animal').

2.2.2 Memory

A very good impression of episodic or autobiographical memory (i.e. memory for personally experienced events) can be gained from the history. Episodic memory can be subdivided into anterograde (i.e. the acquisition of new memories) and retrograde; the latter is best assessed by getting the patient to give a narrative account of their own life. The approach we use is to ask them to recount details of schooling, parents occupation, any moves, employers, marriages, births of children, retirement, grandchildren, and so on. The informant is relied on, not only for pointing out lapses, but also to exclude confabulation.

2.3 Presenting complaint

One should note the mode of onset: sudden or insidious. If sudden, what were the circumstances around the time of onset. For instance, did the symptoms begin after a general anaesthetic; were there features suggestive of encephalitis or subarachnoid haemorrhage. *Note: an important trap is the frequent false attribution by family members of an insidious illness to an acute event. In the early stages patients may compensate such that it is not until a crisis occurs (an accident, inter-current illness, or death of spouse) that problems become evident. One should therefore probe very carefully for subtle evidence of impairment dating from before the acute episode.*

Is the disorder static (stroke, Korsakoff's), stepwise (multi-infarct), or progressive (degenerative)? If progressive, is the duration measured in years (frontotemporal dementia, Alzheimer's disease) or weeks to months (see Table 2.4 for summary of causes of rapidly progressive dementias)? Is the course fluctuating or relentless? A fluctuating course is suggestive of delirium, a non-convulsive seizure disorder, and vasculitides, but also is a prominent feature of dementia with Lewy bodies.

Questions should then be targeted to specific cognitive domain using the same outline as suggested in Table 2.3, but at all times one should endeavour to assess complaints in terms of the impact they are having on the patients lifestyle. The presenting problem and the 'social history' are, therefore, blended: ability to dress oneself, prepare a meal, make a financial transaction, follow directions to an unfamiliar location, etc. will yield greater insights than recording 'cannot concentrate' or 'hopeless at remembering anything', etc.

2.3.1 Memory

The vast majority of cases referred to a memory or cognitive disorders clinic have complaints of 'poor memory'. Some idea of memory performance will have already been gleaned from the patients ability to recount their past life story (Section 2.2.2). When assessing memory complaints it is useful to apply a theoretically-motivated approach to analysing symptoms according to the subcomponent of memory involved (see also Chapter 3). In broad terms assessing memory symptoms can be considered under the following headings:

Working memory: lapses of attention (such as forgetting why you opened the refrigerator door or went into the study, or immediately forgetting a new telephone number) are common everyday symptoms which are increased with anxiety, depression, and also occur more commonly with advancing age. Complaints of this type are also common after head injury and in basal ganglia disorders but should not be used as evidence for an amnesic syndrome.

Table 2.4 Causes of a rapidly progressive dementing illness

Inflammatory	Cerebral vasculitis Multiple sclerosis Sarcoidosis
Neoplastic	Primary CNS tumour Cerebral metastases Paraneoplastic (limbic encephalitis)
Nutritional	Thiamine deficiency (Wernicke-Korsakoff syndrome)
Infectious	Cerebral abscess Herpes encephalitis Progressive multifocal leukoencephalopathy Human immunodeficiency virus Subacute sclerosing panencephalitis Whipple's disease
Prion	Creutzfeldt–Jacob disease
Vascular	Multiple infarcts (e.g. emboli secondary to endocarditis) CADASIL

Episodic memory: difficulty with the acquisition of new event-based memories (such as inability to recall details of a television programme or conversation with a friend despite good attention at the time) is the hallmark of early Alzheimer's disease and other causes of the amnesic syndrome (Table 2.5). Retrograde memory is typically better than anterograde but deteriorates as Alzheimer's progresses.

Semantic memory: loss of memory for words is the usual complaint in patients with progressive fluent aphasia (semantic dementia). It is important, however, to distinguish between the occasional word finding lapse, usually for proper nouns which occurs normally (especially in later life) and the relentlessly progressive loss of vocabulary which occurs in association with left temporal lobe pathology. Low frequency words are the most vulnerable and semantic dementia patients often have some insight into this problem in the early stages. For instance, a carpenter may complain that they can no longer remember the names of tools. Alzheimer's sufferers show a similar phenomenon though it is usually overshadowed by their profound memory deficit.

An often informative question is to ask the patient to rate their overall day-to-day memory on a 0–10 scale (10 being perfectly normal for age, 0 being abysmal). Paradoxically it is typically not the patient with an organic memory deficit who rates themselves as 0/10. In our experience most patients with early Alzheimer's produce self ratings in the 4–8 range with significantly lower scores being given by their spouses.

2.3.2 Language

The overlap between memory and language (semantic memory being the common 'memory' database which underlies our ability to make sense of words, objects, and faces) means that most patients with semantic breakdown actually complain of 'loss of memory for words' or something similar.

Table 2.5 Causes of the amnesic syndrome

Type	Common aetiologies
Transient	Transient global amnesia
	Transient epileptic amnesia
	Closed head injury (may be permanent)
	Post electroconvulsive therapy
	Drugs (esp. ethanol)
Anatomically defined	
Hippocampus (and adjacent mesial temporal structures)	Alzheimer's disease
	Herpes simplex encephalitis
	Limbic encephalitis (paraneoplastic)
	Anoxia (cardiac arrest, CO poisoning, etc.)
	Complicating epilepsy surgery
Diencephalon (dorso-medial thalamus, mammilary bodies)	Korsakoff's psychosis
	Infarction (watershed, deep perforator occlusion, 'top of the basilar' syndrome)
Basal forebrain	Ruptured anterior communicating artery aneurysm
Fornix	Complicating colloid cyst removal from third ventricle
Retrosplenial/posterior cingulate	Various: tumour, haemorrhage, etc.
Psychogenic (non-organic)	

Breakdown in the phonological and/or syntactic aspects of language is more likely to give rise to complaints of impaired speech or communication. Non-fluent language problems are often obvious from the outset of the interview and astute spouses may notice agrammatism and volunteer that the patient has problems with order or endings of words. Inability to decipher syntax in spoken conversation is often described by the patient as difficulty 'hearing', particularly in group situations.

Problems deciphering written language and hence gaining enjoyment from reading should point to dyslexic difficulties. Writing is a late acquired and fragile skill which may breakdown due to problems with composition, spelling, or praxis.

2.3.3 Attention/executive function

Impaired attention is common in frontal dementias and dementia with Lewy bodies but is also a prominent feature of subcortical dementias, delirium, depression, and anxiety states. Attention is normal in very early Alzheimer's disease but deteriorates as the disease progresses. In neuropsychology, attention has diverse meanings including the ability to sustain concentration on external stimuli even when such stimuli occur infrequently, to focus on one particular auditory or visual stimulus when distracted by other irrelevant stimuli, and to divide or partition resources when required to undertake two tasks simultaneously. These abilities require co-ordinated activity of cortical (especially fronto-parietal) and subcortical structures. Patients with attentional deficits complain of difficulty concentrating particularly in distracting environments and maintaining two tasks (e.g. following conversations).

Executive function refers to the ability to plan, set goals, organize subtasks and to shift between them if necessary, to self-monitor cognitive activity, and to inhibit the tendency to distraction. These abilities depend largely upon frontal lobe function. Problems using household appliances, organizing the weekly household, shopping, and maintaining hobbies all suggest pronounced executive dysfunction.

2.3.4 Visuospatial and perceptual function

Complaints of impaired vision are relatively unusual in the primary degenerative dementias. Problems with spatial location causing misreaching for objects or the tendency to miss steps indicate bilateral parietal pathology with interruption of the dorsal ('where?') stream of visual processing. Classic causes of biparietal pathology include watershed infarction, CO poisoning, progressive multifocal leukoencephalopathy and leukodystrophies. Such symptoms are also increasingly recognized in the so-called posterior cortical atrophy (or biparietal) variant of Alzheimer's disease (Mackenzie Ross *et al.* 1996).

Problems with object or face recognition (visual object agnosia and prosopagnosia respectively) occur in the context of severe, usually bilateral temporal pathology with disruption of the ventral ('what?') stream of visual processing. Symptoms of this type may arise in the setting of Alzheimer's disease, but are typically overshadowed by deficits in episodic memory and language. They are more commonly a feature of semantic dementia (the temporal lobe variant of frontotemporal dementia — see Chapter 12).

Visual hallucinations occur late in the course of Alzheimer's disease; presentation with prominent early visual hallucinations suggest a diagnosis of dementia with Lewy bodies (see Chapter 13). They can take the form of frank hallucinations or illusions (misidentifying real objects: usually in the context of poor illumination such as thinking swaying trees at night are people). Whether the patient retains insight into the falsity of such images is of little discriminative value.

Table 2.6 Degenerative dementias which may be dominantly inherited

	Gene	Chromosome
Alzheimer's disease	Amyloid precursor protein (mutations)	21
	Presenilin 1 (mutations)	14
	Presenilin 2 (mutations)	1
Creutzfeldt–Jacob	Prion protein: PRNP (mutations)	20
Frontotemporal demenita	Tau (mutations)	17
Huntington's disease	Huntingtin (CAG trinucleotide expansion)	4

2.4 Family history

A detailed family history, including the ages and causes of death is essential since inherited forms of dementia (Table 2.6) are more common in the presenile than older age group. Even when a positive family history is present, it is common to find that previous generations will not have been given a precise diagnosis: thus it is inadequate to ask if there is a history of 'Pick's disease' etc. One should make more general inquiries into a history of memory problems, sustained behavioural changes, psychiatric illness, chorea, etc. Finally, as in general neurological practice a history of consanguinity raises the possibility of a recessively inherited disorder (e.g. metachromatic leukodystrophy).

2.5 Past medical history

2.5.1 Neurological disorders

Of particular relevance are a past history of seizures, head injury, strokes, or encephalitis. Normal pressure hydrocephalus may be preceded by a past history of bacterial meningitis or subarachnoid haemorrhage. The latter when due to anterior communicating artery aneurysms is also an important cause of an amnesic syndrome.

2.5.2 Non-neurological disorders

Numerous systemic disorders can potentially give rise to cognitive impairment and it is not feasible to inquire directly after all possibilities; a more practical approach is to take a detailed past history to see if any potential candidates turn up. Of particular importance are markers of vasculitis such as rash, arthritis renal disease, etc. and metabolic disorders (e.g. hepatic failure, uraemia, hypercapnia). An association between autoimmune thyroid disease with very high levels of circulating antithyroid microsomal antibodies (Hashimoto's encephalopathy) is being increasingly recognized (see Chapter 17 section 3). Gastrointestinal diseases may be relevant either indirectly through malabsorption (e.g. B12) or via direct CNS involvement (Whipple's disease, coeliac disease). Malignancy may cause cognitive failure by direct spread to the CNS (metastases or leptomeningeal disease) or as a paraneoplastic syndrome: limbic encephalitis, usually associated with small cell lung cancer and causing a rapid onset profound amnesic syndrome (Bak *et al.* in pres). The traditional infection related to cognitive disorders, syphilis is now rare in the western world but still occurs occasionally. Human immunodeficiency virus either *per se* or with an HIV-associated illness (e.g. progressive multifocal leukoencephalopathy) is now the leading infectious cause of chronic cognitive impairment (see Chapter 17 section 4).

2.5.3 Vascular risk factors

Risk factors for vascular disease are sufficiently important to warrant specific inquiry in every case. A past history of vascular events (stroke, myocardial, peripheral), cardiac disease (especially atrial fibrillation), tobacco consumption, hypertension, diabetes mellitus, family history of premature vascular disease, and hypercholesterolemia should be noted.

2.6 Drugs and alcohol

Establishing the patients' level of alcohol intake is crucial. Even if currently abstinent, one should establish if an amnesic patient ever had a period of high intake. Binge drinking combined with poor diet is the usual recipe for causing Korsakoff's. Drug history (prescribed or otherwise) is relevant in suspected delirium. It also offers a useful index to the severity of psychiatric illnesses such as depression or anxiety. For instance, chronic courses of antidepressants usually suggest a more significant illness than one which has not required therapy.

2.7 Psychiatric history

The commonest treatable differential diagnosis of degenerative dementia is psychiatric illness: particularly depression. The importance of a formal psychiatric assessment can not be overstated. Symptoms of mood disturbance (anhedonia, apathy, tiredness, pessimistic ruminations, suicidal ideation) and biological features of depression (anorexia, early morning waking, reduced libido) should be sought in all cases.

In addition, psychiatric symptoms are frequently encountered in degenerative dementias. Hallucinations (particularly visual, Section 2.3.4) and delusional states (such as the Capgras phenomenon) are particularly important. See Chapters 4 and 5 for further discussion.

3 Bedside cognitive test batteries

Cognitive function can be assessed using a problem oriented approach (for example, performing specific language tasks in suspected aphasia), or by using a non-problem oriented 'screening' battery. Ideally, one should incorporate both methods in the assessment of cognitive disorders, the problem oriented approach is the topic of Section 4. Bedside test batteries offer the advantage of providing a numerical score which allows comparison with other patients and monitoring of progress; with experience, the score also enables the examiner to estimate the degree of difficulty at which to pitch subsequent problem oriented tests. For further details see Hodges (1994).

The most universally employed bedside cognitive battery is probably the 'Mini-Mental State Examination' (Folstein *et al.* 1975) (MMSE, Figure 2.2) which provides a score out of 30 and is generally considered abnormal if 24 or less is attained. Whilst a score of ≤ 24 is highly suggestive of a cognitive disorder, it must be realized that scoring above 24/30 does not exclude cognitive dysfunction. For instance, as the test is heavily weighted toward verbal tasks, a patient with a severe disturbance of right hemisphere function may well score 29/30. Likewise, patients with significant frontal pathology frequently score flawlessly; even patients with early Alzheimer's disease may score 27/30 (only failing the recall items) and yet show profound deficits on specific memory tests. The simplicity of the language tasks and the lack of executive components make it particularly insensitive to frontotemporal dementia. Despite these drawbacks, the MMSE is quick and simple to administer, does not require any additional equipment, and its significance is widely appreciated; it is therefore recommended as a minimum screening battery.

Orientation

Year/month/season/day/date
/5

Country/county/town/hospital/floor
/5

Anterograde memory

Registration: I would like you to remember 3 objects (e.g. lemon, key, ball). Ask patient to repeat
/3

Attention:

Starting at 100 can you subtract 7 and keep going down by 7
i.e. 100, 93, 86, 79, 72, 65
OR

Can you spell "WORLD" backwards

(Record best score)
/5

Anterograde memory (cont.)

What were the 3 items I asked you to remember?
/3

Language

Can you tell what this is?
(Show a pen and a watch)
/2

Can you take this piece of paper with your hand, fold it half with both hands, and place it on the floor?
/3

Can you repeat the phrase, "NO IFS ANDS OR BUTS"
/1

Can you read this and do what it says:

CLOSE YOUR EYES
/1

Can you write a sentence about something (any subject)
/1

Visuospatial

Copy this design

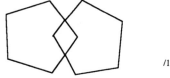

/1

NOTES

Accept date if correct to within 2 days

May be adapted to circumstances: eg country/city/neighbourhood/street/floor

Do not penalise for sequential errors:
Eg "100, 92, 85, 78, 71, 64" scores 4/5

"DRLOW" scores 4/5
"DW" scores 2/5 (i.e. "DW"=D,x,x,x,W)

If the patient deals with the "attention" test very quickly it may be necessary to postpone delayed recall until later in the test.

Must contain a subject, verb and object to score 1 point.

Both pentagons must have 5 sides and be interlocked to score 1 point. Do not penalise for poor artistic quality.

TOTAL: /30

Figure 2.2   Folstein Mini-Mental State Examination (MMSE).

For clinicians who regularly see patients with potential cognitive impairment, a somewhat more expansive screening battery is recommended. Although there are a number of longer standardized batteries, e.g. the CAMCOG (Roth *et al.* 1988) and the Dementia Rating Scale (Mattis 1992), these are not suited to routine 'bedside' clinical practice. Over the past five years, we have evolved the Addenbrooke's Cognitive Examination (ACE: Figures 2.3 and 2.4) for use in the Memory and Early Onset Dementia Clinics which incorporates the MMSE within the total score of 100, takes ten minutes or so to administer, and has been normed on over 100 older control subjects. Derived from our neuropsychological research over the past decade (Greene *et al.* 1996; Gregory *et al.* 1999; Hodges and Patterson 1995; Hodges *et al.* 1992, 1999), the ACE was designed to be sensitive to the early stages of Alzheimer's disease and frontotemporal dementia syndromes. It stresses, therefore, episodic memory, executive function, and language abilities. Based on over 200 cases referred to the clinic, a cut-off score of 83/100 it had a sensitivity of 82% and a specificity of 96% for the detection of early dementia, whilst the MMSE at a cut-off of 24/30 had a sensitivity of 52% and a specificity of 96% in the same population (Mathuranath *et al.* 2000).

The memory tasks on the ACE include learning and delayed recall of a seven-element name and address as well as recall of present and previous heads of state. Language testing is expanded with naming of a further ten mid-frequency line drawings (half living, half artefacts), more comprehension of words and phrases, repetition, and reading (regular and irregular words). Also included is verbal fluency for words beginning with the letter 'P' and from the category animals. In addition to its greater sensitivity in detected dementia it has discriminate value in classifying Alzheimer's and frontotemporal dementia. By summing the scores on the verbal fluency and language sections and dividing by the sum of the orientation and delayed recall sections the VL/OM index is calculated (Figure 2.5). An index of > 3.2 is 58% sensitive and 97% specific to Alzheimer's disease, whilst one of < 2.2 is 58% sensitive and 97% specific to frontotemporal dementia (Mathuranath *et al.* 2000).

4 Problem-oriented cognitive examination

This section will address the examination of higher mental function by cognitive domain but includes some explanation of the subtests included in the ACE. Before beginning, it is important to stress is that one should follow a logical sequence in assessing cognitive function so as to avoid false positive diagnoses due to sequential effects. For example, tests of executive function, which utilize analysis of complex verbal material, would be beyond the grasp of a fluent aphasic, due to the fundamental disorder of language comprehension without needing to implicate frontal lobe damage. Likewise, a patient with an acute delirium may be unable to perform even the most basic memory tasks as a consequence of their attention deficit and therefore ought not to be labelled amnesic.

4.1 Orientation and attention

Assessment of orientation includes details of time and place. Testing personal orientation adds little as, only profoundly aphasic or hysterical patients, are unable to relate their own name. Severe disorientation is not a contraindication to further testing but does call for additional assessment of attention. The attentional component of the MMSE — subtracting backwards by 7 from 100 or spelling WORLD backwards — are both rather flawed since they can be failed due to specific problems with numbers (acalculia) or spelling. Digit span is one of the simplest, yet pure, methods of assessing attention, especially in the backwards condition; normal subjects

MMSE   /30

Anterograde memory

Read the name and address and ask patient to repeat immediately. Repeat this 3 times regardless of score

	Trial:	1	2	3	5 min. delay*
Peter Marshall		——	——	——	——
42 Market Street		———	———	———	———
Chelmsford		—	—	—	—
Essex		—	—	—	—
		Π	Π	Π	Π

subtotal: /28

Retrograde memory

Can you name the...
Prime Minister
Last Prime Minister
Opposition leader
USA President   /4

Verbal fluency
Time 60 seconds for each:
Letter: *Ask the patient to list as many words as possible beginning with the letter "P" (not proper nouns)*   Π
(Score:[after subtracting errors] >17 words=7; 14-17=6; 11-13=5; 8-10=4; 6-7=3; 4-5=2;<4=1)
Animal: *Ask the patient to list as many animals as possible (any letter of the alphabet)*   Π
(Score:[after subtracting errors] >21 words=7;17-21=6; 14-16=5; 11-13=4; 9-10=3; 7-8=2; <7=1)

Naming

Ask patient to name the drawings in figure 4...   /10

Comprehension

Ask the patient to...
Point to the door
Point to the ceiling   /2

Point to ceiling then the door
Point to the door after touching the bed/desk   /2

Repetition

Please repeat the following...
Brown / Conversation / Articulate   /3

The orchestra played and the audience applauded.   /1

Reading

Read the following words...   *Score 1 if all correct*
shed / wipe / board / flame / bridge   /1
sew / pint / soot / dough / height   /1

Visuospatial

Copy this drawing...

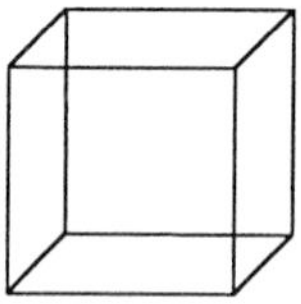

/1

Draw a clockface with numbers and the hands at ten to two...
Score 1 each for circle, numbers and hands   /3

(*Remember to check delayed address recall)

TOTAL   /100

Figure 2.3   Addenbrooke's Cognitive Examination. In 127 normal subjects aged 50–80 years: mean = 93.9, SD = 3.5.

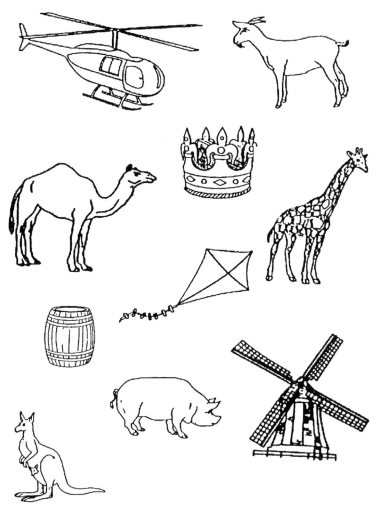

Figure 2.4   Items for use in naming test of the ACE.

have a forward span of at least six digits and a reverse span one or two digits less. Since span is a measure of the ability to temporarily retain a random sequence of *individual* items, the digits must be presented as individual items (read the string to be repeated at a rate of one digit per second). A common pitfall is to cluster digits as one does when reciting telephone numbers.

Maximum:

42

———

17

Figure 2.5   VL/OM ratio for discriminating frontotemporal dementia and Alzheimer's disease.

This inflates span as each cluster becomes an individual item: compare repeating *6953–8127* with *6 … 9 … 5 … 3 … 8 … 1 … 2 … 7.*

Ability to persevere at a given task is another way of considering attention; this can be tested by asking the patient to recite the months of the year in reverse order or to copy an alternating design. Tasks of the latter variety are often completed successfully when copied directly, but degenerate when the patient has to extrapolate the pattern (Figure 2.6). A recent onset of profound disorientation and attention deficit is typical of a delirium and should prompt the examiner to check for asterixis (metabolic flap). It should be noted that many patients with marked episodic memory problems (e.g. early Alzheimer's disease) remain well oriented.

4.2 Language

The analysis of aphasia is complex and here the principles will be considered in the context of the language disorder of Alzheimer's disease and variants of frontotemporal dementia with prominent aphasia (progressive non-fluent aphasia and semantic dementia). Verbal language testing should always include naming, repetition of words and phrases, and comprehension.

Naming is a complex task that requires the integrity of three basic processes: visual analysis, semantic knowledge, and word production (phonology). To exclude a visual deficit, patients can be asked to name to description (*'What do we call the large grey African animal with a trunk?'*). Word production deficits, as well as the production of phonological naming errors, are almost always associated with impaired repetition of multisyllabic words and phrases.

Though Alzheimer's disease is considered primarily a memory disorder, language dysfunction occurs within a few years in most cases. This manifests particularly as word finding difficulty and impairment in naming tasks. Errors on naming tasks are typically circumlocutions (e.g. kite: 'that thing that flies'; kangaroo: 'the Australian one that hops about') or semantically related (co-ordinates such as 'pig' for 'goat' or superordinates such as 'animal' for 'giraffe'). Naming ability is highly related to object familiarity, thus only the most aphasic subject is unable to name the two items on the MMSE (pen and watch). In the ACE we have used ten additional middle range familiarity items (see Figure 2.4).

The characteristics of semantic dementia (progressive fluent aphasia) are fluent speech which is devoid of content with semantic errors but normal phonology and syntax. Comprehension of word meaning is also impaired. In mild cases this can be demonstrated with semantically complex language tasks (e.g. *'Can you point to a source of artificial illumination?'*) or by defining uncommon words (e.g. *'What is an aubergine, accordion …'*). Patients who reply to the question *'do you have any hobbies?'* with *'what's a hobby?'* almost certainly have semantic dementia.

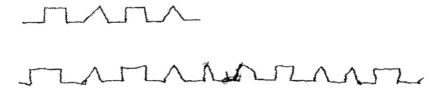

Figure 2.6 Examiners example and patients copy of an alternating pattern. Note that the patients ability to sustain the alternating design degenerates when requested to continue without a template. The patient was a 56-year-old male with delirium secondary to CNS lupus.

In non-fluent aphasia there is derangement of the phonological and syntactic (verb conjugations, prepositions, etc.) aspects of language. In contrast to fluent aphasia, speech is laboured, distorted, and typically littered with phonological errors. Repetition of multisyllabic words and phrases is impaired. Single word comprehension is spared but patients may fail to understand complex grammar such as reversible passive sentences: '*the lion was eaten by the tiger, who survived?*'. Buccofacial apraxia is also a common feature of progressive non-fluent aphasia; patients are unable to perform tasks such as licking lips or blowing out matches to command.

Aphasia is a disorder of language in all modalities thus reading and writing should also be tested. There may be a dissociation between ability to read orthographically regular (pronounced as they are spelt) words such as *mint, flint, hint, etc.* and irregular words such as *pint, cellist, island, etc.* Difficulty reading the latter type is known as surface dyslexia and is one of the hallmarks of semantic dementia (for an irregular word such as 'pint' or 'yacht' to be read correctly, the reader must access knowledge of the word meaning as the graphical representation of the word alone {i.e. its 'surface' structure} will not lead to correct pronunciation. If the semantic knowledge-base breaks down then the word can only be pronounced according to the rules of graphical to phonological translation and thus 'pint' will be pronounced like 'mint'; in other words, analogous to how a normal person would pronounce a non-word e.g. 'rint'): see (Patterson and Hodges 1992).

4.3 Memory

As outlined above, a useful theoretically-based distinction is that between short-term (or working) memory and longer-term memory (in psychology long-term memory refers to anything beyond seconds!). Long-term memory may be subdivided into episodic (autobiographical memory) and semantic (shared knowledge of the world including words, facts, and objects). Working memory can really be regarded as one component of attention and is tested by immediate repetition of strings of words (such as the three items of the MMSE) or digits (see Section 4.1).

Episodic memory impairment is the key deficit in early Alzheimer's disease and in patients with an amnesic syndrome. It is surprising, therefore, that the most commonly used bedside test, the MMSE, contains such inadequate assessment of this domain. In the ACE, we have expanded the episodic memory component by incorporating a name and address learning and recall task: the most critical part being the recall after a five to ten minute delay. Patients with early Alzheimer's disease typically repeat the name address perfectly after two or three trials but show very rapid forgetting and recall little or nothing after a delay. In our normative study of elderly controls, all recalled ⩾ four (the majority between five and seven) elements of the name and address.

Testing semantic memory in terms of knowledge of famous people offers a method of assessing for retrograde amnesia. For instance, asking the patient to list Prime Ministers in reverse chronological order. Breakdown in semantic memory also manifests as inability to name objects or drawings with the production of broad superordinate responses (e.g. 'animal' for 'elephant') and the inability to define the meaning of words. Category fluency (see below) is another sensitive measure of semantic memory.

4.4 Visuospatial

Visual function beyond the primary visual cortex is best evaluated in terms of the distinction between the ventral (occipitotemporal) pathway of 'what' a stimulus is and a dorsal (occipitoparietal) pathway of 'where' it is in space (Ungerleider and Mishkin 1982). As mentioned in Section 2, the former will manifest by disorders of object recognition (visual object agnosia), which may be restricted to loss of ability to recognize previously familiar faces (prosopagnosia). At the bedside, one may be a little restricted in ones ability to detect subtle abnormalities in this domain, though loss of colour recognition (achromatopsia) is often associated, offering a straightforward test.

Dysfunction of the dorsal pathway leads to visuospatial disorganization and difficulty copying complex figures such as the overlapping pentagon and the wire cube. Bilateral pathology causes pronounced deficits with failure to integrate an overall visual seen (simultanagnosia); when asked to describe a complex picture, patients can only describe small individual details. An inability to read large printed words written vertically down a page whilst retaining the ability to read normally printed text is also useful in detecting this sign. Clock-face drawing is another very useful screening test that detects general visuospatial problems as well as neglect secondary to non-dominant parietal pathology.

4.5 Executive function

The term 'executive' refers to aspects of higher-order brain function, such as problem solving, reasoning, and mental abstraction which rely upon the dorso-lateral prefrontal lobes. Frontal lobe disorders are also associated with impulsivity, susceptibility to interference, and failure to persevere with the task at hand. No single test offers foolproof sensitivity in this domain so one should apply as many as possible if the index of suspicion is high.

The combination of letter and category-based verbal fluency provides much useful information. In letter fluency, the patient is asked to generate as many words as they can think of beginning with a given letter in one minute. They are instructed not to use proper nouns and not to just change the endings to create new exemplars ('*go, goes, going, etc.*'). Neuro-psychologists typically use the letters F, A, and S for this test so it is best to choose another letter if it is likely that patients are also going have a formal neuropsychological assessment. In category fluency patients are asked to produce as many exemplars as possible from a given category in one minute. Normal subjects usually generate 15 or more words on letter fluency and do slightly better on the 'animal' category. Patients with executive deficits secondary to frontal or subcortical pathology (Huntington's disease, progressive supranuclear palsy, etc.) show an exaggeration of this relationship doing poorly on category fluency but even worse on letter fluency. Patients with semantic impairments related to temporal lobe diseases such as semantic dementia and Alzheimer's disease typically show the reverse pattern of relatively worse performance on category fluency (Hodges *et al.* 1999; Rosser and Hodges 1994).

The 'go-no go' test offers a way of assessing impulsivity: The patient is asked to tap the desk once if the examiner does so but if the examiner taps twice, he should not tap at all. Patients with frontal pathology are often unable to stop themselves from tapping in both conditions.

Failure to abstract meaning from proverbs ('*What does, "too many cooks spoil the broth" mean*') is a commonly used test but is influenced by background intellectual ability and culture bound. The so-called 'cognitive estimates' test is also useful ('*What is the height of the Post-Office tower in London?*' or '*How fast does a racehorse gallop?*'), as are 'differences and similarities' ('*What's the difference between a child and a dwarf?*' or '*In what way are a sculpture and a piece of music similar?*'). For further discussion of these tasks see Hodges (1994).

5 The general neurological examination

Due to the high prevalence of primary cortical degenerations such as Alzheimer's disease and frontotemporal dementia, the general neurological examination in the demented population is frequently normal. The finding of abnormal signs should, therefore, alert the examiner to an unusual cause of dementia.

5.1 'Neighbourhood' signs to cortical pathology

5.1.1 Occipitoparietal

Visual field testing to confrontation is mandatory since visual field loss or neglect is often asymptomatic. Hemispatial neglect indicates contralateral parietal pathology and may be seen in corticobasal degeneration, atypical cases of Alzheimer's disease, and dementia with Lewy bodies. Severe occipitoparietal pathology can even give rise to cortical blindness. Damage in this area is associated with inability to reach out to a visual target (optic ataxia), to voluntarily direct gaze to a novel visual stimulus (ocular apraxia), and simultanagnosia (see Section 4.4): a triad referred to as the Balint's syndrome.

5.1.2 Frontal

Imitation and utilization behaviour are dramatic phenomena related to ventral frontal lobe damage. The patient with imitation behaviour unconsciously mimics the examiners posture and mannerisms regardless of how absurd they are: raising an arm in the air, placing a leg on the desk, sitting on the floor, etc. Utilization behaviour is more striking still: the patient will use any object placed in their grasp. The classic example is the patient offered multiple pairs of spectacles who attempts to wear them all, one on top of the next. An even more dramatic phenomenon related to utilization behaviour is the alien (or anarchic) hand sign in which the effected limb moves in a semi-purposeful way without conscious control. This sign is virtually pathognomonic of corticobasal degeneration.

The 'primitive release' reflexes are summarized in Table 2.7. Although, non-specific in the elderly, the presence of grasping or pouting are always pathological below the age of 65 and suggest the presence of frontal pathology. Occasionally patients will present with a profile resembling a frontal dementia due to a slow growing tumour in the floor of the anterior cranial fossa. A clue to this is anosmia due to damage to the olfactory nerves.

5.2 Speech

Dysarthria and a marked paucity of language (dynamic aphasia) are commonly associated with progressive supranuclear palsy. Dysarthria in patients with progressive non-fluent aphasia should always raise the possibility of a motor neuron disease associated dementia. Echolalia is sometimes a feature of frontal lobe syndromes whilst palilalia (perseverative utterance of a sound: 'pa, pa, pa, pa …') and palilogia (perseverative utterance of a word or words: 'very good, very good, very good …') are suggestive of progressive supranuclear palsy.

5.3 Eyes

Examination of acuity, fields, fundi, and eye movements should never be omitted. Signs of optic nerve dysfunction (visual failure, afferent pupil defects, disc pallor) point to the possibility of

Table 2.7 Frontal release ('primitive') reflexes

Reflex	Method	Positive response
Grasp	The examiner distracts the patient with conversation then slowly strokes middle and index fingers horizontally across the patients palm.	The fingers involuntarily grasp those of the examiner; the grasp may sometimes increase in intensity according to how hard the examiner attempts to get free.
Palmomental	Using a stimulus with the abrasiveness of an orange-stick, the thenar eminence is briskly stroked.	Brief contraction of the ipsilateral mentalis muscle.
Pout	With the patient's mouth closed but relaxed a tongue depressor is placed across the lips then gently tapped with a tendon-hammer.	Brief 'pouting' movement of the lips.
Glabellar tap	This test is performed by tapping between the patients eyebrows thus causing them to blink. The examiners tapping finger should approach the target from above so as to avoid inducing blinks though visual confrontation.	With repetitive tapping normal subjects will only blink two or three times and then habituate whereas the response is considered pathological if they continue to blink five or more times.

multiple sclerosis or an adult onset leukodystrophy. In younger patients, particularly those with extrapyramidal features a careful search (including slit-lamp examination) for Kayser-Fleischer rings, the hallmark of Wilson's disease is essential.

In addition to testing pursuit eye movements in horizontal and vertical planes, it is important to include testing of rapid (saccadic) eye movements. Slowing of saccades is a feature of progressive supranuclear palsy; impairment of vertical downgoing saccades being the earliest eye sign of this condition.

5.4 Extrapyramidal signs

Parkinsonism is a feature of dementia with Lewy bodies, progressive supranuclear palsy, dementia pugilistica, and idiopathic Parkinson's disease. Compared with idiopathic Parkinson's disease, classic pill-roll tremor is less common in dementia with Lewy bodies and unusual in progressive supranuclear palsy. Prominent truncal rigidity is typical of progressive supranuclear palsy. Parkinsonism may also occur in frontotemporal dementia, particularly the familial form associated with the chromosome 17 mutation (see Chapter 12) but it is seldom a prominent early feature.

Chorea in the context of a dementia is highly suggestive of Huntington's disease. Limb dystonia is one of the major features of corticobasal degeneration, classically having a unilateral onset. Any patient presenting with dystonia and a dementia (especially with psychiatric features) should be investigated for the rare but potentially treatable Wilson's disease.

5.5 Myoclonus

Myoclonus is a hallmark of dementia due to Creutzfeldt–Jacob disease where the jerks are particularly vigorous, but they also occur in corticobasal degeneration, Huntington's disease (especially younger onset), dementia with Lewy bodies, and advanced Alzheimer's disease. Myoclonic jerks (particularly induced by adopting arms outstretched, wrists extended, and fingers spread: 'asterixis') are also a feature of metabolic encephalopathies and thus important to check for in suspected delirium.

5.6 Miscellaneous

As with dysarthria, dysphagia is commonly associated with progressive supranuclear palsy (as pseudobulbar palsy) and motor neuron disease (as either pseudobulbar or bulbar palsy). The presence of a wasted fasciculating tongue being highly suggestive of the latter. Pyramidal weakness may also suggest motor neuron disease as does amyotrophy with muscle fasciculation, though, when motor neuron disease presents with dementia the motor symptoms classically start with bulbar involvement (see Chapter 12). Pyramidal signs also occur in multiple sclerosis, leukodystrophy, or prion disease.

As with pyramidal signs, ataxia is a feature of multiple sclerosis or leukodystrophy. Prion disease in particular can present with cerebellar involvement. Absent deep tendon reflexes (particularly in association with Babinski's signs) may be a clue to a metabolic condition such as a leukodystrophy.

6 Investigations

It is no longer adequate to consider the diagnostic algorithm of dementia as a matter of ruling out a few potentially reversible conditions. The release of the first specific cognition enhancing drugs and many new trials expected or in progress, mean that if responder groups are to be identified then the first step is the most precise diagnosis possible in all cases. In addition, the growing options for genetic counselling and above all, the obligation to provide patients and carers with the best possible information to help them understand and cope with their condition necessitate an effort to reach a positive diagnosis in all instances.

Structural brain imaging studies are mandatory in the investigation of dementia and are discussed in Chapter 6. Although computerized tomography (CAT scanning) is useful in excluding large vascular or space-occupying lesions, magnetic resonance imaging (MRI) offers the potential to detect specific patterns of focal atrophy (such as hippocampal atrophy in early Alzheimer's disease or polar and inferolateral temporal atrophy in semantic dementia) and as such is the imaging study of choice. The extent to which laboratory investigations are persued depends on the clinical setting: for a patient presenting with the classic clinical and neuroimaging findings of, for instance, Alzheimer's disease or semantic dementia, the so-called 'dementia screen' blood tests (Table 2.8) is sufficient. In such circumstances, an abnormal finding (e.g. B12 deficiency or hypothyroidism) will usually not alter the primary diagnosis but is nevertheless an important co-morbidity to recognize and treat.

A more expansive battery of diagnostic tests is indicated where the clinical and imaging findings are either inconsistent with a degenerative dementia or suggest an alternate pathology (e.g. large confluent white matter signal change in a leukodystrophy). Although degenerative conditions still predominate, in the under 65 years age group, as the leading causes of dementia there is certainly a much higher probability of a non-degenerative aetiology, the prevalence of which rises inversely proportional to age. Although a virtually limitless number of both neurological and non-neurological conditions can give rise to cognitive impairment, in many instances the cause will be obvious from other clinical features. Table 2.9 summarizes disorders in which cognitive impairment may occur as a prominent *presenting* feature.

Table 2.8 The minimum laboratory investigations in a dementia

Haematology	Full blood examination
	Erythrocyte sedimentation rate
	B12 and folate
Biochemistry	Urea and electrolytes
	Liver function tests
	Thyroid stimulating hormone
	Calcium, phosphate
Microbiology	Treponemal serology

Table 2.9 Miscellaneous non-degenerative disorders which may present with cognitive decline as a prominent feature

Infections[a]
　Human immunodeficiency virus
　Herpes simplex virus
　JC virus (progressive multifocal leukoencephalopathy)
　Measles (subacute sclerosing panencephalitis)
　Rubella
　Whipple's disease
　Cerebral abscess

Malignancy
　Primary (e.g. glioma, meningioma)
　Metastatic
　Paraneoplastic (esp. small-cell lung, breast, and ovary)

Structural (non-malignant)
　Normal pressure hydrocephalus
　Chronic subdural haematoma

Inflammatory[a]
　Multiple sclerosis
　Sarcoidosis
　Vasculitis (in isolation or with a systemic disease: SLE, etc.)
　Hashimoto's disease

Trauma
　Closed head injury
　Dementia pugilistica

Nutritional
　Thiamine deficiency
　Pellagra (nicotinamide deficiency)

Prion diseases[b]

Mitochondrial encephalomyopathies[a]

CADASIL[c]

Lysosomal and perixosomal storage diseases[c]

Wilson's disease[c]

Heavy metal poisoning
　Arsenic
　Lead
　Mercury

[a] See Chapter 17, [b] see chapter 16, [c] see chapter 18 for further discussion.

One circumstance where comprehensive investigation is always indicated is the patient with a rapidly progressive dementia (see Table 2.4). Lumbar puncture should not be delayed in such cases as an active cerebrospinal fluid is present in many of the potentially reversible diseases (particularly infectious, of which herpes simplex must not be missed and also inflammatory conditions such as cerebral vasculitis). Electroencephalography is often under-utilized in assessing such cases but is an invaluable screen for delirium, as well being diagnostically useful in non-convulsive status epilepticus and conditions associated with period discharges (herpes encephalitis, Creutzfeldt–Jacob, and subacute sclerosing panencephalitis). Finally, for a patient who is rapidly declining, brain biopsy should not be postponed for the sake of outstanding blood tests for which results may take weeks. Where imaging does not point to an obvious lesion, non-dominant frontal biopsy including a leptomeningeal sample is recommended. This is particularly recommended in suspected isolated cerebral vasculitis, where 'blind' treatment with cytotoxic agents is not a satisfactory outcome. Where biopsy is to be undertaken in a rapidly progressive dementia, the surgical team must be forewarned to allow the necessary precautions for prion disease to be implemented.

7 Key points

1   A combination of neurological, psychiatric, and neuropsychological assessment is essential in all cases of early onset dementia.

2   An informant account provides key information particularly concerning changes in personality and behaviour.

3   The patient's ability to relate a logical and complete account of their autobiography and current complaints gives invaluable insights into language, memory, and organizational abilities.

4   The MMSE is an inadequate instrument for the evaluation of patients with early dementia and is particularly insensitive to frontal/executive dysfunction.

5   Where uncertainty exists regarding the presence or absence of a dementing illness, longitudinal follow-up is most useful.

6   Any features atypical for the common causes of degenerative dementia should lead to a thorough search for underlying causes.

7   It is no longer acceptable, particularly in the early onset cases, to consider the assessment of dementia in terms of excluding a few diagnostic possibilities. One of the best ways of ensuring that a treatable condition is not missed is to make a positive diagnosis.

References

Bak, T. H., Antoun, N., Balan, K. K., and Hodges, J. R. (2001). Memory lost, memory regained: Neuropsychological findings and neuroimaging in two cases of paraneoplastic limbic encephalitis with radically different outcomes. *Journal of Neurology, Neurosurgery and Psychiatry.*

Berrios, G. E. and Hodges, J. R. (2000). *Memory disorders in psychiatric practice*. Cambridge: Cambridge University Press.

Cummings, J. L., Mega, M., Gray, K., Rosenberg-Thompson, S., Carusi, D. A., and Gornbein, J. (1994). The neuropsychiatric inventory: comprehensive assessment of psychopathology in dementia. *Neurology*, **44**, 2308–14.

Folstein, M. F., Folstein, S. E., and McHugh, P. R. (1975). 'Mini-mental state'. A practical method for grading the mental state of patients for the clinician. *Journal Psychiatric Research*, **12**, 189–98.

Greene, J. D., Baddeley, A. D., and Hodges, J. R. (1996). Analysis of the episodic memory deficit in early Alzheimer's disease: evidence from the doors and people test. *Neuropsychologia*, **34**, 537–51.

Gregory, C. A., Serra-Mestres, J., and Hodges, J. R. (1999). Early diagnosis of the frontal variant of frontotemporal dementia: how sensitive are standard neuroimaging and neuropsychologic tests? *Neuropsychiatry Neuropsychology and Behavioural Neurology*, **12**, 128–35.

Hodges, J. R. (1994). *Cognitive assessment for clinicians*. Oxford: Oxford University Press.

Hodges, J. R. and Patterson, K. (1995). Is semantic memory consistently impaired early in the course of Alzheimer's disease? Neuroanatomical and diagnostic implications. *Neuropsychologia*, **33**, 441–59.

Hodges, J. R., Patterson, K., Oxbury, S., and Funnell, E. (1992). Semantic dementia. Progressive fluent aphasia with temporal lobe atrophy. *Brain*, **115**, 1783–806.

Hodges, J. R., Patterson, K., Ward, R., Garrard, P., Bak, T., Perry, R., *et al.* (1999). The differentiation of semantic dementia and frontal lobe dementia (temporal and frontal variants of frontotemporal dementia) from early Alzheimer's disease: a comparative neuropsychological study. *Neuropsychology*, **13**, 31–40.

Mackenzie Ross, S. J., Graham, N., Stuart-Green, L., Prins, M., Xuereb, J., Patterson, K., *et al.* (1996). Progressive biparietal atrophy: an atypical presentation of Alzheimer's disease. *Journal of Neurology, Neurosurgery and Psychiatry*, **61**, 388–95.

Mathuranath, P. S., Nestor, P. J., Berrios, G. E., Rakowicz, W., and Hodges, J. R. (2000). A brief cognitive test battery to differentiate Alzheimer's disease and frontotemporal dementia. *Neurology*, **55**, 1613–20.

Mattis, S. (1992). *Dementia rating scale*. Windsor: NFER-Nelson.

Patterson, K. and Hodges, J. R. (1992). Deterioration of word meaning: implications for reading. *Neuropsychologia*, **30**, 1025–40.

Rosser, A. and Hodges, J. R. (1994). Initial letter and semantic category fluency in Alzheimer's disease, Huntington's disease and progressive supranuclear palsy. *Journal of Neurology Neurosurgery and Psychiatry*, **57**, 1389–94.

Roth, M., Tym, E., Mountjoy, C. Q., Huppert, F. A., Hendrie, H., Verma, S., *et al.* (1988). *CAMDEX: The Cambridge examination for mental disorders in the elderly*. Cambridge: Cambridge University Press.

Ungerleider, L. G. and Mishkin, M. (1982). In *Analysis of visual behaviour* (ed. D. J. Ingle, M. A. Goodale, and R. J. W. Mansfield), pp. 544–86. Cambridge, MA: MIT Press.

3 Neuropsychological assessment of early onset dementia

David P. Salmon and John R. Hodges

1 Introduction

Extensive clinical neuropsychological research over the past decade has characterized the various cognitive deficits associated with the dementias and identified the subtle cognitive changes that signal the onset of Alzheimer's disease (AD). These advances have greatly enhanced the ability to diagnose AD in its early stages and to differentiate AD from other dementing disorders. This is particularly important given the development of disease modifying drugs and the fact that there are currently no biological markers for AD.

The neuropsychological deficits associated with AD, and their evolution, is determined by the distribution of the pathology. Alzheimer's disease is a progressive degenerative brain disorder that is characterized by neocortical atrophy, neuron and synapse loss, and the presence of senile plaques and neurofibrillary tangles (see Chapter 10). The hippocampus and entorhinal cortex are involved in the earliest stage of the disease, and cortical association areas become increasingly involved as the disease progresses (Braak and Braak 1991; Hyman *et al.* 1984). In addition to these cortical changes, subcortical neuron loss occurs in the nucleus basalis of Meynert and in the locus coeruleus, resulting in a decrement in neocortical levels of cholinergic and noradrenergic markers, respectively (see Chapter 9).

The extensive pathology that occurs in the limbic system and cortical association areas in AD gives rise to a dementia syndrome that is characterized by severe episodic memory impairment and deficits in semantic knowledge, 'executive' functions, constructional and visuospatial abilities. Because primary sensory and motor cortices and most subcortical structures (e.g. the basal ganglia) are relatively preserved, visual and auditory discrimination and the ability to learn and retain motor skills are unaffected until the latter stages of the disease.

Current conceptualizations of AD presume that the neurodegenerative changes begin well before the clinical manifestations of the disease become apparent. As neuronal degeneration, synapse loss, and the formation of neurofibrillary tangles and neuritic plaques gradually progresses, a threshold for the initiation of the clinical symptoms of the dementia syndrome is eventually reached. Once this threshold is crossed, cognitive deficits become evident and gradually worsen in parallel with continued neurodegeneration. When the cognitive deficits become global and severe enough to interfere with normal social and occupational functioning, established criteria for a clinical diagnosis of AD are met (e.g. DSM-IV; American Psychiatric Association 1994).

Dementia was considered a condition of global intellectual impairment, but in the last 25 years this view has changed as knowledge of the neuropsychological processes affected by various dementing disorders has been gained. It is now known that neuropathologically distinct diseases give rise to diverse dementia syndromes that differ in the patterns of relatively preserved and impaired cognitive abilities they encompass. For example, the dementia syndrome associated with diseases that have their primary locus in subcortical brain structures (e.g. Huntington's disease, progressive supranuclear palsy) differs considerably from that of AD in that it is characterized by relatively mild memory impairment (primarily a retrieval deficit), severe deficits in attention, psychomotor slowing, impairment of 'executive' functions, and little or no aphasia (for review, see Bak and Hodges 1998; Cummings 1990). Similarly, the frontotemporal dementia (FTD) syndromes associated with diseases that primarily affect circumscribed frontal (frontal variant FTD) or temporal (semantic dementia) association cortices differ from the dementia syndrome of AD in that they are characterized by disproportionate deficits in 'executive' functions and semantic knowledge, respectively (see Chapter 12).

The present chapter will review various aspects of the neuropsychological assessment of dementia including the brief examination of mental status, the detection of dementia in its early stages, the detection of 'preclinical' cognitive changes that may presage the development of the dementia syndrome, and the identification of patterns of cognitive deficits that may differentiate among dementing disorders with distinct aetiological and neuropathological bases.

2 Brief assessment of mental status

The most widely used brief global tests of mental status are the Mini-Mental State Examination (Folstein *et al.* 1975), the Information Memory Concentration (IMC) test (Blessed *et al.* 1968), the Mattis (Mattis 1976) Dementia Rating Scale (DRS), and the CAMCOG, the cognitive section of CAMDEX (The Cambridge Mental Disorders of the Elderly Examination) (Huppert *et al.* 1995). Each of these tests briefly assesses a number of the different cognitive domains, and each has been shown to have reasonable sensitivity and specificity for the detection of AD in the relatively early stages of the disease (Folstein *et al.* 1975; Fuld 1978; Monsch *et al.* 1995; Nielsen *et al.* 1999; Salmon *et al.* 1990).

The MMSE was originally designed to provide a brief, standardized assessment of mental status that would serve to differentiate between organic and functional disorders in psychiatric patients. Its major function is now to detect and track the progression of cognitive impairment associated with neurodegenerative disorders such as AD. The MMSE is widely used in clinical practice and has been used as the primary cognitive screening instrument in a number of large scale epidemiological studies of dementia. The MMSE score is often reported in research studies as a benchmark of the severity of dementia that can be used to compare patient cohorts across studies. The MMSE consists of 19 items that assess orientation to place and time, attention and concentration, recall, language, and visual construction. A score of 23 out of a total of 30 points was originally proposed as a cut-off score indicative of cognitive dysfunction. Subsequent investigators reported only moderate sensitivity and specificity for detecting cognitive decline and proposed using cut-off scores of between 25 and 27 (for review, see Tombaugh and McIntyre 1992). With these cut-off scores, sensitivity for the detection of dementia was found to range from 78% to 90% and specificity to range from 70% to 87%. A recent memory clinic based study has confirmed the insensitivity of the MMSE for the early detection of AD and frontotemporal dementia (Mathuranath *et al.* 2000).

The IMC was developed to quantify intellectual deterioration in demented patients so that it could be related to neuropathological manifestations of the underlying disease. The IMC has also been used in case-control and epidemiological studies to screen for cognitive impairment in the elderly and to track the progression of dementia in patients with AD. The IMC is a structured scale with items that assess aspects of orientation, memory, and concentration. The test is scored in terms of errors, with higher scores reflecting poorer performance and greater cognitive impairment. The total score on the 29 item British version of the test ranges from 0 (perfect performance) to 37, while the total score of the 26 item Fuld adaptation ranges from 0 (perfect performance) to 33. In addition, a shortened, 10 item version of the IMC has been developed for dementia screening (Katzman *et al.* 1983). A cut-point of 10 errors has been recommended for detecting cognitive impairment with the IMC (Fuld 1978). Using a cut-point of 10 out of a total of 28 points, another study showed that the short-form of the IMC had 88.6% sensitivity and 94.4% specificity for differentiating between demented patients with probable AD and non-demented elderly individuals (Davous *et al.* 1987).

The DRS was designed to provide a brief assessment of cognitive status in patients who were known to be demented. The role of the DRS has expanded over the years to now include the early detection of cognitive impairment in patients with suspected AD, and the elucidation of patterns of cognitive deficits that distinguish between dementing disorders that differ in their aetiologies and sites of underlying neuropathology. The DRS is a 144 point scale that provides a global measure of dementia derived from subscales for five cognitive capacities: attention, initiation and perseveration, construction, conceptualization, and memory. A cut-off score of 123 was originally suggested for detecting cognitive impairment with the DRS (Mattis 1976), but a recent study that examined the sensitivity and specificity of the DRS for the detection of early AD reported that a cut-off score of 129/130 provided 97% sensitivity and 99% specificity for diagnosis (Monsch *et al.* 1995).

The CAMCOG assesses orientation, language, memory, attention, praxis, calculation, abstraction, and perception with a total score of 107. It incorporates the MMSE and IMC within the battery. A cut-off score of 80 has been suggested for the detection of dementia. Extensive normative data are now available (Huppert *et al.* 1995). Recent work has suggested that patients with AD and dementia with Lewy bodies have distinctive profiles on CAMCOG (Ballard *et al.* 1999; Walker *et al.* 1997).

A brief cognitive battery for use in the clinic or at the bedside has been developed in the Cambridge Memory Clinic, the Addenbrooke's Cognitive Examination or ACE and is described in detail in Chapter 2.

In addition to initially detecting cognitive impairment in the early stages of a dementing illness, mental status tests have some utility for tracking the progression of cognitive decline throughout the course of the disease (Katzman *et al.* 1988; Salmon *et al.* 1990). Studies that have examined the sensitivity of the MMSE to cognitive decline in demented patients report annual rates of change in score that range from –1.8 to –3.2 points per year (Salmon *et al.* 1990; Teri *et al.* 1990). A generally linear decline in score on the IMC has also been reported for patients with AD, with annual rates of decline ranging from 3.0 to 4.4 points. An annual rate of decline of 11.4 points on the DRS has been reported for AD patients (Salmon *et al.* 1990). The DRS appears superior to the other two scales in the more advanced stages of the disease due to its inclusion of a wider range of items that vary in degree of difficulty (Salmon *et al.* 1990).

Although mental status examinations were not designed to discriminate between different dementia aetiologies, several studies have shown that disorders may vary to some extent in the patterns of performance they engender across specific items or subscales of the tests. Brandt *et al.* (1988), for example, found that patients with AD and patients with Huntington's disease (HD) who were matched in terms of the total score on the MMSE performed differently on MMSE items that measure memory and conceptual tracking. Patients with AD were more impaired than those with HD in recalling three words after a five minute delay, whereas HD patients were more impaired than AD patients in counting backwards from 100 by sevens. Salmon and colleagues (Paulsen *et al.* 1995; Salmon *et al.* 1989) found that AD patients were more impaired than HD patients on the Memory subscale of the DRS, but less impaired on the Initiation/Perseveration subscale, even though the two groups were equated in terms of total DRS score. Rosser and Hodges (1994) replicated this finding and demonstrated that patients with progressive supranuclear palsy (PSP) exhibited a pattern of deficits on the DRS subscales that was identical to that of patients with HD. Patients with Parkinson's disease (PD) who were equated to AD patients in total DRS score performed better than the AD patients on the Memory subscale, but worse on the Construction subscale (Paolo *et al.* 1995). Finally, Connor *et al.* (1998) recently demonstrated that patients with the Lewy body variant (LBV) of AD who were matched to patients with 'pure' AD on total DRS score, performed worse than the AD patients on the Initiation/Perseveration and Construction subscales, but better on the Memory subscale.

A number of studies using these tests have shown that there is a strong relationship between the severity of dementia and the degree of neuropathologic abnormality in patients with AD (Blessed *et al.* 1968; DeKosky and Scheff 1990; Mann *et al.* 1988; Terry *et al.* 1991). In one of the first of these studies, Blessed *et al.* (1968) demonstrated that the number of senile plaques in the neocortex of patients with AD correlated mildly, but significantly, with their performance on the IMC test. Several subsequent studies were unable to replicate this finding but did find that large neuron counts correlated significantly with dementia severity (e.g. Mann *et al.* 1988).

Cummings and Cotman (1995) recently argued that the lack of a strong correlation between the number of plaques and dementia severity in patients with AD might be due to an inability to accurately detect and count plaques when they occur with a high density and overlap with one another. Using a more sophisticated immunolabelling technique, a high correlation was obtained between levels of beta-amyloid deposition and severity of cognitive impairment as measured by the IMC test and the MMSE.

The significant correlation between large neuron counts and the severity of cognitive dysfunction in patients with AD reported by Mann *et al.* (1988) led Terry and colleagues (1991) to speculate that extensive synapse loss might also be expected and that this loss might be highly correlated with the severity of dementia prior to death. Terry and colleagues (1991) showed that performance on the three mental status examinations (IMC, MMSE, and DRS) was highly correlated with synaptic density in the midfrontal and inferior parietal regions of the neocortex (see Figure 3.1). Furthermore, a stepwise multiple regression analysis revealed that a model incorporating midfrontal synaptic density, inferior parietal synaptic density, and inferior parietal neuritic plaques accounted for 92% of the variance in test performance.

Although brief mental status tests have been shown to be quite effective for screening for dementia in the clinic and in large scale community-based studies, they cannot substitute for a comprehensive neuropsychological assessment, particularly when attempting to detect a dementing disorder very early in its course (Bondi *et al.* 1999; Petersen *et al.* 1992; Storandt and Hill 1989), when a patient is highly (O'Connor *et al.* 1989) or poorly (Murden *et al.* 1991) educated, or when attempting to identify a pattern of cognitive deficits that may be indicative of a specific dementia aetiology (Mathuranath *et al.* 2000).

3 Detection of neuropsychological deficits in Alzheimer's disease

The neuropsychological assessment of dementia must include a thorough evaluation of a wide range of abilities. In general, the selected assessment procedures should contain tests of verbal and non-verbal episodic memory, language and semantic memory, executive functions, attention, and visuospatial and visuoperceptual abilities.

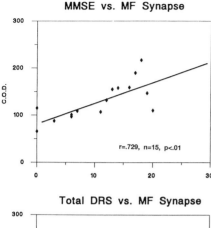

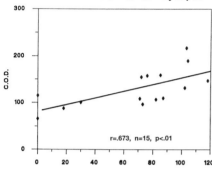

Figure 3.1 The relationship between scores on mental status examinations and the cortical optical density (C.O.D.) of synapses in the midfrontal (MF) cortex of the brains of patients with Alzheimer's disease. The relationship is shown for the Mini-Mental State Exam (MMSE) in the upper panel and for the Dementia Rating Scale (DRS) in the lower panel. (Adapted from Terry *et al.* 1991.)

3.1 Episodic memory

Numerous studies that have shown that measures of the ability to learn and retain new information are most effective in differentiating between mildly demented AD patients and normal older adults (e.g. Bayles *et al.* 1989; Delis *et al.* 1991; Storandt *et al.* 1984). In particular, several studies have shown that measures of the abnormally rapid forgetting exhibited by patients with AD have important clinical utility for the detection and differential diagnosis of the disease (e.g. Butters *et al.* 1988; Locascio *et al.* 1995; Welsh *et al.* 1991, but see Robinson-Whelen and Storandt 1992).

Welsh and colleagues (1991), for example, found that the amount of information recalled after a 10 minute delay differentiated very early AD patients from healthy elderly controls with better than 90% accuracy. This measure was superior in this regard to a number of other verbal memory measures such as immediate recall on each of three learning trials, recognition memory, and the number of intrusion errors produced throughout the test.

Butters and colleagues (1988) similarly found that delayed recall scores and savings scores (i.e. amount recalled after the delay divided by the amount recalled on the third learning trial) on the Logical Memory and Visual Reproduction tests of the Wechsler Memory Scale-Revised (WMS-R) effectively differentiated between mildly demented patients with AD and normal elderly individuals. The utility of delayed recall measures for the early detection of dementia in patients with AD has been confirmed by a number of other investigators (Flicker *et al.* 1991; Knopman and Ryberg 1989; Tröster *et al.* 1993).

The abnormally rapid forgetting exhibited by patients with AD on the clinical memory tests described above suggests that their memory impairment is due to ineffective consolidation of information. A study by Delis and colleagues (1991) addressed this issue by examining the performance of patients with AD on the California Verbal Learning Test (CVLT), a standardized memory test that was developed to assess a variety of memory processes identified through cognitive psychological studies of normal memory (Delis *et al.* 1987). The CVLT assesses rate of learning, retention after short- and long-delay intervals, semantic encoding ability, recognition (i.e. discriminability), intrusion and perseverative errors, and response biases. AD patients were impaired on most measures from the CVLT, but two aspects of their performance suggested that the episodic memory impairment they exhibited was due to ineffective consolidation of information. First, patients with AD were just as impaired on the recognition discriminability trial as they were on the immediate and delayed recall trials of the CVLT. Regardless of the degree of retrieval support provided by the task, patients with AD were unable to effectively recall or recognize the test items. Secondly, savings scores calculated as the amount of information retained after the delay as a function of the amount initially acquired revealed abnormally rapid forgetting of information by AD patients over the 20 minute delay interval.

The possibility that ineffective consolidation or storage contributes importantly to the episodic memory impairment exhibited by patients with AD is supported by studies that have examined the nature of the serial position effect in their free recall performance. When normal individuals are given a list of items to memorize, they typically show a U-shaped serial position curve with better recall for items from the beginning (i.e. primacy effect) and end (i.e. recency effect) of the list than for those from the middle portion. This reflects the operation of two independent types of memory: primary (or short-term) memory which is a passive, time-dependent, limited capacity store that allows the most recent items to be better recalled than other items, and secondary (or long-term) memory which is an actively-accessed, long-lasting store that allows early list items that received the greatest amount of processing to be better recalled than other items.

AD patients have an attenuation of the primacy effect that is evident even in the relatively early stages of the disease (e.g. Bayley *et al.* 2000; Capitani *et al.* 1992; Greene *et al.* 1996). This suggests that information is not adequately maintained in secondary memory, or is not effectively transfered from primary to secondary memory. In contrast, several studies have demonstrated a normal recency effect in mildly demented AD patients (Bayley *et al.* 2000; Capitani *et al.* 1992; Greene *et al.* 1996; Massman *et al.* 1993; Simon *et al.* 1994), a finding that is consistent with preserved primary memory in the early stages of AD.

The impact of this pattern of reduced secondary and relatively preserved primary memory is also evident in the performance of patients with AD on other clinical tests of memory such as the Buschke Selective Reminding Test (SRT) (Buschke 1973).

Another prominent feature of the performance of patients with AD on episodic memory tests is the frequent occurrence of intrusion errors, i.e. when previously learned information is produced during the attempt to recall new material. Butters and colleagues, for example, found that when patients with AD were asked to recall a series of four short stories, facts from the first story intruded into their attempts to recall the second, third, and fourth stories (Butters *et al.* 1987). A similar tendency was observed with a non-verbal episodic memory task when patients with AD incorporated components of a previously remembered geometric form into their drawings of subsequent forms (Jacobs *et al.* 1990).

Although intrusion errors occur commonly in patients with AD, they are not a pathognomonic sign of the disease because they also occur in patients with other forms of dementia (Jacobs *et al.* 1990) and quantitative measures of intrusion errors have not proven to be as sensitive for the detection of dementia as other indices of episodic memory performance (e.g. delayed recall; (Welsh *et al.* 1991, 1992). Intrusion errors can, however, be a useful adjunct to other memory measures in developing clinical algorithms for differentiating AD from other types of dementia (Delis *et al.* 1991; Massman *et al.* 1992).

The episodic memory impairment of AD patients may be exacerbated by a number of ancillary cognitive deficits. For example, an inability to effectively direct and control attentional resources (Baddeley *et al.* 1991; Becker 1988) or a deficient ability to perform semantic encoding may adversely affect AD patients' performance on episodic memory tasks (for review, see Backman and Small 1998; Goldblum *et al.* 1998).

The difficulty patients with AD have in utilizing semantic cues in episodic memory tasks has been taken into account in several recently developed clinical tests of memory. Knopman and Ryberg (1989), for example, developed a Verbal Memory Test that required delayed free recall of semantically-encoded material in order to optimize the possibility of detecting a difference between normal individuals and patients with AD. In a study using this test, normal control subjects and patients with AD were shown a set of ten common nouns, one at a time, and were required to make up a sentence using each word (i.e. sentence generation task). After a five minute delay, free recall of the items was elicited. The results showed that patients with AD were severely impaired in delayed recall on this task and that this measure discriminated them from elderly normal control subjects with better than 95% accuracy.

Buschke and colleagues (1997) recently developed the Double Memory Test which utilizes encoding specificity by presenting the same category cue at initial stimulus presentation and at the time of recall. During initial presentation, a category cue (e.g. bird) is presented in conjunction with a related word (e.g. eagle) and three unrelated words (e.g. scotch, grape, nylon), and the subject must identify the word that is a member of the category. This procedure is repeated until four members are correctly identified from each of four different categories. Immediately following this acquisition phase, one of the category cues is presented and the subject is asked to recall the four items from that category. This procedure is repeated for the remaining three categories. Buschke and colleagues found that this test was highly effective in differentiating between normal elderly individuals and patients with AD, providing 93.3% sensitivity and 98.8% specificity for the detection of the disorder. Furthermore, this version of the test was much more effective for the detection of AD than a version that only provided the category cue at the time of recall, presumably because normal individuals, but not patients with AD, were able to benefit from the encoding specificity procedure.

3.2 Remote memory

In addition to a deficit in learning and remembering new information, patients with AD often have a loss of memory for information acquired prior to the onset of their disease (i.e. retrograde amnesia) (Beatty *et al.* 1988; Graham and Hodges 1997; Greene *et al.* 1995; Hodges *et al.* 1993; Kopelman 1989; Sagar *et al.* 1988). This remote memory loss affects information from all decades of the patients' lives, but is often temporally graded with memories from the more distant past (i.e. childhood and early adulthood) better remembered than memories from the more recent past (i.e. mid and late adulthood) (Beatty *et al.* 1988; Graham and Hodges 1997; Hodges *et al.* 1993). This temporal gradient is similar to the pattern of loss exhibited by patients with circumscribed amnesia and has been attributed to the interruption of a long-term consolidation process that is critically dependent upon the hippocampal-diencephalic memory system (see Graham and Hodges 1997; Zola-Morgan and Squire 1990).

To explore the possibility that the retrograde amnesia of AD is due to a retrieval deficit rather than an inability to adequately consolidate information over time, Hodges and colleagues (1993) examined the performance of patients with AD on an updated version of the Famous Faces test that employed recognition and cueing formats. The results demonstrated that patients with AD were impaired even when retrieval demands were minimized by using a recognition procedure. Furthermore, the retrograde amnesia that was evident on the recognition and cueing formats was temporally graded with information from the distant past better retained than information for the more recent past. These findings were confirmed in a subsequent study using both famous faces and names (Greene and Hodges 1996).

3.3 Semantic memory

Semantic memory that underlies knowledge and language is often disturbed relatively early in the course of AD (for reviews, see Hodges and Patterson 1995; Nebes 1989; Salmon and Chan 1994). This disturbance is evident in AD patients' reduced ability to recall overlearned facts (e.g. the number of days in a year (Norton *et al.* 1997), and in their impairment on tests of confrontation naming (for review see Hodges *et al.* 1991), verbal fluency (Monsch *et al.* 1994), and semantic priming (for review, see Salmon and Fennema-Notestine 1996). Consistent with an impairment of semantic memory, the spontaneous speech of patients with AD is frequently vague, empty of content words, and filled with indefinite phrases and circumlocutions.

The semantic memory deficit of patients with AD has been demonstrated in a number of studies that have examined their performance on tests of verbal fluency (for review see Monsch *et al.* 1994). AD patients are generally more impaired when required to generate exemplars from a particular semantic category (e.g. animals, fruits, or vegetables) than words beginning with a particular letter (e.g. F, A, or S). A comparison of the clinical utility of phonemic and semantic verbal fluency tests for the early detection of AD demonstrated that a cut-off score of 38 on the semantic category fluency test (i.e. animals, fruits, or vegetables) provided 100% sensitivity and 92.5% specificity in differentiating between AD patients and NC subjects, whereas a cut-off score of 31 on the letter fluency test (i.e. F, A, S) provided only 88.8% sensitivity and 84.9% specificity (Monsch *et al.* 1992).

Patients with AD perform poorly on object naming tasks and tend to produce semantically-based errors, such as superordinate or coordinate category responses rather than the specific exemplar (e.g. hippopotamus or animal for rhinoceros) when attempting to name objects (for review see Hodges *et al.* 1996, 1991). A more rigorous assessment of the integrity of semantic memory in patients with AD was provided in studies by Hodges and colleagues (Hodges and Patterson 1995; Hodges *et al.* 1996, 1992) which used an extensive battery of tests to probe for knowledge of particular concepts across different modes of access and output. The various tests in the battery all employed the same 48 stimulus items which were exemplars from three categories of living items (i.e. land animals, birds, and water creatures) and three categories of non-living items (i.e. household items, vehicles, and musical instruments). Knowledge of the items was assessed with fluency tasks, a confrontation naming task, a sorting task designed to test superordinate and subordinate knowledge, a word-to-picture matching task, and a definition task. The results of these studies were consistent with those of a similar study by Chertkow and Bub (1990) and showed that patients with AD were significantly impaired on all measures of semantic memory, regardless of the method of access or output required by the task. An analysis of item-to-item correspondence in performance across a number of the different tests indicated that when a particular stimulus item was missed (or correctly identified) in one test, it was likely to be missed (or correctly identified) in other tests that accessed the information in a different way. These finding were consistent with the notion that semantic knowledge for particular items was actually lost during the course of the disease.

There has been recent interest in the question of whether the breakdown in semantic memory affects all categories of knowledge equally in AD. Category-specific deficits are well documented in the context of focal brain damage: the most commonly observed pattern is loss of knowledge for living things (animals, fruit, and vegetables) which occurs in patients with herpes simplex virus encephalitis. The opposite pattern (i.e. disproportionate impairment for artefacts) has also been documented thus ruling out any explanation based on test difficulty (Garrard *et al.* 1997).

Group studies of AD patients have reached contradictory conclusions with some finding an advantage for living things and others no difference across categories (for review see Garrard *et al.* 1997). A recent comprehensive study has confirmed that a substantial minority do indeed show category effects (usually, but not always, in the direction of worse performance on natural kinds) and that this emerges with increasing degrees of anomia which possibly reflects progressive left temporal lobe pathology (Garrard *et al.* 1998).

Additional evidence for a loss of semantic knowledge in AD patients comes from a series of studies that modelled the organization of semantic memory in patients using multidimensional scaling techniques which generate a graphic representation based on some measurement of the relative association or proximity between concepts (Chan *et al.* 1993, 1997; Salmon and Chan 1994). The resulting models embed the objects under study in a coordinate space or a network where the distances between points are assumed to reflect the psychological proximity between the respective items. The results of these studies showed that proximity data for the category 'animals' (derived using a triadic comparison task) generated cognitive maps that were best represented by three dimensions corresponding to domesticity (i.e. wild versus domestic), predation (herbivore versus carnivore), and size (large versus small). In these network representations, AD patients focused primarily on concrete conceptual information (i.e. size) in categorizing animals, whereas control subjects stressed abstract conceptual knowledge (i.e. domesticity). In addition, a number of animals that were highly associated and clustered together for control subjects were not strongly associated for patients with AD, and AD patients were less consistent than controls in utilizing the various attributes of the animals (predation, domesticity, and size) in categorization. Also, the cognitive maps of AD patients, when compared with those of controls, amnesic patients, or patients with HD, were characterized by atypical strengths of associations and had more unnecessary adjunct links. The severity of these abnormalities increased with increasing dementia severity (Chan *et al.* 1997) suggesting that the structure of semantic knowledge deteriorates in a systematic manner throughout the course of AD.

Several additional studies have shown that semantic memory deteriorates in a systematic fashion throughout the course of AD. Norton and colleagues (1997), for example, found that patients with AD were impaired in the earliest stages of dementia on the Number Information Test, a test designed to assess generic semantic knowledge in a way that minimizes language demands. The NIT consists of 24 general knowledge questions, each of which has a number for an answer (e.g. 'How many days are in a year?'). The impairment exhibited by patients with AD on this test grew as the severity of their dementia increased over time (see Figure 3.2). In addition, patients were highly consistent in the individual items they missed in subsequent test sessions conducted one or two years later, suggesting a true loss of knowledge (rather than deficient retrieval) over the course of the disease.

Longitudinal deterioration of semantic memory in patients with AD was also assessed in a recent study that examined the decline in their performance on semantic category fluency and letter fluency tasks over the course of three years (Salmon *et al.* 1999). Consistent with previous results, AD patients exhibited greater impairment relative to controls on the category than on the letter fluency task. The performance of the patients with AD declined over time on both tasks, but the rate of decline was faster on the category than on the letter fluency task. Furthermore, examination of individual responses across the annual evaluations revealed that when a patient with AD failed to generate a particular response on the category fluency task in a given year, they were unlikely to produce that item in a subsequent year. This consistency suggested that specific exemplars were lost from the category as the disease progressed. These results support the notion that patients with AD suffer a gradual deterioration of the organization and content of semantic memory as the disease progresses.

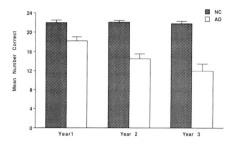

Figure 3.2 The mean number of correct responses produced by patients with Alzheimer's disease (AD) and normal control (NC) subjects on the Number Information Test at each of three annual evaluations. The performance of patients with AD declined significantly over time and was characterized by consistency in the items missed at each evaluation. (Adapted from Norton *et al.* 1997.)

3.4 Reading and writing

Rather surprisingly, given that the ability to read fluently typically develops some years after normal subjects learn to converse, reading is well preserved in the early stages of AD. Indeed the most commonly employed test used to estimate premorbid IQ, the National Adult Reading Test, was based upon this observation (Nelson 1982). In the NART subjects are asked to read aloud irregular words of increasing rarity in the language (*naive.. thyme.. cellist.. placebo*, etc), the correct pronunciation depends upon acquaintance with their meaning. In the early stages of AD, patients perform well on this and other tests of reading but as the disease progresses they do make errors especially with low frequency words (Paque and Warrington 1995; Patterson *et al.* 1994; Strain *et al.* 1998). Writing is more vulnerable than reading since the production of legible and correctly spelt script depends upon the co-ordination of central (spelling) and more peripheral (letter formation) components; either may breakdown in AD, but in the early stages central processes deteriorate leading to problems spelling low frequency irregular words (for review see Graham 2000; Hughes *et al.* 1997).

3.5 Executive function and attention

While episodic and semantic memory deficits are prominent features of the dementia associated with AD, impaired 'executive' functions may also occur early in the course of the disease (for review, see Perry and Hodges 1999; Salmon *et al.* 1998). The 'executive' dysfunction in AD refers to deficits in abilities responsible for concurrent manipulation of information, concept formation, problem solving, and cue-directed behaviour. A recent study by Lefleche and Albert (1995) compared the performance of AD patients on several tests of each of these components of 'executive' functioning and demonstrated that the primary deficit early in the disease is one of concurrent manipulation of information. Mildly demented patients with AD were significantly impaired relative to elderly normal control subjects on tests that required manipulations such as set-shifting, self-monitoring, or sequencing such as the Wisconsin Card Sorting Task (Bondi *et al.* 1993), but not on tests that required cued-directed attention or verbal problem solving. Patients with AD have also been shown to be impaired on problem solving tests (e.g. Tower of London puzzle; Lange *et al.* 1995) and on other tests that involve executive functions such as the Porteus Maze Task, Part B of the Trail-Making Test, and the Raven Progressive Matrices Task (Grady *et al.* 1988).

Considerable experimental research on attentional processes in patients with AD has been carried out over the past decade and has demonstrated that these patients exhibit attentional impairment relatively early in the course of the disease (for reviews, see Parasuraman and Haxby 1993; Perry and Hodges 1999). Recent work has suggested that impairment in attentional processes is second in severity and order of occurrence to the episodic memory deficits in AD (Perry *et al.* 2000). Deficits in performing dual-processing tasks (Grady *et al.* 1989; Greene *et al.* 1995; Morris 1994), tasks that require the disengagement and shifting of attention (Filoteo *et al.* 1992; Oken *et al.* 1994; Parasuraman *et al.* 1992), and aspects of working memory that are dependent upon the control of attentional resources (Baddeley *et al.* 1991; Becker 1988; Collette *et al.* 1999) appear to be affected soon after the onset of AD dementia. In clinical practice, the Stroop test is particularly sensitive to the attentional dysfunction (Perry *et al.* 2000). In contrast, other aspects of attention, such as attentional focusing and sustained attention (Nebes and Brady 1993; Perry *et al.* 2000; Sahakian *et al.* 1989), appear to be affected only in latter stages of the disease.

3.6 Visuoperceptual and spatial abilities

Deficits in visuoperceptual abilities, visuospatial abilities, and constructional praxis occur in patients with AD, but they usually emerge after the early stages of the disease and may have little to contribute to the differentiation of early dementia from normal ageing (e.g. Locascio *et al.* 1995; Storandt *et al.* 1984). Once beyond the early stages of dementia, patients with AD exhibit impaired performance on visuoconstructional tasks such as the Block Design Test (Pandovani *et al.* 1995; Villardita 1993), the Clock Drawing Test (see Figure 3.3; for review, see Freedman *et al.* 1994), or tasks that require copying a complex figure (Locascio *et al.* 1995; Pandovani *et al.* 1995; Villardita 1993). Tests that require visuoperception and visual orientation may also be adversely affected in the later stages of AD. Deficits have been demonstrated in mildly-to-moderately demented AD patients' performance on the Judgement of Line Orientation Test (Ska *et al.* 1990), the Left-Right Orientation Test (Fischer *et al.* 1990), and the Money Road Map Test (Locascio *et al.* 1995).

An attempt has been made to analyse the breakdown in terms of the dorsal 'where' or 'how' versus the ventral 'what' pathway of visual processing (Goodale and Milner 1992; Hodges *et al.* 1996; Ungerleider and Mishkin 1982). Based on the spread of pathology in AD which usually involves regions of the temporal lobes before parietal regions, it might be predicted that the earliest problems would occur in the ventral processing stream causing deficits in colour, object, and letter identification rather than spatial processing. Studies to date have provided partial confirmation of this prediction, but with considerable heterogeneity (Caine and Hodges 2001; Kurylo *et al.* 1996; Mendez *et al.* 1990). Our own study using a wide range of tasks has shown that either pathway can be involved fairly selectively at a relatively early stage of the disease (Caine and Hodges 2001).

3.7 Neuropsychological detection of preclinical dementia

A growing body of evidence suggests that decline in episodic memory may presage the development of the dementia syndrome associated with AD in the elderly (Bondi *et al.* 1994; Fuld *et al.* 1990; Grober and Kawas 1997; Linn *et al.* 1995; Masur *et al.* 1994) and in younger individuals with familial AD (Fox *et al.* 1998). Fuld and colleagues, for example, demonstrated that those elderly individuals in a residential home population who performed poorly on measures of recall from the Fuld Object Memory Test (Fuld *et al.* 1990) or the Selective Reminding Test (Masur *et al.* 1990) were more likely than those who performed well to be subsequently diagnosed with AD within the next five years. Furthermore, continued longitudinal evaluation of this population showed that initial performance on these episodic memory measures, in conjunction with performance on the WAIS Digit Symbol Substitution test and a verbal fluency task, was moderately effective in identifying individuals who would later be diagnosed with AD (32/64; 50%) and provided excellent specificity for identifying individuals who would remain free of dementia (238/253; 94%) over an ensuing 11 year period (Masur *et al.* 1994).

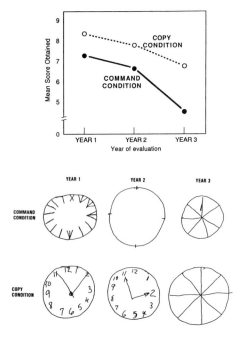

Figure 3.3 The mean scores achieved by patients with Alzheimer's disease on the command and copy conditions of the Clock Drawing Test across three annual evaluations. An example of the deterioration of performance on the Clock Drawing Test in an individual AD patient is shown in the lower portion of the figure. (Adapted from Rouleau *et al.* 1996.)

In a similar study, Linn and colleagues (1995) found that the subsequent development of AD in 55 of 1045 non-demented elderly individuals over a 13 year period was predicted by their initial performance on measures of delayed recall (WMS Logical Memory per cent retained) and immediate auditory attention span (WAIS Digit Span). Interestingly, these neuropsychological tests measures predicted the development of dementia even when the initial screening examination preceded the clinical onset of AD by seven years or more.

Several studies have shown that non-demented elderly individuals with a positive family history for AD (FH+) perform significantly worse than those with a negative family history (FH–) on tests of episodic memory (Bondi *et al.* 1994; Hom *et al.* 1994). Hom and colleagues (1994) demonstrated that a group of non-demented elderly FH+ individuals performed significantly worse than age- and education-matched non-demented FH– individuals on verbal tests of episodic memory and on tests of verbal intelligence. This difference occurred despite the fact that the average performances of both groups on these tests were within normal limits. In a similar study, Bondi and colleagues (1994) compared the performances of non-demented FH+ and FH– elderly subjects on quantitative and qualitative indices derived from the CVLT. Although the groups were carefully matched in terms of demographic variables and performance on standardized mental status examinations, the FH+ subjects recalled significantly fewer items during learning and delayed recall, produced more intrusion errors, and demonstrated a greater recency effect than the FH– individuals. Moreover, five of the non-demented FH+ subjects performed on the CVLT in a manner qualitatively similar to that of a group of mildly impaired AD patients. All five of these subjects were subsequently diagnosed with AD one to two years following their initial evaluation.

A number of recent studies have demonstrated that non-demented elderly subjects who are at risk for developing AD because they carry the ApoE e4 allele perform significantly worse than those without this risk factor on tests of episodic memory (Reed *et al.* 1994). Using the CVLT, Bondi and colleagues (1995) demonstrated that the episodic memory performance of non-demented subjects with the ApoE e4 allele was qualitatively (though not quantitatively) similar to that of early stage patients with AD. The notion that the group with the ApoE e4 allele contained individuals in the preclinical phase of the disease was confirmed by follow-up examinations which revealed that six of the 14 subjects with the ε4 allele subsequently developed either probable or possible AD within an average of three years. None of the 26 subjects without an ε4 allele, in contrast, exhibited any cognitive decline during this interval.

Fox and colleagues (1998) followed a cohort of 63 asymptomatic individuals who were at risk for developing familial early onset AD and identified ten who became demented over the six year course of the study. Examination of the performance of individuals on a battery of neuropsychological tests at the time of their enrollment into the study showed that those who went on to become demented scored significantly lower than those who did not only on a recognition memory test for words and on WAIS-R performance IQ. In addition, symptoms of very mild episodic memory impairment were the most commonly reported problem in the individuals who later developed dementia and were noted by family members an average of six months prior to the first assessment in which they were documented. These results provide further evidence that subtle deficits in memory presage the dementia syndrome by several years, even in early onset familial AD patients who are not subject to the confounding effects of age-related cognitive decline or medical comorbidity.

3.8 Atypical presentations of Alzheimer's disease

The above descriptions of the typical profile of cognitive impairment in AD suggests a homogeneous presentation and progression which mirrors the known distribution of neuropathological changes: first involving the medial temporal lobe and later spreading to the posterior association cortices and basal forebrain areas. There is, however, emerging evidence that patients can present with highly atypical cognitive syndromes: the most clearly documented being (1) progressive aphasia of either fluent or non-fluent type, and (2) so-called posterior cortical atrophy producing either a Balint's like syndrome (optic ataxia, simultanagnosia, and optic apraxia) or an apperceptive visual agnosia (for review see Galton *et al.* 2000 and Chapter 11).

4 Neuropsychological differentiation of dementia aetiologies

Aetiologically and neuropathology distinct disorders give rise to dementia syndromes that differ in the patterns of relatively impaired and preserved cognitive abilities they encompass. Knowledge of the unique patterns of cognitive deficits can aid in the differential diagnosis of various dementing disorders, particularly in the early stages. In addition, comparison of the neuropsychological deficits associated with various disorders allows inferences to be drawn about the brain structure–function relationships. The neuropsychological literature on various non-Alzheimer forms of dementia is now huge. We focus here on studies comparing AD with other dementia and particularly those using traditional 'pen and paper' tests, rather than computer based assessment of cognitive function.

4.1 Alzheimer's disease versus Huntington's disease

Recent studies have shown that AD and HD patients can be differentiated by the nature and pattern of their respective memory deficits. While patients with AD exhibit a severe episodic memory deficit that appears to result from ineffective consolidation (i.e. storage) of new information, the memory disorder of patients with HD is thought to result from a general difficulty in initiating a systematic retrieval strategy when recalling information from either episodic or semantic memory (Butters *et al.* 1985; Delis *et al.* 1991; Moss *et al.* 1986; but see Brandt *et al.* 1992).

   This distinction in the memory deficits associated with the two disorders was illustrated in the study by Delis and colleagues (1991) that compared the performance of patients with AD and patients with HD on the CVLT. The results of this study showed that despite comparable immediate and delayed free- and cued-recall deficits, these patient groups could be distinguished by two major differences (see Figure 3.4). First, patients with AD were just as impaired on the recognition discriminability trial as they were on the immediate and delayed recall trials, whereas patients with HD were less impaired on the recognition discriminability trial than on the various recall trials. The significant improvement shown by the HD patients when memory was tested with a recognition procedure indicates that when the need for effortful retrieval was reduced, their memory impairment was somewhat ameliorated. Secondly, patients with AD exhibited significantly faster forgetting of information over the 20 minute delay interval than did the patients with HD. The potential clinical utility of these different patterns of performance on the CVLT for differential diagnosis was shown when a discriminant function equation based on two key CVLT measures was able to correctly classify the majority of AD and HD cases.

   Although the results of the study by Delis and colleagues (1991) suggest that different processing deficits underlie the episodic memory impairments of patients with AD, a 'cortical' dementia, and patients with HD, a 'subcortical' dementia, a study by Massman and colleagues (1990) indicates that not all so-called 'subcortical' dementing disorders produce identical episodic memory deficits. Massman and colleagues (1990) directly compared the CVLT performance of HD patients and patients with Parkinson's disease (PD). Although these two groups performed similarly on many of the variables that distinguished between HD and AD patients there were also marked differences. Specifically, the HD patients demonstrated slower learning across trials, a larger recency effect during recall, a larger number of perseverative errors, and poorer free and cued recall than the patients with PD. These discrepancies suggest that somewhat different processing deficits may mediate the episodic memory impairments of HD and PD patients, and highlight the insufficiency of the cortical-subcortical distinction even when it is used primarily for heuristic purposes.

   In addition to differences in their ability to learn and retain new information, AD and HD patients differ in their capacity to recall information from the past. As mentioned previously, patients with AD have a severe, temporally-graded retrograde amnesia (i.e. loss of memory for information acquired prior to the onset of their disease) with memories from the more distant

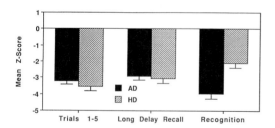

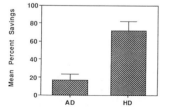

Figure 3.4 The mean z-scores achieved by patients with Alzheimer's disease (AD) and Huntington's disease (HD) on key measures from the California Verbal Learning Test (upper panel). The mean percentage of information retained over the 20 minute delay interval by each patient group is also shown (lower panel). (Adapted from Delis *et al.* 1991.)

past (i.e. childhood and early adulthood) better remembered than memories from the more recent past. Patients with HD, in contrast, suffer only a mild degree of retrograde amnesia that is equally severe across all decades of their lives (Albert *et al.* 1981; Beatty *et al.* 1988). These pattens are consistent with the notion that AD patients have a deficit in consolidating remote memories through repeated processing, rehearsal, or re-exposure, whereas patients with HD have a general retrieval deficit that equally effects the ability to retrieve information from any decade of their lives.

With regard to semantic memory, patients with AD exhibit a significant impairment on tests of object naming (i.e. anomia) whereas, patients with HD often display relatively normal performance. Furthermore, a qualitative examination of the groups' performances shows that patients with AD produce a higher proportion of semantically-based errors (e.g. superordinate errors such as calling a 'camel' an 'animal') than patients with HD, while patients with HD make a higher proportion of perceptual errors (e.g. calling a 'pretzel' a 'snake') than patients with AD (Hodges *et al.* 1991).

Differences in the semantic memory deficits of AD and HD patients have also been noted on tests of verbal fluency. Monsch and colleagues (1994), for example, found that although both HD and AD patients were severely impaired on letter (i.e. F, A, S) and category (animals, fruits, vegetables) fluency tasks, patients with AD exhibited a much greater impairment on the category fluency task than on the letter fluency task, whereas patients with HD were equally impaired on both tasks (see Figure 3.5). Moreover, Rohrer and colleagues (1999) found that mean latency to produce each item in a category fluency task was abnormally fast in patients with AD, as would be expected if retrieval time was normal but the size of the category (i.e. the number of available exemplars) was reduced. In contrast, the mean latency was abnormally slow in patients with HD, as would be expected if all of the category exemplars were available but retrieval was slowed.

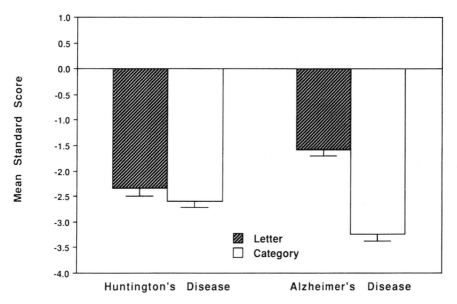

Figure 3.5 The mean standard scores of patients with Alzheimer's disease (N = 44) and Huntington's disease (N = 42) on the letter and category verbal fluency tasks. Patients with Alzheimer's disease were significantly more impaired on the category than the letter fluency task, whereas patients with Huntington's disease were equally impaired on both tasks. (Adapted from Monsch *et al.* 1994.)

Studies that have compared the semantic networks of AD and HD patients also support the position that only the patients with AD suffer a deterioration in the structure and organization of semantic memory (Chan *et al.* 1995).

Differences in semantic memory were also evident when Rouleau and colleagues (1992) examined the visuoconstructive deficits exhibited by AD and HD patients when drawing and copying clocks (see Figure 3.6). In the command condition of this task, subjects are asked to draw a clock, put in all the numbers, and set the hands to 10 past 11. In the copy condition, subjects are asked to copy a drawing of a clock. Both the AD and HD patients were impaired on this task relative to control subjects, but a qualitative analysis of the types of errors produced revealed a dissociation in their performances. Whereas the HD patients made graphic, visuospatial, and planning errors in both the command and copy conditions, the AD patients often made conceptual errors (e.g. misrepresenting the clock by drawing a face without numbers or with an incorrect use of numbers; misrepresenting the time by failing to include the hands; incorrectly using the hands; or writing the time in the clock face) in the command condition but not in the copy condition.

Another form of memory that is differentially affected by AD and HD is implicit memory. Implicit memory refers to the unconscious expression of knowledge through its use in the performance of the specific operations comprising some task. For example, classical conditioning, lexical and semantic priming, motor skill learning, and perceptual learning are all considered forms of implicit memory because in each case, an individuals performance is facilitated 'unconsciously' simply by prior exposure to stimulus material.

Patients with AD have been found to be significantly impaired when lexical (Bondi and Kaszniak 1991), semantic (Salmon *et al.* 1988), or pictorial (Heindel *et al.* 1990) information is activated through prior exposure. Patients with HD exhibit normal priming on each of these tasks (Heindel *et al.* 1989; Salmon *et al.* 1988).

In contrast to these priming results, HD patients are impaired on motor skill learning (Heindel *et al.* 1989), prism adaptation (Paulsen *et al.* 1993), and weight biasing (Heindel *et al.* 1990) tasks that are performed normally by AD patients. All of these tasks involve the generation and refinement (i.e. learning) of motor programs to guide behaviour.

The double dissociation between AD and HD patients on these various implicit memory tasks suggests that different forms of implicit memory are not mediated by a single neurological substrate. Verbal and pictorial priming may both involve the temporary activation of stored representations in semantic memory, and may be dependent on the functional integrity of the neocortical association areas damaged in AD. Motor skill learning, prism adaptation, and the biasing of

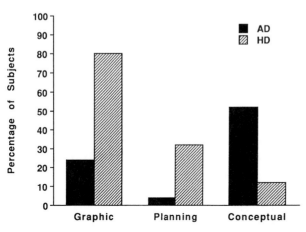

Figure 3.6 The percentage of Huntington's disease (HD) and Alzheimer's disease (AD) patients producing graphic, planning, and conceptual errors on the command condition of the Clock Drawing Test. (Adapted from Rouleau *et al.* 1992.)

weight perception, on the other hand, may all involve the modification of programmed movement parameters that are likely mediated by a corticostriatal system that is severely compromised in HD.

4.2 Alzheimer's disease versus vascular dementia

There is a considerable body of literature which has addressed the question of whether patients with vascular dementia (VaD) can be differentiated from those with AD. This has been reviewed thoroughly elsewhere in the book (see Chapter 14). In brief, it is difficult to draw a firm conclusion since the term VaD has been applied to such a heterogeneous collection of disorders (for instance, a small strategically placed infarction in the thalamus can produce a 'dementia' syndrome which is entirely different to the insidiously progressive and fairly diffuse white matter pathology seen in some patients with chronic hypertension). Even when fairly homogeneous populations have been studied using modern criteria, few have achieved appropriate matching or used a comprehensive battery of neuropsychological tests. Bearing these caveats in mind, the current evidence suggests that patients with VaD are characterized by less marked impairment of episodic memory, greater deficits in attention and executive function, producing relatively worse performance on letter than category fluency, and more prominent neuropsychiatric symptoms.

4.3 Alzheimer's disease versus frontotemporal dementia

The neuropsychological deficits associated with frontotemporal dementia (FTD, the term which is now preferred to Pick's disease) has been much less fully documented than those found in AD. Most studies are concentrated on single cases or small groups that have used patients with FTD to explore the specific theoretically important aspects of cognition, rather than documenting the overall profile found in FTD and there have been very few studies which have compared FTD and AD.

Much of the early literature is marred by a failure to differentiate clearly between the various clinical subtypes of FTD. As described more fully in Chapter 12, patients with FTD may present with one of three major syndromes:

1. Dementia of frontal type also known as frontal variant FTD.
2. Semantic dementia also known as progressive fluent aphasia.
3. Progressive non-fluent aphasia.

Patients with the frontal variant present with prominent changes in personality and behaviour, but despite these profound, and usually socially disabling, alterations patients may perform normally in the early stages of the disease on tests of 'executive' function. Many authors have argued that this reflects the ventromedial locus of pathology in frontal variant FTD and the fact that traditional executive tasks are sensitive to dorsolateral pathology (Gregory *et al.* 1999; Rahman *et al.* 1999).

The semantic dementia syndrome is characterized, by contrast, by a progressive loss of semantic memory resulting in severe anomia, impaired word comprehension, and an impoverished fund of general knowledge evident on verbal and visually based tests of semantic knowledge. This occurs in the face of normal phonology and syntax, and preserved basic perceptual and visuospatial abilities, non-verbal problem solving, digit span, and episodic memory for recent events (see Chapter 12).

Progressive non-fluent aphasia represents, in many ways, the mirror image of semantic dementia in that patients show severe disruption of the phonological and syntactic aspects of speech production, but show preservation of word and picture comprehension. In common with semantic dementia, visuospatial and perceptual skills are retained as is episodic memory, at least if tested using non-verbal tests (Hodges and Patterson 1996).

In view of these gross differences in the three variants of FTD it is rather meaningless to ask the question 'What test differentiates AD from FTD?' without defining the subtype. This explains why earlier studies comparing AD and FTD fail to find substantial differences either using standard neuropsychological or bedside tests (Elfgren *et al.* 1994; Frisoni *et al.* 1995; Gregory *et al.* 1997; Pachana *et al.* 1996).

More recently, two studies from Cambridge (Hodges *et al.* 1999; Perry and Hodges 2000) have attempted to address these shortcomings by comparing well matched groups of patients with frontal variant FTD, semantic dementia and AD using a range of theoretically motivated tests. These studies have confirmed the following distinctive profiles: patients with AD have severe impairment of anterograde episodic memory, less marked but fairly consistent deficits in selective and divided attention, and mild more variable impairment in semantic memory evident particularly on word based tasks; those with semantic dementia have profound and pervasive impairment of semantic memory, show deficits on verbal, but not non-verbal anterograde memory tests, and perform normally on tests of attention and executive function as well as the instructions can be comprehended; frontal variant FTD is characterized by poor performance on tests of executive function and attention, normal semantic memory, and patchy impairment in episodic memory tests most apparent on retrieval based tasks.

4.4 Alzheimer's disease versus dementia with Lewy bodies

The controversial issue of whether dementia with Lewy bodies (DLB) represents a truly distinct clinicopathological entity, a variant or AD, or a number of separate conditions is dealt with more fully in Chapter 13. For simplicity, here we regard DLB as a disease separable from AD and characterized by progressive dementia, parkinsonism, a tendency to marked spontaneous fluctuations with features of delirium, formed visual hallucinations, and neuroleptic sensitivity (McKeith *et al.* 2000). Research on the neuropsychology of DLB is in its infancy and only a handful of studies have systematically compared AD and DLB. The findings to date suggest that the degree of episodic memory deficit is less marked in DLB than in AD. In contrast, patients with DLB have greater impairment in all aspects of attention and working memory and prominent impairment in visuospatial abilities (Calderon *et al.* 2001; Salmon *et al.* 1996). Semantic memory is equivalently impaired in AD and DLB as assessed using verbally based tasks, but patients with DLB make more errors on visual tests such as the Pyramid and Palm Trees test of associative knowledge (Lambon Ralph *et al.* 2001).

5 Summary

Neuropsychological research has identified many of the basic cognitive processes that are adversely affected in AD and other dementing disorders and has provided important information about the brain–behaviour relationships that underlie these deficits. For example, the adverse effects of AD on memory processes such consolidation, retrieval, and semantic encoding have been delineated and their relationship to the degree of structural abnormality in medial temporal lobe structures revealed by magnetic resonance imaging (MRI) has been demonstrated (e.g. Cahn *et al.* 1998; Deweer *et al.* 1995; Fama *et al.* 1997; Kohler *et al.* 1998; Stout *et al.* 1999). Similarly, studies of implicit memory in patients with various dementing disorders have helped to identify the brain structures that may be particularly important for some aspects of this form of memory (for review, see Salmon and Fennema-Notestine 1996). Further advances in our understanding of the neural mediation of these and other cognitive processes should be possible as neuropsychological research continues in the coming years.

6 Key points

1   A number of brief mental status assessment schedules are available which can be used for screening and monitoring populations, but do not substitute for targeted neuropsychological evaluation in the detection of early dementia or for differential diagnosis.

2   Tests of new learning are most effective at differentiating mild AD which reflects poor encoding and consolidation of information. Loss of primacy effect and frequent intrusion errors are also common features on episodic memory tasks in AD.

3   Semantic memory breakdown is a common, but more variable, feature in early AD and is reflected by disproportionate impairment of category, compared to letter-based, verbal fluency and production of semantic errors on naming tasks.

4   Attentional and executive dysfunction can also be detected early in the course of AD.

5   Individuals with a positive family history of AD, those with the ApoE $\varepsilon 4$ allele, and carriers of gene mutations (PS1, APP, etc.) perform worse on tests of episodic memory than normal controls.

6   Huntington's disease (HD) is characterized by impaired systematic retrieval from episodic and semantic memory.

7   Frontotemporal dementia produces a range of distinct cognitive syndromes depending on the predominant locus of pathology. The frontal lobe variant produces gross alterations of social cognition and behaviour followed by breakdown in attentional and executive function. The temporal variant, semantic dementia, causes severe anomia and impaired comprehension with preservation of attention, visually based problem solving, recent memory, and visuospatial function.

8   Vascular dementia is heterogeneous, but compared to AD produces less marked episodic memory impairment, but greater deficits in attention and executive function.

9   Dementia with Lewy bodies can be distinguished from AD by the greater impairment of attention and working memory and particularly early deficits in visuoperceptual ability.

Acknowledgements

This research was supported by NIH grant AG05131 to the University of California, San Diego and by a MRC programme grant to J. R. H.

References

Albert, M. S., Butters, N., and Brandt, J. (1981). Development of remote memory loss in patients with Huntington's disease. *Journal of Clinical and Experimental Neuropsychology*, **3**, 1–12.

American Psychiatric Association. (1994). *Diagnostic and statistical manual of mental disorders* (4th edn). Washington, DC.

Backman, L. and Small, B. J. (1998). Influences of cognitive support on episodic remembering: Tracing the process of loss from normal aging to Alzheimer's disease. *Psychology and Aging*, **13**, 267–76.

Baddeley, A. D., Bressi, S., Della Sala, S., Logie, R., and Spinnler, H. (1991). The decline of working memory in Alzheimer's disease: a longitudinal study. *Brain*, **114**, 2521–42.

Bak, T. and Hodges, J. R. (1998). The neuropsychology of progressive supranuclear palsy — a review. *Neurocase*, **4**, 89–94.

Ballard, C. G., Ayre, G., O'Brien, J., Sahgal, A., McKeith, I. G., Ince, P. G., *et al.* (1999). Simple standardised neuropsychological assessments aid in the differential diagnosis of dementia with

Lewy bodies from Alzheimer's disease and vascular dementia. *Dementia and Geriatric Cognitive Disorders*, **10**, 104–8.

Bayles, K. A., Boone, D. R., Tomoeda, C. K., Slauson, T. J., and Kaszniak, A. W. (1989). Differentiating Alzheimer's patients from the normal elderly and stroke patients with aphasia. *Journal of Speech and Hearing Disorders*, **54**, 74–87.

Bayley, P. J., Salmon, D. P., Bondi, M. W., Bui, B. K., Olichney, J., Delis, D. C., *et al.* (2000). Comparison of the serial position effect in very mild Alzheimer's disease, mild Alzheimer's disease, and amnesia associated with electroconvulsive therapy. *Journal of the International Neuropsychological Society*, **6**, 290–298.

Beatty, W. W., Salmon, D. P., Butters, N., Heindel, W. C., and Granholm, E. L. (1988). Retrograde amnesia in patients with Alzheimer's disease or Huntington's disease. *Neurobiology of Aging*, **9**, 181–6.

Becker, J. T. (1988). Working memory and secondary memory deficits in Alzheimer's disease. *Journal of Clinical and Experimental Neuropsychology*, **10**, 739–53.

Blessed, G., Tomlinson, B. E., and Roth, M. (1968). The association between quantitative measures of dementia and of senile change in the cerebral gray matter of elderly subjects. *British Journal of Psychiatry*, **114**, 797–811.

Bondi, M. W. and Kaszniak, A. W. (1991). Implicit and explicit memory in Alzheimer's disease and Parkinson's disease. *Journal of Clinical and Experimental Neuropsychology*, **13**, 339–58.

Bondi, M. W., Monsch, A. U., Butters, N., Salmon, D. P., and Paulsen, J. S. (1993). Utility of a modified version of the Wisconsin Card Sorting Test in the detection of dementia of the Alzheimer type. *The Clinical Neuropsychologist*, **7**, 161–70.

Bondi, M. W., Monsch, A. U., Galasko, D., Butters, N., Salmon, D. P., and Delis, D. C. (1994). Preclinical cognitive markers of dementia of the Alzheimer type. *Neuropsychology*, **8**, 374–84.

Bondi, M. W., Salmon, D. P., Galasko, D., Thomas, R. G., and Thal, L. J. (1999). Neuropsychological function and apolipoprotein E genotype in the preclinical detection of Alzheimer's disease. *Psychology and Aging*, **14**, 295–303.

Bondi, M. W., Salmon, D. P., Monsch, A. U., Galasko, D., Butters, N., Klauber, M. R., *et al.* (1995). Episodic memory changes are associated with the ApoE-epsilon 4 allele in nondemented older adults. *Neurology*, **45**, 2203–2206.

Braak, H. and Braak, E. (1991). Neuropathological staging of Alzheimer-related changes. *Acta Neuropathologica*, **82**, 239–59.

Brandt, J., Corwin, J., and Krafft, L. (1992). Is verbal recognition memory really different in Huntington's and Alzheimer's disease? *Journal of Clinical and Experimental Neuropsychology*, **14**, 773–84.

Brandt, J., Folstein, S. E., and Folstein, M. F. (1988). Differential cognitive impairment in Alzheimer's and Huntington's disease. *Annals of Neurology*, **23**, 555–61.

Buschke, H. (1973). Selective reminding for analysis of memory and learning. *Journal of Verbal Learning and Verbal Behavior*, **12**, 543–50.

Buschke, H., Sliwinski, M. J., Kuslansky, G., and Lipton, R. B. (1997). Diagnosis of early dementia by the double memory test. *Neurology*, **48**, 989–97.

Butters, N., Granholm, E., Salmon, D. P., Grant, I., and Wolfe, J. (1987). Episodic and semantic memory: A comparison of amnesic and demented patients. *Journal of Clinical and Experimental Neuropsychology*, **9**, 479–97.

Butters, N., Salmon, D. P., Cullum, C. M., Cairns, P., Troster, A. I., Jacobs, D., *et al.* (1988). Differentiation of amnesic and demented patients with the Wechsler Memory Scale-Revised. *The Clinical Neuropsychologist*, **2**, 133–44.

Butters, N., Wolfe, J., Martone, M., Granholm, E., and Cermak, L. S. (1985). Memory disorders associated with Huntington's disease; verbal recall, verbal recognition and procedural memory. *Neuropsychologia*, **23**, 729–43.

Cahn, D. A., Sullivan, E. V., Shear, P. K., Marsh, L., Fama, R., Lim, K. O., *et al.* (1998). Structural MRI correlates of recognition memory in Alzheimer's disease. *Journal of the International Neuropsychological Society*, **4**, 106–14.

Caine, D. and Hodges, J. R. (2001). Evidence for heterogeneity of semantic and spatial deficits in early Alzheimer's disease. *Neuropsychology*, **15**, 155–165.

Calderon, J., Perry, R., Erzinclioglu, S., Berrios, G. E., Dening, T., and Hodges, J. R. (2001). Perception, attention and working memory are disproportionately impaired in dementia with Lewy Body (LBD) compared to Alzheimer's disease (AD). *Journal of Neurology, Neurosurgery and Psychiatry*, **70**, 157–164.

Capitani, E., Della Sala, S., Logie, R., and Spinnler, H. (1992). Recency, primacy, and memory: Reappraising and standardising the serial position curve. *Cortex*, **28**, 315–42.

Chan, A. S., Butters, N., Paulson, J. S., Salmon, D. P., Swenson, M., and Maloney, L. (1993). An assessment of the semantic network in patients with Alzheimer's disease. *Journal of Cognitive Neuroscience*, **5**, 254–61.

Chan, A. S., Butters, N., and Salmon, D. P. (1997). The deterioration of semantic networks in patients with Alzheimer's disease: a cross-sectional study. *Neuropsychologia*, **35**, 241–8.

Chan, A. S., Butters, N., Salmon, D. P., Johnson, S. A., Paulsen, J. S., and Swenson, M. R. (1995). Comparison of the semantic networks in patients with dementia and amnesia. *Neuropsychology*, **9**, 177–86.

Chertkow, H. and Bub, D. (1990). Semantic memory loss in dementia of Alzheimer's type. *Brain*, **113**, 397–417.

Collette, F., Van der Linden, M., Bechet, S., and Salmon, E. (1999). Phonological loop and central executive functioning in Alzheimer's disease. *Neuropsychologia*, **37**, 905–18.

Connor, D. J., Salmon, D. P., Sandy, T. J., Galasko, D., Hansen, L. A., and Thal, L. J. (1998). Cognitive profiles of autopsy-confirmed Lewy body variant vs pure Alzheimer disease. *Archives of Neurology*, **55**, 994–1000.

Cummings, B. J. and Cotman, C. W. (1995). Image analysis of beta-amyloid load in Alzheimer's disease and relation to dementia severity. *Lancet*, **346**, 1524–8.

Cummings, J. L. (1990). *Subcortical dementia*. Oxford University Press.

Davous, P., Lamour, Y., Debrand, E., and Rondot, P. (1987). A comparative evaluation of the short orientation memory concentration test of cognitive impairment. *Journal of Neurology, Neurosurgery, and Psychiatry*, **50**, 1312–17.

DeKosky, S. T. and Scheff, S. W. (1990). Synapse loss in frontal cortex biopsies in Alzheimer's disease: Correlation with cognitive severity. *Annals of Neurology*, **27**, 457–64.

Delis, D. C., Kramer, J. H., Kaplan, E., and Ober, B. A. (1987). *The California Verbal Learning Test*. New York: Psychological Corporation.

Delis, D. C., Massman, P. J., Butters, N., Salmon, D. P., Kramer, J. H., and Cermak, L. (1991). Profiles of demented and amnesic patients on the California verbal learning test: implications for the assessment of memory disorders. *Psychological Assessment*, **3**, 19–26.

Deweer, B., Lehericy, S., Pillon, B., Baulac, M., Chiras, J., Marsault, C., *et al.* (1995). Memory disorders in probable Alzheimer's disease: the role of hippocampal atrophy as shown with MRI. *Journal of Neurology, Neurosurgery and Psychiatry*, **58**, 590–7.

Elfgren, C., Brun, A., Gustafson, L., Johansen, A., Minthon, L., Passant, U., *et al.* (1994). Neuropsychological tests as discriminators between dementia of Alzheimer type and frontotemporal dementia. *International Journal of Geriatric Psychiatry*, **9**, 635–42.

Fama, R., Sullivan, E. V., Shear, P. K., Marsh, L., Yesavage, J. A., Tinklenberg, J. R., *et al.* (1997). Selective cortical and hippocampal volume correlates of Mattis dementia rating scale in Alzheimer's disease. *Archives of Neurology*, **54**, 719–28.

Filoteo, J. V., Delis, D. C., Massman, P. J., Demadura, T., Butters, N., and Salmon, D. P. (1992). Directed and divided attention in Alzheimer's disease: impairment in shifting of attention to global and local stimuli. *Journal of Clinical and Experimental Neuropsychology*, **14**, 871–83.

Fischer, P., Marterer, A., and Danialczyk, W. (1990). Right-left disorientation in dementia of the Alzheimer type. *Neurology*, **40**, 1619–20.

Flicker, C., Ferris, S., and Reisberg, B. (1991). Mild cognitive impairment in the elderly: predictors of dementia. *Neurology*, **41**, 1006–9.

Folstein, M. F., Folstein, S. E., and McHugh, P. R. (1975). 'Mini-mental state': a practical method for grading the mental state of patients for clinicians. *Journal of Psychiatric Research*, **12**, 189–98.

Fox, N. C., Warrington, E. K., Seiffer, A. L., Agnew, S. K., and Rossor, M. N. (1998). Presymptomatic cognitive deficits in individuals at risk of familial Alzheimer's disease: a longitudinal prospective study. *Brain*, **121**, 1631–9.

Freedman, M., Leach, L., Kaplan, E., Winocur, G., Shulman, K. I., and Delis, D. C. (1994). *Clock drawing: A neuropsychological analysis*. New York: Oxford University Press.

Frisoni, G. B., Pizzolato, G., Geroldi, C., Rossato, A., Bianchetti, A., and Trabucchi, M. (1995). Dementia of the frontal type: neuropsychological and [99Tc]- HM-PAO SPECT features. *Journal of Geriatric Psychiatry and Neurology*, **8**, 42–8.

Fuld, P. A. (1978). Psychological testing in the differential diagnosis of the dementias. In *Alzheimer's disease: senile dementia and related disorders* (ed. R. Katzman, R. D. Terry, and K. L. Bick), pp. 185–93. New York: Raven Press.

Fuld, P. A., Masur, D. M., Blau, A. D., Crystal, H., and Aronson, M. K. (1990). Object-memory evaluation for prospective detection of dementia in normal functioning elderly: predictive normative data. *Journal of Clinical and Experimental Neuropsychology*, **12**, 520–8.

Galton, C. J., Patterson, K., Xuereb, J. H., and Hodges, J. R. (2000). Atypical and typical presentations of Alzheimer's disease: a clinical, neuropsychological, neuroimaging and pathological study of 13 cases. *Brain*, **123**, 484–98.

Garrard, P., Patterson, K., Watson, P. C., and Hodges, J. R. (1998). Category-specific semantic loss in dementia of Alzheimer's type: functional-anatomical correlations from cross-sectional analyses. *Brain*, **121**, 633–46.

Garrard, P., Perry, R., and Hodges, J. R. (1997). Disorders of semantic memory. *Journal of Neurology, Neurosurgery and Psychiatry*, **62**, 431–5.

Goldblum, M., Gomez, C., Dalla Barba, G., Boller, F., Deweer, B., Hahn, V., *et al.* (1998). The influence of semantic and perceptual encoding on recognition memory in Alzheimer's disease. *Neuropsychologia*, **36**, 717–29.

Goodale, M. A. and Milner, A. D. (1992). Separate visual pathways for perception and action. *Trends in Neurosciences*, **15**, 20–5.

Grady, C. L., Grimes, A. M., Patronas, N., Sunderland, T., Foster, N. L., and Rapoport, S. I. (1989). Divided attention, as measured by dichotic speech performance, in dementia of the Alzheimer type. *Archives of Neurology*, **46**, 137–320.

Grady, C. L., Haxby, J. V., Horwitz, B., Sundaram, M., Berg, G., Schapiro, M., *et al.* (1988). Longitudinal study of the early neuropsychological and cerebral metabolic changes in dementia of the Alzheimer type. *Journal of Clinical and Experimental Neuropsychology*, **10**, 576–96.

Graham, K. S. and Hodges, J. R. (1997). Differentiating the roles of the hippocampal complex and the neocortex in long-term memory storage: evidence from the study of semantic dementia and Alzheimer's disease. *Neuropsychology*, **11**, 77–89.

Graham, N. L. (2000). Dysgraphia in cortical dementia. *Neurocase*, **6**, 365–377.

Greene, J. D. W., Baddeley, A. D., and Hodges, J. R. (1996). Analysis of the episodic memory deficit in early Alzheimer's disease: evidence from the doors and people test. *Neuropsychologia*, **34**, 537–51.

Greene, J. D. W. and Hodges, J. R. (1996). Identification of famous faces and names in early Alzheimer's disease: Relationship to anterograde episodic and semantic memory impairment. *Brain*, **119**, 111–28.

Greene, J. D. W., Hodges, J. R., and Baddeley, A. D. (1995). Autobiographical memory and executive function in early dementia of Alzheimer type. *Neuropsychologia*, **33**, 1647–70.

Gregory, C. A., Orrell, M., Sahakian, B., and Hodges, J. R. (1997). Can frontotemporal dementia and Alzheimer's disease be differentiated using a brief battery of tests? *International Journal of Geriatric Psychiatry*, **12**, 375–83.

Gregory, C. A., Serra-Mestres, J., and Hodges, J. R. (1999). The early diagnosis of the frontal variant of frontotemporal dementia: how sensitive are standard neuroimaging and neuropsychological tests? *Neuropsychiatry, Neuropsychology and Behavioural Neurology*, **12**, 128–35.

Grober, E. and Kawas, C. (1997). Learning and retention in preclinical and early Alzheimer's disease. *Psychology and Aging*, **12**, 183–8.

Heindel, W. C., Salmon, D. P., and Butters, N. (1990). Pictorial priming and cued recall in Alzheimer's and Huntington's disease. *Brain and Cognition*, **13**, 282–95.

Heindel, W. C., Salmon, D. P., Shults, C. W., Walicke, P. A., and Butters, N. (1989). Neuropsychological evidence for multiple implicit memory systems: a comparison of Alzheimer's, Huntington's and Parkinson's disease patients. *Journal of Neuroscience*, **9**, 582–7.

Hodges, J. R. and Patterson, K. (1995). Is semantic memory consistently impaired early in the course of Alzheimer's disease? Neuroanatomical and diagnostic implications. *Neuropsychologia*, **33**, 441–59.

Hodges, J. R. and Patterson, K. (1996). Nonfluent progressive aphasia and semantic dementia: A comparative neuropsychological study. *Journal of the International Neuropsychological Society*, **2**, 511–24.

Hodges, J. R., Patterson, K., Ward, R., Garrard, P., Bak, T., Perry, R., *et al.* (1999). The differentiation of semantic dementia and frontal lobe dementia (temporal and frontal variants of frontotemporal dementia) from early Alzheimer's disease: a comparative neuropsychological study. *Neuropsychology*, **13**, 31–40.

Hodges, J. R., Patterson, K. E., Graham, N., and Dawson, K. (1996). Naming and knowing in dementia of Alzheimer's type. *Brain and Language*, **54**, 302–25.

Hodges, J. R., Salmon, D. P., and Butters, N. (1991). The nature of the naming deficit in Alzheimer's and Huntington's disease. *Brain*, **114**, 1547–58.

Hodges, J. R., Salmon, D. P., and Butters, N. (1992). Semantic memory impairment in Alzheimer's disease: Failure of access or degraded knowledge? *Neuropsychologia*, **30**, 301–14.

Hodges, J. R., Salmon, D. P., and Butters, N. (1993). Recognition and naming of famous faces in Alzheimer's disease: a cognitive analysis. *Neuropsychologia*, **31**, 775–88.

Hom, J., Turner, M. B., Risser, R., Bonte, F. J., and Tintner, R. (1994). Cognitive deficits in asymptomatic first-degree relatives of Alzheimer's disease patients. *Journal of Clinical and Experimental Neuropsychology*, **16**, 568–76.

Hughes, J. C., Graham, N., Patterson, K., and Hodges, J. R. (1997). Dysgraphia in mild dementia of Alzheimer's type. *Neuropsychologia*, **35**, 533–45.

Huppert, F. A., Brayne, C., Gill, C., Paykel, E. S., and Beardsall, L. (1995). CAMCOG — a concise neuropsychological test to assist dementia diagnosis: socio-demographic determinants in an elderly population sample. *British Journal of Clinical Psychology*, **34**, 529–41.

Hyman, B. T., Van Hoesen, G. W., Damasio, A. R., and Barnes, C. L. (1984). Alzheimer's disease: cell-specific pathology isolates the hippocampal formation. *Science*, **225**, 1168–70.

Jacobs, D., Salmon, D. P., Troster, A. I., and Butters, N. (1990). Intrusion errors in the figural memory of patients with Alzheimer's and Huntington's disease. *Archives of Clinical Neuropsychology*, **5**, 47–57.

Katzman, R., Brown, T., Fuld, P., Peck, A., Schecter, R., and Schimmel, H. (1983). Validation of a short orientation-memory-concentration test of cognitive impairment. *American Journal of Psychiatry*, **140**, 734–9.

Katzman, R., Brown, T., Thal, L. J., Fuld, P. A., Aronson, M., Butters, N., *et al.* (1988). Comparison of rate of annual change of mental status score in four independent studies of patients with Alzheimer's disease. *Annals of Neurology*, **24**, 384–9.

Knopman, D. S. and Ryberg, S. (1989). A verbal memory test with high predictive accuracy for dementia of the Alzheimer type. *Archives of Neurology*, **46**, 141–5.

Kohler, S., Black, S. E., Sinden, M., Szekely, C., Kidron, D., Parker, J. L., *et al.* (1998). Memory impairments associated with hippocampal versus parahippocampal gyrus atrophy: An MR volumetry study in Alzheimer's disease. *Neuropsychologia*, **36**, 901–14.

Kopelman, M. D. (1989). Remote and autobiographical memory, temporal context memory and frontal atrophy in Korsakoff and Alzheimer patients. *Neuropsychologia*, **27**, 437–60.

Kurylo, D. D., Corkin, S., Rizzo J. F., and Growdon, J. H. (1996). Greater relative impairment of object recognition than of visuospatial abilities in Alzheimer's disease. *Neuropsychology*, **10**, 74–81.

Lambon Ralph, M. A., Powell, J., Howard, D., Whitworth, A. B., Garrard, P., and Hodges, J. R. (2001). Semantic memory is impaired in both dementia with Lewy bodies (DLB) and dementia of Alzheimos type (DAT). A comparative neuropsychological study and literature review. *Journal of Neurology, Neurosurgery and Psychiatry*, **70**, 149–156.

Lange, K. W., Sahakian, B. J., Quinn, N. P., Marsden, C. D., and Robbins, T. W. (1995). Comparison of executive and visuospatial memory function in Huntington's disease and dementia of Alzheimer-type matched for degree of dementia. *Journal of Neurology, Neurosurgery and Psychiatry*, **58**, 598–606.

Lefleche, G. and Albert, M. S. (1995). Executive function deficits in mild Alzheimer's disease. *Neuropsychology*, **9**, 313–20.

Linn, R. T., Wolf, P. A., Bachman, D. L., Knoefel, J. E., Cobb, J. L., Belanger, A. J., *et al.* (1995). The 'Preclinical Phase' of probable Alzheimer's disease: a 13-year prospective study of the Framingham cohort. *Archives of Neurology*, **52**, 485–90.

Locascio, J. J., Growdon, J. H., and Corkin, S. (1995). Cognitive test performance in detecting, staging, and tracking Alzheimer's disease. *Archives of Neurology*, **52**, 1087–99.

Mann, D. M. A., Marcyniuk, B., Yates, P. O., Neary, D., and Snowden, J. S. (1988). The progression of the pathological changes of Alzheimer's disease in frontal and temporal neocortex examined both at biopsy and at autopsy. *Neuropathology and Applied Neurobiology*, **14**, 177–95.

Massman, P. J., Delis, D. C., Butters, N., Dupont, R. M., and Gillin, J. C. (1992). The subcortical dysfunction hypothesis of memory deficits in depression: neuropsychological validation in a subgroup of patients. *Journal of Clinical and Experimental Neuropsychology*, **14**, 687–706.

Massman, P. J., Delis, D. C., and Butters, N. (1993). Does impaired primacy recall equal impaired long-term storage?: Serial position effects in Huntington's disease and Alzheimer's disease. *Developmental Neuropsychology*, **9**, 1–15.

Massman, P. J., Delis, D. C., Butters, N., Levin, B. E., and Salmon, D. P. (1990). Are all subcortical dementias alike?: verbal learning and memory in Parkinson's and Huntington's disease patients. *Journal of Clinical and Experimental Neuropsychology*, **12**, 729–44.

Masur, D. M., Fuld, P. A., Blau, A. D., Crystal, H., and Aronson, M. K. (1990). Predicting development of dementia in the elderly with the selective reminding test. *Journal of Clinical and Experimental Neuropsychology*, **12**, 529–38.

Masur, D. M., Sliwinski, M., Lipton, R. B., Blau, A. D., and Crystal, H. A. (1994). Neuropsychological prediction of dementia and the absence of dementia in healthy elderly persons. *Neurology*, **44**, 1427–32.

Mathuranath, P. S., Nestor, P., Berrios, G. E., Rakowicz, W., and Hodges, J. R. (2000). A brief cognitive test battery to differentiate Alzheimer's disease and frontotemporal dementia. *Neurology*, **55**, 1613–1620.

Mattis, S. (1976). Mental status examination for organic mental syndrome in the elderly patient. In *Geriatric psychiatry: a handbook for psychiatrists and primary care physicians* (ed. L. Bellack and T. E. Karasu), pp. 77–121. New York: Grune and Stratton.

McKeith, I. G., Ballard, C. G., Perry, R. H., Ince, P. G., O'Brien, J. T., Neill, D, *et al.* (2000). Prospective validation of consensus criteria for the diagnosis of dementia with Lewy bodies. *Neurology*, **54**, 1050–8.

Mendez, M. F., Mendez, M. A., Martin, R., Smyth, K. A., and Whitehouse, P. J. (1990). Complex visual disturbances in Alzheimer's disease. *Neurology*, **40**, 439–43.

Monsch, A. U., Bondi, M. W., Butters, N., Pauslen, J. S., Salmon, D. P., Brugger, P., *et al.* (1994). A comparison of category and letter fluency in Alzheimer's disease and Huntington's disease. *Neuropsychology*, **8**, 25–30.

Monsch, A. U., Bondi, M. W., Butters, N., Salmon, D. P., Katzman, R., and Thal, L. J. (1992). Comparisons of verbal fluency tasks in the detection of dementia of the Alzheimer type. *Archives of Neurology*, **49**, 1253–8.

Monsch, A. U., Bondi, M. W., Salmon, D. P., Butters, N., Thal, L. J., Hansen, L. A., *et al.* (1995). Clinical validity of the Mattis dementia rating scale in detecting dementia of the Alzheimer type: a double cross validation and application to a community-dwelling sample. *Archives of Neurology*, **52**, 899–904.

Morris, R. G. (1994). Working memory in Alzheimer-type dementia. *Neuropsychology*, **8**, 544–54.

Moss, M. B., Albert, M. S., Butters, N., and Payne, M. (1986). Differential patterns of memory loss among patients with Alzheimer's disease, Huntington's disease, and alcoholic Korsakoff's syndrome. *Archives of Neurology*, **43**, 239–46.

Murden, R. A., McRae, T. D., and Kaner, S. (1991). Mini-mental state exam scores vary with education in blacks and whites. *Journal of the American Geriatric Society*, **39**, 149–55.

Nebes, R. D. (1989). Semantic memory in Alzheimer's disease. *Psychological Bulletin*, **106**, 377–94.

Nebes, R. D. and Brady, C. B. (1993). Phasic and tonic alertness in Alzheimer's disease. *Cortex*, **29**, 77–90.

Nelson, H. E. (1982). *The National Adult Reading Test*. Windsor: NFER-Nelson.

Nielsen, H., Lolk, A., Andersen, K., Andersen, J., and Kragh-Sorensen, P. (1999). Characteristics of elderly who develop Alzheimer's disease during the next two years-a neuropsychological study using CAMCOG. The Odense study. *International Journal of Geriatric Psychiatry*, **14**, 957–63.

Norton, L. E., Bondi, M. W., Salmon, D. P., and Goodglass, H. (1997). Deterioration of generic knowledge in patients with Alzheimer's disease: Evidence from the number information test. *Journal of Clinical and Experimental Neuropsychology*, **19**, 857–66.

O'Connor, D. W., Pollitt, P. A., Hyde, J. B., Miller, N. D., and Fellowes, J. L. (1989). The reliability and validity of the mini-mental state in a British community survey. *Journal of Psychiatric Research*, **23**, 87–96.

Oken, B. S., Kishiyama, S. S., Kaye, J. A., and Howieson, D. B. (1994). Attention deficit in Alzheimer's disease is not stimulated by anticholinergic/anithistaminergic drug and is distinct from deficits in healthy ageing. *Neurology*, **44**, 657–62.

Pachana, N. A., Boone, K. B., Miller, B. L., Cummings, J. L., and Berman, N. (1996). Comparison of neuropsychological functioning in Alzheimer's disease and frontotemporal dementia. *Journal of the International Neuropsycholgical Society*, **2**, 505–10.

Pandovani, A., Di Piero, V., Bragoni, M., Iacoboni, M., Gualdi, G. G., and Lenzi, G. L. (1995). Patterns of neuropsychological impairment in mild dementia: A comparison between Alzheimer's disease and multi-infarct dementia. *Acta Neurologica Scandinavica*, **92**, 433–42.

Paolo, A. M., Troster, A. I., Glatt, S., Hubble, J. P., and Koller, W. C. (1995). Differentiation of the dementias of Alzheimer's and Parkinson's disease with the dementia rating scale. *Journal of Geriatric Psychiatry and Neurology*, **8**, 184–8.

Paque, L. and Warrington, E. K. (1995). A longitudinal study of reading ability in patients suffering from dementia. *Journal of the International Neuropsychological Society*, **1**, 517–24.

Parasuraman, R., Greenwood, P. M., Haxby, J. V., and Grady, C. L. (1992). Visuospatial attention in dementia of the Alzheimer type. *Brain*, **115**, 711–33.

Parasuraman, R. and Haxby, J. V. (1993). Attention and brain function in Alzheimer's disease: A review. *Neuropsychology*, **7**, 242–72.

Patterson, K., Graham, N., and Hodges, J. R. (1994). Reading in dementia of the Alzheimer type: A preserved ability? *Neuropsychology*, **8**, 395–407.

Paulsen, J. S., Butters, N., Sadek, J. R., Johnson, S. S., Salmon, D. P., Swenson, M. R., *et al.* (1995). Distinct cognitive profiles of cortical and subcortical dementia in advanced illness. *Neurology*, **45**, 951–6.

Paulsen, J. S., Butters, N., Salmon, D. P., Heindel, W. C., and Swenson, M. R. (1993). Prism adaptation in Alzheimer's and Huntington's disease. *Neuropsychology*, **7**, 73–81.

Perry, R. J. and Hodges, J. R. (1999). Attention and executive deficits in Alzheimer's disease: a critical review. *Brain*, **122**, 383–404.

Perry, R. J. and Hodges, J. R. (2000). Differentiating frontal and temporal variant frontotemporal dementia from Alzheimer's disease. *Neurology*, **54**, 2277–2284.

Perry, R. J., Watson, P., and Hodges, J. R. (2000). The nature and staging of attention dysfunction in early (minimal and mild) Alzheimer's disease: Relationship to episodic and semantic memory impairment. *Neuropsychologia*, **38**, 252–71.

Petersen, R. C., Smith, G., Kokmen, E., Ivnik, R. J., and Tangalos, E. G. (1992). Memory function in normal aging. *Neurology*, **42**, 396–401.

Rahman, S., Sahakian, B. J., Hodges, J. R., Rogers, R. D., and Robbins, T. W. (1999). Specific cognitive deficits in early frontal variant frontotemporal dementia. *Brain*, **122**, 1469–93.

Reed, T., Carmelli, D., Swan, G. E., Breitner, J. C., Welsh, K. A., Jarvik, G. P., *et al.* (1994). Lower cognitive performance in normal older adult male twins carrying the apolipoprotein E epsilon 4 allele. *Archives of Neurology*, **51**, 1189–92.

Robinson-Whelen, S. and Storandt, M. (1992). Immediate and delayed prose recall among normal and demented adults. *Archives of Neurology*, **49**, 32–4.

Rohrer, D., Salmon, D. P., Wixted, J. T., and Paulsen, J. S. (1999). The disparate effects of Alzheimer's disease and Huntington's disease on semantic memory. *Neuropsychology*, **13**, 381–8.

Rosser, A. and Hodges, J. R. (1994). The dementia rating scale in Alzheimer's disease, Huntington's disease and progressive supranuclear palsy. *Journal of Neurology*, **241**, 531–6.

Rouleau, I., Salmon, D. P., and Butters, N. (1996). Longitudinal analysis of clock drawing in Alzheimer's disease patients. *Brain and Cognition*, **31**, 17–34.

Rouleau, I., Salmon, D. P., Butters, N., Kennedy, C., and McGuire, K. (1992). Quantitative and qualitative analyses of clock drawings in Alzheimer's and Huntington's disease. *Brain and Cognition*, **18**, 70–87.

Sagar, H. A., Cohen, N. J., Sullivan, E. V., Corkin, S., and Growdon, J. H. (1988). Remote memory function in Alzheimer's disease and Parkinson's disease. *Brain*, **111**, 185–206.

Sahakian, B. J., Jones, G. M. M., Levy, R., Gray, J. A., and Warburton, D. M. (1989). The effects of nicotine on attention, information processing, and short-term memory in patients with dementia of the Alzheimer's type. *British Journal of Psychiatry*, **154**, 797–800.

Salmon, D. P., Butters, N., Thal, L. J., and Jeste, D. V. (1998). Alzheimer's disease: Analysis for the DSM-IV task force. In *DSM-IV Sourcebook*, Vol. IV (ed. T. A. Widiger, A. Frances, H. Pincus pp 91–107). Washington, DC: American Psychiatric Association, in press.

Salmon, D. P. and Chan, A. S. (1994). Semantic memory deficits associated with Alzheimer's disease. In *Neuropsychological explorations of memory and cognition: Essays in honor of Nelson Butters* (ed. L. S. Cermak), pp. 61–76. New York: Plenum Press.

Salmon, D. P. and Fennema-Notestine, C. (1996). Implicit memory in Alzheimer's disease: Priming and skill learning. In *The cognitive neuropsychology of Alzheimer's disease* (ed. R. Morris), pp. 105–27. Oxford: Oxford University Press.

Salmon, D. P., Galasko, D., Hansen, L. A., Masliah, E., Butters, N., Thal, L. J. *et al.* (1996). Neuropsychological deficts associated with diffuse Lewy body disease *Brain and Cognition*, **61**, 148–165.

Salmon, D. P., Heindel, W. C., and Lange, K. L. (1999). Differential decline in word generation from phonemic and semantic categories during the course of Alzheimer's disease: implications for the integrity of semantic memory. *Journal of the International Neuropsychological Society*, **5**, 692–703.

Salmon, D. P., Kwo-on-Yuen, P. F., Heindel, W. C., Butters, N., and Thal, L. J. (1989). Differentiation of Alzheimer's disease and Huntington's disease with the dementia rating scale. *Archives of Neurology*, **48**, 1204–8.

Salmon, D. P., Shimamura, A. P., Butters, N., and Smith, S. (1988). Lexical and semantic priming deficits in patients with Alzheimer's disease. *Journal of Clinical and Experimental Neuropsychology*, **10**, 477–94.

Salmon, D. P., Thal, L. J., Butters, N., and Heindel, W. C. (1990). Longitudinal evaluation of dementia of the Alzheimer type: a comparison of three standardised mental state examinations. *Neurology*, **40**, 1225–30.

Simon, E., Leach, L., Winocur, G., and Moscovitch, M. (1994). Intact primary memory in mild to moderate Alzheimer's disease: Indices from the California verbal learning test. *Journal of Clinical and Experimental Neuropsychology*, **16**, 414–22.

Ska, B., Poissant, A., and Joanette, Y. (1990). Line orientation judgement in normal elderly and subjects with dementia of Alzheimer's type. *Journal of Clinical and Experimental Neuropsychology*, **12**, 695–702.

Storandt, M., Botwinick, J., Danziger, W. L., Berg, L., and Hughes, C. P. (1984). Psychometric differentiation of mild senile dementia of the Alzheimer type. *Archives of Neurology*, **41**, 497–9.

Storandt, M. and Hill, R. D. (1989). Very mild senile dementia of the Alzheimer type. II. Psychometric test performance. *Archives of Neurology*, **46**, 383–6.

Stout, J. C., Bondi, M. W., Jernigan, T. L., Archibald, S. L., Delis, D. C., and Salmon, D. P. (1999). Regional cerebral volume loss associated with verbal learning and memory in dementia of the Alzheimer type. *Neuropsychology*, **13**, 188–97.

Strain, E., Patterson, K. E., and Hodges, J. R. (1998). Word reading in Alzheimer's disease: cross-sectional and longitudinal analysis of response-time and accuracy data. *Neuropsychologia*, **36**, 155–71.

Teri, L., Hughes, J. P., and Larson, E. B. (1990). Cognitive deterioration in Alzheimer's disease: behavioural and health factors. *Journal of Gerontology*, **45**, P58–63.

Terry, R. D., Masliah, E., Salmon, D. P., Butters, N., DeTeresa, R., Hill, R., *et al.* (1991). Physical basis of cognitive alterations in Alzheimer's disease: synapse loss is the major correlate of cognitive impairment. *Annals of Neurology*, **30**, 572–80.

Tombaugh, T. N. and McIntyre, N. J. (1992). The mini-mental state examination: A comprehensive review. *Journal of the American Geriatrics Society*, **40**, 922–35.

Tröster, A. I., Butters, N., Salmon, D. P., Cullum, C. M., Jacobs, D., Brandt, J., *et al.* (1993). The diagnostic utility of savings scores: Differentiating Alzheimer's and Huntington's diseases with the logical memory and visual reproduction tests. *Journal of Clinical and Experimental Neuropsychology*, **15**, 773–88.

Ungerleider, L. G. and Mishkin, M. (1982). Two cortical systems. In *Analysis of visual behavior* (ed. D. J. Ingle, M. A. Goodale, and R. J. W. Mansfield), pp. 549–86. Cambridge, MA: MIT Press.

Villardita, C. (1993). Alzheimer's disease compared with cerebrovascular dementia. *Acta Neurologica Scandinavica*, **87**, 299–308.

Walker, A., Allen, R. L., Shergill, S., and Katona, C. L. E. (1997). Neuropsychological performance in Lewy body dementia and Alzheimer's disease. *British Journal of Psychiatry*, **170**, 156–8.

Welsh, K., Butters, N., Hughes, J., Mohs, R., and Heyman, A. (1991). Detection of abnormal memory decline in mild cases of Alzheimer's disease using CERAD neuropsychological measures. *Archives of Neurology*, **48**, 278–81.

Welsh, K. A., Butters, N., Hughes, J. P., Mohs, R. C., and Heyman, A. (1992). Detection and staging of dementia in Alzheimer's disease: use of the neuropsychological measures developed for the consortium to establish a registry for Alzheimer's disease. *Archives of Neurology*, **49**, 448–52.

Zola-Morgan, S. and Squire, L. R. (1990). The primate hippocampal formation: Evidence for a time-limited role in memory storage. *Science*, **250**, 288–90.

4 Neuropsychiatric assessment

Jeffrey L. Cummings and Julia A. Chung

1 Introduction

Neuropsychiatric symptoms, including affective disturbances, personality changes, and psychosis, are common and important in the assessment and treatment of patients with early onset dementia. Early recognition is essential in formulating the differential diagnosis and providing effective interventions that may reduce morbidity and mortality. Single item and multidimensional tools can assist the clinician in evaluating initial symptomatology and monitoring clinical changes. Many illnesses that produce early onset dementia, such as Wilson's disease and the leukodystrophies, have prominent psychiatric features and may be initially misdiagnosed as primary psychiatric disorders such as schizophrenia. This chapter will focus on the neuropsychiatric assessment of disorders that commonly present between the ages of 20 and 65 years. Degenerative disorders will be emphasized, since the psychiatric features of dementias secondary to trauma, cerebrovascular accidents, tumours, and other conditions not generally restricted to this age group are well-characterized elsewhere.

2 Neuropsychiatric assessment

Personality alterations, mood disorders, and psychosis frequently accompany dementing illnesses. These symptoms may cause significant hardship for patients and their caregivers, interfere with medical evaluation and treatment, and lead to untimely mortality through suicide. Neuropsychiatric disturbances in dementia are often more disturbing to caregivers than the cognitive changes. They result in increased medication usage, higher patient care costs, earlier admission to nursing homes, and the need for increased staffing in care facilities.

Patients with dementia may present initially with isolated psychiatric disturbances. The evaluation of all patients should include a thorough history and physical examination, mental status testing, and a careful assessment of past and current neuropsychiatric symptoms. Family history is important because many psychiatric disorders, rare neurodegenerative disorders, and other causes of dementia have genetic influences. Laboratory studies for screening should include a complete blood count, electrolytes, serum glucose, calcium, and phosphorus levels, blood urea nitrogen, liver function tests, thyroid-stimulating hormone, erythrocyte sedimentation rate, vitamin B12 level, folate level, and serologies for syphilis (and HIV, if appropriate). Neuroimaging, including structural imaging (computed tomography [CT] and magnetic resonance imaging [MRI]) and functional imaging (positron emission tomography [PET] and single photon emission computed tomography [SPECT]) also yields important information. Finally, electroencephalography (EEG) and quantitative EEG may be useful in arriving at a diagnosis.

Table 4.1 Neuropsychiatric signs and symptoms

Appearance
  Grooming/dress (dishevelled, flamboyant, bizarre)
  Posture
  Poise
  Behaviour
  Attitude
  Level of psychomotor activity (agitation, psychomotor retardation)

Mood
  Quality (dysphoric, anxious, happy)
  Stability (stable, labile)

Affect
  Mood-congruent
  Range (full, restricted, blunted, flattened)
  Appropriateness

Speech
  Quantity
  Rate (pressured, rapid, slowed)
  Rhythm
  Volume
  Prosody
  Slurring
  Stuttering
  Lack of spontaneous speech

Perceptions
  Hallucinations
    Sensory modality
      Auditory
      Visual
      Tactile (haptic)
      Olfactory
      Gustatory
    Command-type
    Mood-congruent
    Hypnagogic/hypnopompic
    Lilliputian
    Micropsia/macropsia
  Illusions

Thought processes
  Coherence
  Goal-directedness (linear, circumstantial, tangential)
  Perseveration

Thought content
  Delusions
    Mood-congruent
    Paranoid
    Grandiose
    Somatic
    Erotomanic
    Jealous
    Bizarre
    Thought broadcasting
    Thought insertion/withdrawal
    Misidentification syndromes
      Capgras' syndrome
      Fregoli's phenomenon

Table 4.1 (*Continued*)

> Obsessions
> Phobias
> Preoccupations
> Suicidal ideation/plan/intent
> Homicidal ideation/plan/intent
> **Level of insight**

2.1 Definitions

Clinical examination of the patient with suspected neuropsychiatric disturbance should include a psychiatric mental status examination, with careful assessment of mood, affect, speech characteristics, thought content and form of thinking, and perceptions. The mental status examination also includes observation of the patient's appearance and actions, consideration of judgement, insight, impulsivity, and reliability, and evaluation of sensorium and cognition.

2.1.1 Appearance

The patient's general physical appearance should be noted, including an observation of grooming, dress, posture, and poise. Bizarre dress, unusual makeup, dishevelled appearance, body odour, and a tense posture are examples of noteworthy disturbances. The patient's overall behaviour and attitude toward the physician also should be noted; for example, is the patient guarded and paranoid, anxious, seductive, hostile, apathetic, co-operative, or perplexed? Finally, note should be made of the patient's general behaviour and level of psychomotor activity. This includes psychomotor agitation (rocking, pacing, wringing of the hands, etc.), retardation, combativeness, mannerisms, tics, stereotypies, and other abnormal movements.

2.1.2 Mood

The patient's mood should be assessed, preferably by asking the patient directly, although this may not be possible in all patients with dementia (i.e. those with aphasia). Mood is defined by the fourth edition of the *Diagnostic and Statistical Manual of Mental Disorders* (DSM-IV, American Psychiatric Association and American Psychiatric Association. Task Force on DSM-IV 1994) as 'a pervasive and sustained emotion that colours the person's perception of the world'. It is experienced and reported subjectively (as opposed to affect, which is objective). The stability of mood should also be noted; mood that fluctuates rapidly is described as labile. Common mood descriptions include depressed, anxious, euphoric, angry, irritable, expansive, and frightened.

2.1.3 Affect

The patient's affect is defined in DSM-IV as 'a pattern of observable behaviours that is the expression of a subjectively experienced feeling state (emotion)'. In patients with dementia, affect may or may not be mood-congruent or appropriate for the context. The patient should be observed for both the range of affect and its appropriateness. A normal range of affect would include variations in the patient's facial expressions, body movements, and speech. Patients may have a decreased range that is characterized as being restricted (or constricted), blunted, or flat (in order of increasing severity). Patients with parkinsonism may have a flat affect due to masked facies.

2.1.4 Speech

In addition to assessment for aphasia, the patient's speech should be evaluated for quantity, rate, rhythm, and volume. Patients who are depressed may demonstrate slow speech with low volume or monosyllabic answers to questions; manic patients may have loud, pressured (rapid and uninterruptable) speech. Slurred speech may signal intoxication or neurological disease. Prosody (the ability to inflect speech) also should be assessed. Finally, the interviewer should note if the patient lacks spontaneous speech or has impairments such as stuttering and cluttering.

2.1.5 Perceptions

Disturbances of perception include hallucinations and illusions, and may involve any of the sensory systems (although the auditory and visual systems are most commonly affected). Hallucinations are false sensory perceptions that are not associated with true external stimuli. Auditory hallucinations are the most common hallucinations in psychiatric disorders and usually are perceived as voices, although they may also be other noises (such as music). Visual hallucinations may be formed (such as animals or people) or unformed (such as light flashes). Olfactory hallucinations are most common in medical disorders, as are gustatory hallucinations (i.e. in seizure disorders). Tactile (or haptic) hallucinations include phantom limb sensation and formication (crawling sensations). Hallucinations may be mood-congruent or mood-incongruent. Command hallucinations should be noted if present, as well as whether the patient feels obligated to obey them or able to resist them. Hypnagogic and hypnopompic hallucinations occur while falling asleep or awakening, respectively, and may occur at times in healthy individuals. Lilliputian hallucinations occur when objects are perceived as being reduced in size. An illusion is the misperception or misinterpretation of actual external stimuli. Patients may be reluctant to discuss hallucinations, particularly if they are paranoid or afraid of being labelled as 'crazy'. If questions are not successful in eliciting information about perceptual disturbances, observations may still be made as to whether the patient appears to be reacting to internal stimuli (i.e. talking to or looking at people who are not there).

2.1.6 Delusions

Another manifestation of psychosis is the delusion, a false, fixed belief that is not consistent with the patient's intelligence or cultural background. Common delusion types include bizarre, erotomanic, persecutory, jealous, grandiose, somatic, and delusions of reference. Delusions of thought broadcasting, insertion, and withdrawal also are encountered frequently. Misidentification syndromes such as Capgras' syndrome (the delusion that others have been replaced by identical imposters) and Fregoli's phenomenon (the delusion that a persecutor is taking on different faces) are seen in dementia. Delusions may be mood-congruent or mood-incongruent. The examiner should refrain from directly challenging a patient's delusions. Patients may be reluctant to discuss delusional content, so collateral information from a family member or other caregiver is important.

2.1.7 Thought processes and content

The patient's thought processes and content should be evaluated. Thought process is defined as the form in which a person puts together ideas and makes associations. Thoughts are normally coherent and goal-directed. Disturbed thought processes may range from a loosening of associations to frank word salad or incomprehensibility. The quantity of thoughts may be described, from a poverty of thought to overabundance. The speed of thought also may be noted, from slowness to a flight of ideas. Loose associations retain idiosyncratic connections. Thought blocking is interruption in a train of thought. Goal-directedness should be assessed.

Circumstantial speech includes irrelevant details and comments but ultimately returns to the original subject. Tangential speech is a more severe disturbance of goal-directedness, as the patient does not return to the original point. Neologisms, punning, and clang associations (rhyming) may be seen.

Thought content should be evaluated for disturbances such as delusional material, obsessions, compulsions, phobias, preoccupations, and homicidal or suicidal ideation. Overvalued ideas are false beliefs that are not held as firmly as frank delusions. Obsessions are persistent ideas, thought, impulses, or images that are experienced as intrusive and inappropriate and that cause marked anxiety or distress (DSM-IV; American Psychiatric Association and American Psychiatric Association. Task Force on DSM-IV 1994). Compulsions are 'repetitive behaviours or mental acts, the goal of which is to prevent or reduce anxiety or distress, not to provide pleasure or gratification' (American Psychiatric Association and American Psychiatric Association. Task Force on DSM-IV 1994). Phobias involve the persistent, irrational, exaggerated, and invariably pathological dread of a specific stimulus or situation, and result in a compelling desire to avoid the feared stimulus (American Psychiatric Association and American Psychiatric Association. Task Force on DSM-IV 1994). All patients should be questioned about suicidal or homicidal ideation, plans, or intent; patients who represent a danger to themselves or others require immediate intervention.

In addition to the more cognitive aspects of the mental status examination (such as assessment of attention, memory, abstraction, intelligence, and language skills), a psychiatric evaluation should also include assessment of impulsivity, judgement, and insight. An assessment of impulse control can be obtained from the history and from observations of the patient's behaviour during the interview and examination. Judgement and insight are often impaired in patients with dementia. Insight may range from full emotional appreciation to complete denial of illness. A collateral history from family members, friends, or caretakers is an important part of assessment.

2.1.8 Depression

A major depressive episode, as defined by DSM-IV, is characterized by an abnormally and persistently depressed mood (or anhedonia) for at least two weeks. There also must be four or more additional related symptoms (from among changes in appetite or weight, sleep and psychomotor activity; decreased energy; feelings of worthlessness or guilt; difficulty thinking, concentrating, or making decisions; or recurrent thoughts of death or suicidal ideation, plans, or attempts). These symptoms must be present for the majority of the time for at least two weeks, and be accompanied by a change in functioning or clinically significant distress. The mood may be described as sad, depressed, down, hopeless or irritable. Other patients may deny experiencing a depressed mood but have multiple somatic complaints or a telltale demeanour and expression. Insomnia and anorexia are more common than hypersomnia and food craving or weight gain. Depression is often accompanied by anxiety and panic attacks. A major depressive episode may be diagnosed in addition to dementia if it is felt that both have independent aetiologies.

Research criteria have been set forth in DSM-IV for minor depressive disorder, which is similar to a major depressive episode, but with fewer symptoms and less severe impairment. Sad or depressed mood (or loss of interests and pleasure in activities) must be present for a minimum of two weeks, accompanied by two to four of the associated symptoms of depression.

2.1.9 Mania

Mania is an episode of abnormally and persistently elevated, irritable, or expansive mood. To meet DSM-IV criteria for a manic episode, the abnormal mood must persist for at least one week (or less, if the patient is hospitalized), and be accompanied by three or more related symptoms (including significant elevation in self-esteem, decreased need for sleep, pressured speech, racing thoughts or a flight of ideas, distractibility, psychomotor agitation or increased goal-directed activity, and excessive involvement in pleasurable but risky activities such as impulsive gambling or spending sprees). The mood is generally described as euphoric, high, expansive, or cheerful. Labile or irritable moods also are seen.

A hypomanic episode is similar, but less severe than, a full manic episode. DSM-IV criteria specify that a patient's mood must be abnormally and persistently elevated for a minimum of four days. As with mania, at least three of the associated criteria must be met. The presence of associated hallucinations or delusions, or a severity requiring hospitalization, requires the diagnosis of a manic, and not hypomanic, episode.

2.1.10 Apathy

Apathy is a state of reduced motivation. It may coexist with depression or occur independently. Four main subtypes have been described, including motoric, motivational, emotional, and cognitive. Motoric apathy is equivalent to akinesia; the patient has increased response latencies and engages in few activities. Motivational apathy is the absence of motivation to initiate and maintain activity. Emotional apathy is indifference; these patients have decreased or absent emotional interests, and typically display a flat or blunted affect. Finally, cognitive apathy produces an absence of generative ideation. Apathy is a common symptom in a wide variety of neurological conditions.

2.1.11 Personality changes

Personality disorders feature 'an enduring pattern of inner experience and behaviour that deviates markedly from the expectations of the individual's culture, is pervasive and inflexible, has an onset in adolescence or early adulthood, is stable over time, and leads to distress or impairment' (DSM-IV). Personality traits are defined as 'enduring patterns of perceiving, relating to, and thinking about the environment and oneself that are exhibited in a wide range of social and personal contexts'. The pattern of inner experience and behaviour deviates markedly from the expectations of the individual's culture in at least two of the following areas: cognition, affectivity, interpersonal functioning, or impulse control. The pattern is stable and of long duration.

Personality changes may be due to general medical conditions, including dementing illnesses. These are defined as persistent disturbances (representing a change from the patient's previous personality characteristics) in personality that are felt to be secondary to the direct effects of the underlying medical condition. Common manifestations include affective lability or instability, aggressive outbursts, poor impulse control, apathy, and paranoid ideation.

2.1.12 Agitation

The definition of agitation is problematic; there are several definitions in the literature, but one of the most frequently used is that of Cohen-Mansfield: 'Inappropriate verbal, vocal, or motor activity that is not judged by an outside observer to result directly from the needs or confusion of the agitated individual' (Cohen-Mansfield 1996; Cohen-Mansfield and Billig 1986). Agitation may be divided into four subcategories: physically aggressive, physically non-aggressive, verbally aggressive, and verbally non-aggressive behaviours. Examples of physically aggressive agitated behaviours include hitting, kicking, scratching, spitting, pushing, biting, and destroying property. Physically non-aggressive actions include pacing, inappropriate robing or disrobing, handling objects inappropriately, and stereotypies (meaningless repetitive gestures and movements). Verbally aggressive actions include cursing, accusations, threatening, and name calling.

Examples of verbally non-aggressive behaviours are complaining, repetition, screaming, constant requests for attention, and negativism. Patients with dementia may exhibit agitation as a symptom of psychosis or a mood disorder.

2.2 Tools for assessing neuropsychiatric symptoms in dementia

Many rating scales (or rating instruments) have been developed for the assessment and monitoring of neuropsychiatric signs and symptoms. These include specific, single item tools (such as the Hamilton Depression Rating Scale (Hamilton 1960) used in the assessment of depression) and comprehensive, multiple item tools, such as the Neuropsychiatric Inventory (Cummings *et al.* 1994; Cummings 1997) and the BEHAVE-AD (Reisberg *et al.* 1987). These instruments allow neuropsychiatric assessments to be made for both clinical and research purposes.

The development and use of rating scales must take into consideration the type of information assessed, reliability and validity, independence between measures, degree of inference required on items, and presence of agreed-on norms. The method of recording answers (a continuous variable, including severity and/or frequency, or a dichotomous or 'present' or 'absent' variable), the level of judgement required, and the amount of time covered (i.e. a brief period of observation, the past two weeks, or the patient's entire life) are also important.

2.2.1 Single domain instruments

The Hamilton Depression Rating Scale (HDRS) is an example of a widely used instrument that focuses on a specific area of interest. It measures the presence and intensity/frequency of depressive symptoms in 17 areas of interest (including depressed mood; interest in work and activities; 'genital symptoms'; appetite; weight loss; early, middle, and late insomnia; general somatic symptoms; feelings of guilt; suicidal ideation; anxiety; somatic symptoms of anxiety; hypochondriasis; psychomotor retardation and agitation; and degree of insight). There also are four additional items which are rated (diurnal variation, depersonalization/derealization, paranoid symptoms, and obsessional and compulsive symptoms) that are not measures of depression, but which may help in further characterizing the subtype of depression. The scale is administered by means of a structured interview, and patients are rated on either a three point or a five point scale (depending on the particular item).

Table 4.2 Selected assessment instruments

Single item
Hamilton Depression Rating Scale (HDRS)
Cornell Scale for Depression in Dementia
Geriatric Depression Scale (GDS)
Zung Self-Rating Scale for Depression
Cohen-Mansfield Agitation Inventory (CMAI)

Multiple item
Neuropsychiatric Inventory (NPI)
Behavioural Pathology in Alzheimer's Disease Rating Scale (BEHAVE-AD)
Behaviour Rating Scale for Dementia (BRSD)
Alzheimer's Disease Assessment Scale, Non-cognitive Portion (ADAS-noncog)
Brief Psychiatric Rating Scale (BPRS)
Manchester and Oxford Universities Scale for the Psychopathological Assessment of Dementia (MOUSEPAD)
Present Behavioural Examination (PBE)
Revised Memory and Behaviour Problems Checklist (RMBPC) (Teri *et al.* 1992)
Gottfries-Brane-Steen Scale (GBS) (Gottfries *et al.* 1982)

The HDRS was devised for use on patients who have been diagnosed clinically with an idiopathic depressive disorder. Symptoms of depression and dementia frequently overlap, compromising its use in patients with dementia syndromes. Neurovegetative symptoms (such as disturbances in appetite and sleep) important in the assessment of depression are common in dementia. Cognitive abnormalities, psychomotor retardation, agitation, obsessions, delusions, and hallucinations may all be part of a dementia syndrome in the absence of dysphoric mood.

Another single-domain scale that is frequently used is the Cornell Scale for Depression in Dementia (Alexopoulos *et al.* 1988). This instrument was developed specifically for the quantitative measure of depression in patients with dementia and utilizes both patient and caregiver interviews. It includes 19 items (including anxiety, sadness, lack of reactivity to pleasant events, irritability, agitation, retardation, multiple physical complaints, loss of interest, appetite loss, weight loss, lack of energy, diurnal variation, difficulty falling asleep, multiple awakenings, early morning awakening, suicide, self-depreciation, pessimism, and mood-congruent delusions) that are rated mainly on the basis of observation. Symptoms such as phobias and obsessions were purposely excluded from the Cornell Scale because their assessment relies heavily on reliable self-report that may be lacking in these patients. The caregiver is interviewed first and the patient is rated preliminarily on the severity of symptoms during the week prior to evaluation. The patient is then interviewed, and the clinician scores the Cornell Scale based on the information obtained from the two sources. The total time of administration is estimated to be 30 minutes (20 minutes with the caregiver and 10 minutes with the patient). It has been found to be a valid, reliable, and sensitive rating instrument, and appears to be better for rating depressive symptomatology over a wider range of severity than the HDRS.

Other rating scales developed for evaluating depression include the Geriatric Depression Scale (GDS) (Yesavage *et al.* 1982), the Beck Depression Inventory, and the Zung Self-Rating Scale for Depression. The GDS is the most studied of the three and is comprised of 30 (original form) or 15 (short form) items with yes/no responses. Its focus is on the affective and ideational aspects of depression (as opposed to neurovegetative or somatic symptomatology). The GDS has been shown to be valid and reliable in patients with Mini-Mental State Examination scores of 15 (out of a possible 30) or higher (McGivney *et al.* 1994).

The Cohen-Mansfield Agitation Inventory (CMAI) (Cohen-Mansfield *et al.* 1989) is a scale developed for use in measuring agitation in dementia patients. Agitation is difficult to assess because it is a group of heterogeneous behaviours and because patients with dementia often cannot reveal the reasons for their behaviours. Agitation may be assessed in three ways: informant ratings (caregiver information), observational methods, and technological devices (such as pedometers, step sensors, and actigraphs). The CMAI uses caregiver information to assess the frequency and disruptiveness of 29 behaviours in the two weeks prior to evaluation. Various forms of the CMAI exist, including a community version (the CMAI-C) and the nursing home version (using a staff member as the informant).

2.2.2 Multidimensional instruments

The Neuropsychiatric Inventory (NPI) is an instrument which was developed to assess for disturbances in 12 areas known to be common in dementia. These include delusions, hallucinations, dysphoria, anxiety, agitation/aggression, euphoria, disinhibition, irritability/lability, apathy, night-time behaviour disturbances, appetite/eating abnormalities, and aberrant motor activity. Information is gathered from a caregiver who is familiar with the demented patient, and includes a determination of both severity and frequency of the behavioural change. A screening format is used, which allows the ratings to be completed in a minimal amount of time while allowing for the evaluation of a wide range of neuropsychiatric pathology. The NPI has been shown to be a valid and reliable instrument. The NPI also rates the level of caregiver distress produced by each neuropsychiatric symptom. A total NPI and total caregiver distress score can be calculated.

The NPI separates the assessment of dysphoric mood and neurovegetative symptoms in order to differentiate depression and dementia. The dysphoria subscale focuses on the psychological and behavioural aspects of depression, including sadness, tearfulness, feelings of hopelessness, helplessness, and worthlessness, and suicidal ideation or preoccupation about death. Neurovegetative symptoms are separately assessed on the subscales measuring night-time behaviour disturbance and changes in appetite and eating behaviours. Personality changes, such as apathy and irritability or mood lability, are assessed on independent NPI scales.

Different neurological disorders have been found to exhibit characteristic NPI profiles. The NPI includes assessment of abnormalities that are common in a range of dementing disorders, and thus was not designed for use in patients with only one diagnosis (i.e. Alzheimer's disease [AD]). This allows its use in patients with a variety of types of dementia, and makes it potentially useful in differential diagnosis. The NPI is sensitive to treatment effects, and is therefore useful in assessing the efficacy of treatments. It has been used to demonstrate the improvement in behavioural symptoms in Alzheimer's disease patients after treatment with cholinergic agents.

The Behavioural Pathology in Alzheimer's Disease Rating Scale (BEHAVE-AD) is another multiple item instrument which has been used widely in assessing behavioural changes in patients with dementia. It was specifically developed to assess patients with Alzheimer's disease and has been shown to be reliable and valid. The scale is caregiver-based, and evaluates disturbances (over the two weeks prior to evaluation) in seven categories: paranoia and delusional ideation, hallucinations, activity disturbances, aggressiveness, diurnal rhythm disturbances, affective disturbances, and anxieties and phobias. Patients are rated on a four point scale, reflecting the spectrum from absence of the symptom to associated severe behaviours. The Empirical Behavioural Pathology in Alzheimer's Disease Rating Scale (E-BEHAVE-AD; Auer *et al.* 1996) is a related, observationally based assessment that compliments the information obtained by the BEHAVE-AD. This is based on a patient interview and includes 12 items in six dimensions of pathology (paranoid and delusional ideation, hallucinations, activity disturbance, aggressivity, affective disturbance, and anxieties and phobias). These items are scored according to the severity of symptoms observed over the course of the interview. The patient is seen alone in order to prevent any interference from the caregivers. The patient interview is estimated to take 20 minutes.

The Behaviour Rating Scale for Dementia (BRSD) (Tariot *et al.* 1995) is a third commonly used standardized instrument. Like the NPI and BEHAVE-AD, it is caregiver-based. Eight areas are assessed, including depressive features, psychotic features, defective self-regulation, irritability/agitation, vegetative features, apathy, aggression, and affective lability.

The Alzheimer's Disease Assessment Scale (ADAS) (Mohs 1996; Mohs *et al.* 1983) is another multiple item instrument; it has both a cognitive (ADAS-cog) and non-cognitive (ADAS-noncog) portion. It was developed for use in patients with Alzheimer's disease and its reliability and validity have been demonstrated. The cognitive portion assesses disturbances in memory, orientation, language (expressive and receptive), and praxis. The non-cognitive portion includes ten items that are clinician-rated and assesses a variety of symptoms such as depression, psychosis, agitation, changes in appetite, and even tremor.

The Brief Psychiatric Rating Scale (BPRS) is a clinician-rated scale that was originally developed for the evaluation of psychotic symptoms in a general psychiatric population. It has been employed sometimes in studies of dementia patients.

The Manchester and Oxford Universities scale for the Psychopathological Assessment of Dementia (MOUSEPAD) (Allen *et al.* 1996) is a 59 item instrument that is administered by the clinician to the caregiver. It is a semi-structured interview accompanied by a glossary and covers delusions, hallucinations, misidentifications, reduplications, walking, eating, sleep, sexual behaviour, aggression, and other types of behaviour. This instrument rates both the presence of behaviours during the prior month and also during any point after the onset of dementia. Symptoms that occur in the context of physical illness are excluded, and depression is not covered by this scale. Psychotic symptoms such as hallucinations and delusions must be maintained for a minimum of seven days to be rated.

The Present Behavioural Examination (PBE) (Hope and Fairburn 1992) is another multiple item rating scale. Like the MOUSEPAD, the PBE provides a detailed glossary and is based on a clinician interview with the caregiver. The PBE assesses symptoms during the previous four weeks.

2.2.3 Limitations of rating scales

Rating scales are useful tools in assessing and monitoring patients in both clinical and research settings. Nevertheless, their use is limited by several factors. Rating scales may be developed for specific populations (such as geriatric patients with AD), and thus may fail to probe areas of concern in patients with other forms of dementing illnesses. Psychiatric rating scales in general also are subject to bias if the informant distorts or omits information due to paranoia or a perceived stigma of mental illness.

Caregiver-based interviews by definition require a caregiver who is familiar with the patient's behaviour and who is able and willing to participate in the rating process. The caregiver also must speak the same language as the interviewer. The perception of caregivers may be influenced by factors such as guilt, caregiver burden, and related emotional problems. Caregiver information thus can be biased. Symptoms that are common in dementia (such as pacing, agitation, and anxiety) may be stressful to the caregiver, causing depression or precipitating abuse. Caregivers with high burden scores have been found to report more disruptive behaviours than caregivers with lower burden scores (Pearson *et al.* 1993). Caregivers may exaggerate or deny behavioural problems and thus confound assessment and influence treatment decisions. Caregivers who are untrained in behavioural observations may misinterpret symptoms (i.e. interpret delusions, illusions, or confusion in a patient as being hallucinations). There may be more attention paid by caregivers to those behaviours that interfere with care (such as resistance to bathing) than to passive symptoms in later stages of illness. Finally, caregivers may habituate to behaviours after long periods of exposure. They may underreport behaviour out of concern that it would reflect poorly on the patient or the level of care being provided by them.

Patient-based instruments can be of limited use in dementia patients due to such factors as memory disturbances, aphasia, and poor insight, but may be of use early in the course of illness. Patients may have impaired concentration, attention, and judgement that affect their responses to questions. Cognitive disturbance interferes with the use of self-rated scales in patients with severe dementia. Patients may have difficulty answering questions about sleep, appetite, weight loss, and other areas due to impaired memory. Patients may deny, minimize, or explain away their symptoms.

The use of observer-based rating scales is limited by the restricted period of time spent with the patient; subtle changes (such as apathy detectable by the family but not by people who are less familiar with the patient), infrequent but clinically significant behaviours (such as physical aggression), and those disturbances that occur more frequently at other times of the day (i.e. during bathing or at night) can be missed. Other disruptive symptoms may be observable only at home (i.e. the idea that 'one's house is not one's home'). Psychiatric disturbances (such as depression) may be more short-lived in patients with dementia than in typical psychiatric patients without dementia. Therefore, assessment may require observation over a relatively longer period of time in order to capture brief and transient symptomatology. Patients may behave differently in the clinical setting than at home or in the care facility. Cross-cultural aspects also must be taken into account, because the response to illness, particularly psychiatric symptoms, may vary significantly.

3 Psychiatric features of selected early onset dementia syndromes

Characteristic neuropsychiatric symptoms often accompany specific dementia syndromes, although none are pathognomonic. This section will discuss neuropsychiatric features of some of the more common early onset dementia syndromes, with an emphasis on neurodegenerative disorders. Cortical degenerations include familial Alzheimer's disease, frontotemporal dementia, and polioencephalopathies such as Kuf's disease. Subcortical degenerations include Huntington's disease, Wilson's disease, and early onset Parkinson's disease. Leukoencephalopathies include metachromatic leukodystrophy and adrenoleukodystrophy. Other causes of early onset dementia include vascular dementia, multiple sclerosis, and systemic lupus erythematosus.

3.1 Cortical degenerations

Alzheimer's disease (AD), frontotemporal dementias (FTD), and the polioencephalopathies (such as adult neuronal ceroid lipofuscinosis) may have prominent neuropsychiatric features.

3.1.1 Alzheimer's disease

AD is a progressive, neurodegenerative disorder and the most common cause of dementia in the elderly; occasionally it occurs in younger patients. Pathologically, AD is characterized by neurofibrillary tangles, neuritic plaques, neuronal loss, cortical gliosis, granulovacuolar degeneration, and amyloid angiopathy. Early onset is particularly common in patients with Down's syndrome (trisomy 21) and in those with autosomal dominant AD associated with mutations of presenilin 1 on chromosome 14. Neuropsychiatric disturbances are common in AD and include prominent personality changes, mood disturbances, and psychotic symptoms. In the outpatient setting, 88% of patients exhibit behavioural changes (Mega *et al.* 1996).

Personality changes include apathy and disengagement; disinhibition also occurs. Social withdrawal and inappropriate sexual behaviour are less common. Apathy is the most frequent behavioural characteristic of AD.

Mood disturbances are common, but patients rarely meet all DSM-IV criteria for a major depressive or manic episode. Depressive features have been reported in 0–86% of patients with AD (Payne *et al.* 1998; Patterson *et al.* 1990); these rates may be confounded by differences in methodology and the non-specific neurovegetative signs and apathy found in patients with AD that may mimic depression. Major depression is estimated to occur in 5–22% of patients (Borson and Raskind 1997; Payne *et al.* 1998). Less severe depressive symptoms are more common than major depression; dysphoria measured on the NPI increased from 10% in patients with mild AD to 60% in patients with severe disease (Mega *et al.* 1996). Anxiety and phobias occur in approximately 40–50% of patients. Euphoria is uncommon and its presence may suggest an alternate diagnosis such as FTD.

Psychotic symptoms include delusions and hallucinations. A recent review of the literature found prevalence rates for delusions in AD ranging from 10–73% (Rao and Lyketsos 1998). Delusions occur at all stages of AD. Although uncomplicated delusions are the most frequent in AD, patients

Table 4.3 Early onset dementias with neuropsychiatric symptoms

Cortical degenerations
  Alzheimer's disease
  Dementia with Lewy bodies
  Frontotemporal dementias (Pick's disease, frontal lobe degeneration without Pick's bodies,
    amyotrophic lateral sclerosis (ALS)-dementia complex, etc.)

Subcortical degenerations
  Dentatorubral-pallidoluysian atrophy (DRPLA)
  Huntington's disease
  Idiopathic calcification of the basal ganglia (Fahr's disease)
  Parkinson's disease
  Wilson's disease

Neurodegenerative disorders typically seen in childhood and early adulthood
  Adrenoleukodystrophy (ALD) and adrenomyeloneuropathy (AMN)
  Adult onset GM2 gangliosidosis
  Alexander's disease
  Canavan's disease
  Cerebrotendinous xanthomatosis
  Fabry's disease
  Gaucher's disease
  GM_1 gangliosidosis type III
  Hallervorden-Spatz disease
  Krabbe disease (globoid cell leukodystrophy)
  Kufs disease (adult neuronal ceroid lipofuscinosis)
  Lafora's disease
  Metachromatic leukodystrophy (MLD)
  Mitochondrial encephalomyopathies:
    Kearns-Sayre syndrome (KSS)
    Myoclonic epilepsy with ragged-red fibres (MERRF)
    Mitochondrial myopathy, encephalopathy, lactic acidosis, and stroke-like episodes (MELAS)
  Niemann-Pick type II-C
  Pelizaeus-Merzbacher disease
  Progressive myoclonic epilepsy

Demyelinative
  Multiple sclerosis

Vascular
  Binswanger's disease
  Cerebral autosomal dominant arteriopathy with subcortical infarcts and leukoencephalopathy
    (CADASIL)
  Haemorrhage
  Hypotension/hypoperfusion
  Lacunar state
  Multi-infarct
  Strategic infarct

Toxic
  Alcohol
  Medication/drug
  Mercury
  Radiation
  Solvents, including toluene

Metabolic
  Cobalamin (vitamin B12) deficiency
  Dialysis dementia
  Endocrinopathies (including disorders of thyroid, parathyroid, etc.)
  Hypoxia
  Liver disease
  Marchiafava-Bignami disease

Table 4.3 (*Continued*)

Infectious
Bacterial, including neurosyphilis and Lyme disease
Prion diseases, including Creutzfeldt–Jakob disease (CJD) and fatal familial insomnia
Viral, including progressive multifocal leukoencephalopathy (PML), acquired immune deficiency syndrome
(AIDS) dementia complex, post-encephalitic parkinsonism, and subacute sclerosing panencephalitis
Traumatic
Dementia pugilistica
Traumatic brain injury
Neoplastic
Gliomatosis cerebri
Metastatic disease
Primary tumours
Miscellaneous
Leigh disease
Myotonic dystrophy
Neurosarcoidosis
Normal pressure hydrocephalus
Porphyria
Systemic lupus erythematosus

may have more systematized delusions including Capgras syndrome and erotomania. Paranoid delusions are common, identified in 31% of patients in one study (Rubin 1992); delusions of theft were the most common, occurring in 28%. Other delusions seen in AD include delusions of persecution, erotomania, abandonment, spousal infidelity, and misidentification delusions such as the Capgras syndrome. Auditory and visual hallucinations are less common and occur in 3–49% of patients (Patterson *et al.* 1990; Mega *et al.* 1996). Visual hallucinations are more common than auditory hallucinations. Psychosis appears to be associated with greater functional impairment (Rao and Lyketsos 1998).

Agitation is commonplace, disruptive, and may create a significant burden on patients, their families, and their caregivers. Wandering occurs in 10–61%, motor restlessness in 21–60%, and aggression or assaultiveness in 18–25% (Mega *et al.* 1996). Delusions are known to be associated with agitation and aggression, and aggression has been found to increase with the severity of dementia. Disturbances of the sleep cycle are frequent and eventually occur in the majority of patients. Behavioural disturbances, particularly wandering and agitation, tend to persist over time (Devanand *et al.* 1997).

The NPI has been used to characterize patients with AD (Cummings 1997; Mega *et al.* 1996); 86% were found in one study to exhibit neuropsychiatric disturbances, the most common being apathy (72%). Agitation was present in 60% of patients; anxiety in 48%, irritability in 42%, dysphoria in 38%, aberrant motor behaviour in 38%, disinhibition in 36%, delusions in 22%, hallucinations in 10%, and euphoria in only 8%. Agitation, apathy, anxiety, dysphoria, and aberrant motor behaviour increased with dementia severity. Disinhibition was found to decrease with dementia severity.

3.1.2 Frontotemporal dementia

FTD is a neurodegenerative dementia syndrome that has characteristic behavioural and personality changes. Typically, there is relatively symmetrical degeneration in the frontal and temporal lobes, although asymmetrical atrophy may occur. Onset is typically before age 65 and insidious;

Table 4.4 Major neuropsychiatric features of selected dementia syndromes

AD
  Apathy (most common)
  Depressive features
  Psychosis (particularly delusions of theft)
  Agitation
  Anxiety

FTD
  Disinhibition
  Loss of social awareness
  Apathy
  Perseverative behaviours
  Early loss of insight
  Compulsions
  Antisocial behaviour
  Euphoria

HD
  Apathy
  Irritability
  Disinhibition
  Antisocial/violent behaviour
  Emotional lability
  Aggression
  Depression/suicide
  Sexual disturbance
  Obsessive-compulsiveness
  Psychosis

WD
  Irritability
  Depression/suicide
  Psychosis
  Aggression
  Impulsiveness

PD
  Depressed mood
  Anxiety
  Apathy
  Hallucinations/delusions/mania (treatment related)

VaD
  Apathy
  Irritability
  Abulia
  Depression
  Psychosis
  Emotional incontinence

MS
  Depression
  Eutonia (feeling of well-being)
  Euphoria (late in the course)
  Irritability
  Apathy
  Disinhibition
  Psychosis

onset of the disorder in the senium is rare. The Lund and Manchester research criteria include among the core diagnostic features behavioural disorders, affective symptoms, and speech changes (see chapter 12).

Behavioural disturbances are striking and may include disinhibition, loss of personal and social awareness, apathy, mental rigidity, stereotypic and perseverative behaviours, utilization behaviours, impulsivity, distractibility, and impersistence (Mendez *et al.* 1997). There is loss of insight early in the illness. Patients may present with compulsive behaviours such as repetitive checking, cleaning, or self-injury. Symptoms of the Kluver-Bucy syndrome (with compulsive eating, hyperorality, hypersexuality, placidity, and hypermetamorphosis) may result. Compulsive behaviours are more likely to occur in FTD patients than in patients with AD. Compulsions may be due to the inability to inhibit urges to perform compulsive movements associated with damage to the frontal-striatal circuits (Mendez *et al.* 1997). Antisocial behaviours may occur (such as shoplifting, assault, or indecent exposure) and their frequency in FTD patients has been found to be significantly higher than in patients with AD (Miller *et al.* 1997). Apathy occurs earlier in FTD than in AD and is more severe.

Affective symptoms may include depression, anxiety, suicidal ideation, emotional indifference, lack of empathy, and amimia. Speech disturbances include stereotypy, echolalia, perseveration, reduced speech output, or mutism. Euphoria is common in FTD but unusual in AD (Levy *et al.* 1996).

In cases where the degeneration is asymmetrical and the language-dominant cerebral hemisphere is more affected, linguistic symptoms (such as aphasia) may predominate over the behavioural symptoms. Patients with the temporal lobe variant (TLV) of FTD may differ in their clinical presentation depending on the side that is more predominantly affected. In left-sided TLV, patients have prominent aphasia with flat emotional expression; in right-sided TLV, behavioural disturbance is most characteristic with egocentric and socially offensive behaviour, aggression, and sexual disinhibition (Edwards-Lee *et al.* 1997).

The NPI has been used to characterize patients with FTD and to distinguish them from patients with AD (Levy *et al.* 1996). Patients with FTD were found to exhibit significantly higher scores in apathy, euphoria, disinhibition, and aberrant motor behaviour than patients with AD. Using the NPI subscales of disinhibition, depression, and apathy, 77% of patients could be assigned to the correct diagnosis. Table 4.5 shows NPI scores on patients with FTD.

Table 4.5 Neuropsychiatric inventory scores in patients with frontotemporal dementia

	Mean score	Standard deviation	% Affected (n = 22)
MMSE	16.2	10.4	
Delusions	5.2	4.7	23%
Hallucinations	0.0	0.0	0%
Agitation	5.2	4.0	64%
Depression	2.1	2.3	41%
Anxiety	3.8	3.1	59%
Euphoria	3.2	1.7	36%
Apathy	7.1	3.3	95%
Disinhibition	4.9	4.4	68%
Irritability	4.4	2.4	50%
Aberrant motor	6.1	3.9	73%
Age (years)	63.7	8.8	

3.1.3 Polioencephalopathies — Kufs' disease

Kufs' disease, a form of neuronal ceroid lipofuscinosis (NCL),may present as an early onset dementia (see chapter 18). There are four major classifications of the NCLs, based on the age of onset, clinical signs and symptoms, and neuropathological findings. These subtypes include infantile, late infantile, juvenile, and adult cases. All of the subtypes are characterized by the accumulation of autofluorescent cytoplasmic inclusions within neurons and other cells and by cell death, including in the cerebral cortex. The adult form is the rarest type and is further subdivided into two clinical phenotypes, Type A and Type B. Type A is characterized by epilepsy, progressive myoclonus, and neuropsychiatric disturbance; Type B is characterized by behavioural and psychiatric disturbance, dementia, and motor dysfunction (frequently facial dyskinesias). There is, however, overlap between these two forms. Typically, the adult form of the disease has its onset at around age 30 years, and the course is approximately 12.5 years in duration.

Kufs' disease, or late onset neuronal ceroid lipofuscinosis, is differentiated from the more frequently seen childhood onset forms by its lack of the characteristic visual failure and retinal degeneration. Early symptoms include non-specific psychological disturbances that may develop into dementia and psychosis. The clinical picture is heterogeneous, and may include seizures, ataxia, motor disturbances, dysarthria, facial dyskinesias, and other movement disorders.

Kufs' disease may be mistaken for a primary psychiatric disorder such as schizophrenia, multiple personality disorder, or bipolar disorder, particularly early in the disease course when dementia and motor disturbance may not be apparent (Hammersen *et al.* 1998). Facial grimacing and other movement disorders may be confused with tardive dyskinesia after treatment with psychotropic medication. Phobias, anxiety, thought disorder, social withdrawal, apathy, confusion, depressed mood, frank psychosis, and other behavioural changes have been reported (Berkovic *et al.* 1988). Patients may exhibit a labile and inappropriate affect, self-neglect, disinterest, poor attention and concentration, difficulty with abstractions, and other cognitive symptoms of dementia. Visual hallucinations may be elementary or complex and well-formed.

The correct diagnosis is easily missed due to the non-specific clinical symptoms and the need for biopsy and electron microscopy to look for intracellular lipopigments, curvilinear cytosomes, and fingerprint patterns. As with other storage diseases, there are no reliable radiological criteria diagnostic of the illness.

3.2 Subcortical degenerations

Huntington's disease (HD), Wilson's disease (hepatocerebral degeneration), and familial Parkinson's disease (PD) are common subcortical degenerative disorders that may present at an early age and exhibit prominent neuropsychiatric features.

3.2.1 Huntington's disease

HD is an autosomal dominant neurodegenerative disorder characterized by choreoathetosis and subcortical dementia. It is associated with personality changes, mood disorders, and psychosis, as well as cognitive disturbance. The causative genetic defect has been identified as abnormally abundant trinucleotide repeats (cytosine, adenine, and guanine; CAG) on the short arm of chromosome 4. Atrophy occurs at the caudate nuclei, as well as in the putamen, globus pallidus, prefrontal cortex, and other areas. Typically, patients are not diagnosed until they are in their third to fifth decades (see chapter 15).

Psychiatric symptoms and signs (excluding dementia) probably occur in the majority of HD patients, and their course is variable. Rates of psychiatric disturbance range from 21–79% in the literature (Lovestone *et al.* 1996; Zappacosta *et al.* 1996; Mendez 1994; Lauterbach *et al.* 1998). The extent of psychiatric symptomatology may be underestimated due to the frequent use of neuroleptic medications to treat the movement disorder in these patients. Behavioural changes may present initially without evidence of an extrapyramidal syndrome. In some cases, choreo-athetosis is not noted for ten years or more. Most studies have found little association between the emotional and cognitive changes in HD (Cummings 1995), although psychiatric symptoms tend to disappear as patients become increasingly demented. Psychiatric symptoms are not correlated with choreoathetosis (Mendez 1994).

Personality changes are the most common abnormality and include apathy, disinhibition, compulsiveness, irritability, and antisocial or violent behaviour. Such changes may occur in up to 72% of patients with HD (Lauterbach *et al.* 1998). Hospitalization may be required to control explosiveness and emotional lability. One study found apathy in 48% of patients with HD and irritability in 58% (Burns *et al.* 1990). Aggression often accompanies irritability and patients may lash out at others. Violence is more common in the early stages of HD than in later stages (Cummings 1995). Criminal behaviour or antisocial personality traits occur in at least 6% of patients (Mendez 1994), with assault being the most frequent violent crime.

The second most common behavioural disturbance in HD is depression, with major depressive episodes occurring in about 30% of patients and dysthymia in 5% (Cummings 1995). It can occur before either cognitive disturbance or abnormal movements become apparent, sometimes preceding movement disorder by 2–20 years (Cummings 1995). There is controversy over the suggested increased risk of suicide in HD, although most agree that rates are higher in HD patients than in age-matched controls (Cina *et al.* 1996). Some estimate that suicide occurs at rates four times that expected in the general population; others have found slightly higher or lower rates (0.85–12.7%) (Cummings 1995). Disinhibition may contribute to the high number of attempted and completed suicides. Suicide may occur early in the course of the illness, frequently before the patient has even been diagnosed with HD. This may cause the number of known suicides in HD patients to be underreported.

Mania is less common than depression, and is found in only 2–12.5% of patients (Mendez 1994). Hypomania, grandiosity, and euphoria also are reported in HD. Other neuro-psychiatric manifestations of HD include sexual disturbances (including hypersexuality, sexual apathy, and impotence), paraphilias, sleep disturbance, and anxiety disorders. In some cases, HD patients may have marked obsessive compulsive behaviours (Cummings and Cunningham 1992).

HD may cause symptoms of schizophrenia-like psychosis, with hallucinations (usually auditory) and delusions (often persecutory) being fairly common. Psychosis is estimated to occur in 6–25% of patients (Cummings 1995), and is more common in patients with early onset disease. Cognitive decline eventually leads to a remission of symptoms. Psychosis has been correlated with a reduction in anterior hemispheric metabolism and medial caudate pathology (Lauterbach *et al.* 1998).

The advent of presymptomatic genetic testing for at-risk individuals raises questions about the psychosocial impact of predictive testing. In patients with no past psychiatric history, genetic testing has been shown not to result in poor psychological outcome if proper counselling and educational and support services are provided (Mendez 1994). While most people who receive negative results have improvements in their psychological functioning, 10% require support because of difficulty dealing with their decreased risk status (Hayden *et al.* 1995; Wiggins *et al.* 1992). Somewhat surprisingly, patients with test results indicating increased risk for development of HD have been shown to have small decreases in distress and depression in the year following testing (Wiggins *et al.* 1992). This has been attributed to the reduction in uncertainty and the opportunity for informed planning.

The neuropsychiatric symptoms are probably attributable to the caudate pathology and the disruption of connections to limbic structures or of prefrontal-subcortical connections (Mendez 1994). Positron emission tomography (PET) studies in depressed HD patients demonstrate bilateral hypometabolism in caudate nuclei and orbitofrontal/inferior prefrontal cortex. Both depression and mania have been shown to arise from lesions in the caudate. While the length of the CAG repeat sequence has been correlated with the age of onset (inversely) and the severity of motor and cognitive disturbance, no correlation was found between psychiatric symptoms and length of CAG repeats (Zappacosta *et al.* 1996).

3.2.2 Wilson's disease

WD (or hepatolenticular degeneration) is an inherited disorder of copper metabolism with a mean age of onset of 17 years. There is a lack of functional biliary ceruloplasmin, leading to abnormal copper deposition in the liver, brain, and other tissues (including the corneal limbus, producing the typical Kayser-Fleischer ring). The disease is caused by mutations of the ATP7B gene located on chromosome 13q14 (see chapter 18).

Neuropsychiatric symptoms may predominate at initial presentation and may even be seen in isolation. Approximately one-third each of patients present with predominantly hepatic, neurological, or psychiatric symptoms. A recent review of the literature found that the estimated lifetime prevalence of psychiatric features was between 30–100% and that up to one-fifth of WD patients initially present with isolated psychiatric symptomatology (Lauterbach *et al.* 1998). An estimated 50% of patients with WD are psychiatrically hospitalized before the diagnosis is established, and emerging neurological signs and symptoms may be misinterpreted as adverse effects of pharmacotherapy (i.e. tardive dyskinesia from neuroleptic use). As a result, significant delays in diagnosis may occur, interfering with early treatment.

Patients may exhibit mood disturbance, personality changes, and psychosis in addition to cognitive impairment. In a study of 129 patients with WD (Dening and Berrios 1990), the most common psychiatric symptoms found were irritability, depression, incongruous behaviour, and cognitive impairment. Other reported psychiatric symptoms in patients with WD include anxiety disorders, catatonia, and sexual preoccupation and disinhibition (Akil and Brewer 1995).

Studies on mood disorders in this group of patients have focused mainly on unipolar depression. Major depression was found in 27% of patients with WD in one study of 45 patients (Oder *et al.* 1991); seven of these patients had a history of attempted suicide. Depressed mood was correlated with bradykinesia, rigidity, cognitive impairment, and dilatation of the third ventricle on MRI (Oder *et al.* 1993). An estimated 4–16% of patients demonstrate suicidal behaviours at some point in their illness (Lauterbach *et al.* 1998). Little is known about mania in WD, but both mania and hypomania have been reported.

Personality changes are common and frequently include irritability, impulsiveness, emotionality, and aggression. Persistent changes are estimated to occur in 46–71% of patients over their lifetime (Lauterbach *et al.* 1998). In Oder's series of 47 patients, organic personality changes were correlated with dysarthria, dyskinesia, and lesions in the putamen and pallidum evidenced on MRI. A study of 31 cases correlated 'sociopathic' personality features with dysarthria and depressive symptoms with gait disturbance (Dening and Berrios 1989*b*).

Psychosis has long been a subject of interest in patients with WD; organic delusional disorders were once thought to be associated with the disease, but this relationship has not been supported. In fact, a retrospective study of 195 cases suggested that schizophrenia-like psychoses did not occur more frequently in WD patients than in the general population (Dening and Berrios

1989*a*). Hallucinations and catatonia were not found to be increased. Psychosis appears to be slightly (8%) more common in patients with neurologically predominant forms of WD (Brewer and Yuzbasiyan-Gurkan 1992).

3.2.3 Parkinson's disease

PD is a neurodegenerative disorder that is characterized by prominent motor features including resting tremor, bradykinesia, and rigidity. Dementia and other intellectual impairments are common. Depressed mood and anxiety are also common, although suicide and psychotic depression is rare. Proposed biological aetiologies for mood disturbance in PD include degeneration of brain stem monoaminergic afferents, dysfunction of non-motor basal ganglia-thalamo-cortical circuits, and the disruption of mesocortical and mesolimbic dopamine connections to the frontal lobe and the ventral striatum (Mayberg and Solomon 1995). Onset of PD after age 65 is common and shows no hereditary patterns; onset of symptoms before age 55 is typical of autosomal dominant PD (Tanner *et al.* 1999).

The mean frequency of depression in PD is reported to be around 40% (Mayberg and Solomon 1995), but figures range between 20–90% (Hubble and Koller 1995) depending on the study population and diagnostic criteria. Individual premorbid characteristics, psychosocial factors, inferior frontal lobe hypometabolism, and loss of central serotonin have been proposed as associated or contributing factors (Saint-Cyr *et al.* 1995). Fatigue, masked facies, and psychomotor slowing due to PD may cause patients to appear depressed even when they are not, complicating the diagnosis of a major depressive episode. Depression is reported more commonly in patients with left brain dysfunction (right hemiparkinsonism) (Cole *et al.* 1996; Mayberg and Solomon 1995). Often, depression has been reported to begin before motor symptoms are apparent (Mayeux *et al.* 1981). The prevalence of depressive symptoms has been reported to be higher in patients with early onset of PD, but in one study the increased association of mood or anxiety disorders with early onset (defined here as onset before age 55) PD was limited to males (Cole *et al.* 1996), and another study did not find a significant difference in depression between patients with early and late onset of PD (with 50 years as the cut-off age) after controlling for disease duration (Kostíc *et al.* 1994). This same study found that illness severity was not significantly correlated with depression (after controlling for functional impairment), and that in men (but not women) depression predicted impaired physical, social, and role functioning.

Unlike depression, mania and hypomania are not common in untreated patients with PD. Mania and hypomania may result from the use of dopaminergic agents. The incidence of hypomania in patients treated with levodopa is reported as 1.5% (Goodwin 1971).

The reported rate of anxiety disorders ranges from 6.5–38% (Cole *et al.* 1996). Panic attacks were reported in 38% of patients treated with levodopa in one study (Vasquez *et al.* 1993). Anxiety is a common side-effect of anti-parkinsonian medications and is reported to occur in at least 10% of treated patients. Obsessive compulsive behaviour is occasionally seen, particularly with right hemisphere disease (Saint-Cyr *et al.* 1995). All patients who appear anxious and agitated should be evaluated for the presence of akathisia and depression.

Personality changes are described as a deficiency of 'novelty seeking' aspects of behaviour (Saint-Cyr *et al.* 1995); patients are described as being inflexible, rigid, frugal, and orderly. The concept of a 'parkinsonian personality' has existed since the last century and has been the subject of some controversy, although recent authors have reported supportive findings (Hubble and Koller 1995). Damage to the mesolimbic dopaminergic system in PD has been proposed as the aetiology of this personality profile (Menza *et al.* 1993). Assessment of personality in patients with PD is complicated by impairment of motor and cognitive function, as well as comorbid depression. Apathy is the most common personality change in PD. Hypersexuality is reported as a rare side-effect of drug treatment in about 0.9–3% of patients, mostly men (Factor *et al.* 1995). It also has been reported after thalamotomy.

Psychosis is rare in PD but common (occurring in 10–30%) (Factor *et al.* 1995) in patients treated with dopaminergic and anticholinergic agents. Frank delirium may also occur with use of medications for PD. Drug-induced psychosis is most commonly expressed as visual hallucinations (typically human or animal images, described as non-threatening, well formed, and vividly coloured); these are estimated to occur in about 30% of treated patients (Factor *et al.* 1995). Delusions are less common and typically of the paranoid type; prevalence rates range from 3–17% (Roane *et al.* 1998). Early onset of medication-induced hallucinations is atypical for PD and should alert the clinician to investigate for the presence of a non-PD parkinsonian syndrome (such as dementia with Lewy bodies or AD) or a comorbid primary psychiatric disorder (Goetz *et al.* 1998). Pre-existing psychiatric disorders, dementia, cerebral atrophy, advanced age, increased dosage of levodopa, long-term treatment with levodopa, multiple drug therapy, and anticholinergic therapy are reported risk factors for psychosis (Roane *et al.* 1998).

3.3 Leukoencephalopathies

3.3.1 Metachromatic leukodystrophy (MLD)

MLD, an autosomal recessive lysosomal storage disease characterized by the progressive demyelination of both central and peripheral nerves, is the most common of the leukodystrophies. It is associated with a deficiency in the lysosomal acid hydrolase arylsulfatase A and the pathological accumulation of cerebroside sulfate in the nervous system and other selected tissues. MLD is subdivided into three main subtypes, according to the age of onset and clinical picture: the late infantile form (most common), the juvenile form, and the rare adult onset form. The adult form typically becomes symptomatic between age 18 and 30 years of age, and the clinical course is notable for its variability. Generally there is prominent mental deterioration that may be expressed initially as difficulty at work or in school. Psychiatric disturbances may be so serious that the patient is institutionalized in a psychiatric facility. Obvious neurological symptoms may not develop for several years and cognitive impairment can initially be mistaken for the negative symptoms of schizophrenia (see chapter 18).

Some sources claim that very few cases of adult MLD are reported without behavioural or psychiatric symptoms (Fluharty 1990; Baumann *et al.* 1991). A review of published cases (Hyde *et al.* 1992) of MLD found 55 patients considered to have juvenile or adult onset disease (neuropathologically and/or biochemically confirmed), 53% of whom had psychotic symptoms (including 27% with delusions and 18% with hallucinations). However, this number may have included patients who ultimately did not have true MLD (for example, the pseudodeficiency state), as the case reports varied in their extent of biochemical evaluation. Other authors have noted less frequent psychotic features, with one review finding psychosis in only 4 of 24 patients with confirmed MLD (Hageman *et al.* 1995). Hallucinations are predominantly auditory, but visual and olfactory hallucinations are reported. Auditory hallucinations may be described as complex, and can include multiple voices or a running commentary on the patient's behaviour (similar to the hallucinations in schizophrenia). Delusions may be paranoid, bizarre, or include ideas of reference. Psychosis typically disappears when the dementia becomes more prominent.

The wide range of psychiatric symptomatology observed in MLD has led to patients being diagnosed with a variety of primary psychiatric conditions including conduct disorder, schizophrenia, depression, mania, and personality disorders. Behavioural abnormalities in MLD may be characteristic of frontal lobe syndromes, with impulsivity, mood lability, attentional disturbance, impaired judgement, disinhibition, and inappropriate social behaviour. Hypersexuality, aggressiveness, irritability, apathy, suspiciousness, bizarre gesturing, posturing, and hyperactivity also are seen.

3.3.2 Adrenoleukodystrophy (ALD)

ALD is an inherited, progressive, demyelinating disorder characterized by the pathological accumulation of very long chain fatty acids in tissues, particularly the white matter of the brain and the adrenal cortex. It is inherited in an X-linked recessive mode and may present in adulthood, although the childhood form is the most common. Symptoms generally include neurological, psychiatric, and endocrine problems. Adrenomyeloneuropathy (AMN) is a variant of ALD that typically presents at a later age (20 to 30 years); spinal cord symptoms predominate, including peripheral neuropathy and spastic parapesis. AMN patients frequently have mild impairments in cognition, however, with maximal disturbances in memory and frontal-executive functions. Approximately one-third of patients with AMN eventually develop cerebral demyelination. Neuropsychiatric disturbances also are seen in AMN (James *et al.* 1984).

Neuropsychiatric symptoms are common in ALD and may be the initial manifestations. Adults with these disorders may be diagnosed initially with psychiatric disturbances such as schizophreniform psychosis, conversion disorder, schizophrenia, or even Kluver-Bucy syndrome (Aubourg and Mandel 1996). One review found that 39% of patients presented with some type of psychiatric diagnosis (including dementia, psychosis, behavioural changes, nervousness, and social withdrawal) and that 17% presented with psychiatric problems alone (Kitchin *et al.* 1987). Symptoms may include personality changes, anxiety, difficulty with concentration, auditory hallucinations, delusions, paranoia, aggressiveness, flattened affect, social withdrawal, and bizarre or socially inappropriate behaviour. Depression is frequent. The neuropsychological disturbances found in ALD correlate well to the areas of the brain affected by demyelination. Demyelination affecting the frontal lobes leads to typical frontal lobe syndrome symptoms such as disinhibition, apathy, hyperactivity, attentional problems, and other behavioural disturbances. Psychiatric symptoms are relatively common in patients with demyelination affecting the anterior and medial temporal lobes (Aubourg and Mandel 1996).

Heterozygote females may exhibit psychiatric and neurological signs and symptoms; dementia and visual disturbances occur in about 10% of women with neurological symptoms (Moser *et al.* 1991).

3.4 Miscellaneous

Although the focus of this section has been on the degenerative brain disorders, there are numerous other causes of early onset dementia associated with neuropsychiatric disturbances. Examples include vascular dementia, dementia due to multiple sclerosis, and dementia due to systemic lupus erythematosus.

3.4.1 Vascular dementia

Vascular dementia is the second most common cause of dementia in the elderly population and is due to cerebral ischaemia or haemorrhage. An estimated 10–30% of late onset dementias are due to vascular causes. Early onset vascular dementia may differ from the late onset form in having a higher prevalence of cardiac disease and collagen-vascular disorders as causative conditions. Although neuropsychiatric symptoms may be of gradual onset (confusing the differentiation from neurodegenerative processes), the classic picture is that of abrupt onset and stepwise progression related to cerebrovascular events (i.e. within three months of known ischaemic events). Other signs of neurological insult such as incontinence, gait disturbance, and pseudobulbar palsy may be seen. Reflecting the focal lesions caused by ischaemic events, patients classically have a patchy distribution of deficits, with some abilities well preserved and others compromised. In general, the neuropsychiatric disturbances relate to the location and extent of the brain injuries, as well as the premorbid level of functioning.

The category of vascular dementia is heterogeneous and includes dementia due to a variety of underlying lesions. In addition to the classic presentation with multiple cortical infarcts, other aetiologies include haemorrhage, Binswanger's disease, hypotension/hypoperfusion, lacunar state, and strategic infarct (see chapter 14).

Neuropsychiatric symptoms seen with vascular dementia include personality changes, affective disorders, and psychosis. Apathy, irritability, and abulia are the most frequently observed personality changes. Depression is common; mania is rare. Psychotic symptoms include delusions and hallucinations.

Personality changes may be striking and depend in part upon the localization of the lesions. Binswanger's disease may lead to pseudobulbar palsy with emotional incontinence. Younger patients with pseudobulbar palsy tend to exhibit pathological laughter, whereas older patients manifest pathological weeping. Changes in mood and behaviour (including personality changes, apathy, and abulia) and loss of incentive are common (McPherson and Cummings 1996).

In general, depression is common in vascular dementia; prevalence is estimated at 18–54% (Nyenhuis and Gorelick 1998). Compared to patients with AD (matched for severity of dementia, age, and education), patients with VaD have more behavioural retardation, anxiety/depression, and verbal output disturbances as assessed by the Neurobehavioral Rating Scale and the HDRS (Sultzer et al. 1993). In this study, more than a third of the patients with vascular dementia had blunted affect, depressed mood, emotional withdrawal, motor retardation, low motivation, anxiety, unusual thoughts, and somatic concerns; non-cognitive symptoms were not significantly related to the severity of cognitive impairment. Patients may have a major depression, or they may exhibit a minor depression similar to dysthymia. Major depression is not correlated with the degree of disability, whereas minor depression is more closely related to the patient's deficit syndrome. Subcortical lesions are associated with depression; lesions of the head of the caudate may confer the highest risk (Starkstein et al. 1988). Cortical lesions also are reported to result in depression. This may be particularly true of left hemispheric lesions, with more anterior lesions conferring greater risk than left-sided posterior injury (Robinson et al. 1984). However, one recent study found that depression was significantly associated with left hemispheric stroke location only in women (Paradiso and Robinson 1998). Right hemisphere strokes are reported to result in more severe depression when the lesion was more posteriorly located, but only during the immediate post-stroke period. Later in the course (within three to six months of the stroke), severity of depression was associated with anterior lesions. The assessment of depression in right hemisphere stroke may be complicated by anosognosia. Serotonin dysfunction and other alterations in neurotransmitter systems after stroke may be related to the development of depression (Alexopoulos et al. 1997).

Gender differences affect the frequency of post-stroke depression; in one study of 301 patients (Paradiso and Robinson 1998), women were twice as likely as men to develop a major depressive episode in the acute post-stroke period. This study also found that risk factors for depression in women include younger age, a past history of psychiatric disorder, and cognitive impairment. In men, younger age and impairments in social functioning and activities of daily living were associated with major depression.

Mania is less common than depression following stroke. Right hemispheric lesions are associated with mania (Robinson *et al.* 1988); the abnormalities may affect the caudate nucleus, thalamus, inferior medial frontal cortex, or the basal temporal region. Left hemispheric strokes also may produce mania. Patients who develop post-stroke mania frequently have a family history of affective disorder.

Psychosis is uncommon with single strokes and is associated with bilateral cerebrovascular lesions when it occurs. About half of patients have delusions, and hallucinations may occur. Right-sided lesions are often accompanied by visual hallucinations and delusions. Visual hallucinations may follow midbrain lesions (peduncular hallucinosis), lesions of the geniculocalcarine radiations ('release' hallucinations), ischaemic optic neuritis, and retinal ischaemia. Occipital, parietal, and temporal lobe infarcts may result in visual hallucinations as may left hemisphere and subcortical damage. Auditory hallucinations may follow pontine and temporal lobe damage. The risk of organic hallucinosis generally increases with greater lesion burden. Seizures are frequently seen in patients with post-stroke psychosis and may themselves produce visual hallucinations. Patients with Wernicke's aphasia often become paranoid and are a challenge to evaluate because of their language disturbance. Anxiety is relatively common and occurs in about a third of patients.

3.4.2 Multiple sclerosis (MS)

Neuropsychiatric symptoms may predominate at initial presentation and are likely to occur at some point in the majority of patients with MS. These symptoms are linked to the underlying disease process and are not solely accounted for by the psychological stress of chronic neurological disease (see chapter 17). A chart review of 2720 admissions to psychiatric wards found that six of the ten identified patients with MS required psychiatric hospitalization prior to the diagnosis of MS (Pine *et al.* 1995). A Danish study found that 12% of 366 patients with MS had been admitted to a psychiatric unit (Stenager and Jensen 1988). Depression is the most common disturbance, but mania, euphoria, anxiety, psychosis, and personality changes also occur. Cognitive dysfunction is reported to occur in 43–65% of patients, and an estimated 15–30% are severely demented (Rao 1996).

Depression is more common than mania or euphoria, although both unipolar and bipolar affective disorder are more common than in the general population (Rao 1996). Studies have estimated that depression occurs in 27–60% of patients (Diaz-Olavarrieta *et al.* 1999; Mendez 1995). One study of 50 patients with moderate disability from MS found that 54% had met criteria for a major depression during their lifetime (Minden *et al.* 1987). A meta-analysis found rates of depression near 50% (Schubert and Foliart 1993). Evaluation of depression in patients with MS is complicated by the presence of vegetative symptoms in some rating scales. Although findings are mixed, there is evidence that depression is associated with disability in MS. Stenager (Jensen 1989) found a linear relationship between the Kurtzke Disability Status Scale (KDSS) (Kurtzke 1983) and the Beck Depression Inventory (Beck *et al.* 1961) for KDSS ratings of minimal-to-moderate severity; the highest scores were associated with less depression.

Euphoria is less common, despite early reports that patients with MS were usually euphoric and cheerful in spite of their disabilities. When present, it usually occurs late in the course of illness. A study of 87 patients found that euphoria (present in 48% of patients) was related to brain involvement, progressive course, enlarged ventricles on CT, and more severe cognitive impairment (Rabins *et al.* 1986). Another study of 116 patients evaluated with MRI found that elation was significantly correlated with widespread MRI abnormalities (Ron and Logsdail 1989). An older study of over 1000 patients with MS found euphoria in 18.5% (Surridge 1969). A more recent review found a rate of euphoria in MS of 25%, with fewer (10%) having true sustained mood elevation. Mania should be distinguished from euphoria. One study of 100 patients with MS found that 13% met criteria for bipolar illness (Joffe *et al.* 1987).

Anxiety may be more prevalent than originally thought. One study found that anxiety disorders increased after the diagnosis of MS, with only 8% having an anxiety disorder prior to onset and 24% with anxiety disorders afterwards (Minden *et al.* 1987).

Personality changes seen in MS include irritability, apathy, and disinhibition. In the large study above, irritability was found in 40.7% of patients and apathy in 10% (Surridge 1969).

Psychosis is reported, but rare. Delusions and thought disorder have been correlated with degree of pathology in the temporoparietal area on MRI (Ron and Logsdail 1989). Chronic atypical psychosis has been reported as the presenting feature of MS (Kohler *et al.* 1988). Secondary Capgras' delusion (a misidentification syndrome in which the patient believes that a familiar person has been replaced by an imposter) also has been reported (Lebert *et al.* 1994).

A recent study of 44 patients with stable MS (between relapses) utilizing the NPI found that 95% demonstrated neuropsychiatric symptoms in the month prior to assessment (Diaz-Olavarrieta *et al.* 1999). Dysphoria was found in 79%; less common were agitation (40%), anxiety (37%), irritability (35%), apathy (20%), euphoria (13%), disinhibition (13%), hallucinations (10%), aberrant motor behaviour (9%), and delusions (9%). The symptoms that were rated as most severe included dysphoria, agitation, anxiety, and irritability. This study also found few correlations between NPI scores and abnormalities on MRI; hallucinations and euphoria were noted to be more common in those patients with moderately severe frontotemporal changes.

Neuropsychiatric symptoms in MS may be complicated by mood disturbance associated with steroid and β-interferon therapy.

3.4.3 Systemic lupus erythematosus (SLE)

Neuropsychiatric disturbances are common in SLE and may occur at any time in the disease course. They may result from disease in the central nervous system, complications of systemic illness (such as uremia or infection), medication effects (i.e. corticosteroids), or psychological reaction to illness (see chapter 17). Neuropsychiatric symptoms are reported to occur in 33–70% of patients (Moran 1996; Barr and Merchut 1992). A retrospective study of 140 patients found that the majority of neuropsychiatric episodes occurred within the first year of diagnosis or preceded the diagnosis of SLE (Feinglass *et al.* 1976).

The prevalence of psychosis in patients with SLE has been reported to be 17–75%; depressive symptoms have been reported in 6.5–86% of patients (Liang *et al.* 1984; Miguel *et al.* 1994). One study (Miguel *et al.* 1994) found that in 43 hospitalized patients with active SLE, 63% had a psychiatric diagnosis; organic mood disorder (with depressive symptoms) was the most common, followed by delirium and dementia. Another review of 266 patients with SLE found psychosis that could not be accounted for by another known cause in 11 patients (Sibley *et al.* 1992).

Psychosis is reported to occur in 40–67% of encephalopathic patients with SLE (Barr and Merchut 1992). Although the use of corticosteroids has been associated with a variety of psychiatric symptoms, psychosis in SLE is not usually due to steroids. One study (Miguel *et al.* 1994) found a negative correlation between psychosis and current use of corticosteroids; another found that only 2 of 140 patients were considered to have steroid-induced psychosis (Feinglass *et al.* 1976). In some cases it is not clear if psychosis is due to too much steroid therapy or too little; obtaining a thorough chronological history of steroid dosing and symptoms is crucial. Affective disturbance (depression and mania) may be precipitated by steroid use. Antimalarial drugs are another class of medication that may cause psychosis.

Up to two-thirds of the neuropsychiatric symptoms in SLE are estimated to be due to secondary causes (such as medications, metabolic abnormalities, and infections) (Kovacs *et al.* 1993). There is a suggestion that psychiatric symptomatology becomes more frequent as the disease progresses. Psychopathology has been associated with brain calcifications (mainly in the basal ganglia) and ophthalmologic abnormalities (Miguel *et al.* 1994). One study reported that psychosis, insomnia, photosensitivity, incomplete disease control, hypocomplementemia, and tapering steroid doses appear to be risk factors for suicide attempts (Matsukawa *et al.* 1994). Autoantibody titres (such as antibodies to ribosomal P proteins) (Schneebaum *et al.* 1991) have been investigated but are not consistently linked to neuropsychiatric manifestations of SLE.

4 Comment

Early onset dementing illnesses may present with neuropsychiatric disturbances; in some cases, these symptoms initially appear in isolation. Thorough assessment of mental status is essential in the evaluation of patients with dementia; the use of standardized tools can be useful. Early recognition and treatment of these disorders is necessary to reduce morbidity and mortality. Clinicians must maintain a high index of suspicion for the less common forms of early onset dementia. Patients with atypical symptoms, or are treatment-refractory, or have a family history of psychiatric or neurological illnesses warrant further investigation for underlying brain disorders.

5 Key points

1　Neuropsychiatric symptoms, including mood and anxiety disturbance, psychosis, personality changes, and agitation, are common and important in the diagnosis and treatment of patients with early onset dementia.

2　Non-cognitive symptoms may be assessed with standardized tools, including single item instruments (such as the Hamilton Depression Rating Scale) or multiple item instruments (such as the Neuropsychiatric Inventory).

3　Characteristic neuropsychiatric symptoms often accompany specific dementia syndromes, although none are pathognomonic.

4　Apathy is the most common behavioural disturbance seen in AD; depressive symptoms are common, although major depression is rare; euphoria is uncommon and may suggest an alternative diagnosis; psychosis may occur at any stage.

5　Patients with FTD have more apathy, euphoria, disinhibition, and aberrant motor behaviour than do patients with AD.

6　Approximately one-third of patients with WD present with predominantly psychiatric symptoms.

7　Personality changes (such as apathy, irritability, and compulsiveness) are the most common non-cognitive disturbances in HD, followed by depression; suicide is more common than in age-matched controls.

Acknowledgements

This project was supported by a National Institute on Aging (NIA) Alzheimer's Disease Center grant (AG10123), an Alzheimer's Disease Center of California grant, an NIA Fellowship Award (T32–10072), the UCLA General Clinical Research Center (MO1-RR00865), and the Sidell-Kagan Foundation.

References

Akil, M. and Brewer, G. J. (1995). Psychiatric and behavioral abnormalities in Wilson's disease. *Advances in Neurology*, **65**, 171–8.

Alexopoulos, G. S., Abrams, R. C., Young, R. C., and Shamoian, C. A. (1988). Cornell scale for depression in dementia. *Biological Psychiatry*, **23**, 271–84.

Alexopoulos, G. S., Meyers, B. S., Young, R. C., Campbell, S., Silbersweig, D., and Charlson, M. (1997). 'Vascular depression' hypothesis. *Archives of General Psychiatry*, **54**, 915–22.

Allen, N. H. P., Gordon, S., Hope, T., and Burns, A. (1996). Manchester and Oxford Universities scale for the psychopathological assessment of dementia (MOUSEPAD). *British Journal of Psychiatry*, **169**, 293–307.

American Psychiatric Association and American Psychiatric Association. Task Force on DSM-IV. (1994). *Diagnostic and statistical manual of mental disorders*: DSM-IV. American Psychiatric Association, Washington, DC.

Aubourg, P. and Mandel, J. L. (1996). X-linked adrenoleukodystrophy. *Annals of the New York Academy of Sciences*, **804**, 461–76.

Auer, S. R., Monteiro, I. M., and Reisberg, B. (1996). The empirical behavioral pathology in Alzheimer's disease (E-BEHAVE-AD) rating scale. *International Psychogeriatrics*, **8**, 247–66.

Barr, W. G. and Merchut, M. P. (1992). Systemic lupus erythematosus with central nervous system involvement. *Psychiatric Clinics of North America*, **15**, 439–54.

Baumann, N., Masson, M., Carreau, V., Lefevre, M., Herschkowitz, N., and Turpin, J. C. (1991). Adult forms of metachromatic leukodystrophy: clinical and biochemical approach. *Developmental Neuroscience*, **13**, 211–15.

Beck, A., Ward, C., Mendelson, M., *et al.* (1961). An inventory for measuring depression. *Archives of General Psychiatry*, **4**, 561–71.

Berkovic, S. F., Carpenter, S., Andermann, F., Andermann, E., and Wolfe, L. S. (1988). Kufs' disease: a critical reappraisal. *Brain*, **111**, 27–62.

Borson, S. and Raskind, M. A. (1997). Clinical features and pharmacologic treatment of behavioral symptoms of Alzheimer's disease. *Neurology*, **48**, S17–24.

Brewer, G. J. and Yuzbasiyan-Gurkan, V. (1992). Wilson disease. *Medicine*, **71**, 139–64.

Burns, A., Folstein, S., Brandt, J., and Folstein, M. (1990). Clinical assessment of irritability, aggression, and apathy in Huntington and Alzheimer disease. *Journal of Nervous and Mental Disease*, **178**, 20–6.

Cina, S. J., Smith, M. T., Collins, K. A., and Conradi, S. E. (1996). Dyadic deaths involving Huntington's disease: a case report. *American Journal of Forensic Medicine and Pathology*, **17**, 49–52.

Cohen-Mansfield, J. (1996). Assessment of agitation. *International Psychogeriatrics*, **8**, 233–45.

Cohen-Mansfield, J. and Billig, N. (1986). Agitated behaviors in the elderly. I. A conceptual review. *Journal of the American Geriatrics Society*, **34**, 711–21.

Cohen-Mansfield, J., Marx, M. S., and Rosenthal, A. S. (1989). A description of agitation in a nursing home. *Journal of Gerontology*, **44**, M77–84.

Cole, S. A., Woodard, J. L., Juncos, J. L., Kogos, J. L., Youngstrom, E. A., and Watts, R. L. (1996). Depression and disability in Parkinson's disease. *Journal of Neuropsychiatry and Clinical Neurosciences*, **8**, 20–5.

Cummings, J. L. (1995). Behavioral and psychiatric symptoms associated with Huntington's disease. *Advances in Neurology*, **65**, 179–86.

Cummings, J. L. (1997). The neuropsychiatric inventory: assessing psychopathology in dementia patients. *Neurology*, **48**, S10–16.

Cummings, J. L. and Cunningham, K. (1992). Obsessive-compulsive disorder in Huntington's disease. *Biological Psychiatry*, **31**, 263–70.

Cummings, J. L., Mega, M., Gray, K., Rosenberg-Thompson, S., Carusi, D. A., and Gornbein, J. (1994). The neuropsychiatric inventory: comprehensive assessment of psychopathology in dementia. *Neurology*, **44**, 2308–14.

Dening, T. R. and Berrios, G. E. (1989*a*). Wilson's disease. Psychiatric symptoms in 195 cases. *Archives of General Psychiatry*, **46**, 1126–34.

Dening, T. R. and Berrios, G. E. (1989*b*). Wilson's disease: a prospective study of psychopathology in 31 cases. *British Journal of Psychiatry*, **155**, 206–13.

Dening, T. R. and Berrios, G. E. (1990). Wilson's disease: a longitudinal study of psychiatric symptoms. *Biological Psychiatry*, **28**, 255–65.

Devanand, D. P., Jacobs, D. M., Tang, M. X., Del Castillo-Castaneda, C., Sano, M., Marder, K., *et al.* (1997). The course of psychopathologic features in mild to moderate Alzheimer disease. *Archives of General Psychiatry*, **54**, 257–63.

Diaz-Olavarrieta, C., Cummings, J., Velazquez, J., and Garcia de al Cadena, C. (1999). Neuropsychiatric manifestations of multiple sclerosis. *The Journal of Neuropsychiatry and Clinical Neurosciences*, **11**, 51–7.

Edwards-Lee, T., Miller, B. L., Benson, D. F., Cummings, J. L., Russell, G. L., Boone, K., *et al.* (1997). The temporal variant of frontotemporal dementia. *Brain*, **120**, 1027–40.

Factor, S. A., Molho, E. S., Podskalny, G. D., and Brown, D. (1995). Parkinson's disease: drug-induced psychiatric states. *Advances in Neurology*, **65**, 115–38.

Feinglass, E. J., Arnett, F. C., Dorsch, C. A., Zizic, T. M., and Stevens, M. B. (1976). Neuropsychiatric manifestations of systemic lupus erythematosus: diagnosis, clinical spectrum, and relationship to other features of the disease. *Medicine*, **55**, 323–39.

Fluharty, A. L. (1990). The relationship of the metachromatic leukodystrophies to neuropsychiatric disorders. *Molecular and Chemical Neuropathology*, **13**, 81–94.

Goetz, C. G., Vogel, C., Tanner, C. M., and Stebbins, G. T. (1998). Early dopaminergic drug-induced hallucinations in parkinsonian patients. *Neurology*, **51**, 811–14.

Goodwin, F. K. (1971). Psychiatric side effects of levodopa in man. *Journal of American Medical Association*, **218**, 1915–20.

Gottfries, C. G., Brane, G., Gullberg, B., and Steen, G. (1982). A new rating scale for dementia syndromes. *Arch. Gerontol. Geriatr.*, **1**, 311–30.

Hageman, A. T., Gabreëls, F. J., de Jong, J. G., Gabreëls-Festen, A. A., van den Berg, C. J., van Oost, B. A., *et al.* (1995). Clinical symptoms of adult metachromatic leukodystrophy and arylsulfatase A pseudodeficiency. *Archives of Neurology*, **52**, 408–13.

Hamilton, M. (1960). A rating scale for depression. *Journal of Neurology, Neurosurgery, and Psychiatry*, **23**, 56–62.

Hammersen, S., Brock, M., and Cervós-Navarro, J. (1998). Adult neuronal ceroid lipofuscinosis with clinical findings consistent with a butterfly glioma. Case report. *Journal of Neurosurgery*, **88**, 314–18.

Hayden, M. R., Bloch, M., and Wiggins, S. (1995). Psychological effects of predictive testing for Huntington's disease. *Advances in Neurology*, **65**, 201–10.

Hope, R. and Fairburn, C. G. (1992). The present behavioural examination (PBE): the development of an interview to measure current behavioural abnormalities. *Psychological Medicine*, **22**, 223–30.

Hubble, J. P. and Koller, W. C. (1995). The parkinsonian personality. *Advances in Neurology*, **65**, 43–8.

Hyde, T. M., Ziegler, J. C., and Weinberger, D. R. (1992). Psychiatric disturbances in metachromatic leukodystrophy. Insights into the neurobiology of psychosis [see comments]. *Archives of Neurology*, **49**, 401–6.

James, A. C., Kaplan, P., Lees, A., and Bradley, J. J. (1984). Schizophreniform psychosis and adrenomyeloneuropathy. *Journal of the Royal Society of Medicine*, **77**, 882–4.

Jensen, K. (1989). *Mental disorders and cognitive deficits in multiple sclerosis*. Libbey, London.

Joffe, R. T., Lippert, G. P., Gray, T. A., Sawa, G., and Horvath, Z. (1987). Mood disorder and multiple sclerosis. *Archives of Neurology*, **44**, 376–8.

Kitchin, W., Cohen-Cole, S. A., and Mickel, S. F. (1987). Adrenoleukodystrophy: frequency of presentation as a psychiatric disorder. *Biological Psychiatry*, **22**, 1375–87.

Kohler, J., Heilmeyer, H., and Volk, B. (1988). Multiple sclerosis presenting as chronic atypical psychosis. *Journal of Neurology, Neurosurgery and Psychiatry*, **51**, 281–4.

Kostić, V. S., Filipović, S.R., Lečić, D., Momćilović, D., Solić, D. and Šternić, N. (1994). Effect of age at onset on frequency of depression in Parkinson's disease. *Journal of Neurology, Neurosurgery and Psychiatry*, **57**, 1265–7.

Kovacs, J. A., Urowitz, M. B., and Gladman, D. D. (1993). Dilemmas in neuropsychiatric lupus. *Rheumatic Diseases Clinics of North America*, **19**, 795–814.

Kurtzke, J. F. (1983). Rating neurologic impairment in multiple sclerosis: an expanded disability status scale (EDSS). *Neurology*, **33**, 1444–52.

Lauterbach, E. C., Cummings, J. L., Duffy, J., Coffey, C. E., Kaufer, D., Lovell, M., *et al.* (1998). Neuropsychiatric correlates and treatment of lenticulostriatal diseases: A review of the literature and overview of research opportunities in Huntington's, Wilson's, and Fahr's diseases. *The Journal of Neuropsychiatry and Clinical Neurosciences*, **10**, 249–66.

Lebert, F., Pasquier, F., Steinling, M., Cabaret, M., Caparros-Lefebvre, D., and Petit, H. (1994). SPECT data in a case of secondary Capgras delusion. *Psychopathology*, **27**, 211–14.

Levy, M. L., Miller, B. L., Cummings, J. L., Fairbanks, L. A., and Craig, A. (1996). Alzheimer disease and frontotemporal dementias. Behavioral distinctions [see comments]. *Archives of Neurology*, **53**, 687–90.

Liang, M. H., Rogers, M., Larson, M., Eaton, H. M., Murawski, B. J., Taylor, J. E., *et al.* (1984). The psychosocial impact of systemic lupus erythematosus and rheumatoid arthritis. *Arthritis and Rheumatism*, **27**, 13–19.

Lovestone, S., Hodgson, S., Sham, P., Differ, A. M., and Levy, R. (1996). Familial psychiatric presentation of Huntington's disease. *Journal of Medical Genetics*, **33**, 128–31.

Matsukawa, Y., Sawada, S., Hayama, T., Usui, H., and Horie, T. (1994). Suicide in patients with systemic lupus erythematosus: a clinical analysis of seven suicidal patients. *Lupus*, **3**, 31–5.

Mayberg, H. S. and Solomon, D. H. (1995). Depression in Parkinson's disease: a biochemical and organic viewpoint. *Advances in Neurology*, **65**, 49–60.

Mayeux, R., Stern, Y., Rosen, J., and Leventhal, J. (1981). Depression, intellectual impairment, and Parkinson disease. *Neurology*, **31**, 645–50.

McGivney, S. A., Mulvihill, M., and Taylor, B. (1994). Validating the GDS depression screen in the nursing home [see comments]. *Journal of the American Geriatrics Society*, **42**, 490–2.

McPherson, S. E. and Cummings, J. L. (1996). Neuropsychological aspects of vascular dementia. *Brain and Cognition*, **31**, 269–82.

Mega, M. S., Cummings, J. L., Fiorello, T., and Gornbein, J. (1996). The spectrum of behavioral changes in Alzheimer's disease. *Neurology*, **46**, 130–5.

Mendez, M. F. (1994). Huntington's disease: update and review of neuropsychiatric aspects. *International Journal of Psychiatry in Medicine*, **24**, 189–208.

Mendez, M. F. (1995). The neuropsychiatry of multiple sclerosis. *International Journal of Psychiatry in Medicine*, **25**, 123–30.

Mendez, M. F., Perryman, K. M., Miller, B. L., Swartz, J. R., and Cummings, J. L. (1997). Compulsive behaviors as presenting symptoms of frontotemporal dementia. *Journal of Geriatric Psychiatry and Neurology*, **10**, 154–7.

Menza, M. A., Golbe, L. I., Cody, R. A., and Forman, N. E. (1993). Dopamine-related personality traits in Parkinson's disease. *Neurology*, **43**, 505–8.

Miguel, E. C., Pereira, R. M., Pereira, C. A., Baer, L., Gomes, R. E., de Sá, L. C., *et al.* (1994). Psychiatric manifestations of systemic lupus erythematosus: clinical features, symptoms, and signs of central nervous system activity in 43 patients. *Medicine*, **73**, 224–32.

Miller, B. L., Darby, A., Benson, D. F., Cummings, J. L., and Miller, M. H. (1997). Aggressive, socially disruptive and antisocial behaviour associated with fronto-temporal dementia. *British Journal of Psychiatry*, **170**, 150–4.

Minden, S. L., Orav, J., and Reich, P. (1987). Depression in multiple sclerosis. *General Hospital Psychiatry*, **9**, 426–34.

Mohs, R. C. (1996). The Alzheimer's disease assessment scale. *International Psychogeriatrics*, **8**, 195–203.

Mohs, R. C., Rosen, W. G., and Davis, K. L. (1983). The Alzheimer's disease assessment scale: an instrument for assessing treatment efficacy. *Psychopharmacology Bulletin*, **19**, 448–50.

Moran, M. G. (1996). Psychiatric aspects of rheumatology. *Psychiatric Clinics of North America*, **19**, 575–87.

Moser, H. W., Moser, A. B., Naidu, S., and Bergin, A. (1991). Clinical aspects of adrenoleukodystrophy and adrenomyeloneuropathy. *Developmental Neuroscience*, **13**, 254–61.

Nyenhuis, D. L. and Gorelick, P. B. (1998). Vascular dementia: a contemporary review of epidemiology, diagnosis, prevention, and treatment. *Journal of the American Geriatrics Society*, **46**, 1437–48.

Oder, W., Grimm, G., Kollegger, H., Ferenci, P., Schneider, B., and Deecke, L. (1991). Neurological and neuropsychiatric spectrum of Wilson's disease: a prospective study of 45 cases. *Journal of Neurology*, **238**, 281–7.

Oder, W., Prayer, L., Grimm, G., Spatt, J., Ferenci, P., Kollegger, H., *et al.* (1993). Wilson's disease: evidence of subgroups derived from clinical findings and brain lesions. *Neurology*, **43**, 120–4.

Paradiso, S. and Robinson, R. G. (1998). Gender differences in poststroke depression. *Journal of Neuropsychiatry and Clinical Neurosciences*, **10**, 41–7.

Patterson, M. B., Schnell, A. H., Martin, R. J., Mendez, M. F., Smyth, K. A., and Whitehouse, P. J. (1990). Assessment of behavioral and affective symptoms in Alzheimer's disease. *Journal of Geriatric Psychiatry and Neurology*, **3**, 21–30.

Payne, J. L., Lyketsos, C. G., Steele, C., Baker, L., Galik, E., Kopunek, S., *et al.* (1998). Relationship of cognitive and functional impairment to depressive features in Alzheimer's disease and other dementias. *Journal of Neuropsychiatry and Clinical Neurosciences*, **10**, 440–7.

Pearson, J. L., Teri, L., Wagner, A., Truax, P., and Logsdon, R. G. (1993). The relationship of problem behaviors in dementia patients to the depression and burden of caregiving spouses. *The American Journal of Alzheimer's Disease and Related Disorders and Research*, **8**, 15–22.

Pine, D. S., Douglas, C. J., Charles, E., Davies, M., and Kahn, D. (1995). Patients with multiple sclerosis presenting to psychiatric hospitals [see comments]. *Journal of Clinical Psychiatry*, **56**, 297–306; discussion 307–8.

Rabins, P. V., Brooks, B. R., O'Donnell, P., Pearlson, G. D., Moberg, P., Jubelt, B., *et al.* (1986). Structural brain correlates of emotional disorder in multiple sclerosis. *Brain*, **109**, 585–97.

Rao, S. M. (1996). White matter disease and dementia. *Brain and Cognition*, **31**, 250–68.

Rao, V. and Lyketsos, C. G. (1998). Delusions in Alzheimer's disease: a review. *Journal of Neuropsychiatry and Clinical Neurosciences*, **10**, 373–82.

Reisberg, B., Borenstein, J., Salob, S. P., Ferris, S. H., Franssen, E., and Georgotas, A. (1987). Behavioral symptoms in Alzheimer's disease: phenomenology and treatment. *Journal of Clinical Psychiatry*, **48** (Suppl), 9–15.

Roane, D. M., Rogers, J. D., Robinson, J. H., and Feinberg, T. E. (1998). Delusional misidentification in association with parkinsonism. *Journal of Neuropsychiatry and Clinical Neurosciences*, **10**, 194–8.

Robinson, R. G., Boston, J. D., Starkstein, S. E., and Price, T. R. (1988). Comparison of mania and depression after brain injury: causal factors. *American Journal of Psychiatry*, **145**, 172–8.

Robinson, R. G., Kubos, K. L., Starr, L. B., Rao, K., and Price, T. R. (1984). Mood disorders in stroke patients. Importance of location of lesion. *Brain*, **107**, 81–93.

Ron, M. A. and Logsdail, S. J. (1989). Psychiatric morbidity in multiple sclerosis: a clinical and MRI study. *Psychological Medicine*, **19**, 887–95.

Rubin, E. (1992). Delusions as part of Alzheimer's disease. *Neuropsychiatry Neuropsychology Behavioral Neurology.*, **5**, 108–13.

Saint-Cyr, J. A., Taylor, A. E., and Nicholson, K. (1995). Behavior and the basal ganglia. *Advances in Neurology*, **65**, 1–28.

Schneebaum, A. B., Singleton, J. D., West, S. G., Blodgett, J. K., Allen, L. G., Cheronis, J. C., *et al.* (1991). Association of psychiatric manifestations with antibodies to ribosomal P proteins in systemic lupus erythematosus. *American Journal of Medicine*, **90**, 54–62.

Schubert, D. S. and Foliart, R. H. (1993). Increased depression in multiple sclerosis patients. A meta-analysis. *Psychosomatics*, **34**, 124–30.

Sibley, J. T., Olszynski, W. P., Decoteau, W. E., and Sundaram, M. B. (1992). The incidence and prognosis of central nervous system disease in systemic lupus erythematosus. *Journal of Rheumatology*, **19**, 47–52.

Starkstein, S. E., Robinson, R. G., Berthier, M. L., Parikh, R. M., and Price, T. R. (1988). Differential mood changes following basal ganglia vs thalamic lesions. *Archives of Neurology*, **45**, 725–30.

Stenager, E. and Jensen, K. (1988). Multiple sclerosis: correlation of psychiatric admissions to onset of initial symptoms. *Acta Neurologica Scandinavica*, **77**, 414–17.

Sultzer, D. L., Levin, H. S., Mahler, M. E., High, W. M., and Cummings, J. L. (1993). A comparison of psychiatric symptoms in vascular dementia and Alzheimer's disease. *American Journal of Psychiatry*, **150**, 1806–12.

Surridge, D. (1969). An investigation into some psychiatric aspects of multiple sclerosis. *British Journal of Psychiatry*, **115**, 749–64.

Tanner, C. M., Ottman, R., Goldman, S. M., Ellenberg, J., Chan, P., Mayeux, R., *et al.* (1999). Parkinson disease in twins: an etiologic study [see comments]. *Journal of American Medical Association*, **281**, 341–6.

Tariot, P. N., Mack, J. L., Patterson, M. B., Edland, S. D., Weiner, M. F., Fillenbaum, G., *et al.* (1995). The behavior rating scale for dementia of the consortium to establish a registry for Alzheimer's disease. The Behavioral Pathology Committee of the Consortium to Establish a Registry for Alzheimer's Disease. *American Journal of Psychiatry*, **152**, 1349–57.

Teri, L., Truax, P., Logsdon, R., Uomoto, J., Zarit, S., and Vitaliano, P. P. (1992). Assessment of behavioral problems in dementia: the revised memory and behavior problems checklist. *Psychology and Aging*, **7**, 622–31.

Vasquez, A., Jimenez-Jimenez, F., Garcia-Ruiz, P. and Garcia-Urra, D. (1993). 'Panic attacks' in Parkinson's disease, a long-term complication of levodopa therapy. *Acta Neurologica Scandinavica*, **87**, 14–18.

Wiggins, S., Whyte, P., Huggins, M., Adam, S., Theilmann, J., Bloch, M., *et al.* (1992). The psychological consequences of predictive testing for Huntington's disease. Canadian Collaborative Study of Predictive Testing [see comments]. *New England Journal of Medicine*, **327**, 1401–5.

Yesavage, J. A., Brink, T. L., Rose, T. L., Lum, O., Huang, V., Adey, M., *et al.* (1982). Development and validation of a geriatric depression screening scale: a preliminary report. *Journal of Psychiatric Research*, **17**, 37–49.

Zappacosta, B., Monza, D., Meoni, C., Austoni, L., Soliveri, P., Gellera, C., *et al.* (1996). Psychiatric symptoms do not correlate with cognitive decline, motor symptoms, or CAG repeat length in Huntington's disease. *Archives of Neurology*, **53**, 493–7.

5 Psychiatric disorders mimicking dementia

G. E. Berrios and I. S. Marková

1 Introduction

It is a sobering thought that in the new brave world of neuroimaging, neuropsychology, and high power discriminators, on occasions clinicians are not yet able to distinguish between the mental state caused by *echte* 'dementia' from its copies or mimics. It is known that the latter can be generated by a variety of clinical states, ranging from mental symptoms and diseases to iatrogenic states. The diagnosis and management of these mimics is hampered by the fact that little is known about their mechanisms. Indeed, at this stage it is even unclear where the problem really lies, namely whether it is due to fuzziness inherent in the clinical concepts themselves (e.g. dementia, depression, cognitive impairment, confusion) or to a mere lack of sensitivity in current discriminators. If the issue is concepts, then the emphasis should be on understanding the genesis of the concepts involved and the creation of more imaginative operational definitions; if it is a matter of sensitivity, then the effort ought to go into empirical research.

So far, the second option has been preferred but with jejune results: discriminators rarely work, particularly on the borderline case; they exhibit questionable additivity (i.e. two discriminators do not work better than one); and significant group differences are rarely ecologically tangible. All this suggests that the conceptual fuzziness option ought to be followed with more vigour. Before embarking in the required clinical analysis, this chapter will briefly deal with the concepts involved.

2 The word and concept of 'dementia'

Historical analysis suggests that the conceptual boundaries of 'dementia' have been blurred from the start. Travelling in the lexicon of Roman jurisprudence, the adjective '*demens*' ('out of one's mind or senses, mad, raving, foolish'), arrived early into the European vernaculars. The Roman legionnaires brought with them coarser terms: *amens, excors, vecors, insanus, vesanus, delirus*, and *alienatus mente*. By about 500 AC, therefore, a panoply of terms was available to refer to mental deficits be those due to dotage, learning disability, brain damage, toxic states (e.g. deadly nightshade), or puerperal madness. However, by the 13th century, 'dotage' was defined separately ('to dote'): 'to be silly, deranged, or out of one's wits; to act or talk foolishly or stupidly' (OED, 2nd edition) (in French, *radoter*; Rey 1995). Until the 18th century, 'dotage' was used to refer to all types of mental deficit.

By the early 19th century, the semantic baseline of dementia included a *juridical* meaning (synonymous with mental disorder) and a *clinical* meaning (marked mental deficit, regardless of whether it was acquired, irreversible, or terminal). Thus, it was no different from idiocy and other states of congenital defect (Berrios 1987) and could be predicated of chronic madness, cognitive deficits after brain injury, mental retardation, melancholic stupor, senile dementia, etc. By the 1880s specific terms had been found for most of these clinical conditions and for a time dementia had become a veritable 'exogenous psychosis'. Soon, however, the 'cognitive paradigm' of dementia began to be established (Berrios 1989).

Currently, dementia names a *class* of acquired conditions mainly affecting the middle aged and elderly and characterized by progressive and irreversible deterioration of cognitive and other mental functions including personality. This narrow or 'cognitive' definition of dementia encouraged neuropsychological research but delayed the broader clinical analysis. Its lack of clinical detail and variance makes it more susceptible to mimics and copies. It also encourages a definition of 'early' dementia as a 'mini-memory failure' and foments an endless search for ever more sensitive diagnostic instruments. On the other hand, the old paradigm (according to which dementia was an exogenous psychosis affecting all mental functions) conceived of it as a *process* in which no deficit was privileged. Thus, 'early dementia' could be defined, for example, in terms of early affective or personality changes.

2.1 Mimics and phenocopies

The first issue to examine is what is meant by mental states that 'mimic' or 'copy' dementia. Patients suffering from psychoses and neuroses may present as being confused, disorientated, disconnected from reality in various ways or exhibiting functional conversive symptoms that involve language, memory, or other communicational devices. These mental states may thus resemble a clinical picture of dementia. The similarity between such 'functional' mental states and dementia may be partial or more complete. In this chapter, the term *'mimic'* is used to refer to a *partial* copy (Extein and Gold 1986). In the case of dementia, it may just consist of one overriding or predominant symptom (e.g. disorientation). The term *'behavioural phenocopy'* (Berrios and Samuel 1987) is used to refer to a mental state that more completely resembles the full clinical picture of dementia. Linking both these terms with dementia in this context is the notion of *similarity*. In other words, it is through mental states appearing similar to the clinical picture of dementia that 'mimics' and 'phenocopies' are generated. The question then follows, what does 'similar' mean? The analysis of similarity is complex and at least one writer has called it a concept that is 'a pretender, an impostor, a quack' (Goodman 1992). In this chapter we shall use a simple definition: 'two symptoms are similar when they have many but not all properties in common'. A property, in turn, is an 'attribute or quality belonging to a thing or person: in earlier use sometimes, an essential, special, or distinctive quality, a peculiarity; in later use often, a quality or characteristic in general (without reference to its essentialness or distinctiveness)' (OED, 2nd Edition 1992). Properties can be 'essential' and 'accidental'. For example, 'being related to vision' is an *essential* property of a visual hallucination and 'forgetting' is an essential feature of a memory deficit. On the other hand, properties that can change without affecting the class of symptoms involved (e.g. *content*) are called *accidental*. Both types of properties can generate 'similarity' and hence are involved in the production of mimics and behavioural phenocopies.

The question of whether all similarities engender mimics remains to be answered. It is even unclear whether essential or accidental properties are more prone to give the impression of similarity. For example, in a subject with psychomotor slowness and memory deficits, the presence of delusions with a content of ruin (an accidental property) will be more likely to create a copy of depression than a delusion with another content. On the other hand, in a subject with confusion and memory deficits, the presence of visual hallucinations (essential property), regardless of content, may create a copy of 'Lewy body disease' (Perry *et al.* 1996).

Similarity can be predicated of both symptoms and diseases. In regards to the latter, patients are said to have a similar disease X, regardless of whether or not they share all the same symptoms pertaining to X. For example, if X is constituted by symptoms x_1 to x_{10}, in an extreme case, one patient could suffer x_1 to x_5 and the other suffer x_6 to x_{10} and they would still be considered as having the same disease in spite of their phenomenology being different (as per concept of 'family resemblances'; paragraphs 66 and 67; Wittgenstein 1967). In practice, however, not all symptoms x_s have the same weight (e.g. some may be considered as pathognomonic — *sine qua non*) and hence decisions taken concerning similarity depend on more complex judgements relating to patterns and selection of symptoms presented. Alternatively, both patients might have x_1 to x_5 and would thus show very similar presentations of the disease.

2.2 Mechanisms

Before moving on to examine the specific mimics and behavioural phenocopies of dementia, some brief space needs to be given to the question of how such clinical mimics or copies might arise. Again, little research has been done on this and the purpose here is to simply raise some possibilities which may suggest directions for future research.

1   One possibility is that whilst the dementia as a disease is mimicked, the actual symptoms constituting the mimicking mental state (e.g. cognitive impairment) are 'real'. 'Real' in this context means that the symptoms belong to a similar class of symptoms as those obtained in dementia. This might happen in the following ways:

(a)   For example, cognitive impairment may be caused by anticholinergics or by some forms of severe depression. In this case, 'real' cognitive impairment is manifested but, because this has a different aetiology and runs a different course, the mental state is viewed as a behavioural phenocopy and not as a dementia.

(b)   Alternatively, such symptoms may be the non-specific manifestations of general brain insult. Hence, brain disorders other than dementias could again produce such 'real' symptoms. During the late 19th century there was a debate as to whether or not the phenomenology of the organic mental disorders (also called exogenous psychoses) always carried information or a mark that betrayed its underlying aetiology. For example, did the symptomatology of exogenous psychoses produced by hypothyroidism, brain tumours, toxins, meningitis, and brain injury differ from each other in any way? There is no space in this chapter to expand upon this view which was but a remnant of the old medieval theory of 'signatures'. Kraepelin (1899) believed that, in principle, such subtle marks were embedded in the phenomenology of most exogenous psychoses but that not enough research had yet been done to identify them in all cases. By the early 20th century, however, and mainly under the influence of evolutionary theory, views began to change and in the event Bonhoeffer's proposal was accepted that the brain had only a limited number of stereotyped responses to insult and injury (confusion, delirium, coma, stupor, cognitive disorganization, etc.) which were triggered by whatever aetiology. The question that followed, and explored by Bonhoeffer (1910), Redlich (1912), and others, was whether some aetiologies preferentially chose particular stereotyped responses. For example, were toxins and infections more likely to trigger delirium whilst myxoedema gave rise to memory impairment and paranoid ideas?

2   Another possible mechanism underlying clinical mimics/copies is that *both* the symptoms and the consequent dementia are being mimicked by the mental state. In other words, here the symptoms are not 'real' as above but are copies which could, in theory, with finer discriminators, be identified as such. One could speculate that such symptoms arise from heterogeneous aetiology and that they then converge, coincidentally, to give the impression that the patient is suffering from dementia. Many other permutations of this mechanism can be envisaged relating to both the nature of the copies them-

selves (e.g. where the similarities or differences to prototype lie) and their clinical interpretation (e.g. certain types or patterns of mimicking symptoms may predispose to the clinical picture of dementia with a resultant neglect of perhaps other salient symptoms). There is little space here to explore this further but, once again, this is an area demanding conceptual and empirical work.

Examining possible mechanisms as above, raises the role of disease aetiology in this debate. In other words, what part does the aetiology of a disease play in its actual diagnosis? Is it an essential or accidental property? Is it justifiable to describe a mental state as a behavioural phenocopy of dementia when the aetiology is unknown? Such questions remain to be explored.

Returning now to specific clinical copies of dementia, the chapter deals with these in two areas in line with the distinction made earlier. First, *symptoms* mimicking dementia are discussed and, secondly, *disorders* mimicking dementia are described. The latter are further subdivided into (i) 'functional' behavioural phenocopies (conventional psychiatric disorders), (ii) organic behavioural phenocopies (reversible dementias) and, (iii) drug-induced states which likewise show clinical resemblance to dementias (see Table 5.1).

3 Psychiatric symptoms mimicking dementia

In general, psychiatric disorders express themselves in terms of:

(a) *Conventional* or *listed* symptoms (as they appear in the official definitions).

(b) *Unlisted* complaints, which can be unnamed (i.e. not yet described) or discarded (once in list (a) and now considered as obsolete or irrelevant).

Typical of the 'discarded' type are:

(a) Simple and complex *somatic complaints* affecting the inner and outer body and once considered as symptoms of both psychoses and neuroses (shifting and shooting pains; twitching and jerking; sensations of vibration, electric discharge, and of movement inside the head; sudden feelings of hot and cold; 'bluish' hands; hyperaesthesia of the skin; fatigue; etc.) (Dupré 1913, 1925).

(b) Changes in the quality, organization, and rhythm of both *perception* and *consciousness* (the subject 'feels different'; as if he 'can no longer comprehend what is going on'; 'as if the world is moving faster or slower'; as if 'people's faces and the contour of objects are changing all the time' or 'look iridescent or different', etc.).

(c) *Confusion* and *behavioural disorganization*.

Symptoms belonging into some of these subgroups may cause copies of dementia and will be explored further.

Table 5.1 Disorders mimicking dementia

Cause of behavioural phenocopy	Condition
'Functional' disorders	Depression, psychoses, hysteria, fugues, Ganserian answers, Ganser syndrome
'Organic' disorders	B12 deficiency, hypothyroidism, normal pressure hydrocephalus, space occupying lesion
Drug-induced states	Antipsychotics, anticholinergics, tricyclic antidepressants, benzodiazepines

3.1 Disorders of consciousness

The 'disorders of consciousness' exhibited by subjects with functional psychiatric disorders range from subtle to gross (Ey1963). Amongst the former, patients may complain of changes in the perceptual field including increased or decreased opaqueness, brilliancy, strangeness, familiarity, movement, vibration, colouring, tiredness, anxiety, etc. Grosser changes affect not only the content but the structure of consciousness, for example, the subject may feel confused, perplexed, and detached from the world. He may also feel that he no longer can escape his interiority, as if he were trapped in the theatre or box of his own consciousness. When feeling thus, patients may answer incoherently, be unable to enter into a conversation, and appear to the clinician as 'cognitively disorganized'. Disorders of this type are seen in the functional psychoses (schizophrenia, manic depressive illness, cycloid psychoses), anxiety and obsessive compulsive disorders, and somatization and hypochondriacal conditions but they are rarely recorded for they are no longer part of the current diagnostic criteria.

It is important to notice that in Anglo-Saxon psychiatry the clinical phenomena described above would not be classified as 'disorders of consciousness'. The reason for this difference is historical rather than scientific and has to do with the narrow way in which the category in question came to be defined and exclusively related to the 'organic' mental disorders. (This process had been completed by the time Klein and Mayer-Gross (1957) published their famous manual on the clinical examination of patients with 'organic cerebral disease'.) Hence, whenever such mental changes are seen in patients without brain or systemic disease, they have to be explained away as fortuitous or the result of dissociation, conversion, or malingering.

Historically, the same mental changes were once described in relation to all manner of diseases, including the exogenous (organic) and endogenous (functional) psychoses but in the Anglo-Saxon world the decision was taken to link them up exclusively to the organic disorders. Years later, this decision unwittingly helped the reliability and validity claims of systems like DSM-IV (American Psychiatric Association 1994) and provided the basis for neuroimaging of mental symptoms. This is because DSM-IV assumes that:

(a) Subjects suffering from a functional psychosis (say schizophrenia) have no disorder of consciousness and hence can report their subjective experiences objectively (relevant to the reliability of the said systems).

(b) Because there is no pathology of consciousness, all mental symptoms thus reported are independent and stable mental states and not just the result of imagination, reveries, illusions, distorted perceptions or memories (confirming the validity of the mental entities captured by such systems).

Likewise, in order for neuroimaging to make sense, it must be assumed that the tokens or exemplars of mental symptoms that are correlated with the changes in blood flow or in structure actually represent a class of entities which are real and stable in time (Berrios 1999). Lastly, a similar assumption underlies current memory research in schizophrenia as it must be assumed that the results of tests are not affected by a mediating disorder of consciousness.

The two best known disorders of consciousness in Anglo-Saxon psychiatry are confusion and disorientation, and will be dealt with next.

3.1.1 Confusion

On occasions, subjects with confusion may be misdiagnosed as having 'dementia'. Confusion is diagnosed on the basis of information from two sources: observation of a patient who seems to be struggling with his/her physical and social environment, and, the patient's own account whose stereotyped content is usually governed by cultural and generational biases.

Confusion is currently conceptualized as a fundamental disorder of cognition but there was a time when emotions and volitions were also considered as important; indeed, there is much to be said in favour of this broader view. The cognitive bias has influenced the relevant descriptive metaphors: not being able 'to think clearly', 'to see clearly', 'not being with it', etc. These have replaced earlier tropes such as feeling: 'in a cloud', 'muddled up', 'as if one's head was made out of cotton-wool', 'fraught', and even 'out of sorts'.

The nature, composition and mechanisms of confusion remain unknown. Likely to be a final common pathway, it may be caused by a sudden drop in cortical arousal, irruption of REM dreams into wakefulness, failures in the processing of emotions, or subtle perceptual disturbance, and/or memory distortions (Berrios 1981). These ways of talking about the mechanisms of confusion are equally metaphorical for little is known about the neuroscience of confusion.

Confusion can be present during the acute stages of most 'functional' psychoses (Chaslin 1895). Nowadays, this interesting clinical feature is often missed or misdiagnosed: the former for it can be fleeting, occur before the patient has been admitted into hospital, or be masked by the neuroleptics administered by the GPs; the latter for current nosology encourages clinicians to consider confusion as due to some superimposed 'organic' process. Until not long ago, it was otherwise: clinicians and nurses had all had the opportunity to look after unmedicated patients with long periods of confusion. The same clinical phenomenon in our day creates panic all round and diagnoses such as 'frontal lobe syndrome' or 'mild or good prognosis' viral encephalitis are bandied about. Follow-up shows that in most cases there is *restitutio ad integrum* and all investigations prove negative. Nonetheless, these putative diagnoses are rarely revised, particularly when patients actually show periods of veritable organic confusion in response to cyclophosphamide or other cytotoxic agents.

The phenomenology of this type of confusion varies according to the underlying functional psychoses. Usually short-lived and accompanied by obvious bizarre psychotic behaviours, the confusion may on occasions last for weeks and on those cases copy dementia closely. These mimics can be completed by the presence of dyspraxic and dysphasic behaviours that convince everyone that the patient has developed 'acute dementia' and diagnoses such as Creutzfeldt–Jakob disease begin to be mentioned. Particularly prone to producing these copies is the 'excited-inhibited confusion' subtype of the cycloid psychosis (Leonhard 1979):

> 30-year-old female, a high level executive secretary, who after driving her husband to the airport, started feeling 'confused' and as if 'her tongue was heavy'. Within 3 days she had been admitted into a neurological ward with 'dysphasia', 'hyperaesthesia' and 'visual and auditory distortions'. She was diagnosed as having a viral encephalitis and prescribed Acyclovir. All investigations were negative. A month later, she was still confused, with bizarre behaviour, and unruly. Nursing staff demanded 'psychiatric opinion'. The C-L consultant diagnosed conversion hysteria, and the neuropsychiatrist cycloid psychosis (excited-inhibited/confusional type). Transferred to a neuropsychiatric bed, Acyclovir was discontinued and patient was given ECT with dramatic results. Within 4 months she had returned to her old job. At 2 years follow up, there has been no relapse nor is there evidence of any residual deficits.

3.1.2 Disorientation

Persistent disorientation may on occasions lead to the diagnosis of dementia, particularly when it involves time, place, social rules, and the self (Bouchard 1926; Benton *et al.* 1964). Some believe that involvement of the four orientation system signals severity but there is not a great deal of evidence in favour of this claim (Berrios 1982). 'Disorientation' concerns a failure in both 'knowing that' (verbal orientation) and 'knowing what' (behavioural orientation). Before the turn of the century, Sommer (1899) proposed that orientation questions be standardized: What is your name? Your job? Where are you? Where do you live? What year is it? What month?

What date? What day? How long are you here? What town is this? etc., and the same year Finzi (1899) completed outlining the concept of disorientation as a mental symptom. Earlier in the 19th century, it had already been suggested that disorientation was a clinical marker of acute brain syndromes (Sutton 1813; Dupuytren 1834). By the middle of the century, disorientation was seen as a transient memory disturbance (Winslow 1861; Falret 1865); and by the end of the century it had been firmly linked to cerebral arteriosclerosis (Mott 1899) and Parkinson's disease (König 1912).

Wernicke (1906) considered disorientation as 'the real essence of the psychoses' for 'there is no mental patient who is not disorientated in some way. If the symptom is absent, we can conclude that he is not mentally ill in a strict sense. In disorientation one finds reflected the damage caused by (the mostly unknown) disease process.' Wernicke's concept of disorientation was wide: 'in the mentally ill, all abnormal alterations of consciousness, whether transient or chronic, can be brought together under the concept of disorientation.' There were three forms of disorientation: somatopsychic (concerning the body), autopsychic (related to the self, personality, and identity), and allopsychic (pertaining to the environment). Hallucinations did not cause allopsychic disorientation unless the subject was also suffering from mental numbness.

Régis (1906) reported a subgroup of patients suffering from 'dementia praecox' who exhibited confusion and disorientation. Jung (1964) suggested that patients with dementia praecox were distracted by their 'illusions' and this only gave the impression of disorientation. Likewise, Bleuler (1950) believed that in dementia praecox there was no 'primary' failure of temporal orientation. Kraepelin (1919) agreed, although on occasions 'perception of the environment may be disordered in subjects with stupor or in the severely agitated.' Jaspers (1963) recognized four types of disorientation: amnesic, delusional, apathetic, and related to clouding of consciousness. Bleuler (1924) then drew attention to the phenomenon of psychotic 'double orientation'.

4 Psychiatric disorders mimicking dementia:

4.1 Copies produced by functional disorders

4.1.1 Psychosis

Schizophrenia, manic-depressive illness, and the cycloid psychosis are called 'functional psychoses' because no firm organic cause has yet been found for them. From the time of their construction as nosological entities, toxic, infectious, traumatic, genetic, and neurodevelopmental theories have been put forward to explain their origins. Likewise, with each new research technique, hopes are raised that their cause will be found. In relation to schizophrenia, such techniques include the analysis of urine of the 1920s, EEG, pneumoencephalography, early neurotransmitters (pink spot), neurogenetics, neuroimaging, and neuropsychology. Never-theless, this condition (if that is what it is) is currently still diagnosed on phenomenological grounds.

As mentioned above, the Anglo-Saxon view of schizophrenia (in opposition to the classical Continental view) does not countenance any disorders of consciousness as central symptoms. This makes life difficult for those who try to understand why schizophrenia frequently creates copies of dementia. The classical view, on the other hand, allowed for schizophrenia to be accompanied by confusion, e.g. oneirophrenia (Meduna 1950); the inhibition-confusion type of cycloid psychosis (Leonhard 1979); and the puerperal states (Marcé 1858), disorientation, and other persistent disorders of consciousness. This broader view provides a valid explanation and, importantly, the phenomenological elements on the basis of which a differential diagnosis can be developed.

4.1.2 Depression

Anecdotal reports that patients with depression develop 'dementia' have been extant since the 19th century (Berrios 1985) and may explain occasional 'miraculous improvements'. Debates and speculation continue, however, on the relationship between depression and dementia (Bulbena and Berrios 1986; O'Connor *et al.* 1990). A number of unresolved issues remain:

(a) Can 'depressive pseudo-dementia' (DPD) occur in a 'pure form' or is it always the result of an interaction between depression and dementia (Alexopoulos *et al.* 1993; Emery and Oxman 1997)?

(b) Are there types of depression which are more likely to be involved in DPD than others (Bourgeois *et al.* 1989)?

(c) Should 'subjective complaints of dysmnesia without measurable intellectual deficits' also be considered as a subtype of DPD (Yousef *et al.* 1998)?

(d) Is the term 'pseudodementia' appropriate (Reifler 1982; Zapotoczky 1998)?

(e) Is DPD simply a severe form of the well known association between low mood (whether spontaneous or induced) and cognitive deficit (Rapaport 1950; Miller 1975; Strömgren 1977; Jorm 1986; McDonald 1992; Kuiken 1991; Christianson 1992; Bulbena and Berrios 1993)?

(f) Does DPD 'predict' early dementia (Kral and Emery 1989) and early mortality (Arfken *et al.* 1999); and is it a risk factor for Alzheimer's disease (Raskind 1998)?

(g) Can DPD be characterized either in terms of a specific neuropsychological profile (Golinkoff and Sweeney 1989; Hill *et al.* 1993; desRosiers *et al.* 1995; Lachner and Engel 1994) or a biological marker (e.g. temporal lobe atrophy on MRI; O'Brien *et al.* 1994)?

The lack of general agreement in resolving the above issues can, in part, be explained in terms of differences in the samples of patients studied and theoretical perspective, and by the limitations in the sensitivity of current research techniques. Debates on whether DPD is or is not an appropriate term are precious. What matters is whether there is a term vivid enough to keep reminding clinicians of the relevance of mood disorders in the exercise of cognition. The sobriquet DPD remains particularly useful in patients with cognitive impairment, affective symptoms and history of depression, a neuropsychological profile showing scattering and inconsistencies, unhelpful neuroimaging, and good response to antidepressants or ECT. It is also useful in the case of patients in whom the 'short history' of dementia cannot account for the severity of the cognitive impairment. In these cases, and in the permutations that exist in between, the golden rule is to offer energetic treatment of the depressive symptoms as without doing thus it is impossible to evaluate the real level of cognitive impairment. There is no evidence that such treatment (including ECT) increases the risk of dementia (see Table 5.2).

4.1.3 Hysteria

Hysteria was once called the great mimic in psychiatry (Micale 1995; Halligan and David 1999). For reasons which remain obscure, cases of grand hysteria are now less frequent than they were a century ago but the possibility remains that the disease has simply changed configuration. If thus, it could be a plausible explanation for states of sudden onset dementia accompanied by exaggerated behaviours, acting out, histrionism, and occasional hallucinations. When occurring in the middle aged or elderly, syndromes such as the prison psychosis (Nitsche and Wilmanns 1912), Ganser syndrome, and hysterical fugues (see below) may also give rise to mimics of dementia. The neuropsychology of conversion hysteria is difficult to disentangle (Sierra and Berrios 1999).

Table 5.2 Factors complicating the assessment of depressive pseudodementia (DPD)

Terminology	Is the term 'pseudodementia' appropriate?
Nature of relationship between depression, dementia, and DPD	Is DPD a separate syndrome or is it always the result of interaction between depression and dementia?
	Is DPD a severe form of the known association between low mood and cognitive deficit?
Nature of DPD	Are there types of depression which are more likely to be involved in DPD than others?
	Should subjective complaints of memory problems without accompanying measurable objective deficits be considered a subtype of DPD?
	Does DPD predict the onset of early dementia?
	Can DPD be characterized by phenomenology, neuropsychology, or biological markers?

4.1.3a Ganser syndrome and 'Ganserian answers'

The full Ganser syndrome (GS) is currently met with far less frequently than the clinical state called 'Ganserian answers' (GA). In the eyes of the neophyte, both can appear as copies of 'dementia'. GA consists of the production of 'I don't know' or approximate or 'past-the-point' answers to simple questions (e.g. how many ears do you have? Three, etc.). Patients rarely take offence at the childish nature of the questions. Even questions like 'what is your name' or 'what is this' (watch, money, etc.) cause difficulty but stimulate answers which are within the semantic area of the question, showing that the general theme (identity, time, place, etc.) of the question has been understood. Ganser believed that these patients retain the ability to understand questions but have a psychogenic inability to give correct answers (Allen *et al.* 2000).

In addition to GA, patients with GS show clouding of awareness, disorganized sense of space and time, hallucinations (occasionally they re-enact or re-live in a hallucinatory manner traumatic experiences), general or partial analgesia of the body (mouth area included) which may move around according to time of day, and a disorder of consciousness consisting of a subtle, dreamy confusion that has been called 'twilight state'. Interestingly, the patient shows no memory loss for the period before the appearance *en masse* of the symptoms. There may be history of physical trauma (blows about the head, etc.) and patients may be awaiting trial. Ganser believed that both GS and GA occurred in the framework of traumatic or reactive hysteria (Allen *et al.* 2000).

GS has been reported in the wake of brain disease but Latcham *et al.* (1968) believed that it was also mediated by hysteria. Whitlock (1967) suggested that GS be 'restricted to patients who, following cerebral trauma or in the course of an acute psychosis, develop clouding of consciousness …' (p. 28). Heron *et al.* (1991) reported a GS in a patient with history of brain damage and polysubstance abuse; and Sigal *et al.* (1992) conclude that Ganser patients show 'symptoms of premorbid neurological pathology'. GS has also been reported in association with carbon monoxide intoxication (McEvoy and Campbell 1977) and with a left hemisphere tumour (Doongaji *et al.* 1975). The possibility of a GS should be raised in cases of atypical amnesia with GA and history of psychic or physical trauma.

4.1.3b. Hysterical fugues

'Hysterical fugue' refers to a clinical situation where the patient (usually young) claims to have lost autobiographical memory to the point of not knowing who he is. Language and other forms of memory are usually preserved.

'Fugues' were first described during the late 19th century. Charcot (1987) called them 'wandering behaviour' and reported the case of a 23-year-old Hungarian Jew admitted to La Salpêtrière after criss-crossing Europe in a state of fugue. Voisin (1889) likewise observed a case of 'hysterical' automatism in a subject with epilepsy and Meige (1893) created the concept of the 'wandering Jew'. Raymond (1896) concluded that 'fugue states constituted a syndrome' seen in epilepsy, hysteria, and degeneration states.

The early 20th century saw an explosion of publications on the fugue state. Hamelin (1908) classified fugues into:

(a) 'Ambulatory automatisms' as seen in epilepsy, hysteria, and somnambulism.

(b) 'Dromomanes', mainly affected by mental degeneration.

(c) Psychotic fugues, for example, in chronic hallucinatory states, paranoiacs, etc.

Benon and Froissart (1908) defined 'fugue' as: 'a transient, paroxysmal and non-habitual disorder of action during which the patient will displace himself short or long distances under the influence of a psychological abnormal state'. Abeles and Schilder (1935) emphasized the transient loss of autobiographical information (including personal identity). Spontaneous recovery occurred in most cases, and 'behind the superficial conflicts which precipitated the amnesia [many had] deeper motives ...' (p. 609). Stengel (1941) found that his patients had a disturbed childhood, were prone to compulsive lying, and showed a tendency to periodic changes in mood and to developing 'twilight states'. In other papers, Stengel (1943) suggested that 'fugues with an impulse to wander occur in a variety of conditions' and that 'the symbolic meaning of the fugue' was important (Stengel 1943).

Based on the examination of 30 patients, Parfitt and Gall (1944) concluded that:

(a) Both organic and hysterical factors contributed to the development of the fugue states.

(b) 'Personal recall' (their name for autobiographical memory) was more often affected than impersonal recall (semantic memory).

(c) Patients do not forget but refuse to remember.

(d) The difference between hysterical amnesia and malingering was only one of degree.

Berrington *et al.* (1956) suggested that alcoholism, hysterical mechanisms, and brain injury were more important causal factors than 'disturbed childhood'.

Fugue states continue to pose a diagnostic conundrum (Bergeron 1956; Rice and Fisher 1976; Akhtar and Brenner 1979; Behr *et al.* 1985; Riether and Stoudemire 1988; Loewenstein 1996), particularly in older patients when differential diagnosis with 'transient global amnesia' must be made (Hodges 1991).

4.2 Copies produced by organic disorders

The term 'reversible' dementia is a useful misnomer to refer to a group of clinical conditions with insidious onset but rapid progression leading to a state of 'dementia' difficult to distinguish (on the cross-sectional examination) from the conventional forms (Draper 1991). They have been called reversible for, if diagnosed early, can be reversed or arrested. Ideally, this group should be ruled out earlier in the diagnostic process. Although the reversible dementias share clinical features, for example, rapid progression, periods of confusion, fluctuations, lucid periods, early urinary incontinence, psychomotor disorders, there is no reason to believe that the same mechanisms are involved as in the production of 'dementia'.

Under different names, the reversible dementias have been known at least since the beginning of the 20th century. For example, Séglas (1903) wrote: 'The defective expressions 'acute dementia' and 'primitive curable dementia' refer to forms of mental confusion and stupor characterized by a diminution or suspension of psychological activity and a profound obnubilation of consciousness without emotional disorder which only superficially resemble true dementia.' These clinical states were also called 'pseudo-dementias' and the best known was 'primitive mental confusion'. Subjects suffering from this disorder were described as: 'disorientated, unable to recognize familiar persons or objects, unable to remember anything; they may offer vague and incoherent replies often due to a disorder of language due to the loss of the image in certain words, in this case the disorder is called 'pseudo-aphasic mental confusion'. In other occasions linguistic hesitations are due to slowness of thinking. Their attention is always impaired and they are easily distractible. Perception of external objects and internal sensations is defective and this adds to the confusion. Imagination is abolished and voluntary movements may be aimless and disorganized … to these symptoms other are added such as hallucinations and delusions, often sad in content and with the characteristics of dreams. There may also be impulsive gestures and stereotyped acts; in general patients show emotional indifference although, on occasions, they may get anxious in response to their delusions and hallucinations' (Séglas 1903). This clinical description remains unsurpassed.

Some of the 'reversible dementias', such as those caused by melancholia and hysteria, myxoedematous madness, and brain lumps (tumours, clots) have been known since the late 19th century; others, such as vitamin B12 deficiency and normal pressure hydrocephalus, only since the 1960s (although there is historical evidence of earlier reports of similar clinical conditions under a different name). In the rest of this section, the clinical and therapeutic aspects of these states will be described (Draper 1991).

4.2.1 B12 deficiency

Required in the synthesis of myelin, B12 is absorbed by the terminal ileum combined with a transport (intrinsic) factor produced in the parietal cells of the stomach (Lindenbaum 1980). Disorders of either the parietal cells (ulcers and surgical removal) (Buxton *et al.* 1977; Enk *et al.* 1980; Roos 1978) or of the ileum (inflammatory bowel disease) may reduce B12 and folate availability. Another factor is poor nutritional conditions (Carney 1967), particularly in the elderly (Marcus and Freedman 1985). Absorption, however, does not seem to decline with age *per se* (McEvoy *et al.* 1982).

B12 deficiency may cause pernicious anaemia, combined degeneration of the spinal chord, psychosis (Evans *et al.* 1983), and a rapidly progressive form of dementia characterized by marked and intermittent confusion and EEG slowness (Gaymard and Derouesne 1989; Zucker *et al.* 1981). Folate and B12 deficiency syndromes are morphologically indistinguishable (Botez and Reynolds 1979; Marcus and Freedman 1985). The Macrocytic anaemia is not omnipresent marker (Evans *et al.* 1983; Lindenbaum *et al.* 1988). The disorder can be arrested by the administration of cyanocobalamine.

4.2.2 Hypothyroidism

Known at least since the second half of the 19th century, myxoedematous madness (Report 1888) shows, in addition to weight gain, pallor, facial puffiness, dry hair, motor slowness, and bradycardia, a typical torpor and psychological slowness, depression, memory impairment, touchiness, irritability an paranoid ideas (Savage 1892; Goggans *et al.* 1986). If not diagnosed on time, subjects are left with a degree of cognitive impairment. Masked by ageing, the disorder can be easily missed in the elderly.

Mild, moderate, and severe grades of hypothyroidism have been described. Affective symptoms seem more common in the mild form (Bauer *et al.* 1990); and cognitive disorder in the moderate and severe grades (Denicoff *et al.* 1990). There is still some debate as to whether thyroxin replacement should aim at 'biochemical' or 'behavioural' improvement; psychiatrists should favour the latter.

4.2.3 Normal pressure hydrocephalus

NPH refers to a form of communicating hydrocephalus with cognitive impairment (Caltagirone *et al.* 1982; Stambrook *et al.* 1988) which typically develops during the fifth decade of life in subjects with occasional history of encephalitis or meningitis. First reported during the Second World War (David *et al.* 1943), it was rediscovered by Hakim and Adams (1965). Rapidly progressing memory impairment, apraxia of the initiation of gait ('magnetic gait'), early urinary incontinence, absence of festination or other parkinsonian features, and temporary improvement upon removal of CSF are central features (Price and Tucker 1977; Pickard 1982; Grafft-Radford and Godersky 1986; Frank and Tew 1982). It may be associated with affective disorder (Rosen and Swigar 1976). Neuroimaging shows enlarged lateral ventricles and compression of the cortical mantle (Jacobs and Kinkel 1976). The mechanisms involved in this disorder remain obscure but are likely to involve both the circulation of CSF and white matter disorders (Koto *et al.* 1977). When diagnosed correctly, patients respond well to shunting (Ahlberg *et al.* 1988). The main differential diagnosis is other forms of dementia with enlarged ventricles and a motor syndrome.

4.2.4 Space-occupying lesions

Nature, rate of growth, and location of tumour or clot will determine whether they give rise to neurological (Thomas 1983) or psychiatric symptoms (Mulder and Swenson 1974). For example, a meningioma growing slowly in the frontal area is more likely to produce psychiatric symptoms (Angelergues *et al.* 1955) whilst an astrocytoma growing rapidly in a confined area will probably have a 'neurological' presentation. It has been known for a long time that tumours may give rise to a 'dementia-like' state characterized by morosity, motor slowness, memory impairment, episodic disorientation, irritability, and self-neglect (Duret 1905; Dupré 1903; Baruk 1926; Keschner *et al.* 1936).

Volume changes secondary to histopathological changes within the lump may, in turn, cause intermittent changes in intensity of the symptoms and even the occasional 'lucid interval'. This is particularly the case with chronic subdural haematoma when the patient, usually an elderly person, is reported as having developed confusion and/or dementia rather rapidly, without any history of trauma, and which is typically intermittent in nature (Brockelhurst 1982; Patrick and Gates 1984; Windhager *et al.* 1988). When the clot becomes isodense with the brain it might not be seen on CAT scan (Jacobson and Farmer 1979) and in these cases a plain X-ray may be more informative.

4.3 Copies produced by drug-induced states

All psychiatric drugs (e.g. neuroleptics, tricyclic antidepressants, anticholinergics, benzodiazepines) cause side-effects and some of these can mimic aspects of dementia.

4.3.1 Neuroleptics

Traditional neuroleptics such as haloperidol, chlorpromazine, thioridazine, triofluoperazine, etc. cause motor and cognitive symptoms some of which can give the superficial impression of dementia. Excessive slowness, bradykinesia, and bradyphrenia may lock the patient in affect responsiveness. Excessive tranquillization and sedation may in turn lead to slow mentation, reduce cognitive responsiveness, and some memory and attentional impairment. There is no direct dose–effect relationship although large doses are likely to produce more symptoms than smaller ones. Misdiagnosis of dementia is likely to be more common in situations where the neuroleptic has been used to sedate the patient and has accumulated through time and there are no obvious parkinsonian features.

In the elderly, symptoms and signs may continue for two or three months after the medication has been stopped. Of all the conventional neuroleptics listed above, those with higher anticholinergic effect (e.g. thioridazine) tend to cause more cognitive slowing. The newer or atypical antipsychotics are said to cause fewer side-effects related to the dopamine and cholinergic systems. Little is known in regards to long-term side-effects as these drugs have not been around for long enough. In subjects who have received leucotomies, a syndrome of abnormal movements and dementia has been reported caused by treatment with phenothiazines (Hunter *et al.* 1964).

4.3.2 Tricyclic antidepressants

Although effective antidepressants, these drugs have been known for a long time to cause states similar to dementia, particularly in the elderly, and seemingly through their marked anticholinergic effect. Amitriptyline appears to be, in this respect, one of the worst. The anticholinergic syndrome was first described in the 19th century as a result of intoxication with atropa belladona. Whilst the acute syndrome, which includes vivid visual hallucinations (typically of rolling flames), episodic restlessness, confusion, and inversion of the sleeping rhythm, is easily recognizable and unlikely to mimic dementia, the chronic anticholinergic states are more likely to be thus mistaken. These are mainly characterized by memory and attentional impairment and have a neuropsychological profile similar to that seen in Alzheimer's disease (Davis and Berger 1979). Indeed, there was a time when anticholinergic substances were used to cause 'experimental' states of dementia. In the elderly, tertiary tricyclic antidepressants can cause cognitive impairment even when prescribed within 'normal' dosage. Cognitive deficits may persist for weeks after the medication has been stopped.

4.3.3 Benzodiazepines

There has been much debate on the side-effects of the benzodiazepines. Of relevance here, are the so-called 'frontal lobe' changes, chronic drowsiness, and confusion attributed to diazepam and nitrazepam which can, occasionally, mimic dementia.

4.3.4 Other drugs

Reversible cognitive impairment may also be caused by drugs used in neuropsychiatric practice such as those used for cardiovascular disorders, analgesics, antiepileptics, antiparkinsonians, cimetidine, and some antibiotics (Farlow and Hake 1998). Steroids are also known to cause psychoses (Hall *et al.* 1978) and dementia-like states (Varney 1984). Cyclophosphamide and other cytotoxic agents used to treat 'viral encephalitis' may also cause persistent confusion which may persist for days after the drug has been discontinued.

5 Conclusions

Patients suffering from certain mental symptoms and diseases, some organic brain states, and from side-effects of treatment may present with mental states mimicking dementia. Exploration of the reasons and mechanisms causing such similarities shows that both the concepts and boundaries associated with mental symptoms and disorders may be involved and that it is not just a question of identifying further discriminators. Indeed, what 'similarity' means and how it is represented in the context of psychopathology requires clarification.

Tackling such a problem needs both historico-conceptual analysis and clinical exploration. How are these two components to be blended in a chapter whose brief is fundamentally clinical? Playing it the conventional way and invoking evidence-based medicine and Medline searches will not do. The strategy followed in this chapter has been to add historico-conceptual information and treat the past and present as seamless. For only if the reader understands that 'dementia' is not a real and stable object but a historical construction can he/she begin to realize that mimics and behavioural phenocopies are not simply an 'empirical problem' but also the unavoidable consequence of the boundary fuzziness of the notions involved.

It is also clear that empirical research alone cannot resolve the problem. For as it takes place within a 'received' view, such an approach is in most cases tautological. The very methods that make the results more 'reliable', i.e. collecting the same patients with the same instruments and assumptions, cannot but generate yet more empty replications. To understand the problem of mimics, a step back must be taken and the question asked whether the concepts involved in the confusion can themselves generate enough information to be set asunder.

Dementia started as a wide concept. By the late 19th century it suffered much conceptual attrition and the 'cognitive paradigm' was born. Consequently, numerous clinical discriminators were lost. Memory impairment became the only real hard variable in terms of which dementia could be differentiated from other disorders. But memory is not a fixed concept either: models changed and with them the definition of dementia. The worrying thing is that there is no evidence that current views on memory and cognition are any more stable than earlier ones. Hence, the boundaries of dementia as a cognitive disorder are likely to remain inherently unstable. The main lesson to be learned from this is that the compulsive search for discriminators will not solve the clinical problem of copies. A broadening of the concept of dementia to include a gamut of mental symptoms and the concomitant re-mapping of the accompanying clinical categories may be the only solution here. This can only be - undertaken if more research is carried out on the factors that govern the drawing of boundaries around dementia and other clinical categories. In the meantime, the task of differentiating dementia from its copies must continue being based on phenomenology and discriminators. Sufficient information on both these elements has dutifully been offered above (see key points).

6 Key points

1 Dementia can be mimicked or copied by other diseases and mental states.

2 The nature of clinical mimics or copies is poorly understood.

3 Mimics may be due to:
   (i) Conceptual boundary fuzziness.
   (ii) Lack of sensitive discriminators for mental states or symptoms that appear similar.

4 Dementia may be copied:

  (i) By *single* symptoms which may *mimic* the disease.

  (ii) By combinations of symptoms of manifold provenance (*'behavioural phenocopies'*).

5 Crucial to the understanding of mimics and phenocopies is the concept of similarity which also requires conceptual analysis.

6 Symptoms mimicking dementia relate to disorders of consciousness and include confusion and disorientation.

7 Originally considered as intrinsic to all psychoses, disorders of consciousness and confusion are now exclusively linked to the 'organic' disorders. Hence, when met with in the context of a functional psychosis they are either:

  (i) Ignored.

  (ii) Explained on the basis of dissociation/malingering.

  (iii) Taken to indicate the presence of superimposed acute organic disease.

8 Behavioural phenocopies can be produced by:

  (i) 'Functional' disorders (e.g. depression, hysteria, psychoses).

  (ii) 'Organic' disorders (e.g. hypothyroidism, B12 deficiency).

  (iii) Drug-induced states (e.g. antipsychotics, anticholinergics).

9 'Depressive pseudodementia' is a final common pathway to which contribute both genuine cognitive deficits and behavioural phenocopies.

10 Historical research shows that symptoms and disorders (including, memory deficits, dementia, psychosis, etc.) are not conceptually stable. This has consequences for their definition and classification. The nature of, and mechanisms underlying dementia mimics can only be understood if conceptual and empirical research are combined.

References

Abeles, M. and Schilder, P. (1935). Psychogenic loss of personal identity. *Archives of Neurology and Psychiatry*, **34**, 587–604.

Ahlberg, J., Norlen, L., Blomstrand, C., and Wikkelsö, C. (1988). Outcome of shunt operation on urinary incontinence in normal pressure hydrocephalus. *Journal of Neurology, Neurosurgery and Psychiatry*, **51**, 105–8.

Akhtar, S. and Brenner, I. (1979). Differential diagnosis of fugue-like states. *Journal Clinical Psychiatry*, **40**, 381–5.

Allen, D. F., Postel, J., and Berrios, G. E. (2000). The Ganser syndrome. In *Memory disorders in psychiatric practice* (ed. G. E. Berrios and J. R. Hodges), pp. 443–55. Cambridge, Cambridge University Press.

Alexopoulos, G. S., Meyers, B. S., Young, R. C., *et al.* (1993). The course of geriatric depression with 'reversible dementia': a controlled study. *American Journal of Psychiatry*, **150**, 1693–9.

American Psychiatric Association. (1994). *Diagnostic and statistical manual of mental disorders*, 4th edn. Washington, DC, American Psychiatric Association.

Angelergues, R., Hécaen, H., and Ajuriaguerra, J. de (1955). Les Troubles mentaux au cours des tumeurs du lobe frontal. *Annales Médico-Psychologiques*, **113**, 577–642.

Arfken, C. L., Lichtenberg, P. A., and Tancer, M. E. (1999). Cognitive impairment and depression predict mortality in medically ill older adults. *Journal of Gerontology*, **54**, M152–6.

Baruk, H. (1926). *Les Troubles Mentaux dans les Tumeurs Cérébrales*. Paris, Octave Doin.

Bauer, M. S., Whybrow, P. C., and Winokur, A. (1990). Rapid cyclic bipolar affective disorder, I: association with Grade I hypothyroidism. *Archives General Psychiatry*, **47**, 427–31.

Behr, F., Croq, L., and Vauterin, C. (1985). Sémiologie des conduites de fugue. *Encyclopédie Médico- Chirurgicale* (Paris) Psychiatrie, 37113 A10, 2, Paris, Editions Techniques.

Benon, R. and Froissart, P. (1908). Fugue et vagabondage. Définition et étude clinique *Annales Médico-Psychologiques*, **66**, 305–12.

Benton, A. L., Allen, M. W. van, and Fogel, M. L. (1964). Temporal orientation in cerebral disease. *Journal Nervous Mental Disease*, **139**, 110–19.

Bergeron, M. (1956). Fugues. In *Encyclopédie Médico-Chirurgicale*. Psychiatrie, 37140 E10. Paris, Editions Techniques.

Berrington, W. P., Liddell, D. W., and Foulds, G. A. (1956). A Re-evaluation of the fugue. *Journal of Mental Science*, **102**, 280–6.

Berrios, G. E. (1981). Delirium and confusion in the 19th century. *British Journal of Psychiatry*, **139**, 439–49.

Berrios, G. E. (1982). Disorientation states in psychiatry. *Comprehensive Psychiatry*, **23**, 479–91.

Berrios, G. E. (1985). 'Depressive Pseudodementia' or 'Melancholic Dementia': A 19th Century View. *Journal of Neurology, Neurosurgery and Psychiatry*, **48**, 393–400.

Berrios, G. E. (1987). Dementia during the 17th and 18th Century: A Conceptual History. *Psychological Medicine*, **17**, 829–37.

Berrios, G. E. (1989). Non-cognitive symptoms and the diagnosis of dementia. Historical and clinical aspects. *British Journal of Psychiatry*, **154**, 11–16.

Berrios, G. E. (1999). Towards a new descriptive psychopathology. A sine qua non for neurobiological research in psychiatry. *Brain Research Bulletin*, **50**, 457–8.

Berrios, G. E. and Samuel, B. (1987). Affective disorder in the neurological patient. *Journal of Nervous and Mental Disease*, **175**, 173–6.

Bleuler, E. (1924). *Textbook of Psychiatry*. New York, Macmillan.

Bleuler, M. (1950). Psychiatry of cerebral diseases. *British Medical Journal*, **ii**, 1233–8.

Bonhoeffer, K. (1910). *Die symptomatischen Psychosen*. Leipzig, Deuticke.

Botez, M. I. and Reynolds, E. H. (ed.) (1979). *Folic acid in neurology, psychiatry and internal medicine*. New York, Raven Press.

Bouchard, R. (1926). *Sur l'Evaluation du Temps dans Certains Troubles Mentaux*, Thèse de Paris, Vigot frères Editeurs.

Bourgeois, M., Peyre, F., and Verdeux, H. (1989). Mémoire et depression. *Annales Médico-Psychologiques*, **147**, 850–7.

Brockelhurst, G. (1982). Subdural haematoma. *British Journal of Hospital Medicine*, **27**, 170–4.

Bulbena, A. and Berrios, G. E. (1986). Pseudodementia: Facts and Figures. *British Journal of Psychiatry*, **148**, 87–94.

Bulbena, A. and Berrios, G. E. (1993). Cognitive function in the affective disorders: a prospective study. *Psychopathology*, **26**, 6–12.

Buxton, R. A., Collins, C. D., and Phillips, M. J. (1977). Vitamin B12 deficiency following polya gastrectomy. *The British Journal of Clinical Practice*, **31**, 69–72.

Caltagirone, C., Gainotti, G., Masullo, C., and Villa, G. (1982). Neuropsychological study of normal pressure hydrocephalus. *Acta Psychiatrica Scandinavica*, **65**, 93–100.

Carney, M. W. P. (1967). Serum Folate Values in 423 psychiatric patients. *British Medical Journal*, **ii**, 512–16.

Charcot, J. M. (1987). *The Tuesday Lessons* (Translated by C. G. Goetz). New York, Raven Press.

Chaslin, Ph. (1895). *La confusion mentale primitive*. Paris, Asselin et Houzeau.

Christianson, S.-A. (ed.) (1992). *The handbook of emotions and memory*. Hillsdale, New Jersey, Lawrence Erlbaum.

David, Hécaen, and Fouquet, (no initials in original). (1943). Démence, distension ventriculaire, disparition progressive des troubles mentaux après ouverture de la lame optique. *Annales Médico-Psychologiques*, **101**, 435–8.

Davis, K. L. and Berger, P. A. (ed.) (1979). *Brain acetylcholine and neuropsychiatric disease*. New York, Plenum Press.

Denicoff, K. D., Joffe, R. T., Lakshmanan, M. C, Robbins, J., and Rubikow, D. R. (1990). Neuropsychiatric manifestations of altered thyroid state. *American Journal of Psychiatry*, **147**, 94–9.

desRosiers, G., Hodges, J. R., and Berrios, G. E. (1995). The neuropsychological differentiation of patients with very mild Alzheimer's disease and /or major depression. *Journal of the American Geriatric Society*, **43**, 1256–63.

Doongaji, D. R., Apte, J. S., and Bhat, R. (1975). Ganser like state (syndrome), an unusual presentation of a space occupying lesion of the dominant hemisphere. *Neurology India*, **23**, 143–8.

Draper, B. (1991). Potentially reversible dementia: a review. *Australian and New Zealand Journal of Psychiatry*, **25**, 506–18.

Dupré, E. (1903). Tumeurs de l'encéphale. In *Traité de Pathologie Mentale* (ed. G. Ballet), pp. 1164–91. Paris, Doin.

Dupré, E. (1913). Les cénestopathies. *Mouvement Médical*, **23**, 3–22.

Dupré, E. (1925). *Pathologie de l'imagination et de l'émotivité*. Paris, Payot.

Dupuytren Baron, de. (1834). On Nervous Delirium. *Lancet*, **i**, 919–23.

Duret, H. (1905). *Les Tumeurs de L'Encéphale*. Paris, Alcan.

Emery, V. O. and Oxman, T. E. (1997). Depressive pseudo-dementia: a 'transitional' dementia. *Clinical Neuroscience*, **4**, 23–30.

Enk, C., Hougaard, K., and Hippe, E. (1980). Reversible dementia and neuropathy associated with folate deficiency 16 years after partial gastrectomy. *Scandinavian Journal of Haematology*, **25**, 63–6.

Evans, D. L., Gail, M. S., Edelsohn, G. A., and Golden, R. N. (1983). Organic psychosis without anemia or spinal cord symptoms in patients with Vitamin B12 deficiency. *American Journal of Psychiatry*, **140**, 218–21.

Extein, I. and Gold, M. S. (ed.) (1986). *Medical mimics of psychiatric disorders*. Washington, American Psychiatric Press.

Ey, H. (1963). *La conscience*. Paris, Presses Universitaires de France.

Falret, J. Amnesie. (1865). In *Dictionnaire encyclopédique des sciences médicales* (ed. A. Dechambre), Vol. 3, pp. 725–42. Paris, Asselin and Masson.

Farlow, M. R. and Hake, A. M. (1998). Drug-induced cognitive impairment. In *Iatrogenic neurology* (ed. J. Biller), pp. 203–14. Boston, Butterworths-Heinemann.

Finzi, J. (1899). Sul Sintoma Disorientamiento. *Rivista di Patologia Nervosa e Mentale*, **4**, 347–62.

Frank, E. and Tew, J. M. (1982). Normal-pressure hydrocephalus: clinical symptoms, diagnosis, pathophysiology and treatment. *Heart and Lung*, **11**, 321–6.

Gaymard, B. and Derouesne, C. (1989). Démences et syndrome carentiel en vitamine B12. *Gazette Médicale* (Paris), **96**, 35–40.

Goggans, F. C., Allen, R. M. and Gold, M. S. (1986). Primary hypothyroidism and its relationship to affective disorder. In *Medical mimics of psychiatric disorders* (ed. I. Extein and M. S. Gold), pp. 93–110. Washington, American Psychiatric Press.

Golinkoff, M. and Sweeney, J. A. (1989). Cognitive impairment in depression. *Journal of Affective Disorders*, **17**, 105–12.

Goodman, N. (1992). Seven strictures on similarity. In *How classification works* (ed. M. Douglas and D. Hull), pp. 13–23. Edinburgh, Edinburgh University Press.

Grafft-Radford, N. R. and Godersky, J. C. (1986). Normal-pressure hydrocephalus. *Archives of Neurology*, **43**, 940–2.

Hakim, S. and Adams, R. D. (1965). The special clinical problems of symptomatic hydrocephalus with normal cerebrospinal fluid pressure. *Journal of Neurological Science*, **2**, 307–27.

Hall, R. C. W., Popkin, M. K., Stickney, S. K., and Gardner, E. R. (1978). Presentation of the 'steroid psychosis'. *Journal of Nervous and Mental Disease*, **167**, 229–36.

Halligan, P. W. and David, A. S. (ed.) (1999). *Conversion hysteria*. London, Psychology Press.

Hamelin, F. G. (1908). *Contribution à l'Étude des Fugues*. Lille, Le Bigot Frères.

Heron, E. A., Kritchevski, M., and Delis, D. C. (1991). The neuropsychological presentation of Ganser syndrome. *Journal of Clinical and Experimental Neuropsychology*, **13**, 652–66.

Hill, C. D., Stoudemire, A., Morris, R., *et al.* (1993). Similarities and differences in memory deficits in patients with primary dementia and depression-related cognitive dysfunction. *Journal of Neuropsychiatry and Clinical Neurosciences*, **5**, 277–82.

Hodges, J. R. (1991). *Transient amnesia. Clinical and neuropsychological aspects*. London, Saunders.

Hunter, R., Earl, C. J., and Janz, D. (1964). A syndrome of abnormal movements and dementia in leucotomized patients treated with phenothiazines. *Journal of Neurology, Neurosurgery and Psychiatry*, **27**, 219–23.

Jacobs, L. and Kinkel, W. (1976). Computerized axial transverse tomography in normal pressure hydrocephalus. *Neurology*, **26**, 501–7.

Jacobson, P. L. and Farmer, T. W. (1979). The 'hypernormal' CT scan and dementia: bilateral isodense subdural haematomas. *Neurology*, **29**, 1522–4.

Jaspers, K. (1963). *General psychopathology* (Translated by M. Hamilton and J. Hoenig). Manchester, Manchester University Press.

Jorm, A. F. (1986). Cognitive deficit in the depressed elderly. *Australian and New Zealand Journal of Psychiatry*, **20**, 11–22.

Jung, C. G. (1964). The psychology of dementia praecox. In *The collected works*, Vol. 3. London, Routledge and Kegan Paul.

Keschner, M., Bender, M. B., and Strauss, I. (1936). Mental symptoms in cases of tumour of the temporal lobe. *Archives of Neurology and Psychiatry*, **35**, 572–96.

Klein, R. and Mayer-Gross, W. (1957). *The clinical examination of patients with organic cerebral disease*. London, Cassell.

König, H. (1912). Zur Psychopathologie der Paralysis Agitans. *Archives für Psychiatrie und Nervenkrankheiten*, **50**, 285–305.

Koto, A., Rosenberg, G., Zingesser, L. H., *et al.* (1977). Syndrome of normal pressure hydrocephalus: possible relation to hypertensive and arteriosclerotic vasculopathy. *Journal of Neurology, Neurosurgery and Psychiatry*, **40**, 73–9.

Kraepelin, E. (1899). *Psychiatrie. Ein Lehrbuch für Studirende und Aerzte*, 6th edn, Vol. 2. Leipzig, Johann Ambrosius Barth.

Kraepelin, E. (1919). *Dementia praecox and paraphrenia*. Edinburgh, Livingstone.

Kral, V. A. and Emery, O. B. (1989). Long-term follow up of depressive pseudo-dementia of the aged. *Canadian Journal of Psychiatry*, **34**, 445–6.

Kuiken, D. (ed.) (1991). *Mood and memory*. London, Sage.

Lachner, G. and Engel, R. R. (1994). Differentiation of dementia and depression by memory tests. A meta-analysis. *Journal of Nervous and Mental Disease*, **182**, 34–9.

Latchman, R., White, A., Sims A., (1968). Ganser Syndrome: the aetiological argument. *Journal of Neurology*, Neurosurgery and Psychiatry, **41**, 851–854.

Leonhard, K. (1979). *The classification of the endogenous psychoses*. New York, John Wiley.

Lindenbaum, J. (1980). Malabsorption of vitamin B12 and folate. *Current Concepts in Nutrition*, **9**, 105–23.

Lindenbaum, J., Healton, E. B., Savage, D. G., *et al.* (1988). Neuropsychiatric disorders caused by cobalamin deficiency in the absence of anemia or macrocytosis. *New England Journal of Medicine*, **318**, 1720–8.

Loewenstein, R. J. (1996). Dissociative amnesia and dissociative fugue. In *Handbook of dissociation: Theoretical, empirical, and clinical perspectives* (ed. L. K. Michelson and W. J. Ray), pp. 307–36. New York, Plenum Press.

Marcé, L. V. (1858). *Traité de la folie des femmes enceintes, des nouvelles accouchées et des nourrices*. Paris, Baillière.

Marcus, D. L. and Freedman, M. L. (1985). Folic acid deficiency in the elderly. *Journal of the American Geriatric Society*, **33**, 552–8.

McDonald, A. J. D. (1992). Old age depression and organic brain change. In *Recent advances in psychogeriatrics* II (ed. T. Arie). Edinburgh, Churchill and Livingstone.

McEvoy, A. W., Fenwick, J. D., Boddy, K., and James, O. F. W. (1982). Vitamin B12 absorption from the gut does not decline with age in normal elderly humans. *Age and Ageing*, **11**, 180–3.

McEvoy, N. and Campbell, T. (1977). Ganser like signs in carbon monoxide encephalopathy. *American Journal of Psychiatry*, **134**, 453–4.

Meduna, L. J. (1950). *Oneirophrenia: the confusional state*. Urbana, The University of Illinois Press.

Meige, H. (1893). *Études sur certains névropathes voyageurs. Le Juif errant à la Salpêtrière*. Paris, Bataille.

Micale, M. (1995). *Approaching hysteria*. Princeton, Princeton University Press.

Miller, W. R. (1975). Psychological deficits in depression. *Psychological Bulletin*, **82**, 238–60.

Mott, F. W. (1899). Arterial degenerations and diseases. In *A system of medicine* (ed. T. C. Allbutt), Vol. IV, pp. 294–344. London, Macmillan.

Mulder, D. W. and Swenson, W. M. (1974). Psychological and psychiatric aspects of brain tumours. In *Handbook of clinical neurology* (ed. P. J. Vinken and G. W. Bruyn), Vol. 16, pp. 727–40. Tumours of the brain and skull. Amsterdam, North Holland.

Nitsche, P. and Wilmanns, K. (1912). *The history of the prison psychoses*. Monograph N° 13, New York, The Journal of Nervous and Mental Disease Publishing.

O'Brien, J. T., Desmond, P., Ames, D., *et al.* (1994). The differentiation of depression from dementia by temporal lobe magnetic resonance imaging. *Psychological Medicine*, **24**, 633–40.

O'Connor, D. W., Pollit, O. A., Roth, M., *et al.* (1990). Memory complaints and impairment in normal, depressed, and demented elderly persons identified in a community survey. *Archives of General Psychiatry*, **47**, 224–7.

OED (1992). *Oxford English Dictionary*, 2nd edn. Oxford, Oxford University Press.

Parfitt, D. N. and Gall, C. C. C. (1944). Psychogenic amnesia: the refusal to remember. *The Journal of Mental Science*, **90**, 511–31.

Patrick, D. and Gates, P. C. (1984). Chronic subdural haematoma in the elderly. *Age and Ageing*, **13**, 367–9.

Perry, R., McKeith, I., and Perry, E. (ed.) (1996). *Dementia with Lewy bodies*. Cambridge, Cambridge University Press.

Pickard, J. (1982). Adult communicating hydrocephalus. *British Journal of Hospital Medicine*, **27**, 35–44.

Price, T. R. P. and Tucker, G. J. (1977). Psychiatric and behavioural manifestations of normal pressure hydrocephalus. *Journal of Nervous and Mental Disease*, **164**, 51–5.

Rapaport, D. (1950). *Emotions and memory*. New York, International Universities Press.

Raskind, M. A. (1998). The clinical interface of depression and dementia. *Journal of Clinical Psychiatry*, **59** (Suppl 10), 9–12.

Raymond, F. (1896). *Leçons sur les maladies du système nerveux. (Clinique de la Salpêtrière 1894–1895)*. Paris, Doin, Lectures 31 and 32.

Redlich, E. (1912). *Die Psychosen bei Gehirnerkrankungen*. Leipzig, Deuticke.

Régis, E. (1906). *Précis de Psychiatrie*. Paris, Doin.

Reifler, B. V. (1982). Arguments for abandoning the term pseudo-dementia. *Journal of the American Geriatric Association*, **30**, 665–8.

Report (1888). Report of a Committee of the Clinical Society of London on Myxoedema. *Clinical Society Transactions*. Supplement 21.

Rey, A. (1995). *Dictionnaire historique de la langue française*. 2 Vols. Paris, Dictionnaires Le Robert.

Rice, E. and Fisher, C. (1976). Fugue states in sleep and wakefulness: a physiological study. *Journal of Nervous and Mental Disease*, **163**, 7–87

Riether, A. M. and Stoudemire, A. (1988). Psychogenic fugue states: a review. *Southern Medical Journal*, **81**, 568–71.

Roos, D. (1978). Neurological complications in patients with impaired Vitamin B$_{12}$ absorption following partial gastrectomy. *Acta Neurologica Scandinavica*, **59** (Suppl 69), 1–77.

Rosen, H. and Swigar, M. E. (1976). Depression and normal pressure hydrocephalus. *Journal of Nervous and Mental Disease*, **163**, 35–40.

Savage, G. (1892). Myxoedema and insanity. In *Dictionary of psychological medicine* (ed. D. K. Tuke), Vol. 2, pp. 828–30. London, J. & A. Churchill.

Séglas, J. (1903). Séméiologie des afections Mentales. In *Traité de pathologie mentale* (ed. G. Ballet), pp. 74–270. Paris, Doin.

Sierra, M. and Berrios, G. E. (1999). Towards a neuropsychiatry of conversion hysteria. *Cognitive Neuropsychiatry*, **4**, 267–87.

Sigal, M., Altmark, D., Arfici, S., and Gelkopf, M. (1992). Ganser syndrome: a review of 15 cases. *Comprehensive Psychiatry*, **33**, 134–8.

Sommer, T. (1899). *Lehrbuch der psychopathologischen Untersuchungs-Methoden*. Stuttgart, Deuticke.

Stambrook, M., Cardoso, E., Hawryluk, G. A., *et al.* (1988). Neuropsychological changes following the neurosurgical treatment of normal pressure hydrocephalus. *Archives of Clinical Neuropsychology*, **3**, 323–30.

Stengel, E. (1941). On the aetiology of the fugue states. *Journal of Mental Science*, **87**, 572–99.

Stengel, E. (1943). Further studies on pathological wandering (fugues with the impulse to wander). *Journal of Mental Science*, **89**, 224–41.

Strömgren, L. S. (1977). The influence of depression on memory. *Acta Psychiatrica Scandinavica*, **56**, 109–28.

Sutton, T. (1813). *Tracts on delirium tremens, on peritonitis and on the gout*. London, Thomas Underwood.

Thomas, D. G. T. (1983). Brain tumours. *British Journal of Hospital Medicine*, **28**, 148–58.

Varney, N. R. (1984). Reversible steroid dementia in patients without steroid psychoses. *American Journal of Psychiatry*, **141**, 369.

Voisin, J. (1889). Automatisme ambulatoire chez une hystérique. *Annales Médico-Psychologiques*, **46**, 418.

Wernicke, C. (1906). *Grundriss der Psychiatrie*. 2nd edn. Leipzig, Thieme.

Whitlock, F. A. (1967). Ganser syndrome. *British Journal of Psychiatry*, **113**, 19–29.

Windhager, W., Reisecker, F., Huber, H. D., *et al.* (1988). Chronisches Subduralhamatom beim Alterspatienten. Zur Problematik der Diagnose. *Deutschen Medicinischen Wochenschrift*, **113**, 883–8.

Winslow, F. (1861). *On obscure diseases of the brain and disorders of the mind*. London, John W. Davies.

Wittgenstein, L. (1967). *Philosophical investigations*. Translated by G. E. M. Anscombe. Oxford, Basil Blackwell.

Yousef, G., Ryan, W. J., Lambert, T., *et al.* (1998). A preliminary report: a new scale to identify the pseudodementia syndrome. *International Journal of Geriatric Psychiatry*, **13**, 389–99.

Zapotoczky, H. G. (1998). Problems of differential diagnosis between depressive pseudodementia and Alzheimer's disease. *Journal of Neural Transmission*, Suppl 53, 91–5.

Zucker, D. K., Livingston, R. L., Nakra, R., and Clayton, P. J. (1981). B12 deficiency and psychiatric disorders: case report and literature review. *Biological Psychiatry*, **16**, 197–205.

6 Structural imaging

John M. Stevens and Nick C. Fox

1 Introduction

Structural neuroimaging traditionally has been used to exclude potentially treatable surgical causes of dementia, such as neoplasm, subdural haematomas, and hydrocephalus (Moseley 1995; Alexander *et al.* 1995). In recent years, newly recognized entities such as AIDS dementia complex (Barker *et al.* 1995), and venous hypertensive encephalopathy associated with arterio-venous malformations (Deveikis 1998) have entered the list of diagnosable causes, along with a legion of medical conditions which include multiple sclerosis, neurosarcoidosis, and metabolic disorders (Moseley 1995). In most of these conditions, structural neuroimaging plays a central role in confirming central nervous system involvement. However, in patients presenting with dementia alone, the yield of treatable causes is extremely low, so low in fact that the routine use of imaging has not been recommended by some authors (Alexander *et al.* 1995). Nevertheless, it is widely recognized that in routine clinical practice, sufficient doubt about the diagnosis of degenerative dementia exists, especially in its early stages, to fully justify imaging the brain. This is particularly true when the onset of dementia is abrupt, or there is a sudden deterioration, or other clinical features emerge suggesting a non-degenerative cause or superimposed pathology (Lexa *et al.* 1996). Many workers regard imaging as central to the investigation of dementia because of the uncertainty of the clinical diagnosis, and lack of diagnostic laboratory tests (Fox 1998; Black 1999). This chapter concurs with this view. Despite low yields of alternative explanations, structural imaging is strongly recommended as part of the diagnostic work-up of any patient with dementia; and particularly for early onset cases, unusual clinical presentations, or recent or rapid cognitive decline.

Three recent changes have occurred which enhance this recommendation. First, the molecular basis of many of the degenerative dementias is being unravelled, leading to more precise differentiation of disease entities. Secondly, new treatment strategies, including risk factor management, are emerging which necessarily increase the pressure to make an early and more precise diagnosis. Finally, enormous advances in the tools of structural imaging have opened the possibility for imaging to have positive predictive value, the minimum requirement being the ability to discriminate between dementia and normal (and abnormal) ageing, and the desirable bonus being discrimination between different molecular pathologies.

The histological and molecular criteria for diagnosing Alzheimer's disease and other dementias involve mainly subcellular abnormalities such as intracellular inclusions of various types in neurons or glia, amyloid plaques, synaptic loss, and neuronal death (see chapters 8 & 10). Despite advances in structural imaging, changes at this level cannot be visualized directly *in vivo*, and this is likely to remain so for the conceivable future (Benveniste *et al.* 1999; Fox and

Rossor 2000). Moreover, many of these subcellular structural elements are found to some extent in the different types of degenerative dementia as well as in the normally ageing brain, and the pathological criteria defining different entities still depend, in large measure, upon conceptions of relative proportions. The strength of imaging is that it displays the macropathology on a *whole brain basis*. The spatial resolution achievable by structural imaging is comparable to that of the unaided eye, and the contrast resolution between grey and white matter and focal structural changes in the neuropil is generally superior. Modern magnetic resonance imaging can easily acquire over a million data points covering the whole brain in a few minutes, and powerful post-processing tools are becoming increasingly available to enhance structural and statistical analysis, a selection of which will be discussed below.

2 Imaging modalities

2.1 The machines

The main modalities used to produce structural images of the brain are X-ray computed tomography (CT) and magnetic resonance imaging (MRI). CT involves the reconstruction of cross-sectional images of the brain from X-ray attenuation data. CT now is widely available in developed countries, and access is virtually unrestricted. There are no contraindications, the only requirement being the ability of the patient to lie still within the very open doughnut shaped frame of the imaging gantry, for periods which now rarely exceed five minutes, and in the most modern high speed acquisitions, just a few seconds. Contrast between cerebrospinal fluid (CSF) and brain tissues, and between brain and bone is great, permitting high resolution displays of these boundaries and the internal structure of bone. However, contrast discrimination between different tissues within brain substance is considerably lower, and becomes critically dependent on two factors: thickness of the imaging plane, and photon flux. Thicker imaging planes mean greater slice thickness, which greatly reduces spatial resolution perpendicular to the slice plane; and increases in energy flux means increased doses of ionizing radiation. Artefacts are prone to occur next to dense bone, such as the petrous temporal which can obscure parts of the temporal lobe unless special precautions are taken which are only partially effective (Jobst *et al.* 1992).

Magnetic resonance imaging (MRI) utilizes a property of some atomic nuclei, angular momentum, which is polarized in a magnetic field. Polarization can be sampled by creating resonance, achieved by application of radiofrequency electromagnetic radiation of the same-frequency as the precessional frequency of the polarization. The resonance results in the emission of similar radio frequency radiation by the polarized nuclei. Loss of resonance occurs by two main mechanisms, one is thermodynamic (T1 relaxation), and the other is phase dispersal (T2 relaxation). Relaxation times are dependent upon the molecular environment of the polarized nuclei. In medical MRI, resonance is tuned to the precessional frequency of protons, that is hydrogen, and therefore mainly to the most abundant molecule, water. In most brain imaging, tissue visualization and contrast is dependent upon the chemical environment and mobility of water molecules. Historically MRI was devised as a cheaper alternative to CT, but as the much greater versatility, sensitivity, and complexity of MRI became apparent, any notion of it being cheaper than CT rapidly became illusory. Compared to CT, MRI provides superior tissue contrast, higher resolution imagery free from bone hardening artefacts. These features mean MRI is now the gold standard of structured imaging in dementia.

3 Image post-processing

3.1 Visual assessment

Despite the widespread development and application of computer-driven post-acquisition analysis of images in research settings, the eye–brain combination remains the only post-processing actually used in clinical practice. Visual assessment of unenhanced CT or MRI is adequate to exclude the most important treatable causes such as neoplasm and subdural haematoma (Figure 6.1). Imaging is essential whenever there is any doubt about the diagnosis and we recommend that imaging should be performed in all cases of young onset dementia. Clinical neuroradiologists tend to have a perception of the range of normal variation in cerebral structure (e.g. ventricular or sulcal enlargement) which is wider than special interest groups, but both exhibit considerable inter and intra-rater variability. A good example has been semi-quantitative visual scales for rating severity of ischaemic damage in brains of subjects with possible vascular dementia (Scheltens *et al.* 1993; Mantyla *et al.* 1997). At best about 80% of patients received an equivalent white matter grade by different scales, and at worst only 18% (Mantyla *et al.* 1997). It has been a similar story with rating cerebral atrophy, where the variability even between experts has been even higher. These limitations prompted the Consortium to Establish a Register for Alzheimer's Disease (CERAD) to seek quantitative ways of assessing atrophy (Davis *et al.* 1995). These have consisted of linear measurements, planimetry, and volumetry applied either to the whole brain, cerebral ventricles, and other CSF-containing spaces, or to specific regions or structures such as the hippocampus and corpus callosum. These varied attempts at reliably differentiating normal from abnormal atrophy are described below.

3.2 Linear and area measurements

Measurement of the distance between two anatomical boundaries has the advantage of being simple and can usually be applied to routine clinical images, both CT and MRI. Ventricular size

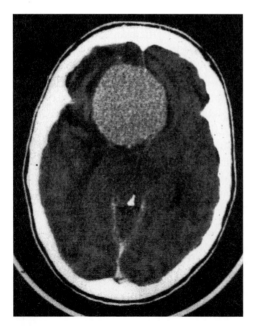

Figure 6.1   Axial, contrast-enhanced CT scan showing a large meningioma.

has been estimated by measuring the maximum width between the frontal horns and dividing by the width of the skull (Evans Index) or the width of the third ventricle (DeCarli *et al.* 1990). Size of subarachnoid spaces has been assessed by measuring the width of the Sylvian fissures at their most antero-inferior point, or the maximum width of the anterior interhemispheric fissure, both of which have regional bias. Regional atrophy has been probed by measuring the interuncal distance (Early *et al.* 1993), minimum temporal lobe width on temporal lobe orientated CT (Jobst *et al.* 1992), height of the hippocampus and parahippocampal gyrus (Pucci *et al.* 1998), and width of the temporal horn (Frisoni *et al.* 1996). A more general index of white matter bulk has been the thickness of the corpus callosum (Vermersch *et al.* 1994).

3.2.1 Planimetry

Neuropathologists often have used this type of evaluation to assess the relative size of gyri and other brain structures from carefully positioned and orientated brain slices (Greenfield 1997). Analogous methods can be applied to computed images, especially MRI. The slice (or slices) need to be carefully defined, and the region of interest outlined by some form of perimetry, and area measured. This approach has been used to estimate the size of the hippocampus (Seab *et al.* 1988), corpus callosum (Yamauchi *et al.* 1993), and individual temporal lobe gyri (Convit *et al.* 1995).

The main advantage of these simple measures should be their reproducibility. The more complex methods address accuracy and thereby increase the chance of detecting biological change, but at the same time may increase the scope for variability. The idea that a simple linear measurement such as the interuncal distance is as robust as a well conducted volumetric study of the hippocampus is an illusion (Early *et al.* 1993).

3.3 Volume of interest based quantitation

In dementia research detection of volume loss has been the commonest goal of quantitation. For most machines the optimal acquisition is a T1-weighted sequence (e.g. IR prepared SPGR or MP-RAGE), ideal slice thickness being 1.0 or 1.5 mm. This acquisition minimizes voxel anisotropy whilst maintaining adequate grey-white matter contrast.

Volume is assessed by measuring the area of a series of equally spaced cross-sections of the object and multiplying by the slice number and interslice distance. The whole volume of the structure of interest should be sampled wherever possible.

Quantities such as ventricular volume, CSF volume, grey and white matter volumes all have been estimated and also the volumes of structures like the hippocampus or amygdala, although the methodology in many instances leaves much to be desired. Some of the problems involved in assessing white and grey matter volumes have been discussed at length (Sisodiya *et al.* 1996). In an effort to reduce inter-subject variability due to differences in head size, volumes of structures are often normalized by factors which take head or brain size into account (Free *et al.* 1995).

3.4 Voxel-by-voxel based comparative quantitation

The volume-of-interest approaches considered above all require varying levels of rater interaction and a good clinical hypothesis. Voxel-by-voxel approaches on the other hand require neither, and thereby permit unbiased evaluation. In these methods MR images of the brain of individual subjects are compared with those of a control group on a voxel-by-voxel basis, each imaging study being normalized to a common standard three-dimensional space, segmented and smoothed using algorithms referred to as statistical parametric mapping (SPM). The resulting voxel values reflect the probability that a given voxel in the subject's brain is like or unlike the equivalent voxel in the statistically pooled brains of controls (Woermann *et al.* 1999; Mummery *et al.* 2000). Although these methods may detect reductions in cortical volume by relative displacement of grey matter, and sometime have seemed to show abnormalities in regions which appear normal to visual inspection, it has proven relatively insensitive to small local changes visible to the eye, such as hippocampal sclerosis (ibid). It is doubtful that SPM as currently applied has much to offer in the diagnosis of early dementia in the individual case.

3.5 Registration

The majority of neuroimaging studies in dementia have been cross-sectional, which has the disadvantage that small changes in brain structure tend to be masked by the large variation between normal individuals. Even with longitudinal studies, detection of small changes remains difficult. The development of automated image registration and subtraction algorithms with subvoxel precision allows small changes to be shown anywhere in the brain without rater interaction. This is achieved by optimization of voxel intensity goodness-of-fit functions which proceed iteratively to produce the best achievable match between an initial and subsequent imaging study (Fox *et al.* 1996; Hajnal *et al.* 1995). Usually change is seen with a subtraction process which reflects displacement of high contrast boundaries, such as between brain and CSF, and tissue loss or gain can be measured from the boundary shift integral (Freeborough and Fox 1997). Separation of early or even presymptomatic AD subjects from controls can be achieved by this method (Fox *et al.* 1999a) (Figure 6.2).

Registration is best performed from MR acquisitions which produce voxels of minimum size and minimum anisotropy. The volume acquisitions used for volumetry usually are the most satisfactory.

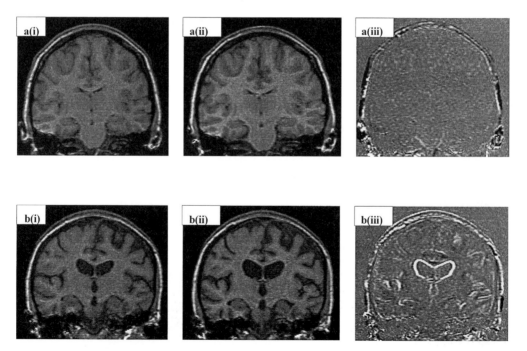

Figure 6.2 Coronal T1-weighted MR scans of an (a) unaffected and (b) affected individual from a family at risk of developing AD. (i) Baseline, (ii) repeat registered, and (iii) subtraction images.

The method has significant limitations. The main one of course is that two examinations are required with an interval amounting to several months, and at present preferably at least a year. Another is closely related. The sensitivity to change is sufficient for the possibility that reversible physiological variation in brain size may be detectable, and this may be particularly relevant when shorter time intervals are used, as would be desirable.

3.6 Other post-processing approaches

Many other strategies have been explored in different clinical contexts. This includes a wide variety of analyses of shape and texture, such as fractals and gyrification index for quantitation of cortical folding patterns, and regional grey-white matter proportionality relationships. None of these seem likely to offer much in earlier onset dementia.

4 Hydrocephalus

Normal pressure hydrocephalus (NPH) is a disorder characterized by a clinical triad of gait disturbance, mental deterioration, and urinary incontinence, which are reversible with ventricular shunting (Hakim and Adams 1965). The imaging signs of NPH include the distinctive morphological change of disproportionately dilated ventricles and absence of cortical atrophy (Wikkelso *et al.* 1989) (Figure 6.3). Neurodegenerative conditions also exhibit ventricular dilation so that volumetry of CSF spaces for NPH diagnosis may not be sufficient. A recent MR study showed CSF volumetry to be successful in identifying shunt-responsive patients (Kitagaki *et al.* 1998). However, an earlier volumetric study had concluded that selective widening of the Sylvian fissures was a discriminating feature of Alzheimer's disease (Sandor *et al.* 1992).

Signal change in the deep cerebral white matter has been variably related to NPH, as well as vascular dementia to be discussed below (George 1991). A role for hypertension and deep white matter ischaemic damages in causing idiopathic NPH has even been proposed (Bradley *et al.* 1991), but the general skepticism felt by many has been expressed rather amusingly: 'With recent reports … water on the brain is probably at its muddiest ever' (Moseley 1995). Neuropathology has nothing to offer either (Greenfield 1997). A consensus seems to be emerging however, that the demonstration of bilateral unequivocally small hippocampi mitigates against expectation of a useful outcome from ventricular shunting (Holodny *et al.* 1998).

5 Ageing

Even in the early onset dementias, the discrimination between the effects of a disorder like Alzheimer's disease from the non-specific effects of ageing alone becomes problematic, as there is overlap between the two groups which increases with age. General clinical experience indicates a wide variation in severity and pattern of non-specific changes in the brain which, because they become more common with increasing age, generally are attributed to ageing. This may affect the validity of control populations selected on the basis of being judged to be normal, both clinically and on brain imaging. Subtle neuropsychological and imaging changes may precede dementia by several years.

Most cross-sectional studies have identified a period in which atrophy accelerates, usually in or after the fifth decade (Greenfield 1997; Blatter *et al.* 1995). Imaging studies suggest that

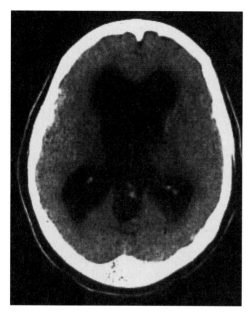

Figure 6.3 CT scan showing hydrocephalus.

the frontal lobes are more susceptible to age-related loss than the temporal lobes (DeCarli *et al.* 1994), but the general lack of adequate longitudinal studies is a major deficiency in these interpretations. Pathological data have suggested that after the age of 50 years, about 3.5% of brain volume is lost per decade, implying a linearity which may not be real.

Some reports have suggested that tissue loss due to ageing is greater in white matter than grey. Data from cell counts have been even more variable: certainly the hippocampus and adjacent regions are not exempt from age-related cell loss; some studies have suggested that the striatum is exempt, others that it is not, and most seem to agree that brain stem nuclei are not affected (Greenfield 1997). The most conspicuous abnormality shown by MRI in the ageing brain is multifocal ischaemic damage in basal grey and white matter. Cortical infarcts are uncommon in the absence of a history of stroke. Distributions and prevalences are widely documented but the range of variation is great. White matter changes will be considered with the discussion of vascular dementia.

6 Alzheimer's disease

Until the molecular pathology of AD can be imaged directly *in vivo*, assessment of cerebral atrophy will remain the main contribution of structural imaging to diagnosis and to measurement of disease progression. Cross-sectional imaging studies of AD, of which there have been many, can be divided into two groups depending on whether they assessed global atrophy or regional, usually medial temporal lobe, atrophy. The level of complexity of the methods used ranges from simple visual assessment to very detailed volumetric measurement. It is salutary for anyone conducting research into the use of atrophy measurements in AD to recognize that despite all the studies claiming diagnostic utility for a particular measure none of these measures has been adopted into routine clinical practice.

6.1 Visual assessment of atrophy

The overlap with normal ageing, and the relative insensitivity of visual inspection, limit the usefulness of atrophy assessment when applied to the individual patient. The overlap with age-related atrophy is less in early onset AD but nonetheless in the early stages of AD scans are often reported as normal for age. The difficulties inherent in assessing atrophy have been recognized in clinical criteria which state that 'the diagnosis of PROBABLE Alzheimer's disease is supported by evidence of cerebral atrophy' ... but a 'normal for age' scan is consistent with this diagnosis (McKhann *et al.* 1984). Various atrophy rating scales have been suggested: for a specificity of 90%, the sensitivity of ratings of atrophy vary from 40–95% (Erkinjuntti *et al.* 1994; Davis *et al.* 1992; Scheltens *et al.* 1992; Horn *et al.* 1996; de Leon *et al.* 1997). Visual assessment of dilatation of the perihippocampal fissures is predictive of cognitive decline in minimally impaired individuals with a sensitivity of 91% and a specificity of 89% (Convit *et al.* 1993; de Leon *et al.* 1993). Assessment of medial temporal lobe atrophy appears more sensitive than assessment of generalized atrophy (Scheltens *et al.* 1997). However, while the presence of hippocampal atrophy on visual inspection makes the diagnosis of AD more likely, apparently normal hippocampi do not exclude the diagnosis.

6.2 Cross-sectional measures of global atrophy

Overall lower brain volumes correlate with gross measures of severity of cognitive impairment. As might be expected, the uncorrected brain volume measurement has little diagnostic value due to the wide range in normal brain size (Murphy *et al.* 1993). The brain normally occupies 85–92% of the intracranial volume and consequently relatively small decrements in brain size lead to large increments in ventricular and/or extraventricular volumes (Matsumae *et al.* 1996). This might imply that the CSF measures would be sensitive markers of disease. However, in addition to large normal variations in CSF volumes the coefficient of variation in CSF measurements has previously been unsatisfactory. Very considerable overlap is present when mildly or even moderately affected patients are studied. Automated tissue segmentation techniques have resulted in variable conclusions on the contribution of white matter losses to cerebral atrophy. Tanabe and colleagues suggested that in mildly affected individuals white matter volumes were unchanged (Tanabe *et al.* 1997). However, such conclusions must be treated cautiously because automated tissue segmentation routines require the signal characteristics of brain tissues to be relatively unaffected by the disease. Certainly significant reductions in the thickness of the corpus callosum in AD have been shown (Vermersch *et al.* 1994). It is likely that both grey and white matter losses contribute to reduced brain volume even in early disease (Rusinek *et al.* 1991; Matsumae *et al.* 1996). As far as making an early diagnosis in an individual patient is concerned, a single measurement of global atrophy is not useful whether total brain, grey matter, white matter or CSF volumes are measured (Fox *et al.* 1999).

6.3 Medial temporal lobe atrophy

Due to their prominent pathological involvement in AD, the temporal lobes and the hippocampal formation are obvious targets as sensitive imaging markers of disease and there is now a considerable imaging literature. Temporal lobe volume reductions are proportionately greater than whole brain volume losses in AD (Rusinek *et al.* 1991; Jernigan *et al.* 1991). MR-based measures have consistently shown that by the time individuals are moderately severely affected the hippocampus has lost 30–40% of its volume (Seab *et al.* 1988; Jack, Jr. *et al.* 1992). Measurements of the amygdala have lower reproducibility but show similar levels of atrophy (Pearlson *et al.* 1992;

Cuenod *et al.* 1993). These structures are best visualized with MRI but temporal lobe orientated CT has been used to measure the minimum width of the medial temporal lobe. This simple measure was effective at differentiating advanced AD from normal controls (Jobst *et al.* 1992). The challenge for imaging in AD is to improve diagnosis when individuals are in the earliest stages of the disease. Even patients described as mildly affected (e.g. MMSE > 21) show hippocampal losses on MRI of around 25% (Killiany *et al.* 1993; Krasuski *et al.* 1998). Claims that MRI measures of interuncal distance are useful for the detection of AD have however not been substantiated (Dahlbeck *et al.* 1991; Howieson *et al.* 1993). In a large and carefully conducted study Jack *et al.* used MR-based volumetry to measure the hippocampus, parahippocampal gyrus, and amygdala in 94 individuals with probable AD and 126 controls. Volumes of each structure declined with increasing age in control subjects. The volume of each of these medial temporal lobe structures was significantly smaller in AD patients than control subjects. The hippocampal measurements were best at discriminating control from AD subjects. Hippocampal volumes declined with disease severity. The mean hippocampal volumes for AD patients relative to control subjects by severity of disease were as follows: 'very mild AD' (CDR 0.5) –1.75 SD below the control mean, 'mild AD' (CDR 1) –1.99 SD, and 'moderate AD' (CDR 2) –2.22 SD (Jack *et al.* 1997). Interestingly, while this cross-sectional study suggests that hippocampal losses are clearly progressive, it is unclear how rates of loss change as the disease progresses. Longitudinal studies are arguably the best way of assessing how rates of atrophy change as the disease progresses. Ideally these studies should include subjects recruited with little in the way of cognitive deficits.

There are very few studies where serial MR-based measurements have been performed in AD and in an appropriate control group. Rates of hippocampal and medial temporal lobe atrophy have been shown to be significantly greater in AD than in normal controls when subjects are rescanned after an interval of a year or more (de Leon *et al.* 1989; Jack *et al.* 1998) and hippocampal losses tend to be symmetrical (Figure 6.4). Hippocampal atrophy predicts subsequent development of dementia in familial AD and may precede symptoms (Fox *et al.* 1996b). By contrast Kaye *et al.* found in a longitudinal study of elderly subjects that volume losses in the temporal lobe, but not the hippocampus, distinguished those individuals who were developing cognitive impairment (Kaye *et al.* 1997). Digital subtraction of registered scans has shown that rates of global cerebral atrophy in mild-to-moderate early onset AD are already tenfold greater than in age matched controls (Fox and Freeborough 1997; Freeborough and Fox 1997) with little overlap with normal ageing. Furthermore rates of whole brain atrophy are already increased in asymptomatic individuals at risk of early onset familial AD who subsequently become clinically affected suggesting that the atrophic process predates declared symptoms and is already widespread at time of diagnosis (Fox *et al.* 1999).

In conclusion, structural imaging in early onset AD suggests that bilateral symmetrical medial temporal lobe atrophy is an early feature of the disease and is predictive of subsequent decline in individuals with isolated memory impairment. The sensitivity of a single measurement is limited by the wide range in cerebral morphology. Sensitivity may be increased by serial imaging but until access to MRI greatly improves serial imaging will not be widely available. As will be seen in the following sections even a typical pattern of hippocampal atrophy is not specific for AD with similar changes also being seen in dementia with Lewy bodies.

7 Frontotemporal lobar degeneration

The imaging features of non-AD dementias have received a fraction of the attention of that devoted to AD and yet, taken together, non-AD pathologies account for the majority of cases of early onset dementia. As will be clear from earlier chapters, cases of frontotemporal lobar degeneration

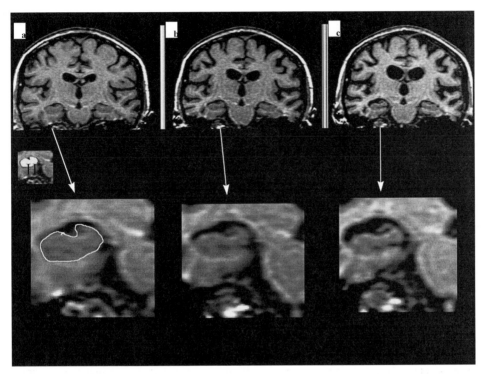

Figure 6.4 Coronal T1-weighted MR scan showing hippocampal atrophy in an early onset familial AD case. (a) Baseline scan when only mildly affected, (b) after 18 months, and (c) after 36 months. The hippocampus appears within normal limits when the patient was first seen (image a) but subsequent imaging shows marked progressive atrophy.

(FTLD) account for a large proportion of non-AD early onset dementia cases (see chapter 1). Unfortunately despite their importance there are several problems associated with reviewing the structural imaging features of FTLD. The term FTLD encompasses cases that were previously described as Pick's disease or complex, semantic dementia, primary progressive aphasia, progressive prosopagnosia, frontal lobe degeneration, frontotemporal dementia (FTD), and frontotemporal dementia and parkinsonism linked to chromosome 17 (FTDP-17). Furthermore published imaging reports have almost entirely been descriptive with a lack of formal quantitation of atrophy. Finally, consensus statements include the presence of frontal and/or temporal lobe atrophy as supportive diagnostic features and therefore unless histological confirmation is obtained there is a risk that descriptions of the imaging features of FTLD become circular (The Lund and Manchester Groups 1994; Neary *et al.* 1998; ECAPD Consortium).

Despite these caveats it is clear that strikingly disproportionate lobar atrophy makes AD much less likely and a focal degenerative disorder such as FTLD probable. The major exception to this rule is focal posterior cortical atrophy where over 50% of cases are found at autopsy to have the pathological features of AD (Victoroff *et al.* 1994; Pantel and Schroder 1996). Other focal atrophy presentations may also rarely be due to AD (Greene *et al.* 1996; Galton *et al.* 2000).

FTLD, including tau mutation cases and cases with histological features of Pick's disease, often have asymmetrical frontal and/or anterior temporal lobe atrophy (Figure 6.5), which may best be assessed with coronal T1-weighted MRI. In general the pattern of atrophy correlates with clinical presentation. Semantic dementia cases tend to show marked, usually asymmetrical, anterior atrophy of the dominant temporal lobe (Hodges *et al.* 1992); primary progressive non-fluent aphasia also shows focal atrophy of the dominant hemisphere but in these cases the atrophy is more anterior and often more focal with peri-sylvian regions bearing the brunt of atrophy (Mesulam 1987); cases with a more frontal presentation, with or without associated motor neuron disease, have a more symmetrical and often less obvious frontal pattern of atrophy (Neary *et al.* 1990, 1998). Interestingly, while temporal lobe atrophy is often bilateral, unilateral right temporal lobe atrophy is much less frequently reported than left temporal lobe atrophy, a disparity that cannot simply be explained by observation bias (Edwards *et al.* 1997; Tyrrell *et al.* 1990). In addition to focal atrophy, diffuse signal change involving one or more frontal or temporal lobes has been described in FTLD on dual echo MRI (Kitagaki *et al.* 1997). For further discussion see chapter 12.

8 Vascular dementia

Structural imaging has become established as an important support to the clinical diagnosis of vascular dementia, which encompasses the overlapping conditions of multi-infarct dementia and subcortical vascular dementia or Binswanger's disease. The former is characterized by evidence of ischaemic damage in the territories of conducting arterial vessels of the brain while the latter involves small vessel damage. The differentiation of vascular dementia (especially small vessel predominant dementia) from primary degenerative dementias such as AD or Lewy body dementia may be problematic due to the fact there is overlap in their clinical features, and that these conditions often coexist as 'mixed dementia' (see chapter 14). Some authors suggest that the diagnosis of vascular dementia should only be made in the presence of relevant vascular changes on CT or MRI (Leys and Scheltens 1996), and both the extent and location of changes are important (Amar and Wilcock 1996; Roman *et al.* 1993). Multiple infarcts and high signal foci in the basal ganglia and thalamus are very supportive of a diagnosis of vascular dementia (Schmidt 1992). Imaging changes in the white matter, 'leukoariosis' on CT or 'white matter hyperintensities' (WMH) on MRI, are common both in AD and in elderly controls; their presence therefore does not preclude a diagnosis of AD. In AD WHMs appear as small foci (< 5 mm) and bilateral

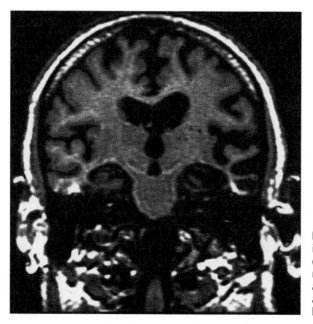

Figure 6.5 Coronal T1-weighted MR image of an individual with semantic dementia (Pick's disease). There is marked asymmetry, with very significant atrophy of the left temporal lobe and almost complete loss of the left hippocampus at this level.

'caps' around the posterior and anterior horns (Bennett *et al.* 1992; Fox *et al.* 1997*b*) (Figure 6.6), whereas extensive, confluent and irregular white matter changes are more suggestive of vascular or mixed dementia (Schmidt 1992). The absence of vascular change on imaging, particular if MRI, essentially excludes a diagnosis of vascular dementia.

9 Creutzfeldt–Jakob disease

Interest in the imaging features of CJD has increased with the appearance of variant CJD (vCJD) in the UK. Traditionally the main role of imaging in CJD has been to exclude other conditions. In sporadic CJD imaging may appear normal, especially on CT (Galvez and Cartier 1984; Zeidler *et al.* 1996) while some cases may show rapidly progressive atrophy (Schlenska and Walter 1989; Fox *et al.* 1997*a*). Increased T2 signal change in the basal ganglia is increasingly recognized as a characteristic and almost pathognomonic feature of CJD (Barboriak *et al.* 1994; Finkenstaedt *et al.* 1996) (Figure 6.7); these signal changes may precede the appearance of atrophy or EEG changes (Tartaro *et al.* 1993). Most commonly in sporadic CJD the signal changes are seen in the caudate or putamen but the globus pallidus and thalamus may be involved and in the cortical ribbon may also show altered signal particularly in the Heidenhain (cortical blindness) variant (de Priester *et al.* 1999). There have been a small number of reports suggesting that diffusion weighted imaging may reveal abnormalities before T2 signal changes appear (Demaerel *et al.* 1999). Given the recent emergence of vCJD and the relatively small numbers of cases to date it is hard to be sure what will constitute the typical imaging features of this condition. Overall it appears that diffuse symmetric high T2 signal in the posterior thalamus is its most characteristic feature (Zeidler *et al.* 1997). In a recent study by Zeidler *et al.* 28 out of 36 cases of vCJD had bilateral posterior thalamic (pulvinar) signal change while in 57 control subjects signal changes were absent or minimal. This suggests that the pulvinar change, best seen on FLAIR imaging, has high specificity for vCJD (> 90%) with reasonable sensitivity (80%) (Zeidler *et al.* 2000).

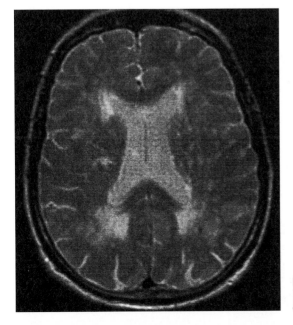

Figure 6.6 Axial T2-weighted MR scan of an individual with vascular dementia, showing extensive white matter hyperintensities.

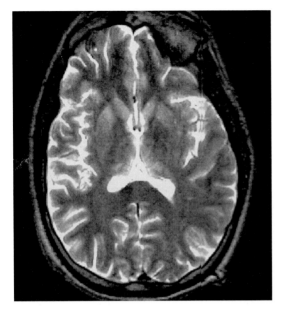

Figure 6.7 Axial T2-weighted MR scan showing high signal intensity in the posterior thalamus characteristic of CJD.

10 Other early onset dementias and the differential diagnosis

The differential diagnosis is wide in a patient with early onset dementia. Imaging is extremely important in the presence of cognitive decline in a patient with AIDS and may show generalized and non-specific atrophy in AIDS associated dementia, white matter changes sparing cortex in progressive multifocal leukoencephalopathy or reveal space occupying lesions due to opportunistic infection or lymphoma. Cerebral atrophy, again without a particularly well-determined pattern, is common in chronic alcoholics with cognitive decline (Lishman 1997). Development of reliable genetic tests has reduced the importance of imaging in diagnosis in Huntington's disease: atrophy of the caudate and putamen are characteristic of the late stages of the disease (Jernigan *et al.* 1991). Dementia with Lewy bodies (DLB) is relatively less prevalent in younger cases of dementia and in the individual imaging is very similar to that seen in AD although the absence of medial temporal lobe atrophy is a pointer towards DLB rather than AD (Barber *et al.* 1999).

11 Key points

1   All patients with early onset dementia should have structural imaging of the brain. Structural imaging, even unenhanced CT, is adequate to exclude the most important treatable causes such as neoplasm and subdural haematoma.

2   The diversity of image contrast techniques possible with modern MRI has not been fully explored in dementia. However, most of the novel techniques have not yielded any breakthroughs in early diagnosis of dementia.

3   Standard MRI of the brain, especially with the addition of coronal volumetric acquisitions, can have positive predictive value for early diagnosis, even in AD.

4   Normal structural imaging of the brain has no negative predictive value in AD, but has important negative predictive value in FTD.

5   Normal structural imaging has strong negative predictive value in vascular dementia.

6   The positive predictive value of structural imaging in the specific diagnosis of NPH remains highly questionable.

7   While hippocampal and medial temporal lobe atrophy are well-established features of AD, it is not proven that measurement increases positive predictive value significantly over visual assessment.

References

Alexander, E. M., Wagner, E. H., Buchner, D. M., *et al.* (1995). Do surgical brain lesions present as isolated dementia? A population-based study. *Journal of the American Geriatrics Society*, **43**, 138–43.

Amar, K. and Wilcock, G. (1996). Vascular dementia. *British Medical Journal*, **312**, 227–31.

Barber, R., Gholkar, A., Scheltens, P., *et al.* (1999). Medial temporal lobe atrophy on MRI in dementia with Lewy bodies. *Neurology*, **52**, 1153–8.

Barboriak, D. P., Provenzale, J. M., and Boyko, O. B. (1994). MR diagnosis of Creutzfeldt–Jakob disease: significance of high signal intensity of the basal ganglia. *American Journal of Roentgenology*, **162**, 137–40.

Barker, P. B., Lee, R. R., and McArthur, J. C. (1995). AIDS dementia complex: evaluation with proton MR spectroscopic imaging. *Radiology*, **195**, 58–64.

Bennett, D. A., Gilley, D. W., Wilson, R. S., *et al.* (1992). Clinical correlates of high signal lesions on magnetic resonance imaging in Alzheimer's disease. *Journal of Neurology*, **239**, 186–90.

Benveniste, H., Einstein, G., Kim, K. R., *et al.* (1999). Detection of neuritic plaques in Alzheimer's disease by magnetic resonance microscopy. *Proceedings of the National Academy of Sciences USA*, **96**, 14079–84.

Black, S. E. (1999). The search for diagnostic and progression markers in AD — So near but still too far? *Neurology*, **52**, 1533–4.

Blatter, D. D., Bigler, E. D., Gale, S. D., *et al.* (1995). Quantitative volumetric analysis of brain MR: Normative database spanning 5 decades of life. *American Journal of Neuroradiology*, **16**, 241–51.

Bradley, W. G. J., Whittemore, A. R., Watanabe, A. S., *et al.* (1991). Association of deep white matter infarction with chronic communicating hydrocephalus: implications regarding the possible origin of normal-pressure hydrocephalus. *American Journal of Neuroradiology*, **12**, 31–9.

Convit, A., de Leon, M. J., Golomb, J., *et al.* (1993). Hippocampal atrophy in early Alzheimer's disease: anatomic specificity and validation. *Psychiatric Quarterly*, **64**, 371–87.

Convit, A., de Leon, M., Hoptman, M. J., *et al.* (1995). Age-related changes in brain: I. Magnetic resonance imaging measures of temporal lobe volumes in normal subjects. *Psychiatric Quarterly*, **66**, 343–55.

Cuenod, C. A., Denys, A., Michot, J. L., *et al.* (1993). Amygdala atrophy in Alzheimer's disease. An *in vivo* magnetic resonance imaging study. *Archives of Neurology*, **50**, 941–5.

Dahlbeck, J. W., McCluney, K. W., Yeakley, J. W., *et al.* (1991). The interuncal distance: a new MR measurement for the hippocampal atrophy of Alzheimer disease. *American Journal of Neuroradiology*, **12**, 931–2.

Davis, P. C., Gearing, M., Gray, L., *et al.* (1995). The CERAD experience, Part VIII: Neuroimaging-neuropathology correlates of temporal lobe changes in Alzheimer's disease. *Neurology*, **45**, 178–9.

Davis, P. C., Gray, L., Albert, M., *et al.* (1992). The Consortium to Establish a Registry for Alzheimer's Disease (CERAD). Part III. Reliability of a standardized MRI evaluation of Alzheimer's disease. *Neurology*, **42**, 1676–80.

de Leon, M. J., George, A. E., Reisberg, B., *et al.* (1989). Alzheimer's disease: longitudinal CT studies of ventricular change. *American Journal of Roentgenology*, **152**, 1257–62.

de Leon, M. J., Golomb, J., George, A. E., *et al.* (1993). The radiologic prediction of Alzheimer disease: the atrophic hippocampal formation. *American Journal of Neuroradiology*, **14**, 897–906.

de Leon, M., George, A. E., Golomb, J., *et al.* (1997). Frequency of hippocampal formation atrophy in normal aging and Alzheimer's disease. *Neurobiology of Aging*, **18**, 1–11.

de Priester, J., Jansen, G. H., de Kruijk, J., *et al.* (1999). New MRI findings in Creutzfeldt–Jakob disease: high signal in the globus pallidus on T1-weighted images. *Neuroradiology*, **41**, 265–8.

DeCarli, C., Kaye, J. A., Horwitz, B., *et al.* (1990). Critical analysis of the use of computer-assisted transverse axial tomography to study human brain in aging and dementia of the Alzheimer type. Review article. *Neurology*, **40**, 872–83.

DeCarli, C., Murphy, D. G., Gillette, J. A., *et al.* (1994). Lack of age-related differences in temporal lobe volume of very healthy adults. *American Journal of Neuroradiology*, **15**, 689–96.

Demaerel, P., Heiner, L., Robberecht, W., *et al.* (1999). Diffusion-weighted MRI in sporadic Creutzfeldt–Jakob disease. *Neurology*, **52**, 205–8.

Deveikis, J. P. (1998). Venous hypertensive encephalopathy. *American Journal of Neuroradiology*, **19**, 1274–5.

Early, B., Escalona, P. R., Boyko, O. B., *et al.* (1993). Interuncal distance measurements in healthy volunteers and in patients with Alzheimer's disease. *American Journal of Neuroradiology*, **14**, 907–10.

ECAPD Consortium, (1998). Provisional clinical and neuroradiological criteria for the diagnosis of Pick's disease. *European Journal of Neurology*, **5**, 519–20.

Edwards, L. T., Miller, B. L., Benson, D. F., *et al.* (1997). The temporal variant of frontotemporal dementia. *Brain*, **120**, 1027–40.

Erkinjuntti, T., Gao, F., Lee, D. H., *et al.* (1994). Lack of difference in brain hyperintensities between patients with early Alzheimer's disease and control subjects. *Archives of Neurology*, **51**, 260–8.

Finkenstaedt, M., Szudra, A., Zerr, I., *et al.* (1996). MR imaging of Creutzfeldt–Jakob disease. *Radiology*, **199**, 793–8.

Fox, N. C. (1998). Magnetic resonance imaging in Alzheimer's disease: from diagnosis to measuring therapeutic effect. Review article. *Alzheimer's Review*, **1(b)**, 1–6.

Fox, N. C. and Freeborough, P. A. (1997). Brain atrophy progression measured from registered serial MRI: validation and application to Alzheimer's disease. *Journal of Magnetic Resonance Imaging*, **7**, 1069–75.

Fox, N. C., Freeborough, P. A., Mekkaoui, K. F., *et al.* (1997*a*). Cerebral and cerebellar atrophy on serial magnetic resonance imaging in an initially symptom free subject at risk of familial prion disease. *British Medical Journal*, **315**, 856–7.

Fox, N. C., Freeborough, P. A., and Rossor, M. N. (1996). Visualisation and quantification of atrophy in Alzheimer's disease. *Lancet*, **348**, 94–7.

Fox, N. C., Kennedy, A. M., Harvey, R. J., *et al.* (1997*b*). Clinicopathological features of familial Alzheimer's disease associated with the M139V mutation in the presenilin 1 gene. Pedigree but not mutation specific age at onset provides evidence for a further genetic factor. *Brain*, **120**, 491–501.

Fox, N. C. and Rossor, M. N. (2000). Seeing what Alzheimer saw — with magnetic resonance microscopy. *Nature Medicine*, **6**, 20–1.

Fox, N. C., Warrington, E. K., Freeborough, P. A., *et al.* (1996). Presymptomatic hippocampal atrophy in Alzheimer's disease: a longitudinal MRI study. *Brain*, **119**, 2001–7.

Fox, N. C., Warrington, E. K., and Rossor, M. N. (1999). Serial magnetic resonance imaging of cerebral atrophy in preclinical Alzheimer's disease. *Lancet*, **353**, 2125.

Free, S. L., Bergin, P. S., Fish, D. R., *et al.* (1995). Methods for normalization of hippocampal volumes measured with MR. *American Journal of Neuroradiology*, **16**, 637–43.

Freeborough, P. A. and Fox, N. C. (1997). The boundary shift integral: an accurate and robust measure of cerebral volume changes from registered repeat MRI. *Ieee Transactions On Medical Imaging*, **16**, 623–9.

Frisoni, G. B., Beltramello, A., Weiss, C., *et al.* (1996). Usefulness of simple measures of temporal lobe atrophy in probable Alzheimer's disease. *Dementia*, **7**, 15–22.

Galton, C., Patterson, K., Xuereb, J. H. and Hodges, J. R. (2000). Atypical and typical presentations of Alzheimers' disease; a clinical, neuropsychological and pathological study of 13 cases. *Brain*, **123**, 484–498.

Galvez, S. and Cartier, L. (1984). Computed tomography findings in 15 cases of Creutzfeld–Jacob disease with histological verification. *Journal of Neurology Neurosurgery and Psychiatry*, **47**, 1244–6.

George, A. E. (1991). Chronic communicating hydrocephalus and periventricular white matter disease: a debate with regard to cause and effect. *American Journal of Neuroradiology*, **12**, 42–4.

Greene, J. D., Patterson, K., Xuereb, J., *et al.* (1996). Alzheimer disease and nonfluent progressive aphasia. *Archives of Neurology*, **53**, 1072–8.

Greenfield, J. G. (1997). *Neuropathology*, 6th edn. Arnold: London.

Hajnal, J. V., Saeed, N., Oatridge, A., *et al.* (1995). Detection of subtle brain changes using subvoxel registration and subtraction of serial MR images. *Journal of Computer Assisted Tomography*, **19**, 677–91.

Hakim, S. and Adams, R. D. (1965). The special clinical problem of symptomatic hydrocephalus with normal cerebrospinal fluid pressure. Observations on cerebrospinal fluid hydrodynamics. *Journal of Neurological Science*, **2**, 307–27.

Hodges, J. R., Patterson, K., Oxbury, S., *et al.* (1992). Semantic dementia. Progressive fluent aphasia with temporal lobe atrophy. *Brain*, **115**, 1783–806.

Holodny, A. I., Waxman, R., George, A. E., *et al.* (1998). MR differential diagnosis of normal-pressure hydrocephalus and Alzheimer disease: significance of perihippocampal fissures. *American Journal of Neuroradiology*, **19**, 813–19.

Horn, R., Ostertun, B., Fric, M., *et al.* (1996). Atrophy of hippocampus in patients with Alzheimer's disease and other diseases with memory impairment. *Dementia*, **7**, 182–6.

Howieson, J., Kaye, J. A., Holm, L., *et al.* (1993). Interuncal distance: marker of aging and Alzheimer disease. *American Journal of Neuroradiology*, **14**, 647–50.

Jack, C. R., Petersen, R. C., Xu, Y., *et al.* (1998). Rate of medial temporal lobe atrophy in typical aging and Alzheimer's disease. *Neurology*, **51**, 993–9.

Jack, C. R., Petersen, R. C., Xu, Y. C., *et al.* (1997). Medial temporal atrophy on MRI in normal aging and very mild Alzheimer's disease. *Neurology*, **49**, 786–94.

Jack, C. R., Jr., Petersen, R. C., O'Brien, P. C., *et al.* (1992). MR-based hippocampal volumetry in the diagnosis of Alzheimer's disease. *Neurology*, **42**, 183–8.

Jernigan, T. L., Salmon, D. P., Butters, N., *et al.* (1991). Cerebral structure on MRI, Part II: Specific changes in Alzheimer's and Huntington's diseases. *Biological Psychiatry*, **29**, 68–81.

Jobst, K. A., Smith, A. D., Szatmari, M., *et al.* (1992). Detection in life of confirmed Alzheimer's disease using a simple measurement of medial temporal lobe atrophy by computed tomography. *Lancet*, **340**, 1179–83.

Kaye, J. A., Swihart, T., Howieson, D., *et al.* (1997). Volume loss of the hippocampus and temporal lobe in healthy elderly persons destined to develop dementia. *Neurology*, **48**, 1297–304.

Killiany, R. J., Moss, M. B., Albert, M. S., *et al.* (1993). Temporal lobe regions on magnetic resonance imaging identify patients with early Alzheimer's disease. *Archives of Neurology*, **50**, 949–54.

Kitagaki, H., Mori, E., Hirono, N., *et al.* (1997). Alteration of white matter MR signal intensity in frontotemporal dementia. *American Journal of Neuroradiology*, **18**, 367–78.

Kitagaki, H., Mori, E., Ishii, K., *et al.* (1998). CSF spaces in idiopathic normal pressure hydrocephalus: morphology and volumetry. *American Journal of Neuroradiology*, **19**, 1277–84.

Krasuski, J. S., Alexander, G. E., Horwitz, B., *et al.* (1998). Volumes of medial temporal lobe structures in patients with Alzheimer's disease and mild cognitive impairment (and in healthy controls). *Biological Psychiatry*, **43**, 60–8.

Leys, D. and Scheltens, P. (1996). *Vascular dementia*. ICG Publications: Dortrecht, Netherlands.

Lexa, F. J., Trojanowski, J. Q., Braffman, B. H., and Atlas, S. W. (1996). The aging brain and neurodegenerative diseases. In Magnetic resonance imaging of the brain and spine (Ed. S. W. Atlas), pp. 803–70, Lippincott Williams and Wilkins: Philadephia.

Lishman, W. A. (1997). *Organic psychiatry*. Blackwell Science: Oxford.

Mantyla, R., Erkinjuntti, T., Salonen, O., *et al.* (1997). Variable agreement between visual rating scales for white matter hyperintensities on MRI. Comparison of 13 rating scales in a poststroke cohort. *Stroke*, **28**, 1614–23.

Matsumae, M., Kikinis, R., Morocz, I., *et al.* (1996). Intracranial compartment volumes in patients with enlarged ventricles assessed by magnetic resonance-based image processing. *Journal of Neurosurgery*, **84**, 972–81.

McKhann, G., Drachman, D., Folstein, M., *et al.* (1984). Clinical diagnosis of Alzheimer's Disease: Report of the NINCDS- ADRDA work group under the auspices of Department of Health and Human Services Task Force on Alzheimer's Disease. *Neurology*, **34**, 939–44.

Mesulam, M.-M. (1987). Primary progressive aphasia: differentiation from Alzheimer's disease. *Annals of Neurology*, **22**, 533–4.

Moseley, I. (1995). Imaging the adult brain. *Journal of Neurology Neurosurgery and Psychiatry*, **58**, 7–21.

Mummery, C. J. Patterson, K., Price, C. J., Azhburner, J., Frackwiak, R. S. J., and Hodges, J. R. (2000). A voxel-based morphometry study of semantic dementia: relationship between temporal lobe atoplay and semantic memory. *Annals of Neurology*, **47**, 36–45.

Murphy, D. G., DeCarli, C. D., Daly, E., *et al.* (1993). Volumetric magnetic resonance imaging in men with dementia of the Alzheimer type: correlations with disease severity. *Biological Psychiatry*, **34**, 612–21.

Neary, D., Snowden, J. S., Gustafson, L., *et al.* (1998). Frontotemporal lobar degeneration: a consensus on clinical diagnostic criteria. *Neurology*, **51**, 1546–54.

Neary, D., Snowden, J. S., Mann, D. M., *et al.* (1990). Frontal lobe dementia and motor neuron disease. *Journal of Neurology Neurosurgery and Psychiatry*, **53**, 23–32.

Pantel, J. and Schroder, J. (1996). Posterior cortical atrophy–a new dementia syndrome or a form of Alzheimer's disease? *Fortschritte Der Neurologie Psychiatrie*, **64**, 492–508.

Pearlson, G. D., Harris, G. J., Powers, R. E., *et al.* (1992). Quantitative changes in mesial temporal volume, regional cerebral blood flow, and cognition in Alzheimer's disease. *Archives of General Psychiatry*, **49**, 402–8.

Pucci, E., Belardinelli, N., Regnicolo, L., *et al.* (1998). Hippocampus and parahippocampal gyrus linear measurements based on magnetic resonance in Alzheimer's disease. *Journal of European Neurology*, **39**, 16–25.

Roman, G. C., Tatemichi, T. K., Erkinjuntti, T., *et al.* (1993). Vascular Dementia: Diagnostic criteria for research studies. Report of the NINDS-AIREN International Workshop. *Neurology*, **43**, 250–60.

Rusinek, H., de Leon, M. J., George, A. E., *et al.* (1991). Alzheimer disease: measuring loss of cerebral gray matter with MR imaging. *Radiology*, **178**, 109–14.

Sandor, T., Jolesz, F., Tieman, J., *et al.* (1992). Comparative analysis of computed tomographic and magnetic resonance imaging scans in Alzheimer patients and controls. *Archives of Neurology*, **49**, 381–4.

Scheltens, P., Barkhof, F., Leys, D., *et al.* (1993). A semiquantitative rating scale for the assessment of signal hyperintensities on magnetic resonance imaging. *Journal of the Neurological Sciences*, **114**, 7–12.

Scheltens, P., Leys, D., Barkhof, F., *et al.* (1992). Atrophy of medial temporal lobes on MRI in 'probable' Alzheimer's disease and normal ageing: diagnostic value and neuropsychological correlates. *Journal of Neurology Neurosurgery and Psychiatry*, **55**, 967–72.

Scheltens, P., Pasquier, F., Weerts, J. E., *et al.* (1997). Qualitative assessment of cerebral atrophy on MRI: Inter- and intra-observer reproducibility in dementia and normal aging. *Journal of European Neurology*, **37**, 95–9.

Schlenska, G. K. and Walter, G. F. (1989). Serial computed tomography findings in Creutzfeldt–Jakob disease. *Neuroradiology*, **31**, 303–6.

Schmidt, R. (1992). Comparison of magnetic resonance imaging in Alzheimer's disease, vascular dementia and normal aging. *European Neurology*, **32**, 164–9.

Seab, J. B., Jagust, W. J., Wong, S. T. S., *et al.* (1988). Quantitative NMR measurements of hippocampal atrophy in Alzheimer's disease. *Magnetic Resonance in Medicine*, **8**, 200–8.

Sisodiya, S. M., Stevens, J. M., Fish, D. R., *et al.* (1996). The demonstration of gyral abnormalities in patients with cryptogenic partial epilepsy using three-dimensional MRI. *Archives of Neurology*, **53**, 28–34.

Tanabe, J. L., Amend, D., Schuff, N., *et al.* (1997). Tissue segmentation of the brain in Alzheimer disease. *American Journal of Neuroradiology*, **18**, 115–23.

Tartaro, A., Fulgente, T., Delli Pizzi, C., *et al.* (1993). MRI alterations as an early finding in Creutzfeld–Jakob disease. *European Journal of Radiology*, **17**, 155–8.

The Lund and Manchester Groups. (1994). Clinical and neuropathological criteria for frontotemporal dementia. The Lund and Manchester Groups. *Journal of Neurology Neurosurgery and Psychiatry*, **57**, 416–18.

Tyrrell, P. J., Warrington, E. K., Frackowiak, R. S., *et al.* (1990). Progressive degeneration of the right temporal lobe studied with positron emission tomography. *Journal of Neurology Neurosurgery and Psychiatry*, **53**, 1046–50.

Vermersch, P., Scheltens, P., Barkhof, F., *et al.* (1994). Evidence for atrophy of the Corpus callosum in Alzheimer's disease. *Journal of European Neurology*, **34**, 83–6.

Victoroff, J., Ross, G. W., Benson, D. F., *et al.* (1994). Posterior cortical atrophy. Neuropathologic correlations. *Archives of Neurology*, **51**, 269–74.

Wikkelso, C., Andersson, H., Blomstrand, C., *et al.* (1989). Computed tomography of the brain in the diagnosis of and prognosis in normal pressure hydrocephalus. *Neuroradiology*, **31**, 160–5.

Woermann, F. G., Free, S. L., Koepp, M. J., *et al.* (1999). Voxel-by-voxel comparison of automatically segmented cerebral gray matter — A rater-independent comparison of structural MRI in patients with epilepsy. *Neuroimage*, **10**, 373–84.

Yamauchi, H., Fukuyama, H., Harada, K., *et al.* (1993). Callosal atrophy parallels decreased cortical oxygen metabolism and neuropsychological impairment in Alzheimer's disease. *Archives of Neurology*, **50**, 1070–4.

Zeidler, M., Sellar, R. J., Collie, D. A., *et al.* (2000). The pulvinar sign on magnetic resonance imaging in variant Creutzfeldt–Jakob disease. *Lancet*, **355**, 1412–18.

Zeidler, M., Stewart, G. E., Barraclough, C. R., *et al.* (1997). New variant Creutzfeldt–Jakob disease: neurological features and diagnostic tests. *Lancet*, **350**, 903–7.

Zeidler, M., Will, R. G., Ironside, J. W., *et al.* (1996). Creutzfeldt–Jakob disease and bovine spongiform encephalopathy. Magnetic resonance imaging is not a sensitive test for Creutzfeldt–Jakob disease. *British Medical Journal*, **312**, 844.

7 Neuroradiological investigation: functional neuroimaging: SPECT/PET

Gene E. Alexander and Pietro Pietrini

1 Introduction

Advances in nuclear medicine technology over the past two decades have significantly enhanced the ability to evaluate the *in vivo* neurophysiological effects of neurodegenerative disease. The development of functional neuroimaging methods such as positron emission tomography (PET) and single photon emission computed tomography (SPECT) have provided the opportunity to assess regional neural activity in the awake human brain. With these advances it has become possible to study with increasing sensitivity and specificity the regional changes that occur in the brain as neurodegenerative diseases progress. Applications of these neuroimaging techniques to investigate the neurophysiological effects of the most common form of age-related dementia, Alzheimer's disease (AD), has increased our understanding of the mechanisms of the progressive cognitive and behavioural dysfunction characteristic of this debilitating illness. Further, studies have illustrated the potential for such functional neuroimaging methods in aiding the early detection of AD, even prior to the onset of clinical symptoms, and in the direct evaluation in the brain of treatment efficacy of pharmacological agents designed to delay or diminish the clinical and pathophysiological effects of this disease. Sensitive and specific markers that identify individuals early in the course of AD offer the opportunity to implement treatments in the very early stages of disease when the intervention may be most beneficial. Thus, the use and further development of such neuroimaging techniques hold great promise in aiding the clinical evaluation and treatment of dementias, such as AD.

In this chapter, we will present a brief description of the basic principles underlying PET and SPECT imaging methodology, followed by a review of the literature illustrating what has been learned from the applications of these functional imaging techniques to the study of AD-related dementia. This includes functional neuroimaging studies performed in the resting state (i.e. with no or minimal sensory stimulation), elucidating the regional distribution of neurophysiological effects of the disease; during cognitive activity and sensory stimulation, providing a cognitive or neurophysiological 'stress' test for neurodegenerative disease; with pharmacological challenge to evaluate treatment efficacy directly in the brain; and with the use of neuroreceptor ligands developed to assess the integrity and progressive dysfunction of neurotransmitter and other biochemical systems altered in AD. Together, these applications of PET and SPECT to the study of the neurophysiological substrate of AD have enhanced our knowledge of the mechanism of cognitive dysfunction, aided efforts at early detection, and have provided a valuable tool to evaluate treatment outcome in the brain of individuals with dementia and those at risk for the development of dementia.

2 Basic principles and methodology

2.1 PET

In PET, positron-emitting radiotracers are utilized to enable three-dimensional reconstruction of functional brain activity. These unstable compounds have an excess of protons in their nucleus. Positrons with the same mass as an electron but with a positive charge are emitted. A positron has the kinetic energy to travel a few millimetres within tissue. When almost at rest the positron interacts with an unbound electron. Since the two particles have an opposite charge, they annihilate each other. This results in two gamma ray photons of 511 keV energy being emitted at 180 degrees from each other. In a PET scanner, the gamma photons are detected by rings of radiation detectors that surround the individual's head. Pairs of these radiation detectors are oriented to face each other at 180 degrees and are connected by an electronic coincidence circuit that detects the photons emitted during the annihilation event when the positron meets an electron. The pairs of coincidence circuits convert light energy into electrical energy to measure the number of photon pairs originating from all angles in the brain. Through a computer reconstruction algorithm, it is possible to determine both the amount and location of radioactivity on a regional basis throughout the brain, with an inherent limitation in spatial resolution due to the few millimetres distance travelled by the positron before the annihilation event occurs.

Since PET requires the use of a local cyclotron to manufacture positron-emitting tracers, its availability has typically been limited to large medical research centres and has made it a relatively expensive functional neuroimaging method to employ.

2.1.1 Regional cerebral blood flow

Using PET, rCBF is commonly assessed with water labelled with ^{15}O. As a freely diffusible tracer, $H_2^{15}O$ quickly equilibrates between brain and blood and provides an excellent indicator of blood flow. Immediately following an intravenous injection of a bolus of $H_2^{15}O$ and after a sufficient number of radioactive tissue counts are observed in brain, a PET scan is acquired that can last from one to four minutes to measure local radioactivity in distinct cerebral regions. Radioactivity can be concurrently measured in the blood by sampling from an indwelling arterial line that is connected to an automatic counter. Using a mathematical model, it is possible to determine absolute rCBF values in terms of ml/100 grams tissue/min.

Since the radioactivity of ^{15}O has a rapid decay (half-life = 2.05 minutes), multiple scans can be performed sequentially in the same individual, ranging from 6–12 minutes apart. This makes it possible to evaluate rCBF repeatedly in a single PET session, while the subject is in the 'resting state' or engaged in performing a variety of tasks. By subtracting a baseline rCBF scan from a task rCBF scan, regions where activity is specifically altered during the task can be identified. In such rCBF studies, arterial blood P_aCO_2 is monitored so that global CBF can be corrected when differences in P_aCO_2 occur.

2.1.2 Regional cerebral glucose metabolism

In PET, the regional brain uptake of $[^{18}F]$-fluoro-2-deoxy-D-glucose (FDG) by neural cells can be measured in an awake individual, providing a measure of rCMRglc. FDG is an analogue of glucose that is labelled with ^{18}F and has a radioactive half-life of 110 minutes. After a bolus intravenous injection, FDG reaches the brain via blood flow and, like glucose, can be transported across the cerebral capillary bed into the neurons by a monosaccharide transport system. Once inside brain cells, FDG is phosphorylated to FDG-6-phosphate (FDG-6-P), but unlike glucose-6-P, FDG-6-P is not further metabolized by glycolytic pathway enzymes. Since brain phosphatase enzyme activity is low, FDG-6-P remains essentially trapped inside brain cells during the duration of the scan.

The quantity of FDG-6-P that has accumulated in a brain region during 45 minutes of uptake after FDG intravenous injection is measured by PET. This PET FDG measurement reflects the rate of phosphorylation of glucose to glucose-6-P and the plasma integral of FDG to which the brain is exposed.

2.2 SPECT

In SPECT imaging, the radiopharmaceuticals use isotopes that emit a single gamma ray photon. This fundamental difference from the radiotracers used in PET, where two photons are emitted, accounts for the principal differences in instrumentation and capabilities for measuring functional brain activity between these two tomographic imaging techniques.

As with PET, SPECT imaging of the brain involves two essential steps: the administration of a radiotracer and the use of a tomographic scanner to measure the regional distribution of the radiotracer in the brain. In SPECT, as in PET, scintillation crystals are used to detect the radioactivity emitted from the tracers. Since only single photons are emitted and travel in all directions, SPECT depends on the use of collimators to determine the point of origin of the emitted photons to localize regional brain activity. These collimators are in the form of lead septa that are positioned in front of the scintillation crystal detectors. The apertures created between the septa serve to limit the exposure of the crystals to gamma ray photons that are arriving at a nearly perpendicular angle to the crystal surface. In PET, such septa are employed for two-dimensional image acquisition, but can be retracted in the new three-dimensional image scanners. With the implementation of multiple head SPECT cameras, sensitivity and spatial resolution have significantly improved. However, SPECT continues to have lower spatial resolution than PET and has greater difficulty in identifying deep brain structures.

The principal radiopharmaceuticals currently used in SPECT to assess neural activity measure rCBF, although agents to assess characteristics of several neuroreceptor systems have also been developed (e.g. Eckelman *et al.* 1984; Kung *et al.* 1990). The most commonly used tracers to measure rCBF in SPECT include [^{99m}Tc]hexamethly-propyleneamine (HMPAO) and [^{99m}Tc]ethyl cysteinate dimer (ECD). The radiotracer, [^{123}I]isopropyl iodoamphetamine (IMP) has also been widely used to measure rCBF with SPECT. Although employed initially in non-tomographic imaging, the use of xenon-133 has continued with SPECT. With a relatively fast clearance, this tracer allows for multiple scans in the same SPECT session, but offers relatively low spatial resolution (Newberg *et al.* 1995).

In general, compared to positron-emitting tracers of PET, the radioisotopes in SPECT emit lower energy photons (i.e. 80–159 keV) that are more susceptible to attenuation as the photons travel through tissue, especially in deeper brain structures. Thus, brain structures like the basal ganglia, which are farther from the detector surface, have poorer resolution than cortical brain regions. This combined with complexities in modelling tracer behaviour makes full regional quantitation of absolute rCBF in SPECT difficult and in practice, as is also often done with PET, regional tissue counts in cortex are typically referenced to global tissue counts or relatively preserved brain regions (e.g. cerebellum) to provide a semi-quantitative measure of cerebral perfusion. Further, the radioactive half-life of 6 hours for [^{99m}Tc] and 13 hours for [^{123}I], as well as the relatively slow washout of the tracers, such as HMPAO and IMP, significantly limit the ability to perform multiple scans to assess rCBF under different test conditions during the same scanning session with these relatively higher resolution SPECT tracers. Importantly, the greater ease of production and the potential for longer storage of these radiotracers compared to positronemitting agents provide the advantage of eliminating the need for an on-site cyclotron as is required with PET.

Despite the technical limitations of SPECT relative to PET, the wide availability and lower cost of this tomographic technique combined with the ability to detect regional reductions in cortical perfusion with a spatial resolution that can approach that of PET has significantly enhanced its role in recent years as a functional imaging method to aid the clinical assessment of neurodegenerative disease.

3 Applications to studies of dementia

As the most common cause of dementia in the elderly, AD has been a major focus of functional neuroimaging research since the early 1980s. AD is characterized by a progressive decline of cognitive functions, in which memory and aspects of attention are typically affected early in the course and are followed by decline in other cognitive abilities, such as language, visuospatial skills, and abstract reasoning (see Chapter 11). The major neuropathological features of AD include the presence of senile plaques, neurofibrillary tangles, and loss of neurons and their synaptic projections (Chapter 10). Although the regional distribution of brain pathology varies among individuals, the areas most commonly affected include the association cortical and limbic regions. In AD, deficits in several neurotransmitter systems have been demonstrated. Dysfunction of the cholinergic system has been implicated in age-related changes in memory and has been a major target in the development of potential therapeutic agents for AD (see Chapter 9).

Here, we will present the main findings from PET and SPECT studies that have examined brain metabolic function under different experimental conditions in AD patients.

3.1 Studies in the resting state

Studies measuring cerebral metabolism and blood flow in a 'resting state', that is with minimal sensory stimulation (e.g. eyes closed and ears occluded), provide the opportunity to evaluate the regional distribution of neurophysiological changes that occur in the context of a neurodegenerative disease, like AD, and monitor changes as the disease progresses (Haxby 1990). The regional pattern of cerebral dysfunction observed in AD patients relative to healthy elderly individuals has been quite consistent across studies and functional imaging methods. Together, these studies have indicated that the association neocortex is prominently affected in AD; the parietotemporal regions, which are typically affected early in the course of the disease, are the brain area most consistently and severely diminished (Frackowiak *et al.* 1981; Foster *et al.* 1983; Duara *et al.* 1986; Kumar *et al.* 1991). Declines in functional activity of other association brain regions, such as frontal and occipital association cortices, are also present, especially as the disease progresses. In contrast, there is a relative preservation of function in regions of the primary sensory cortices, subcortical nuclei, and cerebellum. Further, the number of correlations in functional activity between regions of the association cortex are decreased in patients with AD compared to healthy individuals (Horwitz *et al.* 1987), suggesting disruption of the functional connectivity between brain regions in AD-related dementia.

An association between regional hypometabolism and the distribution of neurofibrillary tangles in AD has been observed post-mortem (DeCarli *et al.* 1992), but this association has not been consistently demonstrated across studies (Mega *et al.* 1997). In general, there have been fewer consistent associations observed between the severity of AD pathology found in the medial temporal lobe brain structures, such as the hippocampus, and the degree of functional neuroimaging abnormalities seen in these regions. This inconsistency may be, in part, due to the limited spatial resolution with PET and SPECT. Spatial resolution of a few millimetres can produce partial volume averaging of functional activity in a brain region that is smaller than the limits of resolution of the scanner. In this case, non-grey matter tissue (i.e. white matter or cerebrospinal fluid) can be included in the determination of the average functional activity for given brain regions. Small structures, like the hippocampus, are particularly vulnerable to this effect with both PET and SPECT, and this can diminish the ability to detect small differences between individuals or groups. Given that brain atrophy also occurs to a greater extent in AD patients than healthy elderly, anatomical information obtained from magnetic resonance imaging has been applied in combination with PET to determine whether the pattern of functional abnormalities observed with functional neuroimaging simply reflect brain atrophy due to cell loss or represent compromised neural synaptic activity (Meltzer *et al.* 1996; Ibañez *et al.* 1998). These studies, using both selected regions of interest and sampling all voxels (i.e. the smallest unit of image volume) in the PET images have indicated that atrophy alone is not sufficient to explain the regional pattern of cerebral dysfunction commonly observed with PET, and that specific patterns of neural dysfunction occur in addition to the cell loss related to atrophy in association neocortex in AD (Figure 7.1). Thus, measures of cerebral metabolism as obtained by PET can be considered a reliable biochemical index of the degree of neuronal functional activity.

3.1.1 Clinical and neurophysiological heterogeneity in AD

Heterogeneity of clinical symptoms in AD has been widely observed. Subgroups in AD have been identified based on patient differences in patterns of neuropsychological impairment, neurological symptoms, and behavioural dysfunction (see Chapter 11). Further, these clinically defined AD subgroups have been shown to differ in regional patterns of cerebral metabolism and perfusion using PET and SPECT. In a study by Grady *et al.* (1990), using a form of principal component analysis, four subgroups were identified in a typical sample of 33 patients with a clinical diagnosis of AD based on differential patterns of cerebral metabolism with PET. One group had a typical pattern of parietotemporal hypometabolism, whereas one subgroup showed reduced metabolism predominantly in frontal regions. Another group had left greater than right hemisphere reductions and one group showed both frontal and parietotemporal hypometabolism.

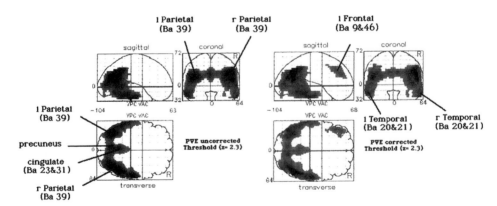

Figure 7.1 Comparison of glucose metabolism between control subjects and Alzheimer's disease (AD) patients before and after partial volume (atrophy) correction. Statistical parametric maps of orthogonal projections for significant voxels are shown. The intercommissural line is set to 0 mm. The anterior commissure (VAC) and the posterior commissure (VPC) are represented in the sagittal and transverse projections. The projections are presented with a Z threshold of 2.3 for uncorrected (left) and partial volume effect (PVE)-corrected (right) values. No area with significant reduction in metabolism became normal after correction. Further, reductions in glucose metabolism in a left frontal area of AD patients became significant only after correction. Ba = Brodmann area; l = left; r = right. (Adapted from Ibañez *et al.* 1998.)

These subgroup differences in PET patterns were subsequently supported in 24 patients with pathologically confirmed AD, indicating that the neurophysiological heterogeneity observed in AD is not related to clinical misdiagnosis or the presence of comorbid neuropathological abnormalities (Strassburger *et al.* 1996).

In addition, regional pattern differences in resting state cerebral activity have been shown in patients with specific behavioural disturbances present in the context of AD-related dementia, such as depression, agitation, disinhibition, delusions, and hallucinations. Mentis *et al.* (1995) showed that 9 AD patients with a delusional misidentification syndrome had lower mean cerebral metabolism in orbitofrontal brain regions compared to 15 AD patients without this behavioural abnormality and 17 healthy controls. Greater reductions of rCBF assessed by SPECT and Tc99 HMPAO in the prefrontal and anterior temporal regions have been demonstrated in AD patients with high ratings of apathy than patients with low apathy scores (Craig *et al.* 1996).

Individual variability in the regional pattern of functional brain abnormalities has also been demonstrated through indices that reflect hemispheric asymmetries in functional brain activity with PET. Greater variability in asymmetries between hemispheres in AD compared to healthy elderly have been well documented (Haxby *et al.* 1985; Duara *et al.* 1986; Waldemar *et al.* 1994) and further, have been correlated with relative differences in performance in cognitive tests that are often associated to a greater degree with right (e.g. visuospatial skills) versus left (e.g. language skills) hemisphere function (Haxby *et al.* 1985).

Although memory impairment is typically the hallmark feature of AD, in a rare subgroup of AD the onset of disease is characterized by visuospatial dysfunction in the absence of prominent memory difficulties (see Chapter 11). Pietrini *et al.* (1996) compared 10 patients with this 'visual variant' of AD, to 22 patients with typical AD and 25 healthy elderly individuals using PET with FDG. Both AD groups showed prominent hypometabolism compared to controls, but the AD patients with early visual complaints had greater reductions of cerebral metabolism in the primary visual and occipital association brain regions than the typical AD patients (Figure 7.2; see Plate 1). Examination of the distribution of histopathology in two of the visual variant AD patients that had come to autopsy showed greater AD pathology in the posterior occipital association and primary visual cortex compared to typical AD patients (Pietrini *et al.* 1997*b*).

AD patients with moderate and severe levels of dementia severity show greater reductions in cerebral metabolism and blood flow than patients with mild dementia (Figure 7.3; see Plate 2) (Frackowiak *et al.* 1981; Haxby *et al.* 1988; Kumar *et al.* 1991). A number of studies have demonstrated correlations between cerebral metabolic and perfusion abnormalities at rest and clinical measures of dementia severity and cognitive performance in AD (e.g. Haxby *et al.* 1988; Buck *et al.* 1997). Using Scaled Subprofile Model analysis, a modified form of principal component analysis, to characterize how regionally distributed brain areas functionally interact, two regional patterns of functional brain activity, as measured by resting rCMRglc were identified whose expression differed between 42 AD patients and 40 healthy elderly individuals. One pattern included a parietotemporal deficit with relative increases of activity in several frontal brain regions. The second pattern was characterized by relatively lower cerebral metabolism in the left frontal association cortex with relatively higher activity in occipital brain regions. Among the AD patients, a greater expression of the parietotemporal deficit pattern was correlated with poorer performance on cognitive tests of visuospatial skills and attention; whereas a greater expression of the frontotemporal deficit pattern was associated with poorer language and verbal memory (Alexander and Moeller 1994).

Demographic and genetic factors have also been associated with the severity of cerebral dysfunction in AD. Stern and colleagues (1995) found that both years of education and ratings of occupational attainment were inversely correlated with parietotemporal perfusion in the AD

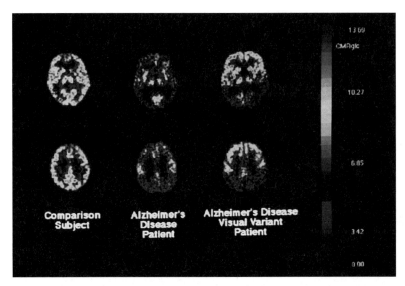

Figure 7.2 Comparison of glucose metabolism for Alzheimer's disease patients with and without prominent visual symptoms and a healthy control subject. Values of CMRglc reported on the colorimetric scale are in units of milligrams per 100 grams of tissue per minute. Relative to the healthy control subject, the patient with Alzheimer's disease (AD) and no visual symptoms shows the typical pattern of reductions in glucose metabolism in frontal, temporal, and parietal association areas, with preservation of metabolic rates in primary sensory regions. In contrast, compared to the AD patient without visual symptoms, the AD patient with visual symptoms shows a prominent glucose hypometabolism in parietal and occipital areas, including primary visual cortex, along with preservation of metabolism in frontal and temporal regions, which is virtually indistinguishable from that of the healthy control subject. CMRglc = cerebral metabolic rate for glucose. (From Pietrini *et al.* 1996.)

group, after they controlled for the degree of dementia severity, providing initial support for a brain reserve that can delay or diminish the clinical symptoms of AD while the pathophysiological effects of the disease progress. This finding was subsequently supported by a study using high resolution, tomographic imaging with PET FDG, in which both years of education and an estimate of premorbid intellectual function were inversely correlated with cerebral metabolism in a parietal association area, as well as several frontal association and subcortical brain regions in a group of 46 AD patients, after dementia severity was controlled for (Figure 7.4) (Alexander *et al.* 1997). Together, these findings indicate that factors such as patient differences in level of education and premorbid intellectual ability may contribute to the clinical and neurophysiological heterogeneity commonly observed in AD.

With recent advances in molecular genetics a number of studies have sought to identify whether differences in patterns or severity of progression of cerebral dysfunction in AD are related to the several genetic factors that have been implicated in the aetiology of this disease. Studies using PET FDG in adults with Down's Syndrome (DS) have shown that the onset of dementia in these individuals is associated with reductions of cerebral metabolism in cortical association areas typically affected in AD in the general population (Dani *et al.* 1996). Similarly, PET studies comparing AD patients with a familiarly inherited mutation of the amyloid precursor protein gene as well as a mutation on chromosome 14 to healthy controls showed similar patterns of hypometabolism observed in non-familial AD (Julin *et al.* 1998; Fox *et al.* 1997; Kennedy *et al.* 1995*b*). Presence of the ε4 allele of the apolipoprotein E gene has been associated with alterations of cerebral metabolism and blood flow in AD patients that may contribute to the neurophysiological heterogeneity observed in AD (Lehtovirta *et al.* 1996; van Dyck *et al.* 1998).

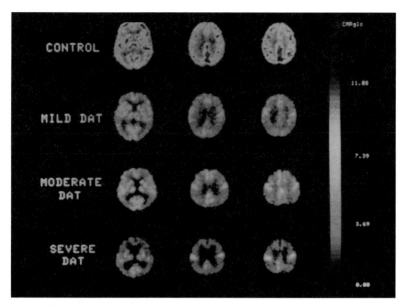

Figure 7.3 Transverse images at three different levels of brain PET scans in a normal control and in Alzheimer's disease (AD) patients with mild, moderate, and severe dementia, respectively (from top to bottom). rCMRglc values reported on the colorimetric scale are in mg/100 g/min. rCMRglc reductions are present mostly in the association areas and become more severe as AD progresses. Primary neocortical areas are relatively spared, even in the latest stages of the disease.

3.1.2 Longitudinal studies

Evaluation of the longitudinal effects of AD on brain function using PET and SPECT assessed in the resting state have shown that the pattern of cerebral dysfunction observed in AD occurs early in the course of dementia and progressively worsens over time (McGeer *et al.* 1990). Studies have also indicated that the hemispheric asymmetries and relative regional pattern differences observed in AD on initial examination tend to remain present as the disease progresses (Grady *et al.* 1986; 1988; Haxby *et al.* 1990). Despite a significant decline in cerebral metabolism in a group of AD patients followed for 26 months, Haxby *et al.* (1990) found stability of right to left metabolic asymmetries in both the relative magnitude and direction of hemispheric differences. Similarly, the relative differences in the pattern of cognitive impairment associated with right versus left metabolic asymmetries were maintained. Measures of rCBF with SPECT have also demonstrated that perfusion in the parietal and temporal brain regions can predict cognitive decline and survival among AD patients that have been followed longitudinally, with greater hypoperfusion in these regions leading to faster mortality (Jagust *et al.* 1998; Claus *et al.* 1999). In a study by Claus *et al.* (1999), 69 patients with AD were followed clinically up to 5.5 years after a baseline SPECT rCBF scan that was obtained at time of initial diagnosis. In their AD sample, relatively lower rCBF in the left temporal and parietal cortices predicted a greater decline over time in measures of language function. Further, those patients in the lowest quartile of left temporal perfusion had a significantly higher risk of mortality over the follow-up period than the AD patients with relatively higher rCBF in this region. These findings provide further support for the use of functional neuroimaging in monitoring the progression of neurodegenerative disease and may assist in the prediction of clinical outcome.

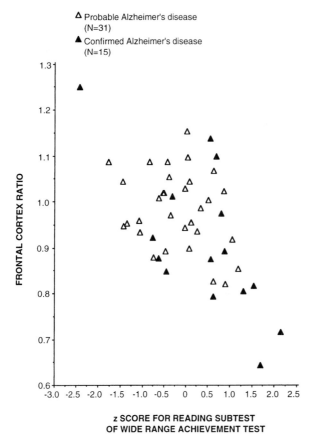

△ Probable Alzheimer's disease (N=31)
▲ Confirmed Alzheimer's disease (N=15)

FRONTAL CORTEX RATIO

z SCORE FOR READING SUBTEST OF WIDE RANGE ACHIEVEMENT TEST

Figure 7.4 Relation between glucose metabolism in the frontal cortex and premorbid intellectual function in Alzheimer's disease (AD) patients. A significant inverse correlation between premorbid intellectual ability and cerebral metabolism in the frontal association region referenced to CMRglc in the left sensorimotor area is observed in 46 AD patients. Premorbid function is measured using standardized residuals (z-scores) of reading performance on the Wide Range Achievement Test, after statistically removing the effects of age, gender, illness duration, and dementia severity with the Mattis Dementia Rating Scale. The open triangles indicate patients with a diagnosis of probable AD according to NINCDS-ADRDA criteria, whereas the filled triangles are patients with autopsy confirmed AD. Frontal cortex ratio = mean of prefrontal and premotor association regions divided by left sensorimotor cortex; CMRglc = cerebral metabolic rates for glucose (mg/100 g/min). (From Alexander *et al.* 1997.)

3.2 Cognitive and sensory stimulation studies

An increasing number of studies have used cognitive and sensory paradigms during the measurement of rCBF or rCMRglc to assess the functional response to brain stimulation in dementia. Whereas resting state studies provide valuable information on the regional distribution of the pathophysiological effects of disease, functional neuroimaging studies during the performance of a cognitive task or exposure to 'passive' sensory stimulation offers a method to directly assess, *in vivo*, how the disease process alters brain systems that are important for specific cognitive and behavioural functions. In general, these studies are conducted by contrasting brain responses during one or more stimulation conditions with a baseline or control condition to determine those brain regions that are significantly increased or decreased from baseline during a specific cognitive process or sensory experience.

3.2.1 Cognitive studies

Several studies have investigated brain responses during the performance of cognitive tasks in AD patients using PET and SPECT. Duara and colleagues (1992) have used cognitive tasks assessing verbal fluency and the reading and recall of memory passages in comparison to the resting state with PET FDG to measure rCMRglc in AD patients and elderly controls. In the study using the verbal fluency task, the AD patients showed a global CMRglc increase that was less than healthy elderly controls, and no significant regional increases were observed in the AD group. The AD patients did, however, show relatively decreased regional metabolism in occipital brain regions relative to rest, which was not observed in the elderly controls. The authors interpreted these findings as suggesting a general increase of brain activity during the task in anterior brain regions with a relative lack of activation in the posterior association cortex, and that this effect was diminished in AD patients compared to healthy subjects. In contrast, the study requiring the reading and recall of memory passages elicited global metabolic increases over rest in 20 AD patients with preferential activation in primary and visual association areas that did not differ from 14 healthy controls (Duara et al. 1992).

In a study in which a continuous visual recognition memory task was used, 21 AD patients were compared to 9 healthy controls with PET FDG to measure the rCMRglc response to the task relative to the resting state (Kessler et al. 1991). In this study, an easier version of the task was administered to the AD group than controls in an effort to equate task performance between the two groups. Despite the attempt to match performance, the AD patients showed poorer task performance than the control subjects and demonstrated a significantly smaller global increase in cerebral glucose metabolism than controls. The relative pattern of regional activation appeared similar in both groups with primary visual cortex showing the greatest relative increase. In a subsequent study, Kessler et al. (1996) compared 17 AD patients performing an auditory continuous recognition task to a group of 18 AD patients receiving the visual recognition task. They found a small increase in global glucose metabolism that did not differ between the two AD groups despite modality specific differences in regional activation with PET FDG for the auditory and visual tasks. These findings suggested that the diminished global activation response previously observed in AD patients compared to healthy controls was not due to the visual modality of the task.

Grady and colleagues (1993) investigated the rCBF response to a visual discrimination task that involved the perceptual matching of faces in a group of 7 AD patients with mild-to-moderate dementia and 8 healthy elderly controls. In this study, the groups did not differ significantly in task accuracy. The AD patients demonstrated increases of rCBF during performance of the face matching task that were equivalent in occipitotemporal regions and higher in occipital brain regions than the control group. In addition, the AD patients showed significant activation in right premotor cortex that was not observed in controls. These findings suggest that the ability to recruit visual association areas during the performance of a visual perceptual discrimination task is preserved despite the presence of reduced rCBF in the resting state in AD with mild dementia. The additional recruitment of the right premotor area in the AD patients may reflect the brain's capacity for functional compensation in the presence of compromised brain function with neurodegenerative disease.

Face matching in healthy young adults has been associated with a widely distributed set of brain regions that are important for object perception and attentional processing (Haxby et al. 1994). Further, individual differences in task performance during the perceptual matching of faces has been directly associated with modulation of this network (Alexander et al. 1999). In AD, the regionally distributed network of brain regions involved in cognitive tasks, like face matching, may be altered early in the course of disease. Indeed, Horwitz and colleagues (1995) applied network path analysis to the same face matching PET data from the AD patients and healthy controls reported in the Grady et al. (1993) study. They found that although the AD patients had the same performance accuracy as controls, they appeared to use a different network of brain regions while performing the face matching task (Horwitz et al. 1995).

In a study by Becker et al. (1996), rCBF was assessed with PET during the performance of auditory-verbal memory tasks in a group of 7 AD patients and 7 healthy controls. They found that the AD group activated brain regions important for auditory and verbal memory processing to a greater extent than the healthy elderly subjects and further, that additional brains regions were activated in the AD patients during the cognitive task conditions compared to the elderly controls. These findings further supported the idea that networks important for cognitive processes are altered by AD and that the brain may compensate for the effects of neurodegeneration through a functional reallocation of neurocognitive resources.

Brain functional responses while performing distinct cognitive tasks in AD patients have also been investigated with SPECT. In a recent study using 133-xenon rCBF and SPECT, Cardebat and colleagues (1998) compared a group of 17 AD patients to 20 healthy controls during a word memory task, passive word listening, and a resting condition. They found no significant rCBF changes during the memory condition compared to listening in the AD group, but a similar pattern of activation as the control subjects was observed in the listening condition relative to rest. Further, they found a significant correlation between right frontal perfusion and memory performance in the AD group.

3.2.2 Sensory stimulation studies

Since patients with moderate-to-severe levels of dementia severity are often unable to reliably perform complex cognitive paradigms, passive sensory stimulation paradigms have been implemented with PET to evaluate the functional brain response in AD patients throughout the full range of dementia severity. Pietrini and colleagues (1999) contrasted the brain response during the presentation of a colour movie with a resting state (i.e. eyes closed, ears occluded) condition using a double-injection PET-FDG technique (Brooks *et al.* 1987) to assess the brain functional metabolic response elicited during audiovisual stimulation in a group of 15 AD patients and 14 healthy elderly control subjects. The AD group ranged from mild to the severe range of dementia severity. The results showed that, as a group, the AD patients were able to activate similar visual and auditory brain regions as the healthy controls. Compared to controls, the AD patients also showed higher metabolism during stimulation than at rest in additional brain regions, including in the parietal cortex, suggesting the possibility of recruitment of brain areas during audiovisual stimulation that are hypometabolic at rest and that are not recruited by healthy controls. In the subgroup of AD patients with mild dementia severity, the degree of brain activation in visual and auditory brain regions was similar to that of healthy controls (i.e. differed by less than 2 standard deviations), whereas the patients with moderate-to-severe dementia showed significantly diminished responses. Further, the degree of cerebral metabolic response in visual association brain regions was highly correlated with dementia severity in the AD group, with the most severely demented patients showing the lowest functional response to stimulation (Figure 7.5).

Mentis *et al.* (1996, 1998) investigated the rCBF response with $H_2^{15}O$ PET during the passive visual presentation of flashing lights that alternated between left and right eyes in a group of AD patients and healthy elderly controls. In these studies, the flash frequency of the lights were parametrically increased from 0 (i.e. eyes open in darkness) to 1, 2, 4, 7, and 14 Hz, acting as a neural 'stress test' to evaluate functional failure of the visual system in AD patients compared to healthy ageing and in relation to dementia severity (Rapoport and Grady 1993). As a group, the AD patients differed from healthy controls in the pattern of brain response to light stimulation as a function of flash frequency. Functional responses to low frequency stimulation was similar for both the AD and healthy control groups, but the AD patients showed smaller rCBF responses than controls at the frequency producing the largest response in the control subjects. Further, the results indicated that functional failure to passive visual stimulation occurs with mild dementia when large neural responses are required and in patients with moderate-to-severe dementia when large and intermediate brain responses are needed compared to healthy elderly controls.

Together, the above studies by Pietrini *et al.* (1999, 2000) and Mentis *et al.* (1996, 1998), indicate that neuronal synaptic viability is progressively affected by the development of a neuropathological process in the course of AD. The greatly diminished synaptic efficiency observed in the later stages of AD could have a role in the lack of response to pharmacological treatment

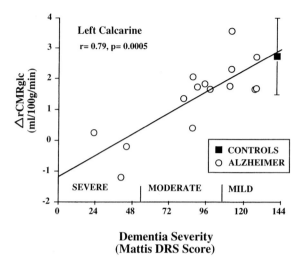

Figure 7.5 Relation between dementia severity and brain metabolic response to audiovisual stimulation in Alzheimer's disease patients. The abscissa represents dementia severity, measured by the Mattis Dementia Rating Scale (DRS) score (maximum score = 144). The ordinate represents regional differences (in absolute rCMRglc in mg per 100 g of brain tissue per minute) between audiovisual stimulation and the resting state for the Alzheimer's disease patients. The mean ± S.D. bar for controls is shown at the right of the figure. Mildly demented patients had rCMRglc increases in visual cortical areas within two standard deviations from the control mean; in contrast, moderate-to-severe dementia patients showed minimal or no response to stimulation. (From Pietrini et al. 1999.)

shown by patients with advanced dementia. As available treatments for AD attempt to augment neurotransmitters in the synaptic cleft, viable synapses are needed for them to be effective (Pietrini et al. 2000).

3.3 Diagnosis and early detection

3.3.1 Differential diagnosis

The use of SPECT and PET to aid clinical diagnosis of neurodegenerative disease is based on the distinctive patterns of cerebral hypometabolism and hypoperfusion typically observed in different forms of progressive dementia. Despite the patient variability previously discussed, AD is typically characterized by dysfunction of parietotemporal brain regions early in the disease course, as well as reductions in other association brain regions like frontal and occipital association cortices as the disease progresses. Although several disorders can be accompanied by a cerebral dysfunction in such regions of the association cortex at different stages of dementia severity, SPECT and PET can provide valuable input to clinical diagnosis by confirming AD when a parietotemporal deficit is observed.

Patients with frontotemporal dementia typically demonstrate prominent reductions in prefrontal and anterior temporal lobe cerebral metabolism and blood flow early in the clinical course (Neary et al. 1988; Alexander et al. 1995; Ishii et al. 1998). Reductions in frontal blood flow and metabolism have been reported in other neurological diseases leading to dementia, including progressive supranuclear palsy (Goffinet et al. 1989; Blin et al. 1990) and motor neuron disease with dementia (Talbot et al. 1995), as well as in disorders like depression (Baxter et al. 1989; Dolan et al. 1992). Symptomatic patients with Huntington's disease demonstrate consistent decrements in metabolism in caudate nucleus (see Chapter 15). Vascular dementia is characterized by widely distributed and varied patterns of cerebral dysfunction that can involve the cerebral cortex, white matter, cerebellum, and subcortical nuclei (Yao et al. 1990; Mielke et al. 1992). In Parkinson's disease with dementia, cortical hypometabolism is observed which can be most pronounced in parietotemporal cortex and can appear similar to the pattern observed in AD (Schapiro et al. 1993). Global hypometabolism together with relatively greater regional decrements in lateral temporal, inferior parietal, and frontal opercular cortex has been reported in corticobasal ganglionic degeneration (Eidelberg et al. 1991).

In general, research studies of resting state rCMRglc and rCBF have shown high degrees of sensitivity and specificity for dementia when compared to healthy elderly individuals. Fewer studies have addressed the ability of PET and SPECT methods to distinguish among neurodegenerative diseases. A recent study including 363 patients with dementia that were followed prospectively with rCBF SPECT showed that functional neuroimaging with SPECT was useful in distinguishing AD from vascular dementia and frontotemporal dementia, but appeared less able to distinguish Lewy body dementia from AD and between vascular dementia and frontotemporal dementia (Talbot *et al.* 1998). Diagnoses in this study were based on clinical criteria and thus, cannot rule out the possibility of misdiagnosis or comorbid neuropathological abnormalities in the sample.

Recent efforts to provide additional advances in diagnostic utility for SPECT and PET have included the development and application of analytical methods, such as Statistical Parametric Mapping, to statistically contrast regional values from individual patient scans to a normative comparison group (Bartenstein *et al.* 1997; Minoshima *et al.* 1995; Signorini *et al.* 1999) and combining information from anatomical imaging with functional imaging (Jobst *et al.* 1998). Further, the use of sophisticated multivariate statistical methods, such as discriminant and principal component-based analyses, has offered the potential to identify combinations of brain regions and patterns of subtle metabolic abnormalities that maximally distinguish patient groups and can subsequently be applied to SPECT or PET scans of patients on an individual basis or aid in the preclinical prediction of individuals who are likely to develop dementia (Azari *et al.* 1993; Johnson *et al.* 1998; Pietrini *et al.* 1993; Alexander and Moeller 1994). The development of diagnostic algorithms that combine functional neuroimaging test results obtained at rest and during cognitive or sensory stimulation with findings from other imaging modalities (e.g. structural MRI, EEG), as well as with clinical and demographic data may ultimately offer the most powerful tool to aid the clinician in the early differential diagnosis of dementia.

3.3.2 Early detection

Recent efforts in identifying the earliest effects of AD on brain function have focused on evaluating individuals at genetic risk for the development of dementia. Decrements in cerebral metabolism in brain regions affected early in AD, such as parietal cortex, have been observed in non-demented individuals with the ApoE ε4 allele (Small *et al.* 1995; Reiman *et al.* 1996). Further, studies of yet clinically unaffected family members in families with mutations on chromosome 14 or mutations in the amyloid precursor protein gene have also shown evidence of resting state hypometabolism in parietotemporal brain regions (Kennedy *et al.* 1995a).

The study of non-demented older adults with DS provides an additional clinical model to assess brain changes that occur prior to the onset of dementia in individuals with a 100% risk for the development of AD pathology (Holland and Oliver 1995). In a longitudinal study of DS adults followed with yearly PET scans for up to 12 years, it has been shown that significant declines in cognitive function and in resting state rCMRglc in the parietotemporal brain regions appears when dementia is diagnosed. However, both cognitive abilities and regional cerebral metabolism at rest remain relatively stable for many years prior to the onset of clinical dementia (Dani *et al.* 1996). This suggests that the development of AD-like neuropathology needs to reach a threshold before triggering a dramatic disruption in brain function.

In an attempt to identify functional brain changes in non-demented DS adults, Pietrini and colleagues (1997a) compared a group of elderly DS individuals to young DS adults using the double injection FDG method with PET during the presentation of passive audiovisual stimulation and in a resting condition. Although rCMRglc at rest did not differ between the two groups (Figure 7.6a), the older DS subjects showed significantly diminished brain responses to stimulation in parietal brain regions compared to the young DS subjects (Figure 7.6b). These findings suggest that despite normal metabolic function at rest, the brain's ability to respond to increased functional demands is impaired by the development of the neuropathological process even before the clinical onset of dementia. These results also indicate that stimulation paradigms with PET may offer greater sensitivity than resting conditions to the earliest effects of AD, acting as a neurophysiological stress test for dementia.

4 Studies with pharmacological probes

Functional neuroimaging methods offer the opportunity to directly evaluate the effects of pharmacological agents in the brain. The use of pharmacological challenge with PET and SPECT has the potential to enhance our understanding of the mechanism and site of action of newly developed treatments, to assist in identifying treatment responders from non-responders, and to evaluate drug efficacy by acting as a neurophysiological outcome measure. Further, by pharmacologically modulating selective neurotransmitter systems, one can investigate the functional role of a given neurotransmitter system in affecting distinct cognitive functions in normal and pathological conditions.

Studies measuring brain response to both long and short-acting cholinesterase inhibition with rCMRglc and rCBF at rest have indicated increased cerebral metabolism and blood flow in some AD patients with treatment that parallels improved cognitive performance (Geaney *et al.* 1990; van Dyck *et al.* 1997). However, other studies have reported decreases in cerebral metabolism with cholinergic enhancement and have suggested that observed increases in rCBF assessed at rest may be related to a non-specific vasodilatory action of neurotransmitter stimulation on large vessels rather than to a direct effect on the neural activity associated with cognitive processing (Blin *et al.* 1997).

In a recent study by Furey and colleagues (1997), rCBF in a group of healthy adults was assessed with PET during the performance of a working memory for faces task while 13 subjects received the cholinesterase inhibitor physostigmine and 8 subjects were given only placebo. Compared to the placebo group, the physostigmine treated group showed a significantly smaller increase of rCBF in a task-related region of the right prefrontal cortex (Figure 7.7; see Plate 3). Further, this relative reduction in rCBF was correlated with improved reaction time performance during the working memory task. These findings suggest that cholinergic enhancement may improve the efficiency of cognition and thus, reduce the need for recruitment of brain regions important for effortful information processing in the frontal cortex. This facilitory effect may be the result of drug induced augmentation of efficiency in stimuli processing in association visual cortical areas (Furey *et al.* 1999). More generally, these results emphasize the value of using functional brain imaging methodologies in conjunction with cognitive stimulation paradigms and pharmacological challenge to more directly evaluate drug effects on neural systems important for specific cognitive processes affected in neurodegenerative disease.

That only a fraction of AD patients demonstrate a clinically detectable improvement to chronic cholinergic enhancement with available treatments has suggested a need for methods to distinguish potential responders from non-responders to pharmacological interventions for dementia. In a study by Riekkinen and colleagues (1997), 9 patients with AD that showed improved performance on cognitive tests of attention with the administration of a single dose of the cholinesterase inhibitor tetrahydroaminoacridine (THA) had higher cortical perfusion assessed at rest in frontal and prefrontal brain regions than 19 AD patients showing no cognitive response to THA. Although limited to the resting baseline condition, these findings are consistent with those of Pietrini *et al.* (1999) and Mentis *et al.* (1996, 1998) in suggesting that impaired synaptic activity may be a contributing factor to the lack of response to pharmacological agents.

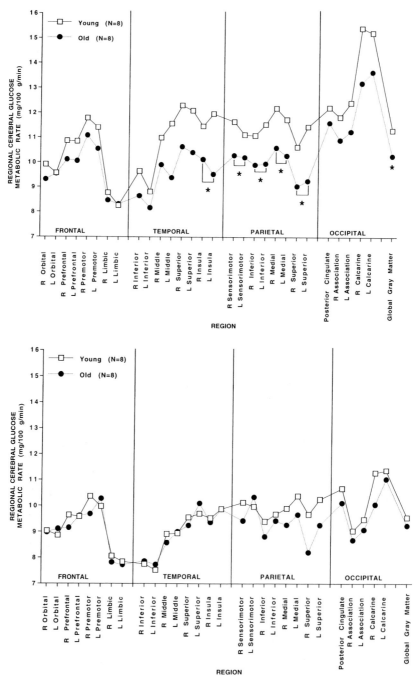

Figure 7.6 Mean absolute rates of regional cerebral glucose metabolism (a) at rest and (b) during audiovisual stimulation in younger and older adults with Down's syndrome. No significant difference between the two groups for any region was observed at rest. The older subjects showed significantly lower glucose metabolism than the younger subjects in regions of the parietal cortex and insula, as well as global grey matter during audiovisual stimulation. Rates for posterior cingulate and global grey matter in younger and older subjects were compared by using t tests. Rates for other areas were compared by using two-factor repeated measures ANOVAs (with hemisphere as the repeated measure). *p < 0.05. (From Pietrini et al. 1997a.)

Testing rCBF effects of cholinergic blockade with anticholinesterase inhibitors, like scopolamine, has shown that AD patients differ from both healthy elderly and young adults in sensitivity to cholinergic depletion (Sunderland *et al.* 1995). Such pharmacological challenge studies may lead to the development of provocative stress tests to aid early detection in the preclinical stages of AD.

PET and SPECT methods have also begun to be implemented in studies evaluating other potential therapeutic interventions in AD, including other neurotransmitter systems (e.g. serotoninergic system), the effect of nerve growth factors, and anti-inflammatory agents (Meltzer *et al.* 1998). Further research is needed to directly evaluate whether and how these potential therapeutic agents alter the function of brain systems important for specific cognitive processes that decline with the progression of AD.

5 Neuroreceptor ligand studies

Studies using radiolabelled ligands to directly image the *in vivo* effects of AD on neurotransmitter systems have mainly focused on the development and implementation of markers for pre- and postsynaptic cholinergic neuroreceptors and acetylcholinesterase activity. Agents such as [^{123}I]iodobenzovesamicol (^{123}I-IBVM) and [^{123}I]iodoquinuclidinyl benzilate (^{123}I-QNB) have been used to evaluate the cholinergic system with SPECT (Weinberger *et al.* 1991; Kuhl *et al.*

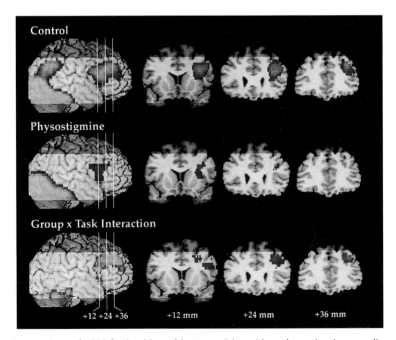

Figure 7.7 Comparison of rCBF for healthy subjects receiving either physostigmine or saline while performing a working memory (WM) task relative to the resting state. For each comparison, the figure shows the result projected onto the right hemisphere and indicates the location for the three coronal sections in frontal cortex, located +12, +24, and +36 mm anterior to the anterior commissure. Z scores that exceeded a threshold of 2.33 (p = 0.01, two-tailed, before correction for multiple comparisons based on spatial extent) and obtained significance after an analysis of spatial extent are shown. Significant rCBF increases during WM task performance relative to rest are shown for the control and physostigmine groups. The group x task interaction shows greater task-related rCBF increases during saline infusion as compared with physostigmine infusion. (From Furey *et al.* 1997.)

1996) whereas radiotracers including [^{11}C]N-methyl-4-piperidyl benzilate (^{11}C-NMPB), N-[^{11}C]methylpiperidin-4-yl proprionate (^{11}CPMP), and N-[^{11}C]methylpiperid-4-yl acetate (^{11}C-MP4A) have been developed for use with PET (Iyo *et al.* 1997; Kuhl *et al.* 1999). Although cholinergic system reductions have been demonstrated, *in vivo*, in several studies with AD patients compared to healthy elderly using both SPECT and PET with such radioligands, the observed reductions, thus far, appear less prominent than those reported in post-mortem *in vitro* studies with biochemical assays. A recent study of five AD patients and eight healthy controls using the ^{11}C-MP4A with PET as an index of acetylcholinesterase activity showed approximately 20–30% reductions in regions of the cerebral cortex in the AD group (Iyo *et al.* 1997). That these preliminary results show reductions which are somewhat less than those observed in *in vitro* post-mortem studies may be related to the assessment of enzyme activity earlier in the course of AD *in vivo* with PET (Frey *et al.* 1998).

Studies to investigate receptor abnormalities in other neurotransmitter systems have begun to be applied to AD. In a study by Blin *et al.* (1993), reductions in the serotoninergic system in AD have been reported using the 5-HT$_2$ receptor ligand, [^{18}F]setoperone with PET in a group of nine AD patients and a comparison group of healthy controls. With recent efforts to develop neuroprotective treatments that can prevent or diminish the inflammatory response observed in AD, there has been much interest in developing ligands that provide markers of microglia formation (Groom *et al.* 1995). Further, recent developments in the measurement of fatty acid metabolism in humans have provided the potential to image, *in vivo*, alterations of cellular signal transduction in AD with PET (Rapoport, 1999). This latter approach provides a unique method to directly test hypotheses concerning the dysfunction of signal transduction mechanisms throughout the course of disease progression.

With continued progress in the development of radioligands providing markers for specific aspects of neurotransmitter and cellular function, functional neuroimaging with PET and SPECT will likely have an increasingly greater role in the evaluation of neurochemical abnormalities in dementia and specifically in evaluating effective treatments that can potentially prevent or delay the onset of cognitive and behavioural symptoms and modify the course of disease.

6 Conclusions and future directions

Studies using PET and SPECT to assess alterations in brain function with dementia can provide important information on mechanism of cognitive and behavioural dysfunction, assist in the early detection of neurodegenerative disease, and aid in the evaluation of pharmacological interventions. In this chapter, we have sought to illustrate what has been learned from applying these functional neuroimaging methods to the study of the most common form of progressive dementia, AD.

Future developments in the application of PET and SPECT will likely lead to greater advances in the evaluation of individuals at risk for dementia and in the selection of appropriate therapies. Combining methodologies to investigate brain response to pharmacological challenge during cognitive or sensory stimulation and with neuroreceptor ligands will advance our understanding of the complexities in treating dementias such as AD. The application of new challenge paradigms, like transcranial magnetic stimulation to temporarily disrupt regional brain function, in conjunction with the information provided by PET and SPECT, will likely offer new insights into the role of specific brain regions in affecting distributed neural systems responsible for complex cognitive processes that are altered by AD and other forms of dementia. The development and wider application of sophisticated statistical analysis methods will likely provide new and more effective ways to characterize the regionally distributed brain systems that become dysfunctional as neurodegenerative diseases progress and to identify differences in brain response to stimulation and pharmacological interventions, potentially leading to increased sensitivity to the effects of disease and incipient dementia. Together, these current and future advances in functional neuroimaging with PET and SPECT will likely lead to significant improvements in the clinical diagnosis and treatment for dementia.

7 Key points

1 Functional neuroimaging with PET and SPECT provide methods to measure, *in vivo*, neural synaptic activity that can identify patterns of cerebral dysfunction associated with dementia.

2 PET and SPECT have enhanced our understanding of the neurophysiological mechanisms associated with cognitive and behavioural dysfunction in the most common form of age-related dementia, Alzheimer's disease (AD).

3 Functional neuroimaging studies of AD at rest evaluates the regional distribution of disease on brain function that is associated with the severity of dementia and patterns of cognitive and behavioural dysfunction.

4 The use of stimulation paradigms in functional neuroimaging studies with PET and SPECT can elicit brain networks associated with complex cognitive processes that become impaired with advancing disease, providing a neurophysiological stress test for dementia.

5 The use of PET and SPECT can aid the differential diagnosis of dementia and assist in early detection of AD among individuals at risk for dementia.

6 Use of pharmacological challenge at rest and during cognitive or sensory stimulation with PET and SPECT provide a method to evaluate drug treatments that delay or diminish the cognitive or neurophysiological effects of dementia.

7 The development of radioligands to measure uptake and turnover of specific neurotransmitters provides an *in vivo* method to evaluate the dysfunction of neurotransmitter systems altered by AD.

References

Alexander, G. E. and Moeller, J. R. (1994). Application of the scaled subprofile model to functional imaging in neuropsychiatric disorders: A principal component approach to modeling regional patterns of brain function in disease. *Human Brain Mapping*, **2**, 79–94.

Alexander, G. E., Prohovnik, I., Sackeim, H. A., Stern, Y., and Mayeux, R. (1995). Cortical perfusion and gray-matter weight in frontal lobe dementia. *Journal of Neuropsychiatry and Clinical Neurosciences*, **7**, 188–96.

Alexander, G. E., Furey, M. L., Grady, C. L., Pietrini, P., Brady, D., Mentis, M. J., *et al.* (1997). Association of premorbid function with cerebral metabolism in Alzheimer disease: Implications for the cognitive reserve hypothesis. *American Journal of Psychiatry*, **154**, 165–72.

Alexander, G. E., Mentis, M. J., Van Horn, J. D., Grady, C. L., Berman, K. F., Furey, M. L., *et al.* (1999). Individual differences in PET activation of object perception and attention systems predict face matching accuracy. *NeuroReport*, **10**, 1965–71.

Azari, N. P., Pettigrew, K. D., Schapiro, M. B., Haxby, J. V., Grady, C. L., Pietrini, P., *et al.* (1993). Early detection of Alzheimer's disease: A statistical approach using positron emission tomographic data. *Journal of Cerebral Blood Flow and Metabolism*, **13**, 438–47.

Bartenstein, P., Minoshima, S., Hirsch, C., Buch, K., Willoch, F., Mosch, D., *et al.* (1997). Quantitative assessment of cerebral blood flow in patients with Alzheimer's disease by SPECT. *Journal of Nuclear Medicine*, **38**, 1095–101.

Baxter, L. R., Schwartz, J. C., Phelps, M. E., Mazziotta, J. C., Guze, B. H., Selin, C. E., *et al.* (1989). Reduction of prefrontal cortex glucose metabolism common to three types of depression. *Archives of General Psychiatry*, **46**, 243–50.

Becker, J. T., Mintun, M. A., Aleva, K., Wiseman, M. B., Nichols, T., and DeKosky, S. T. (1996). Compensatory reallocation of brain resources supporting verbal episodic memory in Alzheimer's disease. *Neurology*, **46**, 692–700.

Blin, J., Baron, J. C., Dubois, B., Pillon, B., Cambon, H., Cambier, J., *et al.* (1990). Positron emission tomography study of progressive supranuclear palsy. Brain hypometabolic pattern and clinicometabolic correlations. *Archives of Neurology*, **47**, 747–52.

Blin, J., Baron, J. C., Dubois, B., Crouzel, C., Fiorelli, M., Attar-Levy, D., *et al.* (1993). Loss of brain 5-HT2 receptors in Alzheimer's disease. In vivo assessment with positron emission tomography and [18F]setoperone. *Brain*, **116**, 497–510.

Blin, J., Ivanoiu, A., Coppens, A., De Volder, A., Labar, D., Michel, C., *et al.* (1997). Cholinergic neurotransmission has different effects on cerebral glucose consumption and blood flow in young normals, aged normals, and Alzheimer's disease patients. *Neuroimage*, **6**, 335–43.

Brooks, R. A., Di Chiro, G., Zukerberg, B. W., Bairamian, D., and Larson, S. M. (1987). Test-retest studies of cerebral glucose metabolism using fluorine-18 deoxyglucose: validation of method. *Journal of Nuclear Medicine*, **28**, 53–9.

Buck, B. H., Black, S. E., Behrmann, M., Caldwell, C., and Bronskill, M. J. (1997). Spatial- and object-based attentional deficits in Alzheimer's disease: Relationship to HMPAO-SPECT measures of parietal perfusion. *Brain*, **120**, 1229–44.

Cardebat, D., Demonet, J.-F., Puel, M., Agniel, A., Viallard, G., and Celsis, P. (1998). Brain correlates of memory processes in patients with dementia of Alzheimer's type: A SPECT activation study. *Journal of Cerebral Blood Flow and Metabolism*, **18**, 457–62.

Claus, J. J., Walstra, G. J. M., Hijdra, A., Van Royen, E. A., Verbeeten, B., and van Gool, W. A. (1999). Measurement of temporal regional cerebral perfusion with single-photon emission tomography predicts rate of decline in language function and survival in early Alzheimer's disease. *European Journal of Nuclear Medicine*, **26**, 265–71.

Craig, A. H., Cummings, J. L., Fairbanks, L., Itti, L., Miller, B. L., Li, J., *et al.* (1996). Cerebral blood flow correlates of apathy in Alzheimer disease. *Archives of Neurology*, **53**, 1116–20.

Dani, A., Pietrini, P., Furey, M. L., McIntosh, A. R., Grady, C. L., Horwitz, B., *et al.* (1996). Brain metabolism and cognition in Down syndrome adults associated with development of dementia. *NeuroReport*, **7**, 2933–6.

DeCarli, C. S., Atack, J. R., Ball, M. J., Kay, J. A., Grady, C. L., Fewster, P., *et al.* (1992). Post-mortem regional neurofibrillary tangle densities but not senile plaque densities are related to regional cerebral metabolic rates for glucose during life in Alzheimer's disease patients. *Neurodegeneration*, **1**, 113–21.

Dolan, R. J., Bench, C. J., Brown, R. G., Scott, L. C., Friston, K. J., and Frackowiak, R. S. (1992). Regional cerebral blood flow abnormalities in depressed patients with cognitive impairment. *Journal of Neurology, Neurosurgery, and Psychiatry*, **55**, 768–73.

Duara, R., Grady, C. L., Haxby, J. V., Sundaram, M., Cutler, N. R., Heston, L., *et al.* (1986). Positron emission tomography in Alzheimer's disease. *Neurology*, **36**, 879–87.

Duara, R., Barker, W. W., Chang, J., Yoshii, F., Loewenstein, D. A., and Pascal, S. (1992). Viability of neocortical function shown in behavioral activation state PET studies in Alzheimer disease. *Journal of Cerebral Blood Flow and Metabolism*, **12**, 927–34.

Eckelman, W. C., Reba, R. C., Rzeszotarski, W. J., Gibson, R. E., Hill, T., Holman, B. L., *et al.* (1984). External imaging of cerebral muscarinic acetylcholine receptors. *Science*, **223**, 291–3.

Eidelberg, D., Dhawan, V., Moeller, J. R., Sidtis, J. J., Ginos, J. Z., Strother, S. C., *et al.* (1991). The metabolic landscape of cortico-basal ganglionic degeneration: Regional asymmetries studied with positron emission tomography. *Journal of Neurology, Neurosurgery, and Psychiatry*, **54**, 856–62.

Foster, N. L., Chase, T. N., Fedio, P., Patronas, N. J., Brooks, R., and DiChiro, G. (1983). Alzheimer's disease: Focal cortical changes shown by positron emission tomography. *Neurology*, **33**, 961–5.

Fox, N. C., Kennedy, A. M., Harvey, R. J., Lantos, P. L., Roques, P. K., Collinge, J., *et al.* (1997). Clinicopathological features of familial Alzheimer's disease associated with the M139V mutation in the presenilin 1 gene: Pedigree but not mutation specific age at onset provides evidence for a further genetic factor. *Brain*, **120**, 491–501.

Frackowiak, R. S. J., Pozzilli, C., Legg, N. J., DuBoulay, G. H., Marshall, J., Lenzi, G. L., *et al.* (1981). Regional cerebral oxygen supply and utilization in dementia: A clinical and physiological study with oxygen-15 and positron tomography. *Brain*, **104**, 753–78.

Frey, K. A., Minoshima, S., and Kuhl, D. E. (1998). Neurochemical imaging of Alzheimer's disease and other degenerative dementias. *Quarterly Journal of Nuclear Medicine*, **42**, 166–78.

Furey, M. L., Pietrini, P., Haxby, J. V., Alexander, G. E., Lee, H. C., VanMeter, J., *et al.* (1997). Cholinergic stimulation alters performance and task-specific regional cerebral blood flow during working memory. *Proceedings of the National Academy of Sciences USA*, **94**, 6512–16.

Furey, M. L., Pietrini, P., Rapoport, S. I., and Haxby, J. V. (1999). Cholinergic modulation improves working memory by enhancing encoding in ventral extrastriate cortex. *Neuroimage*, **9**, S945.

Geaney, D. P., Soper, N., Shepstone, B. J., and Cowen, P. J. (1990). Effect of central cholinergic stimulation on regional cerebral blood flow in Alzheimer disease. *Lancet*, **335**, 1484–7.

Goffinet, A. M., De Volder, A. G., Gillain, C., Rectem, D., Bol, A., Michel, C., *et al.* (1989). Positron tomography demonstrates frontal lobe hypometabolism in progressive supranuclear palsy. *Annals of Neurology*, **25**, 131–9.

Grady, C. L., Haxby, J. V., Schageter, N. L., Berg, G., and Rapoport, S. I. (1986). Stability of metabolic and neuropsychological asymmetries in dementia of the Alzheimer type. *Neurology*, **36**, 1390–2.

Grady, C. L., Haxby, J. V., Horwitz, B., Sundaram, M., Berg, G., Schapiro, M. B., *et al.* (1988). Longitudinal study of the early neuropsychological and cerebral metabolic changes in dementia of the Alzheimer type. *Journal of Clinical and Experimental Neuropsychology*, **10**, 576–96.

Grady, C. L., Haxby, J. V., Schapiro, M. B., Gonzalez-Aviles, A., Kumar, A., Ball, M. J., *et al.* (1990). Subgroups in dementia of the Alzheimer type using positron emission tomography. *The Journal of Neuropsychiatry and Clinical Neurosciences*, **2**, 373–84.

Grady, C. L., Haxby, J. V., Horwitz, B., Gillette, J., Salerno, J. A., Gonzalez-Aviles, A., *et al.* (1993). Activation of cerebral blood flow during a visuoperceptual task in patients with Alzheimer-type dementia. *Neurobiology of Aging*, **14**, 35–44.

Groom, G. N., Junck, L., Foster, N. L., Frey, K. A., and Kuhl, D. E. (1995). PET of peripheral benzodiazepine binding sites in the microgliosis of Alzheimer's disease. *Journal of Nuclear Medicine*, **36**, 2207–10.

Haxby, J. V., Duara, R., Grady, C. L., Cutler, N. R., and Rapoport, S. I. (1985). Relations between neuropsychological and cerebral metabolic asymmetries in early Alzheimer's disease. *Journal of Cerebral Blood Flow and Metabolism*, **5**, 193–200.

Haxby, J. V., Grady, C. L., Koss, E., Horwitz, B., Schapiro, M., Friedland, R. P., *et al.* (1988). Heterogenous anterior-posterior metabolic patterns in dementia of the Alzheimer type. *Neurology*, **38**, 1853–63.

Haxby, J. V. (1990). Resting state regional cerebral metabolism in dementia of the Alzheimer type. In *Positron emission tomography in dementia* (ed. R. Duara), pp. 93–116. New York: Wiley-Liss.

Haxby, J. V., Grady, C. L., Koss, E., Horwitz, B., Heston, L., Schapiro, M., *et al.* (1990). Longitudinal study of cerebral metabolic asymmetries and associated neuropsychological patterns in early dementia of the Alzheimer type. *Archives of Neurology*, **47**, 753–60.

Haxby, J. V., Horwitz, B., Ungerleider, L. G., Maisog, J. M., Pietrini, P., and Grady, C. L. (1994). The functional organization of human extrastriate cortex: A PET-rCBF study of selective attention to faces and locations. *Journal of Neuroscience*, **14**, 6336–53.

Holland, A. J. and Oliver, C. (1995). Down's syndrome and the links with Alzheimer's disease. *Journal of Neurology, Neurosurgery, and Psychiatry*, **39**, 111–14.

Horwitz, B., Grady, C. L., Schlageter, N. L., Duara, R., and Rapoport, S. I. (1987). Intercorrelations of regional cerebral glucose metabolic rates in Alzheimer's disease. *Brain Research*, **31**, 294–306.

Horwitz, B., McIntosh, A. R., Haxby, J. V., Furey, M., Salerno, J. A., Schapiro, M. B., *et al.* (1995). Network analysis of PET-mapped visual pathways in Alzheimer type dementia. *NeuroReport*, **6**, 2287–92.

Ibañez, V., Pietrini, P., Alexander, G. E., Furey, M. L., Teichberg, D., Rajapakse, J. C., *et al.* (1998). Abnormal metabolic patterns in Alzheimer's disease after correction for partial volume effects. *Neurology*, **50**, 1585–93.

Ishii, K., Sakamoto, S., Sasaki, M., Kitagaki, H., Yamaji, S., Hashimoto, M., *et al.* (1998). Cerebral glucose metabolism in patients with frontotemporal dementia. *Journal of Nuclear Medicine*, **39**, 1875–8.

Iyo, M., Namba, H., Fukushi, K., Shinotoh, H., Nagatsuka, S., Suhara, T., *et al.* (1997). Measurement of acetylcholinesterase by positron emission tomography in the brains of healthy controls and patients with Alzhiemer's disease. *Lancet*, **349**, 1805–9.

Jagust, W. J., Haan, M. N., Reed, B. R., and Eberling, J. L. (1998). Brain perfusion imaging predicts survival in Alzheimer's disease. *Neurology*, **51**, 1009–13.

Jobst, K. A., Barnetson, L. P. D., and Shepstone, B. J. (1998). Accurate prediction of histologically confirmed Alzheimer's disease and the differential diagnosis of dementia: The use of NINCDS-ADRDA and DSM-III-R criteria, SPECT, x-ray CT, and apo E4 in medial temporal lobe dementias. *International Psychogeriatrics*, **10**, 271–302.

Johnson, K. A., Jones, K., Holman, B. L., Becker, J. A., Spiers, P. A., Satlin, A., *et al.* (1998). Preclinical prediction of Alzheimer's disease using SPECT. *Neurology*, **50**, 1563–71.

Julin, P., Almkvist, O., Basun, H., Lannfelt, L., Svensson, L., Winblad, B., *et al.* (1998). Brain volumes and regional cerebral blood flow in carriers of the Swedish Alzheimer amyloid protein mutation. *Alzheimer Disease and Associated Disorders*, **12**, 49–53.

Kennedy, A. M., Frackowiak, R. S. J., Newman, S. K., Bloomfield, P. M., Seaward, J., Roques, P., *et al.* (1995*a*). Deficits in cerebral glucose metabolism demonstrated by positron emission tomography in individuals at risk of familial Alzheimer's disease. *Neuroscience Letters*, **186**, 17–20.

Kennedy, A. M., Rossor, M. N., and Frackowiak, R. S. J. (1995*b*). Positron emission tomography in familial Alzheimer disease. *Alzheimer Disease and Associated Disorders*, **9**, 17–20.

Kessler, J., Herholz, K., Grond, M., and Heiss, W.-D. (1991). Impaired metabolic activation in Alzheimer's disease: A PET study during continuous visual recognition. *Neuropsychologia*, **29**, 229–43.

Kessler, J., Ghaemi, M., Mielke, R., Herholz, K., and Weiss, W.-D. (1996). Visual versus auditory memory stimulation in patients with probable Alzheimer's disease: A PET study with 18 FDG. *Annals of the New York Academy of Sciences*, **777**, 233–8.

Kuhl, D. E., Minoshima, S., Fessler, J. A., Frey, K. A., Foster, N. L., Ficaro, E. P., *et al.* (1996). In vivo mapping of cholinergic terminals in normal aging, Alzheimer's disease, and Parkinson's disease. *Annals of Neurology*, **40**, 399–410.

Kuhl, D. E., Koeppe, R. A., Minoshima, S., Snyder, S. E., Ficaro, E. P., Foster, N. L., *et al.* (1999). In vivo mapping of cerebral acetylcholinesterase activity in aging and Alzheimer's disease. *Neurology*, **52**, 691–9.

Kumar, A., Schapiro, M. B., Grady, C. L., Haxby, J. V., Wagner, E., Salerno, J. A., *et al.* (1991). High-resolution PET studies in Alzheimer's disease. *Neuropsychopharmacology*, **4**, 35–46.

Kung, H. F., Ohmomo, Y., and Kung, M. P. (1990). Current and future radiopharmaceuticals for brain imaging with single photon emission computed tomography. *Seminars in Nuclear Medicine*, **20**, 290–302.

Lehtovirta, M., Soininen, H., Laakso, M. P., Partanen, K., Helisalmi, S., Mannermaa, A., *et al.* (1996). SPECT and MRI analysis in Alzheimer's disease: Relation to apolipoprotein E e4 allele. *Journal of Neurology, Neurosurgery, and Psychiatry*, **60**, 644–9.

McGeer, E. G., Peppard, R. P., McGeer, P. L., Tuokko, H., Crockett, D., Parks, R., *et al.* (1990). 18 Fluorodeoxyglucose positron emission tomography studies in presumed Alzheimer cases, including 13 serial scans. *Canadian Journal of Neurological Sciences*, **17**, 1–11.

Mega, M. S., Chen, S. S., Thompson, P. M., Woods, R. P., Karaca, T. J., Tiwari, A., *et al.* (1997). Mapping histology to metabolism: Coregistration of stained whole-brain sections to premortem PET in Alzheimer's disease. *Neuroimage*, **5**, 147–53.

Meltzer, C. C., Zubieta, J. K., Brandt, J., Tune, L. E., Mayberg, H. S., and Frost, J. J. (1996). Regional hypometabolism in Alzheimer's disease as measured by positron emission tomography after correction for effects of partial volume averaging. *Neurology*, **47**, 454–61.

Meltzer, C. C., Smith, G., DeKosky, S. T., Pollock, B. G., Mathis, C. A., Moore, R. Y., *et al.* (1998). Serotonin in aging, late-life depression, and Alzheimer's disease: The emerging role of functional imaging. *Neuropsychopharmacology*, **18**, 407–30.

Mentis, M. J., Weinstein, E. A., Horwitz, B., McIntosh, A. R., Pietrini, P., Alexander, G. E., *et al.* (1995). Abnormal brain glucose metabolism in the delusional misidentification syndromes: A positron emission tomography study in Alzheimer disease. *Biological Psychiatry*, **38**, 438–9.

Mentis, M. J., Horwitz, B., Grady, C. L., Alexander, G. E., VanMeter, J. W., Maisog, J. M., *et al.* (1996). Visual cortical dysfunction in Alzheimer's disease evaluated with a temporally graded 'stress test' during PET. *American Journal of Psychiatry*, **153**, 32–40.

Mentis, M. J., Alexander, G. E., Krasuski, J., Pietrini, P., Furey, M. L., Schapiro, M. B., *et al.* (1998). Effect of Alzheimer disease severity on the functional response throughout the brain to parametric visual stimulation during PET. *American Journal of Psychiatry*, **155**, 785–94.

Mielke, R., Herholz, K., Grond, M., Kessler, J., and Heiss, W. D. (1992). Severity of vascular dementia is related to volume of metabolically impaired tissue. *Archives of Neurology*, **49**, 909–13.

Minoshima, S., Frey, K. A., Koeppe, R. A., Foster, N. L., and Kuhl, D. E. (1995). A diagnostic approach in Alzheimer's disease using three-dimensional stereotactic surface projections of Fluorine-18-FDG PET. *Journal of Nuclear Medicine*, **36**, 1238–48.

Neary, D., Snowden, J. S., Northen, B., and Goulding, P. (1988). Dementia of frontal lobe type. *Journal of Neurology, Neurosurgery, and Psychiatry*, **51**, 353–61.

Newberg, A. B., Alavi, A., and Payer, F. (1995). Single photon emission computed tomography in Alzheimer's disease and related disorders. *Neuroimaging Clinics of North America*, **5**, 103–23.

Pietrini, P., Azari, N. P., Grady, C. L., Salerno, J. A., Gonzales-Aviles, A., Heston, L. L., *et al.* (1993). Pattern of cerebral metabolic interactions in a subject at risk for Alzheimer's disease. *Dementia*, **4**, 94–101.

Pietrini, P., Furey, M. L., Graff-Radford, N., Freo, U., Alexander, G. E., Grady, C. L., *et al.* (1996). Preferential metabolic involvement of visual cortical areas in a subtype of Alzheimer's disease: Clinical implications. *American Journal of Psychiatry*, **153**, 1261–8.

Pietrini, P., Dani, A., Furey, M. L., Alexander, G. E., Freo, U., Grady, C. L., *et al.* (1997*a*). Low glucose metabolism during brain stimulation in older Down's syndrome subjects at risk for Alzheimer's disease prior to dementia. *American Journal of Psychiatry*, **154**, 1063–9.

Pietrini, P., Hof, P., Graff-Radford, N. R., Furey, M. L., Alexander, G. E., Mentis, M. J., *et al.* (1997*b*). Altered regional distribution of brain metabolic and pathological lesions in the visual variant of Alzheimer disease. *Society for Neuroscience Abstracts*, **23**, 2170.

Pietrini, P., Furey, M. L., Alexander, G. E., Mentis, M. J., Dani, A., Guazzelli, M., *et al.* (1999). Association between brain functional failure and dementia severity in Alzheimer's disease: Resting versus stimulation PET study. *American Journal of Psychiatry*, **156**, 470–3.

Pietrini, P., Alexander, G. E., Furey, M. L., Dani, A., Mentis, M. J., Horwitz, B., *et al.* (2000). Cerebral metabolic response to passive audiovisual stimulation in Alzheimer's disease patients and healthy controls assessed by positron emission tomography. *Journal of Nuclear Medicine*, **41**, 575–583.

Rapoport, S. I. (1999). In vivo fatty acid incorporation into brain phospholipids, in relation to signal transduction and membrane remodeling. *Neurochemistry Review*, **24**, 1403–1415.

Rapoport, S. I. and Grady, C. L. (1993). Parametric in vivo brain imaging during activation to examine pathological mechanisms of functional failure in Alzheimer disease. *International Journal of Neuroscience*, **70**, 39–56.

Reiman, E. M., Caselli, R. J., Yun, L. S., Chen, K., Bandy, D., Minoshima, S., *et al.* (1996). Preclinical evidence of Alzheimer's disease in persons homozygous for the e4 allele for apolipoprotein E. *New England Journal of Medicine*, **334**, 752–8.

Riekkinen, P. Jr., Riekkinen, M., Soininen, H., Kuikka, J., Laakso, M., and Riekkinen, P. (1997). Frontal dysfunction blocks the therapeutic effect of THA on attention in Alzheimer's disease. *NeuroReport*, **8**, 1845–9.

Schapiro, M. B., Pietrini, P., Grady, C. L., Ball, M. J., DeCarli, C., Kumar, A., *et al.* (1993). Reductions in parietal and temporal cerebral metabolic rates for glucose are not specific for Alzheimer's disease. *Journal of Neurology, Neurosurgery, and Psychiatry*, **56**, 859–64.

Signorini, M., Paulesu, E., Friston, K., Perani, D., Colleluori, A., Lucignani, G., *et al.* (1999). Rapid assessment of regimal cerebral metabolic abnormalities in single subjects with quatitative and nonquantitative [ISF] FDGPET: A clinical validation of statistical parametric mapping. *NeuroImage*, **9**, 63–80.

Small, G. W., Mazziotta, J. C., Collins, M. T., Baxter, L. R., Phelps, M. E., Mandelkern, M. A., *et al.* (1995). Apolipoprotein E type 4 allele and cerebral glucose metabolism in relatives at risk for familial Alzheimer disease. *Journal of the American Medical Association*, **273**, 942–7.

Stern, Y., Alexander, G. E., Prohovnik, I., Stricks, L., Link, B., Lennon, M. C., *et al.* (1995). Relationship between lifetime occupation and parietotemporal flow: Implications for a reserve against Alzheimer's disease pathology. *Neurology*, **45**, 55–60.

Strassburger, T., Alexander, G. E., Brady, D. R., Mangot, D., Pietrini, P., Mentis, M., *et al.* (1996). Heterogeneity of regional cerebral glucose metabolic (rCMRglc) patterns in neuropathologically confirmed Alzheimer disease (AD). *Neurology*, **46**, A134.

Sunderland, T., Esposito, G., Molchan, S. E., Coppola, R., Jones, D. W., Gorey, J., *et al.* (1995). Differential cholinergic regulation in Alzheimer's patients compared to controls following chronic blockade with scopolamine: A SPECT study. *Psychopharmacology*, **121**, 231–41.

Talbot, P. R., Goulding, P. J., Lloyd, J. J., Snowden, J. S., Neary, D., and Testa, H. J. (1995). Inter-relation between 'classic' motor neuron disease and frontotemporal dementia: Neuopsychological and single photon emission computed tomography study. *Journal of Neurology, Neurosurgery, and Psychiatry*, **58**, 541–7.

Talbot, P. R., Lloyd, J. J., Snowden, J. S., Neary, D., and Testa, H. J. (1998). A clinical role for 99mTc-HMPAO SPECT in the investigation of dementia? *Journal of Neurology, Neurosurgery, and Psychiatry*, **64**, 306–13.

Van Dyck, C. H., Lin, C. H., Robinson, R., Cellar, J., Smith, E. O., Nelson, J. C., *et al.* (1997). The acetylcholine releaser linopirdine increases parietal regional cerebral blood flow in Alzheimer's disease. *Psychopharmacology*, **132**, 217–26.

Van Dyck, C. H., Gelernter, J., MacAvoy, M. G., Avery, R. A., Criden, M., Okereke, O., *et al.* (1998). Absence of an apolipoprotein E e4 allele is associated with increased parietal regional cerebral blood flow asymmetry in Alzheimer disease. *Archives of Neurology*, **55**, 1460–6.

Waldemar, G., Bruhn, P., Kristensen, M., Johnsen, A., Paulson, O. B., and Lassen, N. A. (1994). Heterogeneity of neocortical cerebral blood flow deficits in dementia of the Alzheimer type: A [99mTc]-d,l-HMPAO SPECT study. *Journal of Neurology, Neurosurgery, and Psychiatry*, **57**, 285–95.

Weinberger, D. R., Gibson, R., Coppola, R., Jones, D. W., Molchan, S. E., Sunderland, T., *et al.* (1991). The distribution of cerebral muscarinic acetylcholine receptors in vivo in patients with dementia: A controlled study with 123-IQNB and single photon emission computed tomography. *Archives of Neurology*, **48**, 169–76.

Yao, H., Sadoshima, S., Kuwabara, Y., Ichiya, Y., and Fujishima, M. (1990). Cerebral blood flow and oxygen metabolism in patients with vascular dementia of the Binswanger type. *Stroke*, **21**, 1694–9.

8 Molecular pathology of early onset dementia

Catriona A. McLean, Konrad Beyreuther, and Colin L. Masters

1 Introduction

An understanding of the molecular basis of the more common neurodegenerative diseases of late adulthood has advanced rapidly in the last decade. Accumulation of various proteins either within neurons, glia, or the extracellular space is becoming recognized as a common feature of many of the diverse forms of early onset dementia. These host-encoded proteins accumulate in aggregated insoluble complexes that serve as markers of the underlying molecular pathology. At some stage during the process of protein aggregation, the protein undergoes a 'toxic gain of function' which causes neurodegeneration. While the mechanisms of pathogenesis are only partly understood or remain speculative, the genes encoding these proteins and the mechanisms of the neurodegenerative changes are areas of intense research (Table 8.1).

Table 8.1 Disease-associated protein aggregates and related known pathogenic mutations in the principal neurodegenerative diseases

Neurodegenerative disease	Protein deposit	Pathogenic mutation	Cellular compartment of protein deposition
Alzheimer's disease	Aβ, normal tau isoforms	Amyloid precursor protein Presenilin 1 and 2	Extracellular plaques but evidence of intracellular production
Frontotemporal dementias, Pick's disease, progressive supranuclear palsy, corticobasal degeneration	Abnormal tau isoforms	Tau	Intraneuronal and within glia
Parkinson's disease, dementia with Lewy bodies	α-Synuclein	α-Synuclein	Intracytoplasmic Lewy bodies
Multiple system atrophy	α-Synuclein	Unknown	Intraglial inclusions
Creutzfeldt–Jakob disease	Prion protein (PrP)	PRNP	Extracellular plaques, synapses
Motor neuron disease	Superoxide	SOD 1 dismutase (SOD 1)	Intraneuronal cytoplasmic inclusions
Huntington's disease	Polyglutamine aggregates	Huntingtin gene triplet expansion	Intranuclear and cytoplasmic inclusions

Many of the current advances in molecular pathology of dementia are dependent on brain banks world-wide which provide an invaluable research resource of fresh frozen material from biopsy and autopsy brain tissue. Research using these archival tissues is providing information on the normal cellular proteins and their abnormal insoluble aggregates. Tissue from affected individuals of well-characterized pedigrees is allowing genetic analysis such that risk factors and causative mutations can be established. The development of transgenic mouse lines expressing wild-type and mutant human genes and knockout mice without the functioning gene has led to the production of important models and insights into these neurodegenerative processes. Fully understanding the genes, their associated proteins, and related protein inter-actions will lead to a better understanding of disease pathogenesis. These studies should also uncover the potential for reversibility or slowing of these neurodegenerative processes. A corollary to this molecular approach is that a new nosology of the neurodegenerative diseases will rapidly emerge over the next decade. The molecular definition of dementia will be dependent on both genetic and biochemical parameters, which will complement the traditional morphological approach.

2 Alzheimer's disease

The report by Alois Alzheimer in 1907 of abnormal plaques and tangles in the brain of a patient with early onset dementia was the beginning of the study of this particular entity, as defined by Kraepelin (see chapters 10 and 11). The main protein comprising these extracel-lular plaques, $A\beta$, is also found in vessel walls as a congophilic amyloid angiopathy (CAA) (Glenner and Wong 1984; Masters *et al.* 1985). Other characteristic features in the brains of patients with AD include neurofibrillary changes, synaptic and neuronal loss. An abnormally phosphorylated microtubule associated protein, tau, accumulates within the intracellular compartments of neurons as neurofibrillary tangles (NFT), as neuritic processes within and around some amyloid plaques and as neuropil threads (NT). A complete understanding of the molecular pathology of AD will only come about with the elucidation of the processes through which $A\beta$ deposition is linked with tau-associated neurofibrillary changes and neuronal dysfunction. Our current hypothesis for the pathogenesis of AD is that the produc-tion and accumulation of $A\beta$ leads directly to neuronal degeneration and that accumulation of hyperphosphorylated tau within neurons is a relatively non-specific secondary phenomenon.

Vital clues to the pathogenesis and cause of early onset AD have been found through the genetic study of pedigrees that are well characterized clinically and pathologically and in which the occurrence of the disease has an autosomal dominant pattern. Mutations in three major genes have been found to be causative for AD:

(1) The Alzheimer amyloid precursor protein (APP) on chromosome 21.

(2) The presenilin 1 gene (PS1) on chromosome 14.

(3) The presenilin 2 gene (PS2) on chromosome 1.

Diverse mutations in these three different genes result in an alteration in APP pro-cessing which directly leads to an increase in production of a proteolytic $A\beta$ amyloidogenic fragment of APP. The definition of this biochemical pathway strengthens the hypothesis that the production and accumulation of $A\beta$ is central to the aetiology and pathogenesis of AD (Figure 8.1).

The Amyloidocentric Pathways in Alzheimer's Disease

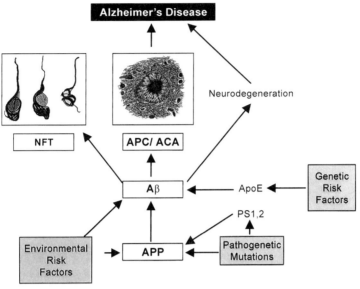

Figure 8.1 A schematic outline of the pathway leading to Alzheimer's disease. The processing of APP into Aβ is modulated by both environmental factors (yet to be identified) and pathogenic mutations in the PS, APP, and possibly other genes. Genetic risk factors identified to date (ApoE, α2M) may operate at the level of Aβ turnover in the brain. Amyloid plaques are the visible result of this pathway, but do not of themselves cause the neurodegeneration of AD. The mechanism of NFT formation remains enigmatic.

2.1 Causative genes

2.1.1 Amyloid precursor protein (APP)

The APP gene on chromosome 21 (Kang *et al.* 1987) comprises 18 exons spanning more than 179 kb. The region encoding the Aβ sequence is included within exons 16 and 17. APP is a ubiquitous type 1 multidomain protein that exists in at least four major alternatively spliced forms. The 695 amino acid isoform (APP 695) is predominantly expressed in neurons and two other major isoforms of APP (APP 751 and 770) contain the 56 residue Kunitz-type serine protease inhibitor (KPI) domain with the longer form containing the OX-2 domain. APP 751 and 770 are predominantly expressed in peripheral tissues and astrocytes. Alternative splicing of exon 15 produces the L-APP isoform found predominantly in lymphocytes and non-neuronal cells (Figure 8.2).

The function of APP remains unknown although the structural domains suggest a role in cell–cell or cell–matrix signalling and transport of Cu/Zn into the interior of the cells. A role in inhibition of platelet aggregation via inhibition of arachidonic acid metabolism has also been described. Secreted APP may play a role in neurite outgrowth during development or during regeneration following injury. Secreted APP (sAPPα) may also have a role in modulation of synpatic plasticity during long-term potentiation.

APP has a short half-life and is processed by at least two pathways. The main pathway in peripheral cells is through the activity of α-secretase at a site corresponding to position 15/16 in the middle of the extracellular portion of the Aβ fragment. Enzymes capable of performing this

(A)

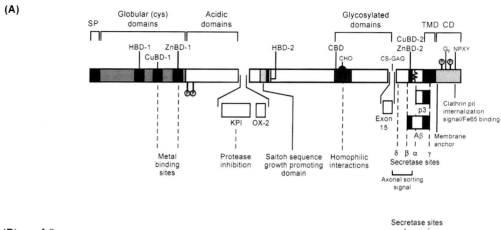

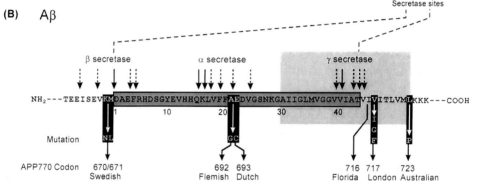

Figure 8.2 The major structural features of (A) APP and (B) Aβ amyloid. The heparin binding domains (HBD1, HBD2), copper and zinc binding domains (CuBD, ZnBD), phosphorylation sites (P), Kunitz protease inhibitor (KPI), growth promoting domain, carbohydrate attachment site (CHO), chondroitin sulfation site (CS-GAG), and the transmembrane (TMD) and cytoplasmic (CD) domains are indicated in (A). In (B), a more detailed picture of the secretase sites is given, together with the pathogenic missense mutations which cause some forms of early onset familial Alzheimer's disease.

function include those responsible for the shedding of tumour necrosis factor α and the angiotensin converting enzyme secretase. This process yields the soluble ectodomain protein sAPPα. The C-terminal fragment, p3CT, remains membrane-bound until the action of γ-secretase that releases p3, a 3 kDa fragment incorporating residues 17–40/42 of Aβ. The alternative pathway involves cleavage of APP at sites corresponding to positions 1 (β-secretase) — an aspartic protease BACE (Vassar *et al.* 1999) and 40 or 42 (γ-secretase) of the Aβ fragment, releasing the amyloidogenic peptide Aβ 1–40/42 (Figure 8.3).

This alternative pathway is a minor pathway of metabolism in non-neuronal cells. Variable cleavage at the C-terminus within different cell compartments produces variable length Aβ molecules: 39, 40, 42, and 43 amino acids long. Production of Aβ 1–40 is dominant and is produced in the post-Golgi compartment whilst Aβ 1–42 cleavage occurs in the endoplasmic reticulum (Haass *et al.* 1995). This postulated compartmentalization of Aβ metabolism suggests that at least two different intracellular pathways may be involved. At which stage Aβ is exteriorized and released into the extracellular space is unknown.

A minor component of full-length APP is also recycled. When APP is inserted into the plasma membrane, it may undergo endocytosis by clathrin-coated pits. Depending on its contribution to

Aβ Amyloidogenesis

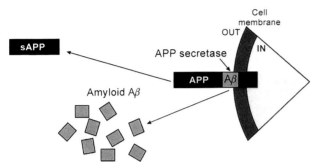

Cell
membrane
OUT

sAPP

APP secretase

IN

APP   Aβ

Amyloid Aβ

Figure 8.3 Schematic depiction of the release of Aβ amyloidogenic fragment from the cell membrane, with the generation of the soluble ectodomain of APP. The pool of Aβ thus generated may exist in a variety of intra- or extracellular compartments (endoplasmic reticulum, secretory vesicle, endosome, lysosome, extracellular space).

Aβ 40:42 ratios, altering the rate of turnover via this pathway may alter the rate of amyloidogenesis. Whether Aβ has a normal function within the cell is also unknown, however the juxta-membranous Aβ domain has a role in axonal transport of APP from neuronal cell bodies to the synapses (Tienari *et al.* 1996). This aspect is important since synaptic degeneration may be a prominent feature of AD. A more detailed understanding of the intra- and extracellular production of Aβ is critical for understanding its role in neurodegeneration.

The six causative mutations in the APP gene account for less than 5% of early onset familial AD (see chapter 11). These mutations produce an increase in Aβ 42 via different mechanisms. Mutations at codon 670/671 (the 'Swedish' mutations) increase β-secretase cleavage and lead to an excess amyloid production. Mutations at codon 717 (the 'London' mutations) at the γ-secretase site lead to an increased ratio of Aβ 42:40 (Figure 8.2). Mutations at 692 and 693 of APP (the 'Dutch' and 'Flemish' mutations) correspond to the α-secretase site, and presumably lead to decreased cleavage by this enzyme and more flux down the β- and γ-secretase pathways; alternatively, the mutations may affect the solubility of Aβ itself (Figure 8.2). Increased APP production in trisomy 21 similarly leads to an increased production of Aβ 42 and is associated with early onset AD. The longer form of Aβ has been found to be highly amyloidogenic, the earliest and most abundant species in neuritic plaques, and generated abundantly within neurons.

2.1.2 Presenilins 1 and 2

The PS1 and PS2 genes are highly homologous. PS1 is located on chromosome 14 and PS2 on chromosome 1. The PS1 gene consists of 12 exons with alternative splicing of exons resulting in variations in transcript length. PS1 is a 463–448 amino acid transmembrane protein comprising six to eight transmembrane domains with a hydrophilic loop between transmembrane domains 6–7 (Figure 8.4). PS1 is expressed in many tissues including the brain. In the CNS, PS1 is found in both neurons and glia. The protein is localized intracellularly, and is membrane-associated within the endoplasmic reticulum and the intermediate compartment of the Golgi complex. Both the N- and C-termini and the hydrophilic loop region are located on the cytosolic face (Figure 8.4). PS2 expression in pancreas and muscle exceeds other sites, including brain (Rogaev 1998).

The PS molecules undergo proteolytic cleavage, regulated by proteases (presenilinases) that are expected to lead to balanced fragment formation and activation of PS function. This 'normal' endoproteolytic processing occurs by cleavage within the large cytoplasmic loop (encoded by exon 9) to produce membrane-associated N- and C-terminal fragments (Thinakaran *et al.* 1996). Once generated these cleavage products can undergo dimerization,

Eight Transmembrane Domain Model of PS1 Structure

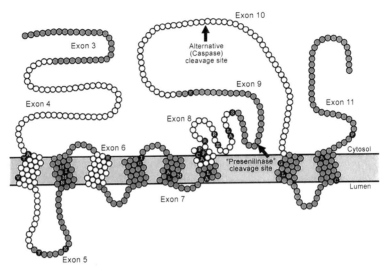

Figure 8.4 A schematic model of the putative eight transmembrane form of PS1. The important 'presenilinase' cleavage site in exon 9 is shown, together with an alternate (caspase) cleavage site further downstream in exon 10. Many of the pathogenic mutations causing early onset familial AD cluster in proximity to the second and sixth transmembrane domains or the presenilinase cleavage site.

and exist at low steady state levels in the brain and peripheral tissues. During apoptosis, or when the presenilins are overexpressed, the holoprotein is diverted into an alternative caspase-3 cleavage pathway that cleaves distal to the normal cleavage site and gives rise to a larger amino-terminal fragment and a smaller C-terminal fragment. Capsase-3 is an apoptosis-related cysteine protease.

In plasma and fibroblasts from patients and at-risk carriers for the presenilin mutations, an increased ratio of Aβ 42:40 has been observed. A similar increase of Aβ 42:40 in transfected cell lines and transgenic mice expressing familial AD forms of PS1 and PS2 has also been observed.

More than 60 mutations in PS1, mostly missense, have so far been found in pedigrees with early onset AD (see chapter 11). A point mutation upstream of a splice-acceptor site that results in the deletion of exon 9 has also been described associated with spastic paraparesis in some EOAD pedigrees (Crook *et al.* 1998). The PS1 mutations correspond to transmembrane areas predominantly with some clustering in transmembrane domains 2 and 6 and the adjacent hydrophilic loop region. The only two known PS2 missense mutations alter residues conserved in PS1.

2.2 Interrelations of APP and presenilins

Mutations in presenilins and APP have common denominators of an increased production of Aβ 42 and the clinical and pathological features of AD may have a role in γ-secretase activity, suggesting that PS1 can facilitate the proteolytic activity involved in cleavage of APP (Ray *et al.* 1999). It is known that an increase in Aβ 42 can also be found in presymptomatic carriers of both PS1 and PS2 mutations and in transgenic mice with mutant presenilins suggesting that an elevation in Aβ 42 precedes the neurodegenerative process and is most likely a primary phenomenom rather then a by-product of the disease process. The finding that Aβ 42 is produced in the endoplasmic reticulum and that PS1 and PS2 have been found to bind directly to immature forms of APP localized in the endoplasmic reticulum, forming APP-PS1 complexes, further links these two proteins.

2.3 Other genetic risk factors in sporadic AD

2.3.1 ApoE

The ApoE gene on chromosome 19 has three major alleles (ε2, ε3, and ε4) that are present in the population as six genotypes. ApoE is a glycoprotein of 299 amino acids. It is a normal constituent of plasma and cerebrospinal fluid lipoprotein particles. The N-terminus contains a receptor binding region (residues 136–150). There is a binding site for lipoproteins near the C-terminus. The protein functions to mediate cholesterol storage, transport, and metabolism.

In AD, the ε4 allele has been found to be associated with an increase in both the extent of Aβ deposition in senile plaques and the relative risk of age of onset of disease in a dose dependent fashion (Roses 1994).

A binding site for Aβ is present near the C-terminus of the ApoE molecule. A recently found polymorphism in the ApoE promoter may correlate with increased expression of the protein and also confer an increased risk of AD. The impact of ApoE on production, aggregation, fibrillogenesis, or amyloid clearance remains unclear.

2.3.2 α2-Macroglobulin (α2M)

The protein is encoded by A2M located on chromosome 12. α2M is a pan-protease inhibitor and a major ligand of the low density lipoprotein receptor-related protein (LRP1). Exon 18 of A2M encodes 'exon II' of the bait domain of α2M which is used to attract and trap proteases. Inheritance of a deletion in the 5′ spice site of exon 18 (A2M-2) confers an increased risk of AD with no effect on age of onset. The deletion bears no relationship to the age of onset of AD (Blacker *et al.* 1998).

α2M is up-regulated during injury along with LRP. It binds tightly to Aβ peptide and attenuates fibrillogenesis and neurotoxicity, and mediates Aβ degradation via endocytosis through the lipoprotein receptor-related protein (LRP1). ApoE and APP are also ligands of LRP1. It is postulated that increased levels of ApoE may confer an increased risk of AD by interfering with α2M-mediated clearance and/or degradation of Aβ by competing with α2M for either Aβ or LRP.

2.4 Aβ in Alzheimer's disease

2.4.1 Aβ plaques

Immunoreactive Aβ reveals a spectrum of plaque morphologies. Diffuse cortical plaques (lacking neuritic processes) (10–100 μm) and poorly defined diffuse sub-pial collections are seen as well as plaques with central strongly immunoreactive amyloidogenic Aβ cores. Aβ plaques incorporating irregular, fragmented, neuritic processes around their periphery are termed neuritic plaques (NP). The temporal, cellular, and extracellular events determining the various plaque forms is poorly understood. Meningeal and intracortical vessels show a variable and often patchy Aβ deposition within their walls.

The presence of neuritic plaques defines AD according to the CERAD neuropatho-logical criteria (Mirra *et al.* 1991). The Aβ plaque load has an uncertain relationship with increasing severity of dementia. This may be due in part to a process of growth and resolution of plaques with the establishment of a plateau phase for plaque production. Neuritic plaques are also frequently seen to be associated with microglia suggesting that processing and clearance of amyloid may be occurring. Astrocytes may also be involved in the degradative process of Aβ.

Monoclonal antibodies have been developed to the variable C-terminus, the N-terminus, and to species truncated at the N-terminus. These antibodies demonstrate that the diffuse senile plaques are immunoreactive with Aβ x–42 epitope and that senile plaques containing a central amyloid core are reactive for both Aβ x–40 and Aβ x–42. Shorter Aβ species, truncated at the N-terminus are also present within the plaques. Antisera to Aβ 1–16 react with a small proportion of plaques, most of which have a dense central core. Further work is needed to establish if p3 has a role in the pathogenesis of plaque formation. The amyloid in CAA is predominantly Aβ 1–40 (Suzuki *et al.* 1994) with some Aβ 1–42, and also contains N-terminal truncated Aβ peptides. Understanding the differential Aβ composition of plaques with varying morphology and CAA may lead to clues concerning the origin and temporal relation of Aβ amyloid production.

2.4.2 Biochemical analysis of Aβ

In conjunction with morphological studies an increasing number of biochemical analyses of brain, CSF and plasma for Aβ have been performed. Methodological differences between investigators are difficult to reconcile, but a pattern is emerging. In brain homogenates form normal individuals the levels of soluble and insoluble Aβ are very low (Teller *et al.* 1996; Kuo *et al.* 1996; McLean *et al.* 1999), although increasing levels of Aβ 1–42 correlate with increasing age. Increased concentrations of insoluble and soluble Aβ correlate with a clinical diagnosis of AD as compared to normal individuals (McLean *et al.* 1999).

Transgenic mice with mutant PS2 also show an age-dependent increase in Aβ 42 and similar changes are seen in mice expressing mutant APP isoforms in association with behavioural deficits with increasing production of amyloid plaques with time, further supporting a role for elevated Aβ 1–42 in plaque deposition.

Aβ is detectable in CSF and plasma. Plasma levels of Aβ are unreliable as a marker of AD. Further work is required to properly assess the diagnostic value of measurements of Aβ in the CSF, however the relative ratio of Aβ 40:42 when combined with the level of tau protein may have some diagnostic value (Kanai *et al.* 1998).

2.4.3 Synthetic Aβ

A further research model for Aβ deposition uses synthetic peptides. These studies have led to an understanding of the structural basis and kinetic processes underlying aggregation. One possible ordered process is a nucleation-dependent polymerization whereby an Aβ nucleus forms from monomers to become an organized structure via the addition of subsequent monomers or oligomers to produce a polymeric chain that then elongates (Jarret and Lansbury 1993). Protofilaments may exist that are oligomeric intermediates (Walsh *et al.* 1997). The principle oligomer appears to be a dimer. The dimeric form of Aβ is also potentially the pathogenic toxic species. Protofilaments are thought to form a tetragonal array and then further mature into fibrils 75–80 Å in diameter, composed of a pentagonal array of filaments. Factors regulating destabilization of the native protein in favour of the partially folded intermediates include: the amino acid sequence and length, the pH, the temperature, the ionic strength, co-solutes, and ligands. Zn(II)and Cu(II) at low μM concentrations induce the rapid aggregation of synthetic Aβ

that is reversible by the use of metal chelators. Other factors include the active proteolysis of the intermediates, the concentration of intermediate forms, interactions with other proteins, and intermolecular cross-linking. Specific studies looking at different lengths Aβ have shown that Aβ 42 aggregates more rapidly than Aβ 40.

2.4.4 Aβ neurotoxicity

Despite these *in vitro* studies the toxic forms of Aβ *in situ* remain uncharacterized. The exact mechanism of Aβ cellular injury is not determined. Aβ *in vitro* has been shown to cause plasma membrane lipid peroxidation, impairment of ion motive ATPases, glutamate uptake, uncoupling of G-protein linked receptors, and generation of reactive oxygen species (Mark *et al.* 1996). These effects may contribute to the loss of intracellular calcium homeostasis reported in cultured neurons. A role for apoptosis is controversial but good supporting evidence is lacking and it seems more likely that apoptosis is far down the cascade of events driven by pathogenic Aβ species. Soluble Aβ may have a physiological role and may interact with receptors. Although it is unclear if a receptor exists, the receptor for advanced glycation end-products (AGE) has been implicated. Studies also suggest that Aβ may bind an intracellular hydrosteroid dehydrogenase known as ERAB (Yan *et al.* 1997). ERAB is overexpressed in neurons of patients with AD. ERAB-Aβ complexes could lead to translocation of Aβ from the endoplasmic reticulum to the plasma membrane and may mediate intracellular deleterious effects. The toxic effect of Aβ *in vitro* is prevented by blocking ERAB. This study links intracellular and extracellular Aβ to neurodegeneration.

2.5 Accumulation of abnormally phosphorylated tau

The gene encoding tau is on chromosome 17 and contains 16 exons. Normal alternative splicing occurs in exons 2, 3, and 10 to create six isoforms. Tau proteins are within the family of micro-tubule associated proteins (MAP). The six tau isoforms range from 352–441 amino acids in length with apparent mass of 45–72 kDa when run on denaturing gels. Exons 9–12 encode four tandem repeat regions (R1, R2, R3, and R4) (Figure 8.5A). Exon 10 encodes a 31 amino acid repeat that is added after the first repeat (R2) to give tau isoforms with four repeats. Splicing out of exon 10 thus results in tau isoforms with only three repeats. The tandem repeat regions and the sequences flanking them are the microtubule binding domains. In normal adult brains the propor-tion of tau with three repeats shows a slight preponderance over those with four repeats. Variability in the length of the N-terminal region due to a 29 or 59 amino acid insert are also observed.

Tau protein mRNA is expressed predominantly in neurons, where it is predominantly present within axons. The normal function of the tau proteins is to promote and stabilize microtubule assembly by binding to tubulin. Microtubules are an integral part of the cytoskeleton and are abundant in nerve cells where they are directly involved in cytoplasmic organisation, especially axonal transport. Relatively little is known about the regulation of normal phosphorylation of tau by specific protein kinases.

2.6 Tau in AD

In AD, tau is hyperphosphorylated. Ultrastructure of NFT reveals paired helical filaments (PHF-tau) predominantly with occasional straight filaments. In AD, immunoreactive PHF-tau is seen almost exclusively within neurons and their processes as flame-shaped neurofibrillary tangles

(A)

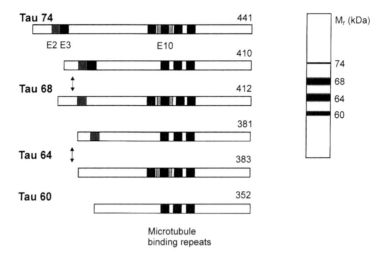

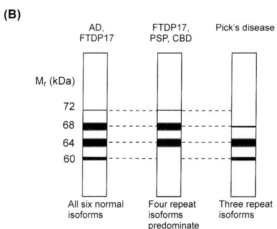

(B)

Figure 8.5 The isoforms of tau and the patterns of occurrence in Western blots of tau in selected diseases. (A) The six normal isoforms of tau with the corresponding normal Western blot pattern. (B) In AD and some pedigrees of FTDP-17 (with mutations outside exon 10), the Western blot pattern is normal. In the majority of FTDP-17, PSP, and CBD cases, the four repeat isoforms predominate. In Pick's disease, the three repeat isoforms predominate (see text for details and references).

(NFT), in the neuropil as threads (NT), and within the dystrophic neurites of neuritic plaques (NP). These changes are concentrated in the neocortical association areas.

It remains unclear whether abnormal phosphorylation of tau is sufficient by itself for PHF formation. It is also unclear whether phosphorylation is the primary event that leads to subsequent aggregation of PHF-tau or whether phosphorylation is a secondary event as a consequence of the aberrant metabolism of tau. Apart from being phosphorylated, PHF-tau shows further biochemical modifications: ubiquitination, oxidation, and glycation. An interaction between tau and sulfated glycosaminoglycans (including heparin) may be a central event in filament formation

(Goedert *et al.* 1996). Hyperphosphorylation of tau inhibits microtubule polymerization. *In vitro* the microtubule assembly-promoting activity of tau can be restored by enzymatic dephosphorylation. The sequelae of the lack of functioning microtubules is compromise of axonal transport and ultimately loss of synpases and retrograde degeneration.

A soluble pool of abnormally phosphorylated tau (P-tau) also exists in AD brains. P-tau may inhibit the function of normal tau due to direct co-aggregation. The co-aggregated P-tau and normal tau may then act as 'seeds' for polymerization of PHF-tau. High molecular weight microtubule associated proteins 1 and 2 (MAP 1 and 2) are also sequestered by P-tau, thus inhibiting MAP 1 and 2 from otherwise maintaining the structure of microtubules, resulting in inhibition of microtubule assembly.

2.6.1 Biochemical analysis of PHF-tau

NFT are not unique to AD and are seen in a number of other neurodegenerative diseases. Biochemical analysis shows the same PHF-tau in Down's syndrome, parkinsonism-dementia complex of Guam, Neimann-Pick disease type C, and Gerstmann-Sträussler-Scheinker (GSS) disease with tangles. In these diseases as well as AD, three major bands ('triplet' PHF-tau) of 60, 64, and 68 kDa as well as a minor 72 kDa band are observed that upon dephosphorylation consist of all six tau isoforms that align with recombinant human brain tau isoforms (Spillantini *et al.* 1997*a*). Some variation in 'triplet' band molecular weights at 55, 64, and 69 kDa are seen (Figure 8.5).

2.7 Interrelation of tau and Aβ

The pathological hallmarks of AD are Aβ amyloid plaque and vessel deposition and tau neurofibrillary changes. Understanding the pathogenesis and disease dynamics from the study of end-stage morphological changes has severe limitations, although providing important information. The processes by which Aβ and/or tau cause neuronal degeneration are made complex by the need to study the *in situ* effects at an early stage of neuronal degeneration. *In vivo*, Aβ is found in a variety of states within both intra- and extracellular compartments. Within separate cellular compartments a diverse array of macromolecules and factors potentially interact with Aβ and tau. An understanding of the potential toxic forms of Aβ and tau and the temporal sequence of events involved in their accumulation are central to current research.

Tau immunoreactive NFT show a hierarchical pattern of involvement commencing in the hippocampus and limbic structures prior to the cortical association areas (Braak and Braak 1991). It has been questioned whether the early stages represent AD as opposed to a 'senile change', when NFT are not seen in association with Aβ plaques in these areas. If the hierarchical progression is correct, and if Aβ is neurotoxic, then the effect of Aβ must be associated with specific pathways and/or neuronal populations, otherwise degeneration would occur throughout the brain in a global manner.

The exact interrelations of Aβ and tau are yet to be determined. The presence of tau aggregates in several neurodegenerative diseases not associated with Aβ accumulation and diseases where Aβ is present in the absence of tau aggregates shows that tau accumulation can be clearly dissociated from Aβ accumulation in some circumstances: Aβ plaques and PHF-tau deposition occur together in AD, Down's syndrome, and dementia pugilistica. Aβ is deposited without evidence of NFT formation in hereditary Dutch type and some sporadic forms of congophilic angiopathy. PHF-tau occurs independent of Aβ formation in a variety of Gerstmann-Sträussler-Scheinker (GSS) disease, amyotrophic lateral sclerosis with parkinsonism and dementia of Guam, Hallevorden-Spatz disease, Niemann-Pick disease (type C), and in a small number of demented elderly with severe neurofibrillary tangle changes in the hippocampus and adjacent cortex ('tangle-only dementia'). In Niemann-Pick disease type C, the cause is a relative deficiency of sphingomyelinase and GSS is caused by mutations in the prion protein. This emphasizes that completely different primary mechanisms can lead to common cytoskeletal changes, with degeneration of specific subsets of neurons and aggregation of hyperphosphorylated tau. This suggests that the production of PHF-tau in AD could be a by-product of the primary cause, initiated at some stage during the process of Aβ production, accumulation, and toxicity.

Studies correlating AD clinical symptomatology with neuritic changes but not with Aβ load have relied on the examination of end-stage disease and the insoluble forms of both tau and Aβ. Biochemical studies now show that there are soluble pools of both Aβ and tau. Increased levels of soluble Aβ may be neurotoxic and provide a source for the toxic dimeric and trimeric forms. Diffusible Aβ oligomers have been detected and found to be neurotoxic *in vitro*. Intracellular insoluble Aβ has also been detected within neurons. Previously it has been presumed that 'plaques are toxic' however studies of the soluble component of Aβ and intracellular insoluble Aβ make it essential to establish the form and site of Aβ neurotoxicity to further our understanding of the pathogenesis of AD (McLean *et al.* 1999).

3 The frontotemporal dementias and related neurodegenerations (Pick's disease, progressive supranuclear palsy, corticobasal degeneration)

Within the concept of frontotemporal dementias (FTD) there is a spectrum of clinicopathological phenotypes. The neuropathological features of these disorders have in common a widespread cerebral cortical neronal loss (more marked in the frontal and temporal lobes with relative preservation of the hippocampus), gliosis, and superficial microvacuolation (greater in laminae 2–3). Variable features allowing pathological subclassifications include the degree of subcortical and substantia nigra neuronal loss, glial and neuronal tau accumulations, classical Pick bodies, and ubiquitin- and β-crystallin immunoreactive inclusions within neurons of the temporal and frontal cortex. Aβ amyloid plaques are not a feature of FTD (see chapters 10 and 12).

More recently, the identification of a subgroup of familial FTD with parkinsonism showing linkage to chromosome 17q21-22 (FTDP-17) has begun the process of a molecular subdivision of this heterogeneous group of diseases. This has simplified the terminology of this group of diseases where previously many of the pedigrees were classified on their dominant clinical symptomatology or neuropathological changes resulting in a plethora of complicated acronyms. Verification of a molecular subdivision of FTDP-17 with detection of several mutations in the tau gene in known pedigrees is now established (Hutton *et al.* 1998; Spillantini *et al.* 1998). The finding of mutations in the tau gene also allows considerable advances to be made in understanding the pathogenesis of FTDP-17 and has furthered understanding in other diseases where tau accumulates as filaments within neurons or glia.

3.1 Tau isoforms in FTDP-17

Molecular analysis of several FTDP-17 families has revealed three groups of mutations: mutations in the intron adjacent the splice site of exon 10 (a predicted stem loop structure involved in regulation of the splice site), missense mutations in exon 10 (a microtubule binding domain), and missense mutations outside exon 10 (in exons 9, 12, and 13) (see Table 8.2).

Table 8.2 Tau mutations related to FTDP-17 frontotemporal degenerations

Mutation type	Mutations	Soluble tau	Tau inclusions	Tau filaments	Glial inclusions
Missense (not exon 10)	G272V, V337M, R406W	Normal ratio of 4:3 repeat	All six isoforms	AD-like PHF	No
Missense (in exon 10)	P301L	Normal ratio of 4:3 repeat[b]	4 repeat predominates	'Twisted ribbons'	Yes
Exon 10 5' splice site	+13, +14, +16, +3[a]	Increased 4 repeat	4 repeat predominates	'Twisted ribbons'	Yes

[a] Exon 10 5' splice site mutations numbered from 3' end of exon 10.
[b] Inferred from unchanged ratio of exon 10 ± RNA.

Several mutations within the intron adjacent to exon 10 have been described, predominantly at the 5' end. In some of these families ballooned neurons rich in tau are described. A further mutation in the 3' end of the intron, just adjacent the splice acceptor site with a G to A transition occurred in a family with abundant nerve cell loss, intraneuronal and glial granular and fibrillar tau deposits within neurons in the cortex, hippocampus, substantia nigra, hypothalamus, and regions in the brain stem. Ultrastructural analysis of these tau filaments reveals they are unlike those of AD and consist of twisted-ribbon filaments of 6–22 nm in diameter and variable 140–300 nm periodicity. The biochemical profile of tau also differs to that of AD and consists of 'doublet' bands at 64 and 69 kDa resulting from an excess of four repeat forms of the tau molecule (Figure 8.5). The mechanism for the excess of four repeat forms is not fully understood but mutations in the predicted stem loop structure may promote recognition of the 5' splice site and inclusion of exon 10 in tau mRNA. The stem loop structure is thought to regulate the splicing in of exon 10. These families have been shown to produce two- to sixfold more tau exon 10+ forms and hence have an equivalent increase in the second tandem repeat resulting in an excess of four repeat structures. This excess of four repeat forms may lead to an increase in native unfolded four repeat tau within the cytoplasm. Subsequent hyperphosphorylation may result in an inability of tau to bind to microtubules. Other factors may then play a role in beginning nucleation of the filaments.

Some pedigrees are described where the mutation is not in exon 10 or in the intron adjacent to it. Two of these are outside microtubule binding domains: R406W in exon 13 and V337M in exon 12. R406W is near key residues involved in phosphorylation and V337M is located in a region involved in an 'inter-repeat' region (IR) between repeat regions 3–4 (R3–4). A further pedigree reveals a mutation (G272V), in exon 9 within a microtubule binding domain. In pedigrees with R406W and V337M, widespread AD-like NFT and NT are reported with no evidence of $A\beta$ deposition. The inclusions in V337M show all six tau isoforms and a normal ratio of three to four repeats with a 'triplet' band pattern at 60, 64, 69, and 72 kDa (Figure 8.5B). The filaments seen in V337M mutations are PHF tau with a diameter of 11–20 nm and a periodicity of 80 nm. These features are identical to those of PHF in AD, however the distribution of the NFT varies compared to AD, with sparing of the hippocampus. There are therefore two main pathological differences between AD and this subgroup of FTDP-17. The first is a lack of $A\beta$ and neuritic plaques in FTDP-17. The second is the topography of the deposition of PHF-tau and associated neuronal loss. It remains to be determined how the R406W and V337M mutations result in the PHF of AD in the absence of typical Aβ accumulations.

3.2 Tau isoforms in Picks disease

Pick's disease (or lobar atrophy) is a rare sporadic and familial cause of frontal lobe dementia. The frequency of the disease is difficult to assess. Some of the original Dutch pedigrees diagnosed as Pick's disease have now been re-categorized as FTDP-17 and have been found to have mutations in the tau gene (Heutink *et al.* 1997). These cases demonstrate the potential for a more accurate epidemiology and molecular subdivision of the frontotemporal dementias (see chapter 12).

Pathological findings in Pick's disease include severe gyral atrophy due to neuronal loss and gliosis in the orbital frontal and anterior and medial temporal lobes. Basal ganglia structures may be involved. Pathognomonic Pick bodies are present within neurons. Pick bodies are round intra-cytoplasmic inclusions that contain hyperphosphorylated tau in straight filaments (15–18 nm diameter) and wide twisted filaments (22–24 nm in diameter). The distribution of Pick bodies is different to the NFT of AD, with areas such as the dentate fasciculus of the hippocampus showing extensive Pick body formation where NFT are not seen. Analysis of tau from Pick's disease brain homogenates reveals that isoforms with only three repeats are seen, resulting in a 'doublet' pattern due to two bands at 60 and 64 kDa (see Figure 8.5B). Neurons of the dentate fasciculus have been shown by *in situ* hybridization experiments to not express tau isoforms with exon 10. The topographic distribution of Pick bodies may therefore relate to areas rich in three repeat. The gene defect in familial Pick's disease remains unknown, although the pattern of three repeat predominance in the insoluble tau suggests that the mutation is directly or indirectly affecting the splicing of exon 10. Supporting this view, immunostaining using a panel of antibodies against peptide sequences of tau isoforms reveals an absence of translated tau isoforms with exon 10 in Pick's disease.

3.3 Tau isoforms in progressive supranuclear palsy (PSP) and corticobasal degeneration (CBD)

Progressive supranuclear palsy (PSP) or Steele-Richardson-Olszewski syndrome and corticobasal degeneration (CBD) are two further diseases with inclusions in neurons of specific areas; overlap in the clinical and pathological features are common (Feany *et al.* 1996). PSP is characterized by supranuclear ophthalmoplegia, pseudobulbar palsy, parkinsonism, and axial dystonia. Dementia is a common end-stage feature. Neuronal loss, gliosis, swollen neurons, and tau positive neurons and glia are seen, as well as globose NFT in selected subcortical, brain stem, and cerebellar nuclei. CBD is characterized by an asymmetrical akinetic-rigid syndrome associated with extrapyramidal motor dysfunction. Neuropathological features include perirolandic atrophy with gliosis, neuronal loss, swollen achromatic neurons, neuritic change, and NFT. Tau-reactive granular neurons, neuropil thread, glial inclusions (glial coils and thorns), and astrocytic clusters are also present. Ultrastructural analysis reveals straight and twisted filaments. Moderate dementia emerges late in the course of the disease.

Genetic variation at or near the tau gene may play a role in pathogenesis. In both CBD and PSP biochemical analyses of tau have revealed a 'doublet' band pattern similar to FTDP-17 mutations with either mutations in or adjacent to exon 10 (Figure 8.5B). This finding further strengthens the morphological association between CBD, PSP, and some cases of FTDP-17. Further analysis of the morphology and biochemistry of tau may help delineate the pathogenesis and correct the nosology of these diseases.

3.4 The general and specific abnormalities of tau in neurodegenerative diseases

The study of diseases in which tau is deposited or accumulates helps to define the pathophysiological significance of tau and the mechanisms of disease specificity. The presence of increased levels of hyperphosphorylated tau in so many neurodegenerative diseases strongly suggests that tau dysfunction is associated with neuronal dysfunction. This is most clearly seen in the FTDP-17 group of diseases where mutations in tau cause it to accumulate in an insoluble form in the neurons in the absence of Aβ. Further abnormalities in tau are seen in other diseases such as Pick's disease, PSP, and CBD in which tau accumulates as abnormal filaments. The variation in the proportion of the three and four repeat isoforms in association with tau mutations has confirmed that several distinct mechanisms for tau accumulation exist. In AD, tau is abnormally phosphorylated and forms PHF within neurons, however all six normal tau isoforms are present. The primary abnormality of Aβ accumulation is postulated to occur prior to abnormal tau accumulation and degeneration of neurons, but the link between Aβ accumulation and tau remains uncertain. The presence of PHF tau in other diseases where Aβ does not accumulate suggests that the final common pathway leading to PHF tau may contain distinct processes arising from different primary stimuli.

4 Dementia with Lewy bodies

Large numbers of Lewy bodies characteristically occur in two diseases: dementia with Lewy bodies (DLB) and idiopathic Parkinson's disease (PD). DLB and PD are predominantly sporadic, and rarely familial but recently described mutations in the gene encoding α-synuclein (α-SN) in several PD pedigrees has provided new information into the pathogenesis of a wider variety of diseases (Polymeropoulos et al. 1997; Kruger et al. 1998). Causative genes for DLB are not yet identified, but as a nosologic entity, DLB is relatively recent. Differentiation from AD can be difficult clinically and family histories may well be inaccurate (McKeith et al. 1996). SPECT scanning has also been unable to provide significant differentiation. DLB and AD may occur concurrently, further complicating nosology and understanding of pathogenesis. An unresolved controversy also exists over the relationship between DLB and idiopathic PD with or without dementia. Clinical features favouring diagnosis of DLB include fluctuation in cognition, visual hallucinations, and extrapyramidal signs (see chapter 13). Pathognomonic findings include the presence of Lewy bodies (LB) and Lewy neurites (LN) in the cortical and limbic areas. LB are intracytoplasmic round eosinophilic bodies that show a radiating halo in neurons within the substantia nigra and other pigmented nuclei of the brain stem in idiopathic Parkinson's disease.

In DLB, LB predominate in lower cortical laminae of the cingulate, transentorhinal, and insular cortex and are also frequently seen in the diencephalon, substantia nigra, and locus ceruleus. Further pathological features include irregular neuritic processes, prominent in the CA2 region of the hippocampus and scattered within the same cortical regions as the LB, microvacuolation, and synapse loss of the medial temporal cortex (see chapter 10). Cortical LB and LN are immunoreactive with ubiquitin and microtubule-associated protein five, and more recently have been shown to react with antisera to α-synuclein (α-SN) (Figure 8.6) (Baba et al. 1998; Spillantini et al. 1997b). Modified neurofilament subunit proteins may also be components of LB, although cross-reactivity with α-SN has not been excluded. Ultrastructural examination of LB reveals masses of aggregated 25 nm diameter filaments that appear similar to neurofilaments and are associated with α-SN reactivity on immunogold labelling. Biochemical analysis of the LB shows full-length, partially truncated, and high molecular weight aggregates

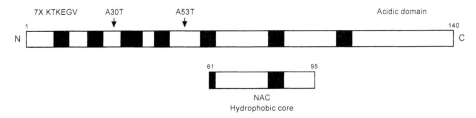

Figure 8.6 Schematic outline of the α-synuclein protein, with the two mutations (A30P, A53T) indicated, and the hydrophobic 'non-amyloid component' (NAC) core region. The shaded areas represent the seven KTKEGV repeat motifs.

of α-SN with ubiquitin. The latter suggests that aggregated α-SN is in the process of being targeted for 26S proteosome destruction. Loosely filamentous, ubiquitin negative, pale bodies within neurons of the substantia nigra, possible LB precursors, and thread-like filaments within the neuronal perikarya also immunoreact with α-SN. If these filamentous collections are precursor forms of LB, then ubiquitination appears to be a later modification of α-SN filaments within LB. That the α-SN changes from an unfolded protein to an aggregated insoluble form in association with ubiquitin suggest that the cell is unable to dispose of these protein aggregates.

Recombinant C-terminally truncated α-SN assembles into filaments resembling those of LB, suggesting that truncation by proteolysis may also play a role in the process. Mutations in α-SN may accelerate LB formation, as seen in *in vitro* studies. These aggregates also induce apoptotic cell death in human neuroblastoma cell lines. More recent studies showing the presence of α-SN immunoreactive LB in FAD and α-SN co-localizing with NFT suggest that diverse factors may further predispose neurons to accumulate LB.

The role of LB *per se* in the pathogenesis of LBD and PD remains unknown. A correlation between cortical LB numbers and dementia remains controversial, although a correlation of LB in the temporal cortex and cognitive impairment has been recorded. Loss of synapses may also be a substrate of cognitive impairment in DLB. The significance of LN both in terms of neurodegeneration and clinical phenotype is also unclear. Why certain cells accumulate α-SN, what the factors are in the cascade from a soluble protein to an insoluble amyloid-like aggregate, and at what stage the process is neurotoxic are yet to be determined. Thus the recent work on α-SN and LB formation has provided a close parallel with other neurodegenerative diseases in which accumulation of proteins or fragments of proteins occur, including Aβ mutations in AD and tau mutations in FTDP-17. These studies provide an important framework for future research.

4.1 α-Synuclein (α-SN)

α-SN has been mapped to chromosome 4q21-23. Known mutations include Ala53Thr and Ala30Pro occurring in familial PD (Polymeropoulos *et al.* 1997; Kruger *et al.* 1998).

α-SN is a small soluble protein, 140–143 amino acids in length (19 kDa), with a central hydrophobic 35 residue domain (Figure 8.6). Other names for α-SN include; non-Aβ component of AD (NACP), synelfin, and PNP-14. Other members of the synuclein family include β- and γ-SN and persyn. Synelfin has been implicated in synaptic events associated with learning and memory in birds and synaptic modulation. All synuclein proteins have considerable structural homology and are highly conserved across many species, implying functional evolutionary constraints. β- and γ-SN are encoded by genes on chromosomes 5q35 and 10q23 respectively. α- and β-SN differ in the central hydrophobic region. Immunoreactive β-SN is not present within

LB. The full-length α-SN protein is relatively unfolded, without significant secondary structure, while the hydrophobic core has a strong tendency to form β-pleated sheets.

α-SN is found abundantly in the neuronal cytosol and is enriched at presynaptic terminals. α-SN mRNA and protein are found in embryonic mouse brain from day 12–15 and appear to precede the appearance of synaptophysin, indicating α-SN may play a role in CNS development. In adult human brain α-SN co-localizes with synaptophysin in the synaptic terminals and subcellular fractionation studies suggest an association with membranous structures in synaptic vesicles as well as a cytosolic component. More recent studies suggest α-SN has a function in lipid binding through its hydrophobic core and it has been found to bind small diameter vesicles (20–25 nm) containing acidic phospholipids. Brain vesicle binding of α-SN is abolished by familial PD mutation *in vitro*. It is likely that α-SN becomes structured upon binding to vesicles. These findings suggest a role for α-SN in vesicle function at the presynaptic terminal.

4.1.1 Multiple system atrophy (MSA) — a further α-synucleinopathy?

MSA is a largely sporadic neurodegenerative disease that is now linked to aberrant α-SN metabolism. Extensive neuronal loss in the striatum, substantia nigra, pons, inferior olivary nucleus, cerebellar Purkinje cells, and neurons of the intermediolateral column of the spinal cord are found. In this disease, the pathognomonic hallmarks of oligodendroglial (GCI) and neuronal (NCI) cytoplasmic inclusions and degenerating neuritic processes have been recently found to be immunoreactive with antisera to α-SN (Gai *et al.* 1998; Tu *et al.* 1998). These inclusions had previously been shown to be strongly immunoreactive to ubiquitin and β-crystallin. Overexpression of β-crystallin occurs secondarily to cell stress and is one of the heat shock proteins. GCI inclusions are composed of loosely packed granular filaments 30–50 nm in diameter. The major component of the filaments, present in both the cytoplasm and nuclei of both nerve and glial cells, is α-SN. As α-SN is not normally expressed in oligodendrocytes in detectable quantities, it is proposed that either selective up-regulation of expression needs to occur in oligodendrocytes in MSA or that degradation of α-SN is impaired (Tu *et al.* 1998). As with the α-SN LB inclusions, understanding pathogenesis of MSA now requires further studies to establish whether the aggregated α-SN within inclusions is directly associated with the primary cause or only a marker of the disease process.

5 Prion diseases

Transmissible spongiform encephalopathies (TSE) are a group of rare neurodegenerative diseases with common pathological features of cortical and subcortical spongiform change, neuronal loss, gliosis, and a variable load of aggregated prion protein (PrP), most easily seen as a type of amyloid plaque formation. Human TSE are either sporadic, acquired, or familial in type. TSE are not unique to humans and are well-recognized in other animals including diseases such as scrapie in sheep (endemic in the United Kingdom for more than 100 years), and bovine and feline spongiform encephalopathies (BSE, FSE) (occurring since the mid 1980s) (Table 8.3). The most common sporadic human subtype presents as a rapidly dementing disorder, Creutzfeldt–Jakob disease (CJD). Acquired forms of the disease include kuru (acquired through endocannabalism of infected tissue), and CJD acquired through iatrogenic transmission of contaminated cornea, dura mater, and pituitary hormone extracts (Bilette de Villemeur *et al.* 1996; Weller *et al.* 1986). There is now also compelling evidence that the new variant of CJD (vCJD) is acquired through the zoonotic transmission of (BSE) (Will *et al.* 1996; Hill *et al.* 1997; Bruce *et al.* 1997). About 10% of the human TSE are familial and

Table 8.3 Transmissible spongiform encephalopathies

Disease	Natural host
Scrapie	Sheep and goat
Transmissible mink encephalopathy (TME)	Mink
Chronic wasting disease (CWD)	Mule, deer, and elk
Bovine spongiform encephalopathy (BSE)	Cattle
Exotic ungulate encephalopathy (EUE)	Nyala
Kuru	Humans-fore
Creutzfeldt–Jakob disease (CJD)	Humans
Gerstmann-Sträussler-Scheinker (GSS) syndrome	Humans
Fatal familial insomnia	Humans

have causative mutations in the prion protein gene (PRNP). These infectious genetic conditions include fatal familial insomnia (FFI), Gerstmann-Sträussler-Scheinker syndrome (GSS), and familial forms of typical CJD (see chapter 16).

5.1 The prion protein

The open reading frame of the gene encoding the prion protein (PRNP) is contained within a single exon on chromosome 20q. It is constitutively expressed in the adult brain and appears to be regulated during development, with highest expression in neurons, although many other cells synthesize PrP^C. PrP is a glycolipid (GPI) anchored membrane protein comprising a structured C-terminal three α-helical domains, two β-strands, and five random N-terminal octarepeats within codons 51–91. Two asparagine-linked oligosaccharide side chains yield different glyco-forms (Figure 8.7). The normal function of PrP is unknown, although it may influence the activity of other membrane receptors or ion channels.

There are five non-pathogenic polymorphisms: an octapeptide repeat deletion (–8), a Met-Val at codon 129 (M129V), a Glu-Lys at codon 219, a Ala-Val at codon 117, and a Asn-Ser at codon 171 (Table 8.4).

5.1.1 PrP^{CJD}

The disease-associated isoforms of PrP (PrP^{CJD}) have a similar molecular weight, the same amino acid sequence, and the same glycolipid anchor as the normal membrane-bound prion protein (PrP^C). However, PrP^{CJD} differs from PrP^C in its relative protease resistance, β-sheet content, and ability to be recycled within the cell. Limited proteolysis of PrP^{CJD} produces a N-terminal truncated protease-resistant fragment of 27–30 kDa, whilst the PrP^C is completely degraded. PrP^C contains 40% α-helix and little β-sheet, whereas PrP^{CJD} contains 30% α-helix and 45% β-sheet. Residues 90–112 are important for the major conformational changes that occur during conversion from PrP^C to PrP^{CJD} (Figure 8.7). Many different mutations in the human PRNP gene, resulting in non-conservative substitutions, have been found that segregate with inherited prion diseases. All known point mutations in PRNP with biological significance occur or are adjacent to regions of secondary structure and may therefore destabilize the struc-

PrP Structure

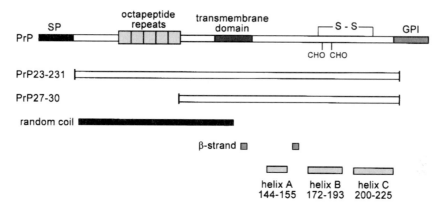

Figure 8.7 Schematic outline of the prion (PrP) protein. A signal peptide (SP) is followed by the octapeptide repeat region, within the N-terminal random coil half of the protein. A possible transmembrane domain is indicated, but it remains to be determined whether this is functional *in vivo*. A disulfide bridge (S–S) and two glycosylation sites occur within the C-terminal half, in which three alpha-helices (A, B, C) have been defined by NMR studies. Normal processing removes the signal peptide and adds a glycolipid anchor (GPI) to yield PrP 23–231. Partial proteolysis of the abnormal isoform yields PrP 27–30 which is truncated at the N-terminus. The areas of increased β-sheet structure in the abnormal isoforms are not yet defined.

ture of PrP^C (Collinge *et al.* 1992; Goldfarb *et al.* 1991) (Table 8.4). Normal cycling of PrP^C occurs subsequent to its passage through the Golgi. PrP^C attaches to the cell surface by its GPI anchor, then undergoes a process of internalization through caveolae, recycling within endosomes, and then is completely degraded within six hours. In contrast, PrP^{CJD} has a much longer half-life and accumulates within the cell, probably in secondary lysosomes.

Table 8.4 Mutations and non-pathogenic polymorphisms in the human prion protein gene (PRNP)

	Missense	Deletion	Insertion
Normal polymorphisms	M129V, E219K, N171S	Single octapeptide at codon 81	
Mutations associated with GSS	P102L, P105L, A117V, Y145 stop*, F198S, Q217R, Q212P		8 octapeptide repeat at codon 84, 8 octapeptide repeat at codon 76
Mutations associated with CJD	D178N, V180L, E200K, R209H, V210I, M232R		2, 4, 5, 6, 7 octapeptide repeat at codons 51–91
Mutations associated FFI	D178N, E200K		
Mutations associated with less specific phenotypes	T183A		6 octapeptide repeat at codons 51–91

* = The mutation Y145 stop terminates on a stop codon.

5.1.2 PrP^{CJD} initiation and replication

Although mutations in PRNP that destabilize the secondary and tertiary structure of PrP explain the pathogenesis of a minority of TSE, the sporadic forms of the disease with no mutations in PRNP form the bulk of human TSE. In acquired disease, the incubation period is dependent on the route of inoculation, the dose (concentration of PrP^{CJD}), and various strain differences. Direct intracerebral transmission via contaminated electrodes and dura mater grafts leads to shorter incubation periods (1–14 years) compared to CJD acquired peripherally through cadaveric human growth hormone (3–20 years). The concentration of PrP^{CJD} in the brain increases progressively throughout the incubation period. Other variables determining the concentration of PrP^{CJD} in the brain include local factors such as the rate of clearance from the extracellular space. The lymphoreticular system may play an important role in acquired TSE (Blattler *et al.* 1997). A further aspect contributing to the rate of conversion of PrP^C to PrP^{CJD} and its spread within the brain relates to its strain. Various strains of disease-associated PrP in mice (PrP^{Sc}) were initially defined on variations in incubation times and topography of lesions in the CNS. Variation in the pattern and distribution of PrP deposition was also noted as a strain-dependant variable (DeArmond *et al.* 1987). Physical and chemical differences in strains are thought to be due to the tertiary structure; the role of differential glycosylation is not yet established.

It is unclear how PrP^C converts to PrP^{CJD} in sporadic disease. It is postulated that once the initiation of PrP^C to PrP^{CJD} has occurred in the CNS in either sporadic or acquired TSE, subsequent amplification of PrP^{CJD} occurs via a template-assisted conformational change of the normal PrP^C through a series of rate limiting intermediate steps. The transitional process may require the presence of additional molecules (species specific 'protein X'). The nature of these interacting molecules is unknown although, PrP has been shown to interact with Bcl2, heat shock protein 60, and the laminin receptor.

5.1.3 Neurotoxicity and mechanisms of neurodegeneration induced by PrP^{CJD}

Experiments with null mice (Prnp$^{0/0}$) engrafted with PrP^C expressing tissue, then inoculated with PrP^{Sc}, suggest that PrP^{CJD} may only be toxic when formed within PrP^C expressing cells, or when presented from the outside to a cell already expressing PrP^C. Therefore, conversion of PrP^C to PrP^{CJD} ensues either at the cell surface or in an internalized compartment (Brandner *et al.* 1996). Propagation of infection across neural pathways also requires the presence of PrP^C. The mechanism of neurotoxicity is unknown although oxidative stress and the production of free radicals may be implicated. PrP^C may directly or indirectly regulate the activity of Cu/Zn super-oxide dismutase.

5.1.4 Determinants of clinicopathological phenotype

The human TSE present a wide spectrum of clinical and pathological phenotypes. However, at the centre is the typical picture of sporadic CJD with a rapidly progressive myoclonic dementia, with widespread cortical spongiform change associated with neuronal loss and gliosis, with less pronounced changes in the subcortical structures and cerebellum. In typical sporadic CJD, PrP deposition is also seen by immunohistochemistry to have a fine 'synaptic' pattern in areas where the spongiform change is present. In less than 10% of sporadic CJD, PrP^{CJD} also aggregates as deposits in amyloid plaques. By contrast, and at one end of the spectrum, FFI presents with insomnia, dysautonommia, disruption of circadian rhythms, and motor dysfunction with localized thalamic gliosis as the predominant pathological change (Goldfarb *et al.* 1992). PrP deposition is not evident by immunocytochemistry in FFI. Kuru presents a further clinicopathological subtype with prominent cerebellar symptoms and chronic emotional lability with dementia occurring only late in the clinical course. Prominent PrP plaque deposition is seen in the cerebellum with a fine synaptic deposition in the lower cortical laminae associated with gliosis and neuronal loss (McLean *et al.* 1998). The recently identified vCJD lacks the chronic emotional lability of kuru, and is characterized by psychiatric and sensory symptoms at onset with subsequent myoclonus and other movement disorders followed by dementia and akinetic mutism (Will *et al.* 1996). The neuropathological lesions are characterized by widespread severe and 'florid' PrP plaques deposited throughout the brain. The variables determining the extent and distribution of the microscopic pathological lesions are largely unknown; the strain of agent, route of agent entry, host factors, incubation period, and length of illness are all possible contributing factors.

Experimentally, the strain of agent is known to have a dominant effect when the host genotype is held constant. Scrapie and BSE transmission studies have also shown maintenance of phenotypic characteristics throughout ten or more serial passages, implying that various isolates maintain their strain-specific properties (Bruce *et al.* 1997). The mechanisms by which the prion strain modifies the pattern of disease may relate to glycosylation of PrP^C affecting either the rate of deposition or clearance of PrP^{CJD}. Regional differences in the ratio of deposition or clearance could then result in specific patterns of PrP^{CJD} accumulation. The accumulation of PrP^{CJD} concentrated within areas exhibiting spongiform degeneration and reactive gliosis suggests that the synthesis and distribution of PrP^{CJD} has a central role in the impairment of neuronal function in these diseases.

The host genotype, particularly the naturally occurring polymorphism on codon 129 in the human PRNP gene, is thought to influence incubation period and disease phenotype, particularly the presence of PrP^{CJD} plaques. All vCJD cases reported so far have been homozygous for methionine at codon 129, and a high frequency of homozygous V129 is seen in cases with iatrogenic disease. In kuru, PRNP allelic variations are seen in a distribution similar to that of a non-affected control population. This acquired TSE has occurred over a long time-frame compared to vCJD, with significantly larger numbers available for study (McLean *et al.* 1998), and these PRNP findings suggest that the host encoded codon 129 is not the main determinant of the phenotype. It remains to be determined if homozygosity at codon 129 dictates a shorter incubation period in vCJD. The presence of methionine at codon 129 is also thought to dictate the phenotype in FFI, where a D178N mutation is present (Goldfarb *et al.* 1992). If a valine is present at codon 129, then the inherited mutation presents as CJD. At least one exception to this has been reported in an Australian kindred where the D178N mutation was present with methionine at codon 129, with considerable clinicopathological heterogeneity present within the family, including cases typical of both CJD and typical FFI (McLean *et al.* 1997).

6 Conclusions

An understanding of the pathogenesis of many diverse neurodegenerative diseases associated with early onset dementia is evolving. A common trend is emerging in which accumulation of an abnormal form of a normal cellular protein is associated with a toxic gain of function. Causative mutations in the gene encoding the protein, although uncommon, are providing essential insights into the sporadic forms of the disease. These findings also have the potential to move the current nosology of these neurodegenerative diseases towards a molecular-based classification. This has already occurred by consensus of opinion in FTDP-17. Biochemical parameters may further refine a new nosology and have potential to be useful in guiding therapy and assessment of severity of the disease. Ongoing research, encompassing many technologies, is providing a wider understanding of the production of the abnormal protein forms. However, the many recent molecular insights have also served to strengthen the need for continuous revision of our concepts of neurodegenerative diseases using the classical traditional morphological approaches. The molecular pathology of this group of diseases is likely to remain dependent on these approaches for some time yet.

7 Key points

1   Accumulation of proteins either within neurons, glia, or the extracellular space is a common feature in many of the diverse forms of early onset dementia. Host-encoded proteins accumulate as aggregated insoluble complexes and serve as molecular markers of underlying disease. The mechanism of neurotoxicity is poorly understood, but may result from an increase in an abnormal form of a cellular protein resulting in a 'toxic gain of function'.

2   Mutations in the amyloid precursor protein (APP) gene and in presenilin genes 1 and 2 (PS1 and PS2) can lead to Alzheimer's disease. The mechanism of neurotoxicity is debated but probably due to an increase in the product of metabolism of APP — the amyloid, Aβ. Aβ accumulates as extracellular plaques within the brain and within vessel walls as a congophilic amyloid angiopathy (CAA). In AD, an insoluble, hyperphosphorylated, microtubule binding protein called tau, accumulates within neurons as neurofibrillary tangles. The interrelation of Aβ and tau is yet to be determined.

3   Mutations in the tau gene can result in frontotemporal dementia with parkinsonism (FTDP-17). Mutations in or upstream from exon 10 of the tau gene result in an excess of isoforms of the tau protein with four repeat microtubular binding domains which leads to accumulation of insoluble tau within neurons and glia.

4   The presence of aggregated, insoluble, α-synuclein (α-SN) protein within neurons, as a pathognomonic marker (Lewy body) of two diseases, Parkinson's disease (PD) and dementia with Lewy bodies (DLB), and the finding that mutations in the gene encoding α-synuclein result in familial PD, highlights a potential neurotoxic function for accumulating α-synuclein.

5   Transmissible spongiform encephalopathies (TSE) are due to accumulations of an abnormal form of a normal cellular protein — the prion protein (PrP). The acquired form of TSE is hypothesized as being due to an abnormal form of the prion protein (PrP^{CJD}) causing a template driven conformational change of the normal cellular prion protein (PrP^{C}). Accumulation of the abnormal PrP may be seen in tissue sections.

6   The variables determining the regional vulnerability and the temporal sequence of events remain largely unknown in most neurodegenerative diseases, but rapidly increasing knowledge and research into the disease-associated proteins is likely to elucidate this aspect and the potential for reversibility.

References

Baba, M., Nakajo, S., Tu, P. H., Tomita, T., Nakaya, K., Lee, V. M., *et al.* (1998). Aggregation of α-synuclein in Lewy bodies of sporadic Parkinson's disease and dementia with Lewy bodies. *Am. J. Pathol.*, **152**, 879–84.

Billette de Villemeur, T., Deslys, J. P., Pradel, A., Soubrie, C., Alperovitch, A., Tardieu, M., *et al.* (1996). Creutzfeldt–Jakob disease from contaminated growth hormone extracts in France. *Neurology*, **47**, 690–5.

Blacker, D., Wilcox, M. A., Laird, N. M., Rodes, L., Horvath, S. M., Go, R. C. P., *et al.* (1998). α-2 macroglobulin is genetically associated with Alzheimer disease. *Nat. Genet.*, **19**, 357–60.

Blattler, T., Brandner, S., Raeber, A. J., Klein, M. A., Voigtlander, T., Weissmann, C., *et al.* (1997). PrP expressing tissue required for transfer of scrapie infectivity from spleen to brain. *Nature*, **389**, 69–73.

Braak, H. and Braak, E. (1991). Neuropathological stageing of Alzheimer related changes. *Acta Neuropathol. Berl.*, **82**, 239–59.

Brandner, S., Isenmann, S., Raeber, A., Fischer, M., Sailer, A., Kobayashi, Y., *et al.* (1996). Normal host prion protein necessary for scrapie induced neurotoxicity. *Nature*, **379**, 339–43.

Bruce, M. E., Will, R. G., Ironside, J. W., McConnell, I., Drummond, D., Suttie, A., *et al.* (1997). Transmissions to mice indicate that 'new variant' CJD is caused by the BSE agent. *Nature*, **389**, 498–501.

Collinge, J., Brown, J., Hardy, J., Mullan, M., Rossor, M. N., Baker, H., *et al.* (1992). Inherited prion disease with 144 base pair gene insertion. 2. Clinical and pathological features. *Brain*, **115**, 687–710.

Crook, R., Verkkoniemi, A., Pereztur, J., Mehta, N., Baker, M., Houlden, H., *et al.* (1998). A variant of Alzheimer's disease with spastic paraparesis and unusual plaques due to deletion of exon 9 of presenilin 1. *Nat. Med.*, **4**, 452–5.

DeArmond, S. J., Mobley, W. C., DeMott, D. L., Barry, R. A., Beckstead, J. H., and Prusiner, S. B. (1987). Changes in the localization of brain prion proteins during scrapie infection. *Neurology*, **37**, 1271–80.

Feany, M. B., Mattiace, L. A., and Dickson, D. W. (1996). Neuropathologic overlap of progressive supranuclear palsy, Pick's disease and corticobasal degeneration. *J. Neuropathol. Exp. Neurol.*, **55**, 53–67.

Gai, W. P., Power, J. H., Blumbergs, P. C., and Blessing, W. W. (1998). Multiple system atrophy: a new alpha synuclein disease? *Lancet*, **352**, 547–8.

Glenner, G. G. and Wong, C. W. (1984). Alzheimer's disease and Down's syndrome: sharing of a unique cerebrovascular amyloid fibril protein. *Biochem. Biophys. Res. Commun.*, **122**, 1131–5.

Goedert, M., Jakes, R., Spillantini, M. G., Hasegawa, M., Smith, M. J., and Crowther, R. A. (1996). Assembly of microtubule-associated protein tau into Alzheimer-like filaments induced by sulphated glycosaminoglycans. *Nature*, **383**, 550–5

Goldfarb, L. G., Brown, P., McCombie, W. R., Goldgaber, D., Swergold, G. D., Wills, P. R., *et al.* (1991). Transmissible familial Creutzfeldt–Jakob disease associated with five, seven, and eight extra octapeptide coding repeats in the PRNP gene. *Proc. Natl. Acad. Sci. USA*, **88**, 10926–30.

Goldfarb, L. G., Petersen, R. B., Tabaton, M., Brown, P., LeBlanc, A. C., Montagna, P., *et al.* (1992). Fatal familial insomnia and familial Creutzfeldt–Jakob disease: disease phenotype determined by a DNA polymorphism. *Science*, **258**, 806–8.

Haass, C., Lemere, C. A., Capell, A., Citron, M., Seubert, P., Schenk, D., *et al.* (1995). The Swedish mutation causes early onset Alzheimer's disease by β secretase cleavage within the secretory pathway. *Nat. Med.*, **1**, 1291–6.

Heutink, P., Stevens, M., Rizzu, P., Bakker, E., Kros, J. M., Tibben, A., *et al.* (1997). Hereditary frontotemporal dementia is linked to chromosome 17q21 q22: a genetic and clinicopathological study of three Dutch families. *Ann. Neurol.*, **41**, 150–9.

Hill, A. F., Desbruslais, M., Joiner, S., Sidle, K. C., Gowland, I., Collinge, J., *et al.* (1997). The same prion strain causes vCJD and BSE. *Nature*, **389**, 448–50.

Hutton, M., Lendon, C. L., Rizzu, P., Baker, M., Froelich, S., Houlden, H., *et al.* (1998). Association of missense and 5′ splice site mutations in tau with the inherited dementia FTDP 17. *Nature*, **393**, 702–5.

Jarrett, J. T. and Lansbury, P. T. (1993). Seeding 'one dimensional crystallization' of amyloid: a pathogenic mechanism in Alzheimer's disease and scrapie? *Cell*, **73**, 1055–8.

Kanai, M., Matsubara, E., Isoe, K., Urakami, K., Nakashima, K., Arai, H., *et al.* (1998). Longitudinal study of cerebrospinal fluid levels of tau, Aβ1–40, and Aβ1–42(43). in Alzheimer's disease—a study in Japan. *Ann. Neurol.*, **44**, 17–26.

Kang, J., Lemaire, H., Unterbeck, A., Salbaum, J. M., Masters, C. L., Grzeschik, K., *et al.* (1987). The precursor of Alzheimer's disease amyloid A4 protein resembles a cell-surface receptor. *Nature*, **325**, 733–6.

Kruger, R., Kuhn, W., Muller, T., Woitalla, D., Graeber, M., Kosel, S., *et al.* (1998). Ala30Pro mutation in the gene encoding α-synuclein in Parkinson's disease. *Nat. Genet.*, **18**, 106–8.

Kuo, Y. M., Emmerling, M. R., Vigo-Pelfrey, C., Kasunic, T. C., Kirkpatrick, J. B., Murdoch, G. H., *et al.* (1996). Water soluble Aβ (N-40, N-42) oligomers in normal and Alzheimer disease brains. *J. Biol. Chem.*, **271**, 4077–81.

Mark, R. J., Blanc, E. M., and Mattson, M. P. (1996). Amyloid β-peptide and oxidative cellular injury in Alzheimer's disease. *Mol. Neurobiol.*, **12**, 211–24.

Masters, C. L., Simms, G., Weinman, N. A., Multhaup, G., McDonald, B. L., and Beyreuther, K. (1985). Amyloid plaque core protein in Alzheimer disease and Down syndrome. *Proc. Natl. Acad. Sci. USA*, **82**, 4245–9.

McKeith, L. G., Galasko, D., Kosaka, K., Perry, E. K., Dickson, D. W., Hansen, L. A., *et al.* (1996). Consensus guidelines for the clinical and pathologic diagnosis of dementia with Lewy bodies (DLB): report of the consortium on DLB international workshop. *Neurology*, **47**, 1113–24.

McLean, C. A., Storey, E., Gardner, R. J., Tannenberg, A. E., Cervenakova, L., and Brown, P. (1997). The D178N (cis 129M). 'fatal familial insomnia' mutation associated with diverse clinicopathologic phenotypes in an Australian kindred. *Neurology*, **49**, 552–8.

McLean, C. A., Ironside, J. W., Alpers, M. P., Brown, P. W., Cervenakova, L., Anderson, R. M., *et al.* (1998). Comparative neuropathology of Kuru with the new variant of Creutzfeldt–Jakob disease: evidence for strain of agent predominating over genotype of host. *Brain Pathol.*, **8**, 429–37.

McLean, C. A., Cherny, R. A., Fraser, F. W., Fuller, S. J., Smith, M. J., Beyreuther, K., *et al.* (1999). Soluble pool of Ab amyloid as a determinant of severity of neurodegeneration in Alzheimer's disease. *Ann. Neurol.*, **46**, 860–6.

Mirra, S. S., Heyman, A., McKeel, D., Sumi, S. M., Crain, B. J., Brownlee, L. M., *et al.* (1991). The Consortium to Establish a Registry for Alzheimer's Disease (CERAD). Part II. Standardization of the neuropathologic assessment of Alzheimer's disease. *Neurology*, **41**, 479–86.

Polymeropoulos, M. H., Lavedan, C., Leroy, E., Ide, S. E., Dehejia, A., Dutra, A., *et al.* (1997). Mutation in the alpha-synuclein gene identified in families with Parkinson's disease. *Science*, **276**, 2045–7.

Ray, W. J., Yao, M., Mumm, J., Schroeter, E. H., Saftig, P., Wolfe, M., *et al.* (1999). Cell surface presenilin-1 participates in the γ-secretase-like proteolysis of Notch. *J. Biol. Chem.*, **274**, 36801–7.

Roses, A. D. (1994). Apolipoprotein E affects the rate of Alzheimer disease expression: βamyloid burden is a secondary consequence dependent on APOE genotype and duration of disease. *J. Neuropathol. Exp. Neurol.*, **53**, 429–37.

Spillantini, M. G., Goedert, M., Crowther, R. A., Murrell, J. R., Farlow, M. R., and Ghetti, B. (1997a). Familial multiple system tauopathy with presenile dementia: a disease with abundant neuronal and glial tau filaments. *Proc. Natl. Acad. Sci. USA*, **94**, 4113–18.

Spillantini, M. G., Schmidt, M. L., Lee, V. M., Trojanowski, J. Q., Jakes, R., and Goedert, M. (1997b). α-Synuclein in Lewy bodies. *Nature*, **388**, 839–40.

Spillantini, M. G., Murrell, J. R., Goedert, M., Farlow, M. R., Klug, A., and Ghetti, B. (1998). Mutation in the tau gene in familial multiple system tauopathy with presenile dementia. *Proc. Natl. Acad. Sci. USA*, **95**, 7737–41.

Suzuki, N., Iwatsubo, T., Odaka, A., Ishibashi, Y., Kitada, C., and Ihara, Y. (1994). High tissue content of soluble β1–40 is linked to cerebral amyloid angiopathy. *Am. J. Pathol.*, **145**, 452–60.

Teller, J. K., Russo, C., DeBusk, L. M., Angelini, G., Zaccheo, D., Dagna-Bricarelli, F., *et al.* (1996). Presence of soluble amyloid β-peptide precedes amyloid plaque formation in Down's syndrome. *Nat. Med.*, **2**, 93–5.

Thinakaran, G., Borchelt, D. R., Lee, M. K., Slunt, H. H., Spitzer, L., Kim, G., *et al.* (1996). Endoproteolysis of presenilin 1 and accumulation of processed derivatives in vivo. *Neuron*, **17**, 181–90.

Tienari, P. J., De Strooper, B., Ikonen, E., Simons, M., Weidemann, A., Czech, C., *et al.* (1996). The β amyloid domain is essential for axonal sorting of amyloid precursor protein. *EMBO J.*, **15**, 5218–29.

Tu, P. H., Galvin, J. E., Baba, M., Giasson, B., Tomita, T., Leight, S., *et al.* (1998). Glial cytoplasmic inclusions in white matter oligodendrocytes of multiple system atrophy brains contain insoluble α-synuclein. *Ann. Neurol.*, **44**, 415–22.

Vassar, R., Bennett, B. D., *et al.* (1999). β-Secretase cleavage of Alzheimer's amyloid precursor protein by the transmembrane aspartic protease BACE. *Science*, **286**, 735–41.

Walsh, D. M., Lomakin, A., Benedek, G. B., Condron, M. M., and Teplow, D. B. (1997). Amyloid β protein fibrillogenesis. Detection of a protofibrillar intermediate. *J. Biol. Chem.*, **272**, 22364–72.

Weller, R. O., Steart, P. V., and Powell-Jackson, J. D. (1986). Pathology of Creutzfeldt–Jakob disease associated with pituitary derived human growth hormone administration. *J. Neuropathol. Appl. Neurobiol.*, **12**, 117–29.

Will, R. G., Ironside, J. W., Zeidler, M., Cousens, S. N., Estibeiro, K., Alperovitch, A., *et al.* (1996). A new variant of Creutzfeldt–Jakob disease in the UK. *Lancet*, **347**, 921–5.

Yan, S. D., Fu, J., Soto, C., Chen, X., Zhu, H. J., Almohanna, F., *et al.* (1997). An intracellular protein that binds amyloid-β peptide and mediates neurotoxicity in Alzheimer's disease. *Nature*, **389**, 689–95.

9 Neurochemical pathology in degenerative dementias

Elaine Perry, Rose Goodchild, and Margaret Piggott

1 Introduction

The focus of this chapter on transmitter abnormalities in dementia is: how transmitter deficits contribute to cognitive and non-cognitive/neuropsychiatric clinical features; how these can be targeted by specific pharmacotherapies; and, if such therapies are of clinical value, whether diagnostic markers of relevant transmitter disturbances (such as *in vivo* neuroimaging) can be developed to facilitate disease management.

1.1 Relevant neurotransmitter systems

Chemical messengers involved in CNS signalling can be divided into two groups. There are neurotransmitters, released at synapses that operate via ionotropic receptors, designed to rapidly and accurately mediate the transfer of information between neurons — the so-called 'executive' transmitters such as glutamate (GLU, excitatory) and GABA (inhibitory). In contrast, a large number of neuromodulatory transmitter systems exist whose predominant action is to alter the responsiveness of a neuron to this fast neurotransmission. These include noradrenergic, serotonergic, dopaminergic, cholinergic, and histaminergic together with the neuropeptide systems. These transmitters utilize volume transmission and generally operate via G-protein coupled (metabotropic), rather than ionotropic, receptors (exceptions are the nicotinic gated and 5-HT$_3$ ion channels which mediate fast synaptic transmissions). Activation of metabotropic receptors produces changes in the electrical characteristics of a neuronal membrane by indirect coupling, often via soluble intracellular second messenger systems, to target ionic channels. Neuromodulatory transmitters produce changes in synaptic excitability that follow a slower time-scale and are often longer lasting than those produced by direct activation of ionotropic receptors. Both excitatory and inhibitory actions are mediated by different mechanisms depending on coupling to various second messenger systems. Neuromodulators are not thought to be directly involved in information transfer between neurons, but instead to modify the efficacy or characteristics of synaptic transmission.

Neurons in the brain utilizing GLU or GABA are ubiquitous, with all areas of the brain sending or receiving GLU projections and containing GABA local circuit neurons (in some instances GABA neurons are also projection neurons). By comparison neuromodulatory transmitter systems are discretely localized, in keeping with their role in modulating specific brain functions or mode. It has been customary to ascribe specific global functions to these modulators. Examples include: the role of dopamine in drive/reinforcement/intention; acetylcholine in selective attention; noradenaline in arousal; and 5-HT in mood. However current theories depend largely on parallel views of relevant drug actions and on experimental or neuropathological models. It is likely that individual transmitters have both overlapping and distinct functions, depending on interactions in particular brain areas or pathways.

Noradrenergic (NE) and serotonergic (5-HT) systems share the common characteristics of originating in discrete brain stem nuclei (locus coeruleus and raphé) with widespread projections to almost all other cortical and subcortical regions, including spinal cord. The dopaminergic nuclei, situated in the mid brain substantia nigra and ventral tegmental nuclei, have more restricted projections to basal ganglia and specific cortical areas (see also Sections 3 and 4). Histaminergic neurons are confined to the hypothalamus with extensive projections throughout the brain, distributed more or less evenly. The distributions of and projections for neuropeptide containing neurons is generally more complex, and are not discussed in detail in view of the present lack of clear-cut correlations with symptoms of dementia and (with the exception of opioid peptides) relevant CNS therapies. Cholinergic systems are described in greater detail (below) in view of the development of anti-dementia drugs targeted to cholinergic mechanisms, implicated in many but not all of the different types of dementia under discussion (Sections 2–6).

1.2 Cholinergic systems

Acetylcholine is a widely distributed neurotransmitter, not only at peripheral neuromuscular and ganglionic synapses but also in the CNS. It is likely to be one of the most important neuro-modulatory (as opposed to executive) transmitter systems in the brain where it is distributed in a more complex and anatomically diverse fashion than other modulators such as noradrenaline, 5-HT, and dopamine. There are two major distally projecting cholinergic pathways: one originating in the basal forebrain (including septal, diagonal band, and Meynert nuclei), innervating all cortical and archicortical areas with particularly dense terminations in hippocampal and amygdaloid regions; the other in the brain stem (pedunculopontine and tegmental nuclei), innervating in parti-cular the thalamus but also other brain stem areas (e.g. reticular formation and substantia nigra) and select cortical regions including those in frontal and, as most recently identified, also occipital (Higo et al. 1996) lobes. 90% of the input to the thalamus from the brain stem is cholinergic (Bentovoglio and Steriade 1990), and neuronal firing in brain stem cholinergic neurons is asso-ciated with both waking and REM sleep/dreaming cortical activation. This pathway is thought to contribute to processes such as arousal and attention.

The forebrain cholinergic system is the principal ascending pathway that maintains the cerebral cortex in its operative mode. According to Mesulam (1995) the size of nucleus basalis cholinergic projections to the cortex indicates that 'this pathway is likely to constitute the single most substan-tial regulatory afferent system of the cerebral cortex'. Based on the maintenance of cortical activa-tion during REM sleep in the absence of monoaminergic (e.g. noradrenergic and 5-HT) activity, but continued firing of cholinergic nucleus basalis neurons, Buzsaki et al. (1988) concluded that 'it appears that the ascending cholinergic system alone is capable of keeping the neocortex in its operative mode'. Basal forebrain cholinergic neurons project not only to all cortical areas but also to select thalamic nuclei, including the reticular nucleus (Heckers et al. 1992), which has also been implicated in selective attention. These forebrain cholinergic projections are widely impli-cated in cognition on the basis of experimental animal and human pathological evidence. Views of the function of this pathway have evolved from its being primarily involved in memory, towards a more general role in modifying cortical responsiveness (e.g. in evaluating and discriminatory processes). Acetylcholine facilitates the synaptic action of other transmitters such as glutamate so enhancing signal selection (Metherate et al. 1987). The consensus view on the role of these cholinergic projections is that they control selective attention (Voytko 1998). Current concepts of the role of cortical acetylcholine include: affecting discriminatory processes; modulating the efficiency of cortical processing of sensory and association information; controlling the reception and evaluation of stimuli for their level of significance; modifying cortical responsiveness in terms of the relevance and novelty; confining the contents of the conscious stream; and discriminating between independent sensory stimuli (for review see Everitt and Robbins 1997; Perry *et al.* 1999). Cortical acetylcholine thus governs the many brain functions associated with different cortical regions (perception, learning, cognition, affect, judgement, and so on).

A third cholinergic system in the brain consists of interneurons in the striatum which, although only a small proportion (10%) of the neurons in this region, contribute to the striatum being the most active of all brain areas in the terms of overall cholinergic activity (with the striatum having the highest densities of the presynaptic markers, choline acetyltransferase (ChAT), and acetylcholinesterase (AChE), and of postsynaptic, muscarinic receptors). The role of these striatal cholinergic neurons in basal ganglia circuitry, which controls extrapyramidal movement, is relevant to the use of antimuscarinic medication in treating motor disorder in Parkinson's disease. The broader function of corticostriatal loop circuitry, whereby information from all cortical areas is funnelled through the striatum and, via the basal ganglia, back to the frontal cortex represents (indirect) cholinergic modulation of the frontal cortex. A direct cholinergic input to the frontal cortex and basal ganglia also arises from the brain stem pedunculopontine nucleus.

This anatomical complexity of cerebral cholinergic systems is relevant to their potential role in cognition, involvement in Alzheimer's and Lewy body (Sections 2 and 3) diseases and pharmacotherapy.

2 Alzheimer's disease

A broad spectrum of neurotransmitter systems is affected in Alzheimer's disease (AD), raising questions concerning their individual or co-ordinate contributions to specific clinical symptoms, role in the pathological cascade, and potential relevance in diagnosis and pharmacotherapy.

Where transmitter abnormalities have been compared between early and late onset AD, these have been found to be greater than the early onset cases. Cholinergic, 5-HT, and noradrenergic (NE) markers are more severely depleted in early onset cases (Arai *et al.* 1992; Perry *et al.* 1981). There are several potential explanations for this: normal age related reductions lead to diminishing differences in older AD cases; disease duration is shorter in late onset cases and pathology less advanced; with increasing age and multiple pathological contributions, smaller transmitter deficits may precipitate clinical symptoms; or there may be intrinsic, biological differences between early and later onset forms of AD.

2.1 The cholinergic system

2.1.1 Neurochemical pathology

The importance of acetylcholine in cognitive impairment in ageing and dementia was first recognized over 20 years ago. In the 1970s two converging lines of evidence generated the then novel cholinergic hypothesis of geriatric cognitive impairment. Antimuscarinic agents, such as scopolamine, were found to induce memory and related impairments in normal individuals similar to those in ageing and AD. In AD itself neurochemical deficits of cortical cholinergic activity were identified in autopsy brain tissue, correlating with the degree of cognitive impairment to a greater extent than other neurotransmitter abnormalities (Perry *et al.* 1978, 1981). As a result of these

Table 9.1 Cholinergic systems in Alzheimer's disease

Presynaptic marker, choline acetyltransferase	Reduced in most cortical areas, related to cognitive and non-cognitive impairments. Also reduced in striatum, especially ventral, and select thalamic nuclei.
Acetylcholinesterase	Reduced in conjunction with loss of cholinergic axons in cortex.[a] Increased in plaques.
Vesicular acetylcholine transporter (presynaptic)	Loss related to severity cognitive impairment.[a]
Muscarinic receptors	
M1	Generally unchanged in cortex, until late stage when reduced M1 receptor uncoupling also apparent.
M2	Decreased in cortex.[a]
Nicotinic receptors $\alpha_4 \beta_2$	Reductions in α_4 subunit to greater extent than α_3 or α_7 reflected in loss of nicotine,[a] cytisine, and epibatidine binding.
Butyrylcholinesterase	Increases as diseases progresses, especially in neuritic plaques.
Cholinergic neurons in nucleus basalis	Variable loss, especially prominent in posterior section of CH4.
Pedunculopontine cholinergic neurons	Generally reported unchanged, although these neurons develop neurofibrillary tangles.

[a] Denotes information available from *in vivo* imaging, in addition to autopsy studies.

findings, together with animal experimentation demonstrating the functional importance of the cholinergic system in behaviour dependent on cognition, new therapies for AD based on increasing synaptic levels of acetylcholine have now been developed.

The clinical relevance of the cholinergic deficit in AD (see Table 9.1) was until recently considered to be limited to cognitive dysfunction with parallel experiments in non-human primates or rodents demonstrating disruptive effects of basal forebrain cholinergic lesions on cognitive functions. Transmitter deficits in AD occur to the greatest extent in cortical areas primarily concerned with memory and cognition — the hippocampus, adjacent temporal lobe regions, and select parietal and frontal areas (Geula and Mesulam 1996).

Neuropathologically, loss of neurons from the cholinergic nucleus of Meynert (CH 4) is well documented in AD, although the extent of the loss reported varies from moderate to severe, and it has been suggested that in AD cholinergic dysfunction exceeds degeneration (Perry *et al.* 1982).

While it is clear that dysfunction or degeneration of the basal forebrain cholinergic projections to the cerebral cortex is the primary manifestation of disrupted cholinergic transmission in AD, based on loss marker enzymes such as ChAT and AChE, the precise involvement of other key cholinergic proteins is less clear. For example, the vesicular acetylcholine transporter, which is coded by the first intron of the ChAT gene (Cervini *et al.* 1995; Misawa *et al.* 1995), has not been comprehensively analysed due to the lack of a specific pharmacoligand. However, using a more specific vesamical analogue (benzytrozamicol), Efange *et al.* (1997) have detected a loss of vesicular acetylcholine transporter binding in ageing and AD, which is correlated with ChAT activity.

It is generally agreed on the basis of autopsy studies, that the M1 subtype is unchanged until later in the disease when it may decline, probably in relation to cholinoceptive (postsynaptic) neurodegeneration. The M2 subtype is generally reported to be modestly reduced. The status of the other subtypes is not clearly established. With respect to muscarinic receptor coupling, most studies using a variety of investigative procedures have identified some degree of uncoupling, especially with respect to the M1 receptor subtype (reviewed, Robinson and Harrell 1997).

A highly consistent receptor abnormality in AD is the loss of the nicotinic receptor (Aubert *et al.* 1992; Court and Perry 1994; Perry *et al.* 1995) which appears to primarily reflect loss of nicotinic receptors containing the $\alpha4$ subunit (generally associated with the $\beta2$ subunit) as opposedo of to $\alpha3$ or $\alpha7$ subtypes. Immunohistochemically, loss of $\alpha4$ and $\beta2$ reactive fibres has been observed in temporal cortex, associated with reactive neuropil threads, tangles, and plaques (Sparks *et al.* 1998). The possibility that $\alpha4$ $\beta2$ receptor abnormality is an early, aetiopathogenic event in AD and that therapy targeted to this or a related nicotinic receptor may be protective is discussed below.

2.1.2 Clinical correlates

With respect to clinical correlates of regional cholinergic deficits, these have recently been reported to be strongest between dementia scores and transmitter changes in parietal and temporal cortex. In the recent study of Dournaud *et al.* (1995) there was a significant correlation (r = 0.66, n = 12) between choline acetyltransferase (ChAT) activity in middle frontal gyrus and intellectual status assessed by the Blessed Mental Test Score, but correlation coefficients were greater in parietal and temporal lobe areas (0.91 and 0.68). Similar derangements of the cholinergic system occur in a variety of other diseases of the brain affecting cognitive function — Parkinson's disease, Down's syndrome in middle age, progressive supranuclear palsy, cerebrovascular dementia, and more recently head injury and dementia with Lewy bodies (DLB). In DLB, cortical cholinergic deficits correlate with cognitive impairment, independently of Alzheimer-type pathology (Samuel *et al.* 1997).

There has been a recent shift of emphasis regarding the clinical significance of such cholinergic deficits. Non-cognitive or neuropsychiatric symptoms, in addition to cognitive impairment, also to have a cholinergic component. For example visual hallucinations, which are common in DLB, relate to neocortical cholinergic deficits (Perry *et al.* 1993), such deficits (e.g. loss of ChAT) being greater than in AD (Perry *et al.* 1994) in which hallucinations are less common. Other symptoms which may have a cholinergic basis, to judge from beneficial effects of cholinotherapy in AD (see below), include delusions, apathy, and agitation. It has also been suggested that acetylcholine is centrally involved in the process of conscious awareness (Perry *et al.* 1999), and that the variety of clinical symptoms associated with cholinergic dysfunction in AD and related disorders reflects disturbances in the conscious processing of information. There is evidence that implicit memory for example (which does not involve conscious awareness) is relatively intact in AD (see Perry *et al.* 1999).

To further complicate the question of clinical correlates of cholinergic abnormalities, non-cortical brain regions are also affected in diseases such as AD and DLB. Other areas include striatum (particularly ventral areas) and thalamus (including the reticular nucleus) where reductions in ChAT positive neurons or projections occur (Perry *et al.* 1998). Since the thalamus receives joint cholinergic input from the basal forebrain and pedunculopontine neurons (Heckers *et al.* 1992), abnormalities in AD could reflect pathology in one or both of these projections. In addition to basal forebrain pathology in AD, tangles and neuron loss also occur in the cholinergic brain stem nuclei (Mufson *et al.* 1988). A thalamic involvement could be important in relation to both cognitive and non-cognitive abnormalities and also control of REM sleep. A decade before the cholinergic 'hypothesis' of geriatric cognitive impairment, a cholinergic 'hypothesis' of

REM/dreaming sleep was proposed (Jouvet 1972), and it is now well established that excitation of brain stem pedunculopontine cholinergic neurons induces wakefulness and REM sleep (Datta and Siwek 1997). However, it is only relatively recently that abnormalities in sleep architecture, including changes in REM latency, frequency, and/or density have been recorded in AD (see Bahro *et al.* 1993). It has been suggested that abnormalities in REM sleep could in turn contribute to both cognitive deficits and psychiatric symptoms such as delusions and hallucinations (Christos 1993). Cholinergic mechanisms may thus contribute to cognitive decline in a variety of ways depending on the pathways involved and also to a range of non-cognitive symptoms. This diversity is important in relation to cholinergic pharmacology — interpreting effects of cholinergic drug treatment in disease and also drug effects in normal individuals, which in turn provide clues about disease mechanisms.

2.1.3 Acetylcholine: beta-amyloid interactions

Since the earliest observations that senile plaques in both AD and normal old age are reactive for acetylcholinesterase (AChE) with respect to both the amyloid core and plaque neurites, and that plaque densities correlate with the loss of choline acetytlansferase (Perry *et al.* 1978), it has been evident that cholinergic dysfunction and β-amyloid deposition are closely related. The important but as yet unanswered question is whether defects in cholinergic transmission precede or result from β-amyloidosis. Ageing primate studies have shown that AChE may be deposited in plaques during the early stages of amyloid formation (Struble *et al.* 1982), and transgenic overexpression of human AChE induces progressive cognitive deterioration in mice (Beeri *et al.* 1995). Evidence that muscarinic receptor (M1 or M3) stimulation alters APP metabolism in favour of the α secretase (as opposed to the Aβ pepide generating) pathway (Nitsch *et al.* 1996), and that nicotinic receptor stimulation is associated with reduced plaque densities in human brain (Ulrich *et al.* 1997; Court *et al.* 1998), suggests that APP processing is regulated by neuronal activity and that promoting cholinergic transmission may be protective against the pathological process of Aβ deposition or toxicity. Acetylcholine is known to regulate neurite outgrowth (Owen and Bird 1995). However, cholinergic deficits in a number of diseases in which β-amyloidosis is not invariable (such as Parkinson's disease, DLB, head injury, or vascular dementia) suggests that impaired cholinergic transmission may not *per se* trigger β-amyloidosis.

In recent publications linking β-amyloid and cholinergic dysfunction, the emphasis has mainly been on the cholinotoxicity of β-amyloid and related peptides (reviewed, Perry 2000). Both *in vivo* and *in vitro*, exposure to a variety of Aβ peptides (1–40, 1–42, 25–35, 1–28) is followed by dysfunction or degeneration of the cholinergic system, as indicated by loss of cholinergic markers, altered acetylcholine synthesis, or release. In a minority of reports an aetiopathological role for cholinergic dysfunction in APP mismetabolism has been inferred. No doubt future experimental data and, most importantly, the longer-term consequences in patients of chronic cholinotherapy on progressive pathology, will resolve the relation between cholinergic dysfunction and β-amyloidosis. Such data will be of greatest value in patients treated at the earliest stages of AD, before tau pathology and neuronal loss are substantial. Since AChE - histochemical activity is evident in the early stages of plaque formation and is associated (in contrast to butyrylcholinesterase, Guillozet *et al.* 1997) with diffuse Aβ plaques, another intriguing question is whether treatment with AChE inhibitors will specifically influence the pathology occurring in the vicinity of the plaque. This could be investigated in transgenic amyloid mice models which develop β-amyloid plaques that are, as in human brain, AChE positive (Nordberg *et al.* 1995).

2.1.4 Nicotinic receptor role in aetiopathology

Marked regional variations in nicotinic cholinergic receptor (nAChR) abnormalities in AD (consistently and extensively reduced in cortex and hippocampus with variable less extensive losses in subcortical regions), as well as receptor reductions in the absence of a general decrease in the number of neurons (Schröder *et al.* 1991), suggest that nAChR abnormalities may occur at an early stage of the pathological process before irreversible neuronal degeneration takes place. This is supported by the fact that mRNA for the $\alpha4$ nicotinic subunit in the frontal cortex of AD patients is not reduced, whereas $\alpha4$ protein levels are reduced (Schröder *et al.* 1995), thus indicating that the decrease in the number of receptors may be due to alterations in translational or post-translational processes, and not to diffuse cell death. This suggestion is further supported by the absence of nAChR changes in head injury (Murdoch *et al.* 1998). If the hypothesis of an early involvement of nAChR in AD is correct, then administration of nicotinic agonists may be protective. Whilst there is not as yet any evidence that nAChR stimulation in patients is protective, preventing, or slowing disease progression, there are supportive data based on nicotine effects in animal models and on effects of tobacco use in man.

The question of whether there is an inverse association between tobacco smoking and AD, indicated in earlier studies (Lee 1994), has not been resolved by more recently published epidemiological analysis (Ott *et al.* 1998), and thus remains controversial. By contrast, such an association is more consistent in Parkinson's disease (reviewed Clementi *et al.* 2000). Almost all the epidemiological evidence suggests that tobacco smoking reduces the risk of developing PD, and that this relationship is not due to any obvious confounding factors. The reason for differences between PD and AD with respect to protective effects of tobacco smoking may be that in AD, but not in PD, there is a vascular component, and that smoking adversely affects cardiovascular and cerebrovascular function.

Direct evidence of protective effects of tobacco smoking based on autopsy human brain analyses is available from the results of two studies. Ulrich *et al.* (1997) reported a highly significant difference in the density of cortical senile plaques in the brains of female smokers compared to age-matched non-smokers; the density being lower in the smokers. These cases were not selected for clinical history, including both normal and AD for example. In an analysis restricted to normal elderly individuals (Court *et al.* 1998), a similar difference in β-amyloid plaque densities was apparent. However, in neither of these studies was the density of neurofibrillary tangles lower in smokers. This is thus limited evidence that nicotine may be protective against β-amyloidosis in the human brain, and this is consistent with the finding that nicotine protects against experimentally induced β-amyloid induced cell death.

Other experimental data supporting a protective effect of nicotinic agonists such as nicotine *in vivo* or *in vitro* are reviewed elsewhere (Clementi *et al.* 2000), and include reductions in toxic (including ischaemic, age-related, or neurotrophic deprived, as well as Aβ induced) cell death. Whether this protective effect is mediated via a particular nAChR subtype and what the mechanism might be — channel opening or desensitization (with alterations in Ca^{2+} gating and intracellular calcium-dependent mechanisms, for example), is not established. Alterations in the production or function of nerve growth factors is another possible consequence. In rat brain, acute intermittent nicotine treatment leads to increased levels of the neurotrophin, fibroblast growth factor 2, in cortex, striatum, and mid brain (Belluardo *et al.* 1998).

2.1.5 Diagnostic markers

There is not yet a satisfactory biological marker for the diagnosis of AD, based on blood or CSF measurements. Advances in PET or SPECT imaging of the human brain *in vivo* progressively provide the prospect of determining whether the cholinergic system is affected. The vesicular acetylcholine transporter has been monitored using iodobenzovesamicol reductions in binding of this ligand in AD correlating with MMSE, and being more pronounced in demented compared to non-demented PD patients (Kuhl *et al.* 1996). An inhibitor of AChE (*N*-methyl-4-piperidyl acetate) has been used *in vivo* to demonstrate consistent reductions of the enzyme in AD, more prominent in parietal and temporal than frontal, occipital, and sensorimotor cortex (Iyo *et al.* 1997). Iodinated quinuclidinyl benzilate binding ($[^{123}I]$QNB SPECT), which *in vivo* is thought to reflect M1 receptor sites, is reduced in advanced but not moderate AD cases (Wyper *et al.* 1993). In one SPECT study, reduced iododexetimide (a muscarinic antagonist that has preferential M2 specificity) binding has been demonstrated in temporal and parietal cortex in mild, probable AD (Claus *et al.* 1997). Administration of the muscarinic antagonist scopolamine, while resulting in decreased $[^{123}I]$QNB binding in controls, induced the opposite effect in AD patients, indicating a differential receptor sensitivity in the disease (Sunderland *et al.* 1995). Reductions in $[^{11}C]$nicotine binding in temporal cortex of AD patients, reversed by tacrine, have been reported in PET studies (Nordberg *et al.* 1995). Other potential cholinergic markers are in development (reviewed Maziere 1995), and alterations in cerebral perfusion resulting from treatment with cholinergic drugs are also being investigated.

In vivo cholinergic imaging, while thus being relevant to determining whether a patient may be suitable for cholinergic therapy, may not readily differentiate AD from other disorders which affect the cholinergic system — DLB, PD, and vascular dementia for example. Presynaptic markers such as the vesicular acetylcholine transporter, and also AChE, may however differentiate AD on the basis of distinct regional patterns of change. In addition, muscarinic receptors, particularly M1 and M2, may also distinguish AD from Lewy body disorders since in the latter cortical M1 levels are increased (Perry *et al.* 1994) and M2 levels may be more extensively reduced than in AD (Section 3).

While chemical neuroimaging appears to offer the best prospect for detecting cerebral cholinergic abnormalities *in vivo*, blood or CSF measurements of cholinergic markers such as AChE remain inconsistent (reviewed in McQueen 1995).

2.1.6 Therapy

Since the introduction of cholinesterase inhibitors, for the treatment of AD, moderate improvements versus placebo in cognitive function and/or a slowing of further cognitive decline have been reported (see Chapter 19). If therapy could be targeted to the CNS, particularly to brain areas most affected, more effective enhancement of cholinergic functions at higher drugs levels might be predicted to result in a greater clinical response. Such therapy is not yet available, although new nicotinic agonists, agents modulating the NGF–trk A receptor interaction, or cerebral implantation of cholinergic enriched cells (Winkler *et al.* 1998) may offer such a prospect.

It has only recently been appreciated that response to cholinergic therapy can be detected not only in terms of cognitive outcome measures but also, and perhaps more extensively, in relation to non-cognitive measures (Cummings 1997). The cholinesterase inhibitors physostigmine, tacrine, rivastigmine, and metrifonate have variously been reported in placebo controlled trials to decrease psychoses (hallucinations and delusions), agitation, apathy, anxiety, disinhibition, pacing and aberrant motor behaviour, and lack of co-operation in AD (Cummings *et al.* 1993; Kaufer *et al.* 1995; reviewed in Cummings 1997) and in both PD and DLB (Section 3).

Another intriguing aspect of cholinergic therapy is whether increasing regional blood flow, associated with cholinergic drug treatment in AD (e.g. linopiridine, a releaser of acetylcholine) (Van Dyck *et al.* 1997), is an important component of the therapeutic effect. This raises the further question of the extent to which cholinergic dysfunction in AD is related to regional perfusion abnormalities, and how these in turn may contribute to the pathological cascade.

2.2 Non-cholinergic systems

Non-cholinergic modulatory transmitter systems affected in AD include: noradrenergic (NE), serotonergic (5-HT), histaminergic (HA), and a variety of peptidergic (e.g. somatostatin and CRF). Abnormalities include neurofibrillary tangle formation and/or cell loss in the relevant perikarya containing nuclei and/or neurochemical deficits in the respective target zones. Evidence for abnormalities of the principal 'executive' systems, glutamate (GLU) or GABA, is primarily based on loss of neurons presumed to use these transmitters (e.g. hippocampal and neocortical pyramidal neurons), and less on neurochemical indices since there are not as yet reliable and specific, quantifiable biochemical pre-synaptic markers applicable to autopsy tissue. Evidence so far indicates that in comparison to the cholinergic system, non-cholinergic abnormalities occur at a later stage in AD and are not so strongly correlated to cognitive impairment. They may relate more closely to non-cognitive aspects of the disease, for example noradrenergic dysfunction to depression, and 5-HT to aggression and also depression. For summary of non-cholinergic changes in AD see Table 9.2.

Table 9.2 Non-cholinergic systems in Alzheimer's disease

Noradrenergic	
Locus coeruleus nucleus	Neuron population extensively reduced
Noradrenaline and metabolite (MPHG)	Reduced in cortex and some subcortical areas
Dopamine-β-hydroxylase	Reduced
MAO-B	Increased
Serotonergic	
Dorsal raphé nucleus	Neurofibrillary tangles, and varying degrees of neuron loss
5-HT and metabolite (5-HIAA)	Reduced in cortex and various subcortical areas
5-HT transporter	Reduced in some cortical areas, related to depression
5-HT$_2$ receptor	Reductions, related to aggression
Dopaminergic	
Substantia nigra	Neuron population normal, or near normal
Dopamine and metabolite (HVA)	Unchanged, or inconsistently reported reduced in striatum
Dopamine transporter	No change or minimal reduction in striatum[a]
D$_2$ receptor	Normal although reported to be slightly reduced *in vivo*[a]
Histamine	
Nuclei in the hypothalamus	Affected by tangles
Histamine	Reduced
Histidine decarboxylase	Reduced
Histamine receptors H$_1$ H$_2$ H$_3$	No changes
Neuropeptidergic	
Somatostatin	Loss of immunoreactivity in cortex
Galanin	Increased in nbM

Glutamate and GABA systems: loss of glutamate neurons is inferred from the loss of pyramidal cells in the hippocampus, although reliable presynaptic markers remain to be established; subpopulations of GABA neurons (e.g. containing peptides) may be affected but there is no overall loss of the transmitter.
[a] Denotes imaging data available, in addition to autopsy findings

2.2.1 Noradrenaline and adrenaline

Early observations on the loss of locus coeruleus noradrenergic neurons, together with cortical reductions of NE, its metabolites (e.g. MHPG), its synthesizing enzyme (dopamine-β-hydroxylase), and increases in MAO B, clearly implicated NE in AD neurochemical pathology. Recent investigations of autopsy tissue have continued to demonstrate reductions in cortical NE, and also in subcortical areas including striatum, globus pallidus, and amygdala (Storga *et al.* 1996). Psychosis in AD has been associated with a relative preservation of NE in the substantia nigra, and similar non-significant trends in cortical regions (Zubenko *et al.* 1991). In keeping with transmitter changes, the NE transporter is reduced in the locus coeruleus (Tejani-Butt *et al.* 1993). The α_2 adrenergic receptor is also reduced in cortex, hypothalamus, and cerebellum (Meana *et al.* 1992), which may reflect its presynaptic localization.

Measurement of CSF NE originally indicated reductions in AD patients, not affected by L-deprenyl administration, although more recently in advanced cases increased NE, compared to mild cases or controls was reported (Elrod *et al.* 1997), with a negative correlation with MMSE (Oishi *et al.* 1996). Results of CSF MHPG measurements have been equally inconsistent with no change (Liu *et al.* 1991), increases (Sheline *et al.* 1998), associated with declining MMSE (Oishi *et al.* 1996). In plasma the NE metabolites DOPAC and DOPEG are unchanged (Ahlskog *et al.* 1996), and increases in MHPG have been correlated with increases in cognitive impairment (Lawler *et al.* 1995). Decreased plasma and CSF NE has been measured following treatment with the cholinesterase inhibitor physostygmine (Peskind *et al.* 1995). No doubt the great need for biological markers has driven these CSF and plasma analyses, although it could be argued that they do not directly reflect cerebral NE pathology and that alterations may be a consequence of non-specific factors such as decreased mobility.

With respect to drug treatments focused on the noradrenergic system, clonidine (an $\alpha 2$ adrenergic agonist) has been reported in a small open label trial to induce no significant alterations in ADAS (Bierer *et al.* 1994), and in a previous study L-deprenyl induced no changes in CSF NE or adrenaline (Martignoni *et al.* 1991).

Apart from the above isolated reports of CSF or plasma adrenaline, there have been few studies of the central adrenergic system in AD. Burke *et al.* (1994) reported reductions in size, and degenerative changes such as abnormal tau, in the CI region of the rostral ventral lateral medulla which contains adrenergic neurons that represent the tonic vasomotor centre of the brain.

2.2.2 Serotonin

In conjunction with neurofibrillary tangle formation and varying degrees of cell loss in the dorsal raphé nuclei, the 5-HT innervation to the cortex and to lesser extent striatum is compromised in AD, reflected in the loss of 5-HT markers (reviewed in Palmer and Dekosky 1993). Halliday *et al.* (1992) have differentiated between cases with and without raphé neuropathology, the former being associated with symptoms of dementia only and the latter with other features. This is consistent with the proposal that relative preservation of 5-HT markers in the cortex is associated with psychosis (hallucinations) in DLB (Perry *et al.* 1990*a, b*). Reductions in 5-HT and or its metabolite (5-HIAA) continue to be reported in a variety of brain areas including cortical, amygdaloid, and striatal (Nazarali and Reynolds 1992); nucleus basalis of Meynert, raphé nucleus, and substantia nigra (Storga *et al.* 1996). Impaired axonal transport in raphé neurons has been inferred from elevated levels of both tryptophan hydroxylase (the 5-HT synthesizing enzyme) and of 5-HT and 5-HIAA in the raphé, and decreased transmitter and metabolite areas in the cortex (Burke *et al.* 1990).

In terms of clinical correlates, loss of the 5-HT uptake site in temporal but not frontal cortex is associated with the incidence of depression in AD (Chen *et al.* 1996). Lower cortical 5-HT and 5-HIAA in AD patients treated with neuroleptics suggest that neurochemical data need to be interpreted carefully in terms of potential drug effects. Psychosis in AD has been correlated with decreased 5-HT in the prosubiculum and to a lesser extent other cortical and subcortical regions (Zubenko *et al.* 1991). Reductions in the $5-HT_2$ receptor subtype have been consistently reported in AD (Cheng *et al.* 1991) and related to symptoms of aggression (Proctor *et al.* 1992).

Reductions in CSF 5-HT and tryptophan have been reported (Tohgi *et al.* 1992) and 5-HIAA levels reported to be non-significantly (Liu *et al.* 1991) and significantly (Mashige *et al.* 1994) reduced. Platelet abnormalities have been more consistently reported for 5-HT than for NE (above). Reduced platelet levels of 5-HT (Kumar *et al.* 1995) reduced 5-HT uptake levels (Inestosa *et al.* 1993), and altered affinity of the uptake site (Kumar *et al.* 1995) indicate an involvement of peripheral 5-HT systems which may also include lymphocytes in which 5-HT binding is reduced (Singh *et al.* 1990). Physiologically, the prolactin response to oral D-fefluramine (which stimulates cerebral 5-HT function) is greater in AD compared to normal (McLoughlin *et al.* 1994), a response that has been linked to sweet food craving.

In relation to therapy, serotonin reuptake blockade by citalopram may be one of the few effective non-cholinergic pharmacological interventions in AD in terms of reducing emotional disturbance (Schneider and Sobin 1992). In more recently published open label trials of citalopram in elderly demented or mostly demented patients with behavioural disturbances, there were significant reductions in irritability, depression, anxiety, restlessness, and disruptive vocalizations (Ragneskog *et al.* 1996; Pollock *et al.* 1997). Citalopram also reverses the CSF 5-HT deficit (Tohgi *et al.* 1995).

2.2.3 Dopamine

Despite early observations on the normality of the substantia nigra in AD and absence of consistent abnormalities in neurochemical indices of dopaminergic function, the possible involvement of DA in AD continues to be investigated. This may reflect the advent of *in vivo* imaging markers such as beta-CIT as well as the lack of a satisfactory neurochemical substrate for extrapyramidal features emerging at later stages of AD (Stern *et al.* 1996; Lopez *et al.* 1997).

While no significant loss of substantia nigra neurons is generally observed (Perry *et al.* 1990), a loss of neurons positive for tyrosine hydroxylase (the DA synthesizing enzyme) in the ventral tegmental area has been reported by one group (Kastner *et al.* 1993) but not by others (Joyce *et al.* 1997). While some groups have reported dopaminergic abnormalities in AD — reduced caudate HVA (a dopamine metabolite) (Nazarali and Reynolds 1992) and much more extensively reduced DA and its other metabolites DOPA and DOPAC not only in striatum but also in cortex, amygdala, substantia nigra, and raphé (Storga *et al.* 1996) — others have found DA and HVA to be normal in striatum (Langlais *et al.* 1993). Elevated DA content in putamen, and lower than normal HVA in caudate has been noted (Piggott *et al.* 1999). Where clinical correlates of brain tissue abnormalities have been sought, no correlation between psychosis, depression, or agitation and temporal lobe DA, HVA, or DOPAC have been found (Bierer *et al.* 1993).

The dopamine uptake site is reported reduced in putamen (Allard *et al.* 1990) and selectively in nucleus accumbens (Murray *et al.* 1995), but also to be normal with significant decline with increasing age of onset of AD, perhaps reflecting increased EPS in older onset AD patients (Piggott *et al.* 1999). Reduced striatal D2 receptors have been reported *in vivo* IBZM-SPECT (Pizzolato *et al.* 1996), but at autopsy unchanged D2 receptors have been observed (consistent with unchanged dopamine uptake sites), in contrast to the loss of D2 receptors in DLB (Section

3). Dopamine D3 receptors in dorsal striatum are moderately elevated in AD (Piggott *et al.* 1999), perhaps as a consequence of neuroleptic medication.

CSF measurement have included: normal HVA (Soininen *et al.* 1992); reduced HVA related to extrapyramidal symptoms and depression (Wolfe *et al.* 1990) reversed by L-deprenyl and associated with cognitive improvement (Martignoni *et al.* 1991); and DA levels inversely correlated with MMSE scores (Oishi *et al.* 1996).

In vivo neuroimaging data on the possible role of DA in AD are equally inconsistent. No change in fluoro-18-dopa PET scans was reported by Tyrrell *et al.* (1990), although Meguro *et al.* (1997) reported a correlation with cognitive function. In PET studies a 20% loss dopamine uptake sites, detected using [^{11}C]CFT was noted by Rinne *et al.* (1998), which correlated with the severity of EPS. Some of the variability in dopaminergic activities in AD may be due to heterogeneity within the cases selected and the symptoms displayed (Förstl *et al.* 1994), and also to the inclusion of patients with DLB.

In relation to treatment in AD, L-deprenyl has been reported to provide a global amelioration of cognitive dysfunction in an open label trial, unexpectedly associated with diminished CSF DA (Martignoni *et al.* 1991), but no detectable benefit on behaviour, neuropsychiatric symptoms for cognitive function after six months (Freedman *et al.* 1998), and no effect on disease progression (Kuhn and Muller 1996).

2.2.4 Neuropeptides

Abnormalities in over six different neuropeptides (somatostatin, corticotrophin releasing factor (CRF), neuropeptide Y, galanin, neurotensin, and substance P) have been reported in AD (Auchus *et al.* 1994). The most consistent observations relate to loss of cortical somatostatin-like immunoreactivity and CRF, which may reflect degeneration of cortical GABA neurons in which these peptides coexist. Considerable interest has also been generated by the finding that galanin levels are increased in the nucleus of Meynert (Beal *et al.* 1990), since this peptide is the only one coexisting with acetylcholine in these neurons, and intracerebral galanin impairs learning and memory in rodents (McDonald and Crawley 1997). Clinical correlates of these peptide abnormalities detected in brain tissue are not established, nor are there yet relevant pharmacotherapies.

2.2.5 Histamine

Neuropathology of the hypothalamus in AD, implicating the histaminergic system, includes the presence of numerous neurofibrillary tangles in the tuberal and posterior hypothalamus which contain the highest densities of histamine neurons (Airaksinen *et al.* 1991). Neurochemical findings include reductions (around 50%) in levels of histamine in the hypothalamus, hippocampus, and both frontal and temporal cortex, reflecting loss or dysfunction of histaminergic fibres originating in the hypothalamus (not mast cell changes, since there are no histamine positive mast cells in the brain) (Panula *et al.* 1998). The enzyme controlling histamine synthesis, histamine decarboxylase is also reduced in frontal cortex (Schneider *et al.* 1997).

Elevations in blood histamine, related to cognitive deficits and inversely related to depression have been reported in AD and also occur in vascular dementia (Alvarez *et al.* 1996).

2.2.6 Adenosine

Clinical trials of propentofylline (Kittner *et al.* 1997), which is thought to act on cAMP regulation of microglial apoptosis, so limiting secondary nerve cell damage (Schubert *et al.* 1997), have re-focused attention on earlier studies of adenosine receptors in AD. Although originally no changes in cortical adenosine receptors were reported, reductions in A_1 receptor numbers but not coupling have been reported in the hippocampus (Kalaria *et al.* 1990; Jaarsma *et al.* 1991) and in striatum in which reductions correlated with reduced ChAT activity (Ikeda *et al.* 1993).

2.2.7 Cannabinoids

Although cannabinoid systems are implicated in memory and learning, they have not been the focus of attention in AD. There is one report of reductions in cannabinoid receptor binding, but not in mRNA, in hippocampus and striatum, and to a lesser extent in globus pallidus and substantia nigra (Westlake *et al.* 1994).

2.2.8 Glutamate

The loss of hippocampal and cortical pyramidal neurons presumed to include those using glutamate as a neurotransmitter, together with glutamate induced excitotoxic mechanisms in general, have long implicated this transmitter in AD (Palmer *et al.* 1996). It has however been a continuing challenge to identify a glutamate involvement neurochemically, due primarily to the absence of specific neuronal markers of presynaptic glutamate function. Moreover the possibility of compensatory hyperactivity in surviving glutamate neurons cannot be excluded.

Measurements of glutamate levels have not consistently demonstrated reductions in AD. Levels in autopsy samples of the nucleus of Meynert have for example been reported unchanged (Beal *et al.* 1990). *In vitro* or *in vivo* imaging using 1H MR spectroscopy have demonstrated no change in cortical areas (Mohanakrishan *et al.* 1995; Ernst *et al.* 1997). Immunoreactivity of the dipeptide, *N*-acetylaspartyl-glutamate (NAAG), a potential glutamate protransmitter, has recently been reported reduced in temporal cortex, with reactivity in microglia and plaques (Passani *et al.* 1997). Deficits in the glutamate transporter, EAAT2 protein but not mRNA expression have recently been identified correlating with changes in the amyloid precursor protein, APP (Li *et al.* 1997). No consistent glutamate receptor abnormalities have been identified in AD despite a prolific early literature. However, elevated NMDA receptor binding has recently been reported in the striatum (Ulas *et al.* 1994), which may reflect impaired function of corticostriatal glutamate projections.

In relation to peripheral markers, the enzyme alpha-ketoglutarate dehydrogenase, which is reduced in brain, is also reduced in fibroblasts in AD, although in the absence of abnormalities in glutamate metabolism (Cooper *et al.* 1996). In terms of aetiopathology, Aβ25–35 has been shown to induce cell death in cortical or hippocampal cell culture in the presence but not absence of glutamate (Gray and Patel 1995). Despite such tenuous neurochemical evidence, and parallel effects of the transmitter on cognition and neurotoxicity, pharmacotherapy targeted to specific glutamate receptors has been advocated in AD (Cacabelos *et al.* 1999). Non-competitive NMDA antagonists such as memantine are neuroprotective and cognitive enhancing in animal models, without inducing adverse effects, and apparently lead to clinical improvements in patients with dementia of various aetiologies (Muller *et al.* 1995). Cholinergic therapy itself may also enhance glutamate function since cholinesterase inhibitors or M1 receptor agonists lead to increases extracellular glutamate in the striatum (Dijk *et al.* 1995), presumably as a result of activation of corticostriatal glutamate projections.

2.2.9 GABA

Compared with glutamate, there is less evidence of abnormalities of the major inhibitory transmitter, GABA, in AD. Increased GABA levels have been reported in extracted autopsy tissue (Marczynski 1998), although 1H MR spectroscopy has identified no change in

GABA levels (Mohanakrishan *et al.* 1995). No alterations in CSF GABA levels were reported by Oishi *et al.* (1996). If GABA neurons are relatively spared in AD this would be consistent with the relative resistance of GABA neurons *in vitro* to β-amyloid toxicity (Pike and Cotman 1993).

3 Lewy body disorders: dementia with Lewy bodies and Parkinson's disease

In dementia with Lewy bodies (DLB) or Parkinson's disease developing cognitive impairment, transmitter abnormalities occur in the cortex and subcortical areas such as striatum in the absence of gross pathological changes. In contrast to AD, cortical neurofibrillary tangles are rare and β-amyloidosis occurs to a lesser extent. Postsynaptic cholinergic mechanisms (receptor coupling) appear to be preserved (see below). Paradoxically, conventional anti-parkinsonism therapy may be less effective in DLB than in PD due to postsynaptic striatal abnormalities in DLB (see below). There is thus good reason to believe that transmitter oriented anti-dementia therapy may be more effective than in AD, and similar in efficacy to anti-parkinsonism therapy in PD. Table 9.3 summaries the neurotransmitter changes seen in PD and DLB.

3.1 Dopamine

3.1.1 Dopamine presynaptic markers

Parkinson's disease (PD) and dementia with Lewy bodies (DLB) both exhibit neurochemical derangement of striatal dopaminergic transmission. *In vivo* measurements show reductions of striatal dopamine uptake sites, marking dopaminergic terminals, in PD progressively with disease duration (Booij *et al.* 1997), and such losses correlate with increasing motor disability (Antonini *et al.* 1995). Increased reductions in substantia nigra neurons, dopamine levels, and uptake sites have been identified in post-mortem tissue and related to disease severity (Perry *et al.* 1993; Wilson *et al.* 1996). Dopamine loss in PD occurs at early stages of the disease in posterior putamen, with reductions extending to associative and limbic rostral striatal regions as the disease progresses, which may represent neurochemical correlates of non-motor symptoms that develop later (Kish *et al.* 1988; Chinaglia *et al.* 1992). Cognitive changes including mild visuospatial deficits and impairment of planning and episodic memory do however occur in early stages of PD and these may have different neurochemical (e.g. cholinergic and serotonergic) and pathological substrates to the dementia that may occur later (McFadden *et al.* 1996). PD patients also frequently experience depression, 20–60% having affective changes at some stage (see Chapter 4).

Dementia with Lewy bodies (DLB) is a common neurodegenerative dementia with visual hallucinations, disturbances of consciousness, and spontaneous parkinsonian features (McKeith *et al.* 1996). The extrapyramidal features may be mild and include masked faces, stooped posture, slow gait, and rigidity, and are distinguished from PD by less tremor and more myoclonus (see Chapter 13). Striatal dopamine losses, which are less extensive than in PD, have been reported (Langlais *et al.* 1993; Piggott *et al.* 1998). Recent measures of dopamine content and turnover at different coronal levels of the striatum in the rostrocaudal axis (Piggott *et al.* 1999) have demonstrated that dopamine is reduced in DLB to a lesser extent than in PD, and with a different pattern of loss, being uniform in the caudate in DLB, but much greater at posterior levels in PD. DLB and PD also differ in that there is no significant increase in dopamine turnover (as indicated by HVA:dopamine ratios) in DLB, whereas dopamine turnover in PD is

Table 9.3 Neurotransmitter systems in dementia with Lewy bodies compared to Parkinson's disease

	Parkinson's disease	Dementia with Lewy bodies
Dopaminergic		
Dopamine concentration	Severely reduced in caudal striatum, especially putamen	Moderate-to-severe loss in caudal putamen
	Moderately reduced in rostral striatum, with greater loss in putamen	Moderately reduced in caudate and rostral putamen, with caudate reduction as great as putamen
	Moderate loss in cortex	Moderate loss in cortex
Substantia nigra cell loss	Extensive	Moderate
Dopamine transporter	Very extensively reduced in caudal putamen	No reduction rostral striatum
	Moderately reduced in rostral putamen and posterior caudate	Moderate reduction in posterior putamen
	Slight loss in rostral caudate	Slight reduction in posterior caudate
D2 receptors	Elevated by up to 70% in rostral striatum	Slight reduction of about 10% in rostral striatum
	Increased by about 25% in caudal striatum, greater increase in putamen	Moderate reduction of up to 25% in posterior striatum, with greater reduction in caudate
D1 receptors	No change or slight elevation in caudal striatum	No change
D3 receptors	Slightly reduced in ventral striatum	No change
Cholinergic		
Choline acetyltransferase	Cortical cholinergic deficits are greater in PD cases with compared to without dementia	Extensive loss in cortex, especially in temporal, parietal, and cingulate
	Normal in striatum	Moderately reduced in striatum
M1 receptors	Elevated in cortex	Elevated in cortex
Nicotinic receptors	Moderately reduced in striatum, especially putamen	Moderately reduced in striatum, especially in putamen and neuroleptic treated cases
Serotonin		
Serotonin concentration	Moderate loss in striatum	Moderate loss in striatum and frontal cortex
	Slightly reduced in frontal cortex	
Raphé nucleus cell loss		
Serotonin transporter		Moderately reduced in temporal association cortex
5-HT$_{2A}$ receptors		Moderately reduced in temporal cortex
Norepinephrine		
Norepinephrine concentration	Slightly reduced in striatum	Extensively reduced in putamen
		Variable losses reported in cortex
Locus coeruleus cell loss	Extensive	Extensive

increased by more than sixfold in caudate and up to thirteen times in putamen. Dopamine uptake sites are moderately reduced in DLB, consistent with dopaminergic denervation (Piggott *et al.* 1998), with most extensive reductions in the posterior striatum (Perry *et al.* 1998; Piggott *et al.* 1999) — similar in extent to that in early stage PD (Tissingh *et al.* 1998). SPECT imaging with [^{123}I]β-CIT has demonstrated lower dopamine uptake sites in DLB compared to Alzheimer's disease (Donnemiller *et al.* 1997) and Costa *et al.* (1998) have shown dopamine uptake site loss in DLB using [^{123}I]FP-CIT.

Although clinical pathological data are not yet available, the reduction in striatal dopamine innervation is the most likely explanation for the mild extrapyramidal motor symptoms in DLB. Reduced dopamine in the caudate may in addition contribute to non-motor features. Rostral caudate receives input from the frontal cortex, and lesions or dopamine loss in this circuit have been related to cognitive impairment and depression (Brown *et al.* 1997; Lawrence *et al.* 1998). Dopamine concentrations are reduced in the cerebral cortex in DLB (Ohara *et al.* 1998) particularly in cingulate cortex, and anterior cingulate cortical abnormalities may contribute to cognitive impairments in PD (Grossman *et al.* 1992). Non-significant reductions in dopamine, and its metabolite HVA, in frontal, temporal, and parietal cortex have been reported in DLB (Langlais *et al.* 1993) and significant reductions have previously been reported in frontal and cingulate cortex and hippocampus in PD (Scatton *et al.* 1983). In contrast, dopamine uptake sites are reduced in frontal cortex in DLB but not in PD. Mesocortical dopamine is thus compromised in DLB, as in PD, and may relate to non-motor cognitive features in both disorders (Torack and Morris 1988).

3.1.2 Dopamine receptors

Elevated levels of striatal D2 receptors are frequently reported in PD, especially in early and unmedicated cases, and this has now been detected *in vivo* at the time of diagnosis and for several years thereafter (Antonini *et al.* 1997; Hierholzer *et al.* 1998). The increase in D2 receptors is probably a compensatory mechanism in response to dopaminergic denervation. Low D2 receptor density is reported in 'parkinson-plus' syndromes such as multiple system atrophy and progressive supranuclear palsy. It has been suggested that this is an aid to diagnosis in these conditions, and may explain why such patients derive little benefit from L-dopa medication (Tissingh *et al.* 1997). In DLB, striatal D2 receptors are not elevated (Piggott *et al.* 1998; 1999), despite presynaptic dopaminergic loss in posterior putamen of sufficient magnitude to induce such elevation in PD. In select striatal regions D2 receptors are reduced in DLB (Piggott *et al.* 1999). In caudal putamen D2 receptors are significantly lower than controls in DLB (Perry *et al.* 1998, Piggott *et al.* 1999).

DLB patients react adversely to typical and atypical neuroleptic administration, which in many cases results in severe rigidity, confusion, and increased mortality (McKeith *et al.* 1995; 1992). This neuroleptic sensitivity may be a consequence, at least in part, of the low level of D2 receptors with increased susceptibility to D2 antagonistic neuroleptic drugs.

Postsynaptic striatal D1 receptors are unchanged in DLB (Piggott and Marshall 1996; Piggott *et al.* 1999), and in an AD subgroup with parkinsonism (Joyce *et al.* 1998). The possible mechanism of selective vulnerability of D2-bearing compared to D1-bearing striatal neurons in DLB is unknown. There may be specific intrinsic striatal pathology or modifications elsewhere in the cortico-striato-thalamic circuit. In PD, D1 receptors are elevated (Pearce *et al.* 1990; Seeman *et al.* 1987), especially at posterior striatal levels (Piggott *et al.* 1999). These differences in striatal D1 receptor involvement may relate to distinctions in motor symptoms between PD and DLB. In frontal cortex D1 receptors are unchanged in DLB with a non-significant tendency to be increased in PD.

D3 receptors are normal in DLB (Piggott *et al.* 1999) but reduced at least in early-tomoderate stages of PD (Ryoo *et al.* 1998; Piggott *et al.* 1999). D3 receptors are concentrated in limbic areas of striatum and abnormalities may relate to motivational aspects of striatal function (Morissette *et al.* 1998).

The clinical distinction between patients with PD who develop dementia and DLB patients (who often present with dementia) is arbitrary based on motor symptoms preceding cognitive symptoms by more than one year (McKeith *et al.* 1996). Characteristics of the motor features of PD and DLB do vary, however, with tremor and greater laterality being seen in PD, and postural instability, gait disturbance, and myoclonus encountered more often in DLB (see chapter 13). It may be that as PD patients develop dementia, at any stage after disease onset, the dopaminergic neurochemical profile progressively resembles that in DLB with non-motor areas of substantia nigra, ventral tegmental area, striatum, and cortex becoming affected, D2 receptor levels decreasing, and reduced benefit of L-dopa and neuroleptic sensitivity emerging with cognitive decline. D2 up-regulation has been reported to be less persistent in PD presenting bilaterally (Wenning *et al.* 1998). Whether it is possible to predict which PD patients will become demented, based on characteristics of motor dysfunction (gait and laterality), neuropsychiatric features, fluctuations, and hallucinations, and whether the dementia is identical to that in DLB requires further investigation.

3.2 Acetylcholine

Cholinergic deficits in DLB are profound, as indicated by neocortical activities of choline acetyltransferase (ChAT), which are lower than in Alzheimer's disease (Dickson *et al.* 1987; Langlais *et al.* 1993; Perry *et al.* 1994). Such deficits correlate with cognitive impairment in AD and DLB (Samuel *et al.* 1997) but in DLB, where more extensive loss is seen in the cingulate, temporal, and parietal cortex, clinical correlates also include neuropsychiatric features such as hallucinations. Cholinergic activity is even lower in hallucinating compared to non-hallucinating DLB cases (Perry *et al.* 1990*b*). In PD, neuronal loss in the cholinergic nucleus basalis of Meynert is greater in demented than non-demented PD cases. Neuronal loss in cholinergic nuclei and ChAT loss in cortical areas in PD may not be equivalent (Mohr *et al.* 1995) and the latter may be a better parameter with which to seek correlates of dementia. The extent and pattern of cholinergic deficits in PD, with and without dementia, differs from that in AD and in DLB. Not only are cortical areas affected by cholinergic dysfunction in DLB, but also in subcortical areas such as striatum and thalamic nuclei. ChAT in the thalamic reticular nucleus is reduced in DLB but not AD (Perry *et al.* 1998), which may relate to disturbances in consciousness and or REM sleep abnormalities. In the striatum, ChAT reduced in DLB and AD, but not PD and it has been suggested that underactivity of intrinsic striatal neurons in DLB may offset nigrostriatal dopaminergic degeneration and account for less severe clinical parkinsonism.

In both DLB and PD cortical muscarinic M1 receptors are elevated and in DLB not uncoupled as they are in AD (Perry *et al.* 1998). This is consistent with the integrity of cholinoceptive mechanisms in the cortex and provides a basis for more positive responses to cholinergic therapy (see also Sections 2.1.7 and 3.6). Nicotinic receptors are, however equally affected in DLB and AD (Perry *et al.* 1990*a, b*) with reductions in nicotine or epibatidine binding in both, related to synapse loss in AD but not DLB (Sabbagh *et al.* 1998). Clinical correlates of nicotinic receptor abnormalities are unknown but may include alterations in consciousness (Section 2).

3.3 Serotonin

Serotonergic (5-HT) deficits in DLB and PD are consistent with the involvement of this transmitter system in depression, and high frequency of depression in both diseases (Gnanalingham *et al.* 1997; Kuhn *et al.* 1996). Lewy bodies occur in the serotonergic dorsal raphé nucleus in PD and DLB and Langlais *et al.* (1993) reported that serotonin levels are significantly reduced (60–70%) in striatum in DLB but not in cortex. Neocortical serotonin was however reported to be reduced (70%) and also in putamen (80%) in the five DLB cases examined by Ohara *et al.* (1998). Serotonin levels were found to be significantly reduced in DLB in frontal cortex (60–70%), to a greater extent than PD, and equally in cases which did and did not experience hallucinations, but the metabolic index of serotonin release (5-hydroxyindole acetic acid/serotonin is higher in hallucinating cases than in PD or non-hallucinating DLB cases (Perry *et al.* 1993). 5-HT$_2$ binding in temporal cortex is also lower in non-hallucinating than hallucinating DLB cases (Perry *et al.* 1990*b*). Consistent with these findings, serotonin reuptake inhibitor therapy has been reported to induce hallucinations in demented patients, although alleviation of depressive symptoms was effective (Omar *et al.* 1995). Recently, extensive (50–60%) reductions in serotonin transporter binding has been identified in secondary visual cortical areas in DLB (Ballard *et al.* in press). Reductions in striatal serotonin of (60%) also occur in typical PD (Scatton *et al.* 1983) with less extensive reductions (40–50%) in frontal cortex, cingulate, and hippocampus.

3.4 Norepinephrine

Degeneration of the locus coeruleus is extensive in PD, especially in cases with dementia, implying that depletion of cortical norepinephrine may be a factor in dementia in this group. Moreover, norepinephrine metabolism is lower in demented PD compared to non-demented patients (Cash *et al.* 1987). A loss of norepinephrine of 40–80%, independent of dopaminergic reductions, was however reported in PD without dementia, and suggested as a factor in mood disorder and more cognitive subtle changes (Scatton *et al.* 1983). In DLB, norepinephrine is reduced in putamen (> 90%), which combined with lower ChAT in DLB striatum than in PD, has been suggested to contribute to the milder parkinsonism and absence of tremor in DLB (Langlais *et al.* 1993). Alterations in norepinephrine are also likely to contribute, depending on degeneration of other transmitter systems, to: expression of depressive symptoms in limbic areas; cognitive decline in neocortex; and movement disorder characteristics in basal ganglia. For example in a group of AD patients with depression low neuron numbers in the locus coeruleus combined with higher than usual neuron density in the nucleus basalis of Meynert were reported (Förstl *et al.* 1994).

3.5 Glutamate

In the basal ganglia circuit, excitatory amino acid transmission occurs between several components: cortico-striatal, thalamo-cortical, thalamo-striatal, and sub-thalamic nucleus to substantia nigra and other targets. In PD, enhanced glutamatergic output from the sub-thalamic nucleus (due to dopamine deficiency), increasing inhibition of the thalamus is considered to be an essential aspect of the neurochemical pathology of the movement disorder (DeLong 1990), and glutamate antagonists have been used as treatment in PD (Starr 1995). In addition excitotoxic mechanisms have been implicated in the progress of PD and other neurodegenerative diseases (Kornhuber and Weller 1997). However reports of transmitter derangements at the receptor level are sparse. An investigation of NMDA receptor MK-801 binding in the striatum in DLB and PD failed to reveal any disease-related differences (Piggott, M. A. unpublished observation). Gerlach *et al.* (1996) reported in contrast reductions in MK-801 binding in the caudate but no change in glutamate content. NMDA receptor immunoreactivity is unaltered in AD and DLB in hippocampus and entorhinal cortex, while GluR2/3 AMPA receptor subunit immunoreactivity is decreased (Thorns *et al.* 1997).

3.6 Treatment implications

Since non-cognitive/neuropsychiatric features in AD respond as well, if not better than cognitive symptoms to cholinergic therapy (Section 2.1), and since intrinsic cortical pathology is less or minimal, patients with DLB have been predicted to respond well to such treatment. This prediction is supported by the findings of an open-label trial of the cholinesterase inhibitor, rivastigmine (Exelon) in which 9/11 DLB patients improved with respect of reductions in NPI (Neuropsychiatric Inventory) scores of agitation, delusions, and hallucinations (McKeith *et al.* 2000). Such therapy did not exacerbate, but slightly diminished extrapyramidal symptoms, which is similar to the experience of Hutchinson and Fazzini (1996) in demented patients with PD. Conversely anti-parkinsonism medication such as L-dopa may be less effective in patients with DLB compared with PD and novel pharmacological approaches to basal ganglia dysfunction are indicated which depend less on the integrity of D2 dopaminergic receptors. Nicotinic cholinergic drugs may be particularly appropriate to DLB since these alleviate both cognitive (primarily attentional) and motor disorders.

4 Huntington's disease

The neuropathological hallmark of Huntington's disease (HD) is severe degeneration of the striatum (see chapter 15). However there is also a generalized reduction in brain volume, shrinkage of the cortical ribbon, a decrease in white matter volume, and expansion of the ventricular system (De La Monte *et al.* 1988). It is the striatal lesion and neurochemical abnormalities within the basal ganglia that have been most extensively characterized, particularly with regard to providing an anatomical/neurochemical basis for the choreic movements of HD. A variety of psychiatric and cognitive symptoms also accompany the disorder, which may relate to cortical and white matter changes (see Chapter 15). For summary of the neurotransmitter changes in HD see Table 9.4

Table 9.4 Neurotransmitter systems in Huntington's disease

GABA and glutamate decarboxylase	Extensively lost in striatum and in both external and (later in the disease process) internal sections of the globus pallidus Variable losses in cortex
Enkephalin	Severely reduced in striatum and external globus pallidus
Substance P	Reduction in internal globus pallidus greater as disease progresses Increased in cortex
Choline acetyltransferase	Moderate-to-severe reduction in striatum Unchanged or mild loss in cortex
Dopamine receptors	Severely reduced in striatum
Glutamate receptors	AMPA and Kainate decreased in lower laminae of frontal cortex

4.1 Basal ganglia abnormalities and the neural bases of chorea

The striatum is the area of the brain particularly effected in Huntington's disease, with up to 80% neuronal loss (Vonsattel and DiFiglia 1998). The vast majority of striatal neurons are GABAergic projection neurons, which coexist with both larger cholinergic and smaller GABAergic local circuit interneurons (Kawaguchi *et al.* 1995). Different populations of intrinsic striatal neurons express different neuropeptides, which has facilitated examination of differential neuronal susceptibility in HD. Neurochemical measurements have indicated an extensive decrease in levels of striatal GABA, and its synthesizing enzyme glutamate decarboxylase, reflecting the loss of GABAergic neurons (Storey and Beal 1993). Since the concentration of neuropeptides expressed by interneurons is unchanged, or even increased at post-mortem (Vonsattel and DiFiglia 1998), it appears that a relatively selective loss of striatal projection neurons occurs. However, some interneurons are undoubtedly also lost, as for example, striatal ChAT activity is decreased in HD striatum which indicates a probable loss of intrinsic striatal cholinergic interneurons (Wu *et al.* 1979). Densities of neurotransmitter receptors, including ionotropic GABA and glutamate receptors and also dopamine, histamine, 5-HT, muscarinic acetylcholine, and metabotropic glutamate receptors, are universally decreased in the striatum probably due to dysfunction and degeneration of intrinsic striatal neurons (Dure *et al.*1991; Goodchild *et al.* 1999; Whitehouse *et al.* 1985; Young *et al.* 1988). In addition to the striatum, GABA and glutamate decarboxylase levels are also reduced in target nuclei of striatal efferents, namely the globus pallidus and SN (Storey and Beal 1993).

Different, although not necessarily mutually exclusive, theories exist to explain the development of the typical akinetic chorea (Albin *et al.* 1989; Hedreen and Folstein 1995). It is suggested that neurons of the *indirect* movement pathway are selectively lost in comparison to those of the *direct* pathway, thus decreasing this pathway's inhibitory influence upon movement. Whilst neurons of both the direct and indirect pathways, projecting to the internal globus pallidus/SN (pars reticulata) and external globus pallidus, respectively, are GABAergic, they differentially co-express certain neuropeptides; substance P is associated with the direct and enkephalin with the indirect pathway (Albin *et al.* 1989; Graybiel 1990). Both of these neuropeptides are decreased in the HD striatum and pallidum (Storey and Beal 1993). However, whilst enkephalin levels in the external globus pallidus are reduced early in the disease process, it is not until later stages where this is accompanied by losses of substance P in the internal globus pallidus (Albin *et al.* 1990; Reiner *et al.* 1988). Furthermore, comparison of post-mortem GABA concentrations in the external and internal segments of the globus pallidus has shown that a greater imbalance exists in choreic as compared with rigid HD cases (Storey and Beal 1993).

An alternative suggestion to selective vulnerability of the *indirect* movement pathway is hyperactivity of the nigro-striatal dopamine projection, whereby hyper-stimulation of D1- and D2-receptors produces an imbalance in the activity of the direct and indirect pathways in the reverse manner to that which results in the bradykinesia of Parkinson's disease (Albin *et al.* 1989; Hedreen and Folstein 1995). Dopamine receptor densities are decreased very early in HD, with losses described in pre-symptomatic carriers who exhibit no clear neuronal loss (Augood *et al.* 1997) and dopamine receptor antagonists are efficacious in reducing chorea (Hedreen and Folstein 1995). This hypothesis was rejuvenated recently when it was found that inhibitory GABAergic projections from the striatum to the dopaminergic neurons in the pars compacta of the SN (SNpc) are the first striatal neurons to be lost HD (Hedreen and Folstein 1995). It is therefore possible that decreased inhibition in the SNpc in early HD results in increased striatal dopamine release, with changes in the expression of neuropeptides then paralleling changes in neuronal activity (Hedreen and Folstein 1995). However, when HD cases with differing degrees of chorea have been examined it is GABA concentrations, and not those of dopamine or its metabolites, which vary with the severity of motor symptoms (Hedreen and Folstein 1995).

Nevertheless, whether chorea results from a selective loss of striatal projections to the external globus pallidus and/or an increase in striatal dopamine levels, both theories centre around an imbalance of GABA release in the external and internal globus pallidus leading to decreased inhibitory output from the basal ganglia to the motor thalamus (Albin *et al.* 1989). In an extension to this hypothesis of chorea, it is has been suggested that the rigidity of later disease stages, and the akinetic-rigid variant of HD, result from non-selective pathology involving both pathways to the output nuclei of the basal ganglia (Storey and Beal 1993).

4.2 Correlates of dementia

In addition to the striatal lesion, other brain areas are often, although more variably, involved (Vonsattel and DiFiglia 1998). Other nuclei of the basal ganglia, the thalamus, and limbic structures may be affected in later stages of the disease. Frontal lobe atrophy is reported in approximately 80% of cases (Vonsattel and DiFiglia 1998) and loss of pyramidal neurons from the deep cortical layers, with sparing of layer IV, occurs consistently in many regions of neocortex (Heinsen *et al.* 1994). Decreases in neocortical GABA and glutamate concentrations have been found, though reports are conflicting (Ellison *et al.* 1987; Storey *et al.* 1992). In addition, concentrations of some interneuron expressed neuropeptides, including substance P, are increased at post-mortem examination (Beal *et al.* 1988), suggesting that as in the striatum, there is neuronal loss accompanied by selective sparing of local circuit interneurons in the neocortex (Pearson and Reynolds 1994). However, in contrast to striatum, ChAT activity is not significantly decreased in frontal cortex (Wu *et al.* 1979), consistent with the absence of abnormalities in the nucleus basalis (Clark *et al.* 1983; Mann 1989). Indeed, in contrast to other dementias, such as AD, neuronal loss is not found in nuclei of ascending neuromodulator systems (Mann 1989) and furthermore, evidence exists for increased activity of cortically projecting dopaminergic and serotonergic systems (Pearson and Reynolds 1994).

A range of neurotransmitter receptors have been examined in a variety of neocortical regions with the vast majority found unchanged (Dure *et al.*1991; Whitehouse *et al.* 1985; Young *et al.* 1988). However, glutamatergic AMPA and kainate receptors are selectively decreased in lower laminae of the frontal cortex, consistent with the pathology in these layers (Wagster *et al.* 1994). Breakdown of cortical lamination has also been described in the entorhinal cortex and subiculum (Braak and Braak 1992) and GABA and glutamate concentrations are reduced in the hippocampus (Reynolds *et al.* 1987).

The neuropathological and neurochemical correlates of the neuropsychiatric and cognitive abnormalities of HD are still a matter of debate (Lawrence *et al.* 1998). CT scans have demonstrated that cognitive and visual-spatial impairments correlate with structural changes in the striatum (Sax *et al.* 1983) and post-mortem neurochemical analyses have found that striatal, rather than cortical, deficits of GABA, glutamate, and ChAT differ when severely demented and non-demented HD cases are compared (Reynolds *et al.*1990). However, the characterization of cortical pathology has lead to discussion of the origin of the non-motor features (Cammarata *et al.* 1993). Glucose metabolism is reduced in many regions in HD, and whilst striatal deficits correlate with severity of chorea, the degree of dementia has been found to correlate with decreased cortical metabolism (Kuwert *et al.* 1990).

The nuclei of the basal ganglia are increasingly considered as components of integrated cortico-basal ganglia-thalamo-cortical circuitry. Several segregated loops have been identified whereby information derived from functionally separate cortical regions is processed in parallel through the basal ganglia, outputted to distinct thalamic nuclei and relayed back to separate cortical regions. Evidence exists for the presence of separate circuits concerned with motor, affective, visual, associative information (Alexander and Crutcher 1990; Lawrence *et al.* 1998). It is likely that the breakdown of information processing through these wider loops, with contributions from both cortical and striatal pathology, is responsible for motor and cognitive symptoms of HD (Lawrence *et al.* 1998).

5 Frontotemporal dementia

Frontotemporal dementia (FTD) generally presents at a younger age (45–60 years) than the majority of AD cases. Loss of personal awareness, disinhibition, extreme eating habits, perseverative behaviour, and progressive reduction of speech are the features that most clearly distinguish FTD from AD (see Chapter 12). Parkinsonian signs of rigidity, gait disturbance, and flat facies may occur during the course of the disease, with dysphagia and mutism later.

Cortical pathology is most apparent in the second and deep cortical layers which coincides with the localization of select receptor subtypes, for example dopamine D2 (Goldsmith *et al.* 1997) and 5-HT$_1$, but not GABA$_A$, M1, M2, or glutamate binding (Zilles and Schleicher 1995). Other pathological features include, to varying degrees, degeneration in the substantia nigra (SN), hippocampus, medial thalamus, striatum, amygdala, and locus coeruleus, in descending order of frequency and severity of involvement (see chapter; Yats *et al.* 1980). Analyses of neurochemical correlates of clinical symptoms in FTD based on autopsy tissue have been few and usually involved limited numbers of subjects (Bettendorff *et al.* 1997; Francis *et al.* 1993; Gilbert *et al.* 1988; Nagaoka *et al.* 1995; Sjogren *et al.* 1998; Sparks and Markesbery 1991; Yates *et al.* 1980). For summary of neurotransmitter changes in FTD see Table 9.5.

5.1 Dopamine

Basal ganglia involvement, with substantia nigra and ventral tegmental area dopaminergic cell loss (as well as severe intrinsic striatal pathology in some patients) occurs in most patients and is a likely cause of parkinsonian symptoms. Mesocortical dopamine loss may also contribute to non-motor features of dementia and depression (Knopman *et al.* 1990). Homovanillic acid (HVA) and 5-hydroxyindoleacetic acid (5-HIAA) have been reported to be reduced by about 30% in the CSF of FTD cases (especially with increased apathy), indicative of degeneration in central dopaminergic and serotonergic systems (Sjogren *et al.* 1998). However Francis *et al.* (1993) reported that HVA was not reduced in CSF from four FTD cases. Dopamine content has been reported to be unchanged in several cortical areas (Yates *et al.* 1980), but also to be severely deficient (98–99% loss) in the striatum of one patient, especially in the caudate (Gilbert *et al.* 1988) — an extent greater than might be expected from the apparent cell loss in the substantia nigra. A study of one young case of FTD with prominent behavioural changes and emergent motor symptoms (Nagaoka *et al.* 1995) identified the loss of dopamine as the principal neurochemical deficit, with greater than 60% reductions in substantia nigra, nucleus basalis, locus coeruleus, raphé nucleus, lateral nucleus of the thalamus and occipital cortex, as well as striatum, with caudate loss greatest. In three non-familial FTD cases examined neurochemically (Perry, R. in preparation), with a typical constellation of symptoms but generally older age of onset (52, 67, and 80 years) and longer disease duration (25, 13, and 10 years), dopamine was severely reduced in striatum, with a greater loss in the caudate, and was also reduced in hippocampus and frontal cortex (Brodmann area 8). Other dopaminergic abnormalities included reduced dopamine re-uptake site density (greater in the caudate and at posterior striatal levels), and elevated D2 receptors. Possible clinical correlates of reduced striatal dopamine include rigidity and flat facies and also (particularly in caudate) depression (Bhatia and Marsden 1994).

Table 9.5 Neurotransmitter systems in frontotemporal dementia

Serotonin	
5-HT concentration	Moderately reduced in basal ganglia and cortex (frontal and temporal)
5-HT transporters	Reduced in frontal cortex
5-HT$_{1A}$ receptors	Moderately reduced in temporal and slightly reduced in frontal cortex, but not reduced in parietal cortex
5-HT$_{2A}$ receptors	Extensively reduced in frontal cortex, and moderately reduced in temporal, parietal, and cingulate cortex. Slightly reduced in striatum
Dopamine	
DA concentration	Extensively reduced in striatum, especially caudate, and may be reduced in frontal cortex
DA transporters	Reduced in striatum, especially caudally and in caudate
D2 receptors	Elevated in striatum
D1 receptors	Unchanged
Acetylcholine	No change in cholinergic parameters generally reported
Norepinephrine	May be reduced
Glutamate receptors	Moderate reduction in AMPA receptors in frontal and temporal cortex with no change in NMDA or Kainate receptors

5.2 Acetylcholine

Cholinergic systems are generally reported to be normal in FTD, with a relative sparing of the nucleus basalis of Meynert (Foster *et al.* 1998), although Sparks and Markesbery (1991) reported reduced ChAT and AChE in the nucleus basalis. No reduction in temporal lobe ChAT has been reported (Francis *et al.* 1993; Knopman *et al.* 1990). Reductions in ChAT (about 50%) were noted in the striatum of one FTD case with no reductions in cortex (Gilbert *et al.* 1988). We (Perry, R. *et al.* in preparation) found no loss of ChAT in cingulate cortex or striatum, although there were reduced (40%) levels in the anterior and ventral posterolateral nuclei of the thalamus in two cases. Reduced ChAT in these thalamic nuclei may affect the function of the cingulate cortex and sensory cortex, with which they have reciprocal connections. Preserved striatal cholinergic markers may contribute to a dopamine/cholinergic imbalance and exacerbate extrapyramidal features. Total muscarinic receptor binding has been reported to be reduced (by up to 50%) in temporal cortex but not in frontal cortex (Francis *et al.* 1993; Hansen *et al.* 1988).

5.3 Serotonin

Serotonergic dificits are the most frequently reported neurochemical abnormality in FTD. In one case of FTD serotonin concentration was reduced by 40% or more in substantia nigra caudate and putamen, medial, and lateral thalamus, nucleus basalis, raphé nucleus, locus coeruleus, and frontal and temporal cortex (Nagaoka *et al.* 1995), reductions which were difficult to reconcile with the mild pathology seen in the dorsal raphé nucleus. Gilbert *et al.* (1988) also found serotonin to be reduced by 30–50% in the substantia nigra, striatum, and hypothalamus. Postsynaptic 5-HT$_1$ receptors have been reported to be low in frontal cortex in the absence of changes in 5-HT$_2$ receptors (Francis *et al.* 1993). Serotonin binding was also reduced by about 50% in the hypothalamus together with temporal and frontal cortex (but not in the nucleus basalis) (Sparks and Markesbery 1991). Francis *et al.* (1993) found no indication of reduced serotonin concentration in temporal lobe, but Sparks and Markesbery (1991) identified reduced imipramine binding in frontal cortex suggestive of reduced serotonin uptake sites. In the study of Perry *et al.* (in preparation) 5-HT$_2$ receptors were reduced by about 30% in caudate, putamen, and cingulate cortex. Clinical consequences of these serotonin deficits may be stereotyped compulsive behaviours and increased sweet and carbohydrate consumption (Miller *et al.* 1995).

5.4 Other transmitter abnormalities

Norepinephrine was found to be reduced by 30% or more in one FTD case in the nucleus basalis, lateral and medial thalamus, locus coeruleus, and amygdala (Nagaoka *et al.* 1995), although pathological changes in the locus coeruleus appeared mild. CSF levels of neuropeptide Y-like immunoreactivity (NPY-LI) correlated with clinical symptoms of suspiciousness, anxiousness, restlessness, and irritability in both FTD and AD (Minthon *et al.* 1996), with a decline in NPY-LI with disease duration in AD but not in FTD. Somatostatin-like immunoreactivity correlated with NPY-LI in CSF in FTD but not in AD (Minthon *et al.* 1997). Bettendorff *et al.* (1997) reported thiamine diphosphate content in a series of 16 FTD patients post-mortem to be reduced by 40–50% in cortex, with increases in thiamine monophosphate and suggested that this indicated reduced mitochondrial oxidative metabolism. The concentration of GABA was normal in all brain areas examined in one FTD case (Gilbert *et al.* 1988), and the concentration of glutamic acid was also normal except in frontal cortex and amygdala where slight reductions occurred (Gilbert *et al.* 1988).

5.5 Therapeutic implications

FTD patients are often reported to experience food cravings, especially for sweet and carbohydrate foods, with weight gain, and also to exhibit compulsive behaviour (Miller *et al.* 1995). These symptoms may be caused to some extent by the serotonin deficit (Miller *et al.* 1995; Sparks and Markesbery 1991), since selective serotonin reuptake inhibitors tend to decrease appetite. Some of the behavioural symptoms in FTD are reported to improve with serotonin reuptake inhibitor treatment (Miller *et al.* 1995; Swartz *et al.* 1997), in particular disinhibition, depression, carbohydrate craving, and compulsions.

   In view of the dopamine and possible norepinephrine deficits in FTD, combined reuptake inhibitors in these systems may also be beneficial (see Chapter 19). Dopamine replacement therapy with agonists or L-dopa may be useful if postsynaptic receptors are intact. An alternative treatment for motor symptoms might be the use of antimuscarinic drugs, to restore striatal cholinergic-dopaminergic balance.

6 Conclusion

Whist there is no lack of identified neurotransmitter derangements in the different types of dementia discussed, no obvious unitary transmitter hypothesis of dementia applicable to the different diseases is apparent. A cholinergic hypothesis of cognitive, and as more recently recognized also non-cognitive dysfunction, can be sustained in AD, PD, DLB, and perhaps also vascular dementia, on the basis of clinical correlates and/or response to therapy. However other neurochemical and molecular pathological changes no doubt contribute to the clinical picture in these disorders to varying degrees. Cholinergic therapy is likely to be of greatest value either early in the disease or in those cases (e.g. DLB) in which cortical pathology is minimal.

In HD and FTD there are no obvious cholinergic correlates of dementia, unless striatal (HD) or thalamic (FTD) cholinergic abnormalities are relevant. In these diseases, dementia is more likely related to non-cholinergic cortical abnormalities and/or to basal ganglia pathology and the future development of non-cholinergic anti-dementia agents directed towards glutamate, GABA, or dopamine systems is likely to be relevant as both protective and symptomatic. It will also be of interest to determine the general applicability of anti-dementia therapies being developed based on nicotinic cholinergic receptors since:

(a) These receptors promote the release or enhance the action of wide a range of transmitters in addition to acetylcholine (including cortical GABA and glutamate, and striatal dopamine).

(b) Nicotinic agonists are neuroprotective in a variety of ageing, lesioned, and neurotoxic model situations (reviewed Clementi *et al.* 2000).

As *in vivo* chemical probes of the different neurotransmitter systems such as dopamine, 5-HT, and acetylcholine are progressively developed, neuroimaging may assist in the differential diagnosis of those dementing disorders which continue to present the clinician with diagnostic difficulty.

Whether new advances in understanding pathogenesis in dementing diseases will emerge from transgenic or gene knockout animal models remains to be determined.

7 Key points

1   Interest in the involvement of neurotransmitter systems in degenerative dementia is three fold:

  (i) Many of these systems are primarily modulatory and particular transmitter disturbances relate to specific cognitive and non-cognitive/neuropsychiatric symptoms.

  (ii) As yet most of the drugs currently available for treatment aim to relieve specific symptoms as a result of manipulating one particular transmitter system.

  (iii) New *in vivo* neuroimaging chemical probes of transmitter function continue to emerge which are expected to be of diagnostic value and, in relation to treatment response, prognostic value.

2   The transmitter systems that are currently most relevant in the context of all of the above respects are primarily cholinergic, dopaminergic, and serotonergic, and also, in at least one respect, glutamate, GABA, noradrenergic, and a minority of neuropepidergic systems.

3   Alzheimer's disease is associated with an involvement of cholinergic systems, primarily pathways from the basal forebrain projecting to the cortex, but also to a lesser extent striatal and thalamic systems. There is a loss of presynaptic more than postsynaptic cholinergic markers and the nicotinic receptor is centrally involved. Non-cholinergic systems affected include noradrenergic, serotonergic, histaminergic, and the peptides: somatostatin, galanin, and CRF. Evidence suggests that disturbances in cholinergic function relate to both cognitive and neuropsychiatric features of the disease and that both are relieved to some extent by cholinergic therapy. Symptoms such as depression however are more likely associated with disturbances in monaminergic (5-HT and noradrenaline) transmission and these symptoms are alleviated by antidepressive medication.

4   In the Lewy body disorders PD and DLB, the nigrostriatal dopaminergic system is affected (more so in PD than DLB) in conjunction with degeneration of substantia nigra neurons. The striatal dopamine receptor D2 is up-regulated to a greater extent in PD than DLB which, together with the loss of striatal cholinergic activity, is indicative of more striatal pathology in DLB. In both of these conditions, loss of cortical cholinergic activity is thought, as in AD, to contribute to declining cognitive function and also to psychotic symptoms such as hallucinations.

5   Neurotransmitter pathology in Huntington's disease is most notable in basal ganglia regions such as the striatum and globus pallidus, where there are multiple abnormalities of GABA, glutamate, peptidergic (enkephalin and substance P), and in more advanced stages also reduced cholinergic activities reflecting loss of these interneurons. In contrast few consistent abnormalities of the cerebral cortex have been reported with the exception of diminished numbers of AMPA and kainate receptors.

6   In contrast to AD, PD, and DLB, cortical cholinergic innervation is spared in FTD although, from the limited literature available, it is apparent that there are reductions in the striatal dopaminergic and serotonergic innervation and also of the cortical serotonergic input.

7   The cholinergic system is affected in two other types of dementia or cognitive impairment arising from primarily non-degenerative conditions — cerebrovascular disease and head injury. It is not yet clear why this transmitter system should be vulnerable in many but not all types of cerebral disease which can give rise to dementia.

Acknowledgements

Thanks to Secretarial Staff at the MRC Unit Newcastle upon Tyne for the manuscript preparation and Dr Jenny Court for information on the nicotinic receptor.

References

Ahlskog, J. E., Uitti, R. J., Tyce, G. M., O'Brien, J. F., Petersen, R. C., and Kokmen, E. (1996). Plasma catechols and monoamine oxidase metabolites in untreated Parkinson's and Alzheimer's disease. *J. Neurol. Sci.*, **136**, 162–8.

Airaksinen, M. S., Paetau, A., Paljarvi, L., Reinikainen, K., Riekkinen, P., Suomalainen, R., *et al.* (1991). Histamine neurons in human hypothalamus: anatomy in normal and Alzheimer diseased brains. *Neuroscience*, **44**, 465–81.

Albin, R. L., Young, A. B., and Penney, J. B. (1989). The functional neuroanatomy of basal ganglia disorders. *Trends Neurosci.*, **12**, 366–75.

Albin, R. L., Young, A. B., Penney, J. B., Handelin, B., Balfour, R., Anderson, K. D., *et al.* (1990). Abnormalities of striatal projection neurones and NMDA receptors in presymptomatic Huntington's disease. *N. Engl. J. Med.*, **322**, 1293–8.

Alexander, G. E. and Crutcher, M. D. (1990). Functional architecture of basal ganglia circuits: neural substrates of parallel processing. *Trends Neurosci.*, **13**, 266–71.

Allard, P., Alafuzoff, I., Carlsson, A., Erikson, E., Gottfries, C. G., Marcusson, J. O. 1990. Loss of dopamine uptake sites labeled with [3H]GBR-12935 in Alzheimer's disease. *Eur Neurol* **30**, 181–185.

Alvarez, X. A., Franco, A., Fernandez-Novoa, L., and Cacabelos, R. (1996). Blood levels of histamine, IL-1 beta, and TNF-alpha in patients with mild to moderate Alzheimer disease. *Mol. Chem. Neuropathol.*, **29**, 237–52.

Antonini, A., Schwarz, J., Oertel, W. H., Pogarell, O., and Leenders, K. L. (1997). Long-term changes of striatal dopamine D2 receptors in patients with Parkinson's disease: a study with positron emission tomography and [11C]raclopride. *Mov. Disorders*, **12**, 33–8.

Antonini, A., Vontobel, P., Psylla, M., Gunther, I., Maguire, P. R., Missimer, J., *et al.* (1995). Complementary positron emission tomographic studies of the striatal dopaminergic system in Parkinson's disease. *Arch. Neurol.*, **52**, 1183–90.

Arai, H., Ichimiya, Y., Kosaka, K., Moroji, T., and Iizuka, R. (1992). Neurotransmitter changes in early- and late-onset Alzheimer-type dementia. *Prog. Neuropsychopharmacol. Biol. Psychiatry*, **16**, 883–90.

Aubert, I., Araujo, D. M., Cécyre, D., Robitaille, Y., Gauthier, S., and Quirion, R. (1992). Comparative alterations of nicotinic and muscarinic binding sites in Alzheimer's and Parkinson's diseases. *J. Neurochem.*, **58**, 529–41.

Auchus, A. P., Green, R. C., and Nemeroff, C. B. (1994). Cortical and subcortical neuropeptides in Alzheimer's disease. *Neurobiol. Aging*, **15**, 589–95.

Augood, S. J., Faull, R. L. M., and Emson, R. C. (1997). Dopamine D1 and D2 receptor gene expression in the striatum in Huntington's disease. *Ann. Neurol.*, **42**, 215–21.

Bahro, M., Riemann, D., Stadtmuller, G., Berger, M., and Gattaz, W. P. (1993). REM sleep parameters in the discrimination of probable Alzheimer's disease from old age depression. *Biol. Psychiatry*, **34**, 482–6.

Ballard, C., Johnson, M., Piggott, M., Perry, R., O'Brien, J., Rowan, E. and Perry, E. A. (2001). A positive association between 5HT reuptake sides and depression in dementra with Lewy bodies. *Journal of Affective Disorders*.

Beal, M. F., Ellison, D. W., Mazurek, M. F., Swartz, K. J., Malloy, J. R., Bird, E. D., *et al.* (1988). A detailed examination of substance P in pathologically graded cases of Huntington's disease. *J. Neurol. Sci.*, **84**, 51–61.

Beal, M. F., MacGarvey, U., and Swartz, K. J. (1990). Galanin immunoreactivity is increased in the nucleus basalis of Meynert in Alzheimer's disease. *Ann. Neurol.*, **28**, 157–61.

Beeri, R., Andres, C., Lev-Lehman, E., Timberg, R., Huberman, T., Shani, M., *et al.* (1995). Transgenic expression of human acetylcholinesterase induces progressive cognitive deterioration in mice. *Curr. Biol.*, **5**, 1063–71.

Belluardo, N., Blum, M., Mudo, G., Andbjer, B., and Fuxe, K. (1998). Acute intermittent nicotine treatment produces regional increases of basic fibroblast growth factor messenger RNA and protein in the tel- and diencephalon of the rat. *Neuroscience*, **83**, 723–40.

Bentivoglio, M. and Steriade, M. (1990). Brainstem-diencephalic circuits as a structural substrate of the ascending reticular activation concept. In *The diencephalon and sleep* (ed. M. Mancia and M. Marini), pp. 7–29. Raven Press: New York.

Bettendorf, L., Mastrogiacomo, F., Wins, P., Kish, S. J., Grisar, T., Ball, M. J. 1997. Low thiamine diphosphate levels in brains of patients with frontal lobe degeneration of the non-Alzheimer's type. *J. Neurochem.*, **69**, 2005–2010.

Bhatia, K. P., Marsden, C. D. 1994. The behavioural and motor consequences of focal lesions of the basal ganglia in man. *Brain* **117,** 859–876.

Bierer, L. M., Aisen, P. S., Davidson, M., Ryan, T. M., Schmeidler, J., and Davis, K. L. (1994). A pilot study of clonidine plus physostigmine in Alzheimer's disease. *Dementia*, **5**, 243–6.

Bierer, L. M., Knott, P. J., Schmeidler, J. M., Marin, D. B., Ryan, T. M., Haroutunian, V., *et al.* (1993). Post-mortem examination of dopaminergic parameters in Alzheimer's disease: relationship to non-cognitive symptoms. *Psychiatr. Res.*, **49** (3), 211–17.

Booij J., Tissingh, G., Boer, G. J., Speelman, J. D., Stoof, J. C., Janssen, A. G., *et al.* (1997). [^{123}I]FP-CIT SPECT shows a pronounced decline of striatal dopamine transporter labelling in early and advanced Parkinson's disease. *J. Neurol. Neurosurg. Psychiatry*, **62**, 133–40.

Braak, H. and Braak, E. (1992). Allocortical involvement in Huntington's disease. *Neuropathol. Appl. Neurobiol.*, **18**, 539–47.

Brown, L. L., Schneider, J. S., and Lidsky, T. I. (1997). Sensory and cognitive functions of the basal ganglia. *Curr. Opin. Neurobiol.*, **7**, 157–63.

Burke, W. J., Galvin, N. J., Chung, H. D., Stoff, S. A., Gillespie, K. N., Cataldo, A. M., *et al.* (1994). Degenerative changes in epinephrine tonic vasomotor neurons in Alzheimer's disease. *Brain Res.*, **66**, 35–42.

Burke, W. J., Park, D. H., Chung, H. D., Marshall, G. L., Haring, J. H., and Joh, T. H. (1990). Evidence for decreased transport of tryptophan hydroxylase in Alzheimer's disease. *Brain Res.*, **537**, 83–7.

Buzsaki, G., Bickford, T. G., Ponomareff, G., Thai, L. J., Mandel, R. J., and Gage, F. H. (1988). Nucleus basalis and thalamic control of neocortical activity in the freely moving rat. *J. Neurosci.*, **26**, 735–44.

Cacabelos, R., Takeda, M., and Winblad, B. (1999). The glutamatergic system and neurodegeneration in dementia: preventative strategies in Alzheimer's disease. *Int. J. Geriatr. Psychiatry*, **14**, 3–47.

Cammarata, S., Caponnetto, C., and Tabaton, M. (1993). Ubiquitin-reactive neurites in cerebral cortex of subjects with Huntington's chorea: a pathological correlate of dementia? *Neurosci. Lett.*, **156**, 96–8.

Cash, R., Dennis, T., Raisman, R., Javoy-Agid, F., and Scatton, B. (1987). Parkinson's disease and dementia: norepinephrine and dopamine in locus ceruleus. *Neurology*, **37**, 42–6.

Cervini, R., Houhou, L., Pradat, P. F., Béjanin, S., Mallet, J., and Berrard, S. (1995). Specific vesicular acetylcholine transporter promoters lie within the first intron of the rat choline acetyltransferase gene. *J. Biol. Chem.*, **270**, 24654–7.

Chen, C. P., Alder, J. T., Bowen, D. M., Esiri, M. M., McDonald, B., Hope, T., *et al.* (1996). Presynaptic serotonergic markers in community-acquired cases of Alzheimer's disease: correlations with depression and neuroleptic medication. *J. Neurochem.*, **66**, 1592–8.

Cheng, A. V., Ferrier, I. N., Morris, C. M., Jabeen, S., Sahgal, A., McKeith, I. G., *et al.* (1991). Cortical serotonin-S2 receptor binding in Lewy body dementia, Alzheimer's and Parkinson's diseases. *J. Neurol. Sci.*, **106**, 50–5.

Chinaglia, G., Alvarez, F. J., Probst, A., and Palacios, J. M. (1992). Mesostriatal and mesolimbic dopamine uptake binding sites are reduced in Parkinson's disease and progressive supranuclear palsy: a quantitative autoradiographic study using [^{3}H]mazindol. *Neuroscience*, **49**, 317–27.

Christos, G. A. (1993). Is Alzheimer's disease related to a deficit or malfunction of rapid eye movement (REM) sleep? *Med. Hypotheses*, **41**, 435.

Clark, A. W., Parhad, I. M., and Folstein, S. E. (1983). The nucleus basalis in Huntington's disease. *Neurology*, **33**, 1262–7.

Claus, J. J., Dubois, E. A., Booij, J., Habraken, J., de Munck, J. C., Van Herk, M., *et al.* (1997). Demonstration of a reduction in muscarinic receptor binding in early Alzheimer's disease using iodine-123 dexetimide single-photon emission tomography. *Eur. J. Nucl. Med.*, **24**, 602–8.

Clementi, F., Court, J., and Perry, E. (2000). Involvement of neuronal nicotinic receptors in disease. In *Handbook of experimental pharmacology* (ed. F. Clementi, D. Fornasari, C. Golti) **144**, 751–812.

Cooper, A. L., Sheu, K. F., and Blass, J. P. (1996). Normal glutamate metabolism in Alzheimer's disease fibroblasts deficient in alpha-ketoglutarate dehydrogenase complex activity. *Dev. Neurosci.*, **18**, 499–504.

Costa, D. C., Walker, Z., Walker, R. W. H., Gacinovic, S., Janssen, A. G. M., and Katona, C. L. E. (1998). FP-CIT and SPET reveals severe dopaminergic degeneration in dementia with Lewy bodies and drug-naive Parkinson's disease compared with Alzheimer's disease and controls. *Nucl. Med. Commun.*, **19**, 378–9.

Court, J. A., Lloyd, S., Thomas, N., Piggott, M. A., Marshall, E. F., Morris, C. M., *et al.* (1998). Dopamine and nicotinic receptor binding and the levels of dopamine and homovanillic acid in human brain related to tobacco use. *Neuroscience*, **87**, 63–78.

Court, J. A. and Perry, E. K. (1994). CNS nicotinic receptors: possible therapeutic targets in neurodegenerative disorders. *CNS Drugs*, **2**, 216–33.

Cummings, J. L., Gorman, D. G., and Shapira, J. (1993). Physostigmine ameliorates the delusions of Alzheimer's disease. *Biol. Psychiatry*, **33**, 536–41.

Cummings, J. T. (1997). Changes in neuropsychiatric symptoms as outcome measures in clinical trials with cholinergic therapies for Alzheimer's disease. *Alz. Dis. Assoc. Disorders*, **4**, 51–9.

De La Monte, S. M., Vonsattel, J.-P., and Richardson, E. P. (1988). Morphometric demonstration of atrophic changes in the cerebral cortex, white matter and neostriatum in Huntington's disease. *J. Neuropathol. Exp. Neurol.*, **47**, 516–25.

DeLong, M. R. (1990). Primate models of movement disorders of basal ganglia origin. *Trends Neurosci.*, **13**, 281–5.

Dickson, D. W., Davies, P., Mayeux, R., Crystal, H., Horoupian, D. S., Thompson, A., *et al.* (1987). Diffuse Lewy body disease: neuropathological and biochemical studies of six patients. *Acta Neuropathol.*, **75**, 8–15.

Dijk, S. N., Francis, P. T., Stratmann, G. C., and Bowen, D. M. (1995). Cholinomimetics increase glutamate outflow via an action on the corticostriatal pathway: implications for Alzheimer's disease. *J. Neurochem.*, **65**, 2165–9.

Donnemiller, E., Heilmann, J., Wenning, G. K., Berger, W., Decristoforo, C., Moncayo, R. *et al.* 1997. Brain perfusion scintigraphy with 99mmTc-HMPAO or 99mmTC-ECD and 123I-beta-CIT single-photon emission tomography in dementia of the Alzheimer-type and diffuse Lewy body disease. *Eur. J. Nucl. Med.* **24**, 320–325.

Dournaud, P., Dalaere, P., Hauw, J. J., and Epelbaum, J. (1995). Differential correlation between neurochemical deficits, neuropathology and cognitive status in Alzheimer's disease. *Neurobiol. Aging*, **16**, 817–23.

Dure, L. S., Young, A. B., and Penney, J. B. (1991). Excitatory amino acid binding sites in the caudate nucleus and frontal cortex of Huntington's Disease. *Ann. Neurol.*, **30**, 785–93.

Efange, S. M., Garland, E. M., Staley, J. K., Khare, A. B., and Mash, D. C. (1997). Vesicular acetylcholine transporter density and Alzheimer's disease. *Neurobiol. Aging*, **18**, 407–13.

Ellison, D. W., Beal, M. F., Mazurek, M. F., Malloy, J. R., Bird, E. D., and Martin, J. B. (1987). Amino acid neurotransmitter abnormalities in Huntington's disease and the quinolinic acid animal model of Huntington's disease. *Brain*, **110**, 1657–73.

Elrod, R., Peskind, E. R., DiGiacomo, L., Brodkin, K. I., Veith, R. C., and Raskind, M. A. (1997). Effects of Alzheimer's disease severity on cerebrospinal fluid norepinephrine concentration. *Am. J. Psychiatry*, **154**, 25–30.

Ernst, T., Chang, L., Melchor, R., Mehringer, C. M. 1997. Frontotemporal dementia and early Alzheimer disease: differentiation with frontal lobe H-1 MR spectroscopy. *Radiology* **203**, 829–836.

Everitt, B. J. and Robbins, T. W. (1997). Central cholinergic systems and cognition. *Annu. Rev. Psychol.*, **48**, 649–84.

Forstl, H., Levy, R., Burns, A., Luthert, P., and Cairns, N. (1994). Disproportionate loss of noradrenergic and cholinergic neurons as cause of depression in Alzheimer's disease; a hypothesis. *Pharmacopsychiatry*, **27**, 11–15.

Foster, N. L., Sima, A. A. F., Minoshima, S., and Kuhl, D. E. (1998). Clinical and neuropathological correlations with PET in FTDP-17 and sporadic frontal dementia. *Neurobiol. Aging*, **19**, S296.

Francis, P. T., Holmes, C., Webster, M. T., Stratmann, G. C., Procter, A. W., and Bowen, D. M. (1993). Preliminary neurochemical findings in non-Alzheimer dementia due to lobar atrophy. *Dementia*, **4**, 172–7.

Freedman, M., Rewilak, D., Xerri, T., Cohen, S., Gordon, A. S., Shandling, M., *et al.* (1998). L-deprenyl in Alzheimer's disease: cognitive and behavioural effects. *Neurology*, **50**, 660–8.

Gerlach, M., Gsell, W., Kornhuber, J., Jellinger, K., Krieger, V., Pantucek, F., *et al.* (1996). A post mortem study on neurochemical markers of dopaminergic, GABA-ergic and glutamatergic neurons in basal ganglia-thalamocortical circuits in Parkinson syndrome. *Brain Res.*, **741**, 142–52.

Geula, C. and Mesulam, M. M. (1996). Systematic regional variations in the loss of cortical cholinergic fibres in Alzheimer's. *Cerebral Cortex*, **6**, 165–77.

Gilbert, J. J., Kish, S. J., Chang, L. J., Morito, C., Shannak, K., and Hornykiewicz, O. (1988). Dementia, parkinsonism, and motor neuron disease: neurochemical and neuropathological correlates. *Ann. Neurol.*, **24**, 688–91.

Gnanalingham, K. K., Byrne, E. J., Thornton, A., Sambrook, M. A., Bannister, P. 1997. Motor and cognitive function in Lewy body dementia: comparison with Alzheimer's and Parkinson's disease. *J. Neurol. Neurosurg. Psych.* **62**, 243–252.

Goldsmith, S. K., Shapiro, R. M., and Joyce, J. N. (1997). Disrupted pattern of D2 dopamine receptors in the temporal lobe in schizophrenia — A postmortem study. *Arch. Gen. Psychiatry*, **54**, 649–58.

Goodchild, R. E., Court, J. A., Hobson, I., Piggott, M. A., Perry, R. H., Ince, P., *et al.* (1999). Distribution of histamine H3-receptor binding in the normal human basal ganglia: comparison with Huntington's and Parkinson's disease cases. *Eur. J. Neurosci.*, **11**, 449–56.

Gray, C. W. and Patel, A. J. (1995). Neurodegeneration mediated by glutamate and beta-amyloid peptide: a comparison and possible interaction. *Brain Res.*, **691**, 169–79.

Graybiel, A. M. (1990). Neurotransmitters and neuromodulators in the basal ganglia. *Trends Neurosci.*, **13**, 244–53.

Grossman, M., Crino, P., Reivich, M., Stern, M. B., and Hurtig, H. I. (1992). Attention and sentence processing deficits in Parkinson's disease: the role of anterior cingulate cortex. *Cerebral Cortex*, **2**, 513–25.

Guillozet, A. L., Smiley, J. F., Mash, D. C., and Mesulam, M. M. (1997). Butyrylcholinesterase in the life cycle of amyloid plaques. *Ann. Neurol.*, **42**, 909–18.

Hansen, L. A., Deteresa, R., Tobias, H., Alford, M., and Terry, R. D. (1988). Neocortical morphometry and cholinergic neurochemistry in Pick's disease. *Am. J. Pathol.*, **131**, 507–18.

Heckers, S., Geula, C., and Mesulam, M. M. (1992). Cholinergic innervation of the human thalamus: dual origin and differential nuclear distribution. *J. Comp. Neurol.*, **325**, 68–82.

Hedreen, J. C. and Folstein, S. E. (1995). Early loss of neostriatal striosome neurones in Huntington's disease. *J. Neuropathol. Exp. Neurol.*, **54**, 105–20.

Heinsen, H., Strik, M., Bauer, M., Luther, K., Ulmar, G., Gangnus, D., *et al.* (1994). Cortical and striatal neurone number in Huntington's disease. *Acta Neuropathol.*, **88**, 320–33.

Hierholzer, J., Cordes, M., Venz, S., Schelosky, L., Harisch, C., Richter, W., *et al.* (1998). Loss of dopamine-D2 receptor binding sites in parkinsonian plus syndromes. *J. Nucl. Med.*, **39**, 954–60.

Higo, S., Matsuyama, T., and Kawamura, S. (1996). Direct projections from the pedunculopontine and laterodorsal tegmental nuclei to area 17 of the visual cortex in the cat. *Neurosci. Res.*, **26**, 109–18.

Hutchinson, M. and Fazzini, E. (1996). Cholinesterase inhibition in Parkinson's disease. *J. Neurol. Neurosurg. Psychiatry*, **61**, 324–6.

Ikeda, M., Mackay, K. B., Dewar, D., and McCulloch, J. (1993). Differential alterations in adenosine A1 and kappa 1 opioid receptors in the striatum in Alzheimer's disease. *Brain Res.*, **616**, 211–17.

Inestosa, N. C., Alarcon, R., Arriagada, J., Donoso, A., and Alvarez, J. (1993). Platelet of Alzheimer patients: increased counts and subnormal uptake and accumulation of [^{14}C]5-hydroxytryptamine. *Neurosci. Lett.*, **163**, 8–10.

Iyo, M., Mamba, H., Fukushi, K., Shinotoh, H., Nagatsuka, S., Suhara, T., *et al.* (1997). Measurement of acetylcholinesterase by positron emission tomography in the brains of healthy controls and patients with Alzheimer's disease. *Lancet*, **349**, 1805–9.

Jaarsma, D., Sebens, J. B., and Korf, J. (1991). Reduction of adenosine A1-receptors in the perforant pathway terminal zone in Alzheimer hippocampus. *Neurosci. Lett.*, **121**, 111–14.

Jouvet, M. (1972). Some monoaminergic mechanisms controlling sleep and wakening. In *Brain and human behaviour* (ed. A. G. Karczmar and J. C. Eccles), pp. 131–60. Springer–Verlag: Berlin.

Joyce, J. N., Smutzer, G., Whitty, C. J., Myers, A., and Bannon, M. J. (1997). Differential modification of dopamine transporter and tyrosine hydroxylase mRNAs in midbrain of subjects with Parkinson's, Alzheimer's with parkinsonism, and Alzheimer's disease. *Movement Dis.*, **12**, 885–97.

Kalaria, R. N., Sromek, S., Wilcox, B. J., and Unnerstall, J. R. (1990). Hippocampal adenosine A1 receptors are decreased in Alzheimer's disease. *Neurosci. Lett.*, **118**, 257–60.

Kastner, A., Hirsch, E. C., Herrero, M. T., Javoy-Agid, F., and Agid, Y. (1993). Immunocytochemical quantification of tyrosine hydroxylase at a cellular level in the mesencephalon of control subjects and patients with Parkinson's and Alzheimer's disease. *J. Neurochem.*, **61**, 1024–34.

Kaufer, D. L., Cummings, J. L., and Christine, D. (1995). Effect of tacrine on behavioural symptoms in Alzheimer's disease: an open label study. *J. Geriatr. Psychiatry Neurol.*, **9**, 1–6.

Kawaguchi, Y., Wilson, C. J., Augood, S. J., and Emson, P. C. (1995). Striatal interneurones: chemical, physiological and morphological characterization. *Trends Neurosci.*, **18**, 527–35.

Kish, S. J., Shannak, K., Hornykiewicz, O. 1988. Uneven pattern of dopamine loss in the striatum of patients with idiopathic Parkinson's disease. Pathophysiologic and clinical implications. *N. Engl. J. Med*, **318**, 876–880

Kittner, B., Rossner, M., and Rother, M. (1997). Clinical trials in dementia with propentofylline. *Ann. N. Y. Acad. Sci.*, **826**, 307–16.

Knopman, D. S., Mastri, A. R., Frey, W. H. D., Sung, J. H., Rustan, T. 1990. Dementia lacking distinctive histologic features: a common non-Alzheimer degenerative dementia. *Neurology* **40**, 251–256.

Kornhuber, J. and Weller, M. (1997). Psychotogenicity and N-methyl-D-aspartate receptor antagonism: implications for neuroprotective pharmacotherapy. *Biol. Psychiatry*, **41**, 135–44.

Kuhl, D. E., Minoshima, S., Fessler, J. A., Frey, K. A., Foster, N. L., Ficaro, E. P., *et al.* (1996). *In vivo* mapping of cholinergic terminals in normal aging, Alzheimer's disease and Parkinson's disease. *Ann. Neurol.*, **40**, 399–410.

Kuhn, W. and Muller, T. (1996). The clinical potential of Deprenyl in neurologic and psychiatric disorders. *J. Neural Transm.*, **48**, 85–93.

Kuhn, W., Muller, T., Gerlach, M., Sofic, E., Fuchs, G., Heye, N., *et al.* (1996). Depression in Parkinson's disease: biogenic amines in CSF of 'de novo' patients. *J. Neural Transm.*, **103**, 1441–5.

Kumar, A. M., Kumar, M., Sevush, S., Ruiz, J., and Eisdorfer, C. (1995). Serotonin uptake and its kinetics in platelets of women with Alzheimer's disease. *Psychiatr. Res.*, **59**, 145–150.

Kuwert, T., Lange, H., Langen, K.-J., Herzog, H., Aulich, A., and Feinendegen, L. (1990). Cortical and subcortical glucose consumption measured by PET in patients with Huntington's disease. *Brain*, **113**, 1405–23.

Langlais, P. J., Thal, L., Hansen, L., Galasko, D., Alford, M., Masliah, E. 1993. Neurotransmitters in basal ganglia and cortex of Alzheimer's disease with and without Lewy bodies. *Neurology* **43**, 1927–1934.

Lawlor, B. A., Bierer, L. M., Ryan, T. M., Schmeidler, J., Knott, P. J., Williams, L. L., *et al.* (1995). Plasma 3-methoxy-4-hydroxyphenylglycol (MHPG) and clinical symptoms in Alzheimer's disease. *Biol. Psychiatry*, **38**, 185–8.

Lawrence, A. D., Sahakian, B. J., and Robbins, T. W. (1998). Cognitive functions and corticostriatal circuits: insights from Huntington's disease. *Trends Cognitive Sci.*, **2**, 379–87.

Lee, P. N. (1994). Smoking and Alzheimer's disease: a review of the epidemiological evidence. *Neuroepidemiology*, **13**, 131–44.

Li, B., Mallory, M., Alford, M., Tanaka, S., and Masliah, E. (1997). Glutamate transporter alterations in Alzheimer's disease and possibly associated with abnormal APP expression. *J. Neuropathol. Exp. Neurol.*, **56**, 901–11.

Liu, H. C., Yang, J. C., Chang, Y. F., Liu, T. Y., Chi, C. W. 1991. Analysis of monoamines in the cerebrospinal fluid of Chinese patients with Alzheimer's disease. *Annals. NY. Acad. Sci.*, **640**, 215–218.

Liu, Y., Stern, Y., Chun, M. R., Jacobs, D. M., Yau, P., and Goldman, J. E. (1997). Pathological correlates of extrapyramidal signs in Alzheimer's disease. *Ann. Neurol.*, **41**, 368–74.

Lopez, O. L., Wisnieski, S. R., Becker, J. T., Boller, F., and DeKosky, S. T. (1997). Extrapyramidal signs in patients with probable Alzheimer disease. *Arch. Neurol.*, **54**, 969–75.

McDonald, M. P. and Crawley, J. N. (1997). Galanin-acetylcholine interactions in rodent memory tasks and Alzheimer's disease. *J. Psychiatry Neurosci.*, **22**, 303–17.

McFadden, L., Mohr, E., Sampson, M., Mendis, T., and Grimes, J. D. (1996). A profile analysis of demented and nondemented Parkinson's disease patients. *Adv. Neurol.*, **69**, 339–41.

McKeith, I. G., Ballard, C. G., and Harrison, R. W. (1995). Neuroleptic sensitivity to risperidone in Lewy body dementia. *Lancet*, **346**, 699.

McLoughlin, D. M., Lucey, J. V., and Dinan, T. G. (1994). Central serotonergic hyperresponsivity in late-onset Alzheimer's disease. *Am. J. Psychiatry*, **15**, 1701–3.

McQueen, M. J. (1995). Clinical and analytical considerations in the utilisation of cholinesterase measurements. *Clin. Chim. Acta*, **237**, 91–105.

Mann, D. M. A. (1989). Subcortical afferent projection systems in Huntington's chorea. *Acta Neuropathol.*, **78**, 551–4.

Marczynski, T. J. (1998). GABAergic deafferentation hypothesis of brain aging and Alzheimer's disease revisisted. *Brain Res. Bull.*, **45**, 341–79.

Martignoni, E., Blandini. F., Petraglia, F., Pacchetti, C., Bono, G., Nappi, G. 1992. Cerebrospinal fluid norepinephrine, 3-methoxy-4-hydroxyphenylglycol and neuropeptide Y levels in Parkinson's disease, multiple system atrophy and dementia of the Alzheimer type. *J. Neurol. Transm. - Parkinson's Disease & Dementia Section*, **4**, 191–205.

Mashige, F., Takai, N., Matsushima, Y., Ito, A., Takano, M., Tsuchiya, E., *et al.* (1994). Simultaneous determination of catecholamines, serotonin, and their precursors and metabolites in body fluid by an HPLC system with multi-electrode electrochemical detector. *Jpn. J. Clin. Pathol.*, **42**, 591–9.

Maziere, M. (1995). Cholinergic neurotransmission studied *in vivo* using position emission tomography or single photon emission computerized tomography. *Pharmacol. Ther.*, **66**, 83–101.

McKeith, I. G., Grace, J. B., Walker, Z., Byrne, J., Walkinson, D., Stevens, T. L., Perry, E. K. (2000). Rivastigmine in the treatment of dementia with Lewy bodies: preliminary findings from an open trial. International *Journal of Geriatic Psychiatry*, **15**, 387–392.

Meana, J. J., Barturen, F., Garro, M. A., Garcia-Sevilla, J. A., Fontan, A., and Zarranz, J. J. (1992). Decreased density of presynaptic alpha 2-adrenoceptors in postmortem brains of patients with Alzheimer's disease. *J. Neurochem.*, **58**, 1896–904.

Meguro, K., Yamaguchi, S., Itoh, M., Fujiwara, T., and Yamadori, A. (1997). Striatal dopamine metabolism correlated with frontotemporal glucose utilization in Alzheimer's disease: a double-tracer PET study. *Neurology*, **49**, 941–5.

Mesulam, M. M. (1995). Cholinergic pathways and the ascending reticular activating system of the human brain. *Ann. N. Y. Acad. Sci.*, **757**, 169–79.

Metherate, R., Tremblay, N., and Dykes, R. W. (1987). Acetylcholine permits long term enhancement of neuronal responsiveness in cat primary somatosensory cortex. *Neuroscience*, **22**, 75–81.

Miller, B. L., Darby, A. L., Swartz, J. R., Yener, G. G., and Mena, I. (1995). Dietary changes, compulsions and sexual behavior in frontotemporal degeneration. *Dementia*, **6**, 195–9.

Minthon, L., Edvinsson, L., and Gustafson, L. (1996). Correlation between clinical characteristics and cerebrospinal fluid neuropeptide Y levels in dementia of the Alzheimer type and frontotemporal dementia. *Alz. Dis. Assoc. Disorders*, **10**, 197–203.

Minthon, L., Edvinsson, L., and Gustafson, L. (1997). Somatostatin and neuropeptide Y in cerebrospinal fluid: correlations with severity of disease and clinical signs in Alzheimer's disease and frontotemporal dementia. *Dementia Geriatr. Cogn. Disorders*, **8**, 232–9.

Misawa, H., Takahashi, R., and Deguchi, T. (1995). Coordinate expression of vesicular acetylcholine transporter and choline acetyltransferase in sympathetic superior cervical neurones. *NeuroReport*, **6**, 965–8.

Mohanakrishnan, P., Fowler, A. H., Vonsattel, J. P., Husain, M. M., Jolles, P. R., Liem, P., *et al.* (1995). An *in vitro* 1H nuclear magnetic resonance study of the temporoparietal cortex of Alzheimer brains. *Exp. Brain Res.*, **102**, 503–10.

Morissette, M., Goulet, M., Grondin, R., Blanchet, P., Bedard, P. J., Di Paolo, T., *et al.* (1998). Associative and limbic regions of monkey striatum express high levels of dopamine D3 receptors: effects of MPTP and dopamine agonist replacement therapies. *Eur. J. Neurosci.*, **10**, 2565–73.

Mufson, E. J., Mash, D. C., and Hersh, L. B. (1988). Neurofibrillary tangles in cholinergic pedunculopontine neurons in Alzheimer's disease. *Ann. Neurol.*, **24**, 623–5.

Muller, W. E., Mutschler, E., and Riederer, P. (1995). Non-competitive NMDA receptor antagonists with fast open-channel blocking kinetics and strong voltage-dependency as potential therapeutic agents for Alzheimer's dementia. *Pharmacopsychiatry*, **28**, 113–24.

Murdoch, I., Perry, E. K., Court, J. A., Graham, D. I., Dewar, D. 1998. Cortical cholinergic dysfunction after human head injury. *Journal of Neurotrauma* **15**, 295–305.

Nagaoka, S., Arai, H., Iwamoto, N., Ohwada, J., Ichimiya, Y., Nakamura, M., *et al.* (1995). A juvenile case of frontotemporal dementia: neurochemical and neuropathological investigations. *Prog. Neuro-Psychopharmacol. Biol. Psychiatry*, **19**, 1251–61.

Nazarali, A. J., Reynolds, G. P. 1992. Monoamine neurotransmitters and their metabolites in brain regions in Alzheimer's disease: a postmortem study. *Cell & Mol. Neurobiol* **12**, 581–287.

Nitsch, R. M., Deng, M., Growdon, J. H., and Wurtman, R. J. (1996). Serotonin 5-HT2a and 5-HT2c receptors stimulate amyloid precursor protein ectodomain secretion. *J. Biol. Chem.*, **271**, 4188–94.

Nordberg, A., Lundqvist, H., Hartvig, P., Lilja, A., and Langstrom, B. (1995). Kinetic analysis of regional (S) (-) 11C-nicotine binding in normal and Alzheimer brains — *in vivo* assessment using positron emission tomography. *Alz. Dis. Assoc. Disorders*, **9**, 21–7.

Ohara, K., Kondo, N., Ohara, K. 1998. Changes of monoamines in post-mortem brains from patients with diffuse lewy body disease. *Prog. Neuro-Psychopharmacol and Biol. Phychiay.* **22**, 311–317.

Oishi, M., Mochizuki, Y., Yoshihashi, H., Takasu, T., and Nakano, E. (1996). Laboratory examinations correlated with severity of dementia. *Ann. Clin. Lab. Sci.*, **26**, 340–5.

Omar, S. J., Robinson, D., Davies, H. D., Miller, T. P., and Tinklenberg, J. R. (1995). Fluoxetine and visual hallucinations in dementia. *Biol. Psychiatry*, **38**, 556–8.

Ott, A., Slooter, J. C., Hofman, A., van Harskamp, F., Witterman, J. C. M., van Broeckhoven, C., *et al.* (1998). Smoking and risk of dementia and Alzheimer's disease in a population — based cohort study; the Rotterdam study. *Lancet*, **351**, 1840–4.

Owen, A. and Bird, M. (1995). Acetylcholine as a regular of neurite outgrowth and motility in cultured embryonic mouse spinal cord. *NeuroReport*, **6**, 2269–72.

Palmer, A. M. 1996. Neurochemical studies of Azheimer's disease. *Neurodegeneration* 5(**4**), 381–391.

Palmer, A. M., DeKosky, S. T. 1993. Monoamine neurons in aging and Alzheimer's disease. *J Neurol Transm* **91**, 135–159.

Panula, P., Rinne, J., Kuokkanen, K., Eriksson, K. S., Sallmen, T., Kalimo, H., *et al.* (1998). Neuronal histamine deficit in Alzheimer's disease. *Neuroscience*, **82**, 993–7.

Passani, L. A., Vonsattel, J. P., and Coyle, J. T. (1997). Distribution of N-acetylaspartylglutamate immunoreactivity in human brain and its alteration in neurodegenerative disease. *Brain Res.*, **772**, 9–22.

Pearce, R. K., Seeman, P., Jellinger, K., and Tourtellotte, W. W. (1990). Dopamine uptake sites and dopamine receptors in Parkinson's disease and schizophrenia. *Eur. Neurol.*, **30**, 9–14.

Pearson, S. J. and Reynolds, G. P. (1994). Neocortical neurotransmitter markers in Huntington's disease. *J. Neural Transm.*, — *General Section*, **98**, 197–207.

Perry, E. (2000). The cholinergic system in Alzheimer's disease. In *Dementia* (ed. J. O'Brien D. Aries, A. Burus Arnold London pp. 417–432).

Perry, E., Walker, M., Grace, J., and Perry, R. (1999). Acetylcholine in mind: a neural correlate of consciousness. *Trends Neurosci.*, **22**, 273–280.

Perry, E. K., Blessed, G., Tomlinson, B. E., Perry, R. H., Crow, T. J., Cross, A. J., *et al.* (1981). Neurochemical activities in human temporal lobe related to ageing and Alzheimer-type changes. *Neurobiol. Aging*, **2**, 251–6.

Perry, E. K., Court, J., Goodchild, R., Griffiths, M., Johnson, M., Lloyd, S., *et al.* (1998). Clinical neurochemistry: Developments in dementia research based on brain bank material. *J. Neural Transm.*, **105**, 915–33.

Perry, E. K., Haroutunian, V., Davis, K. L., Levy, R., Lantos, P., Eagger, S., *et al.* (1994). Neocortical cholinergic activities differentiate Lewy body dementia from classical Alzheimer's disease. *NeuroReport*, **5**, 747–9.

Perry, E. K., Kerwin, J., Perry, R. H., Irving, D., Blessed, G., and Fairbairn, A. (1990*a*). Cerebral cholinergic activity is related to the incidence of visual hallucinations in senile dementia of Lewy body type. *Dementia*, **1**, 2–4.

Perry, E. K., Marshall, E., Kerwin, J., Smith, C. J., Jabeen, S., Cheng, A. V., *et al.* (1990*b*). Evidence of a monoaminergic-cholinergic imbalance related to visual hallucinations in Lewy body dementia. *J. Neurochem.*, **55**, 1454–6.

Perry, E. K., Marshall, E., Thompson, P., McKeith, I. G., Collerton, D., Fairbairn, A. F., *et al.* (1993). Monoaminergic activities in Lewy body dementia: relation to hallucinosis and extrapyramidal features. *J. Neural Transm.*, **6**, 167–77.

Perry, E. K., Morris, C. M., Court, J. A., Cheng, A., Fairbairn, A., McKeith, I. G., *et al.* (1995). Alteration in nicotine binding sites in Parkinson's disease, Lewy body dementia and Alzheimer's disease: possible index of early neuropathology. *Neuroscience*, **64**, 385–95.

Perry, E. K., Tomlinson, B. E., Blessed, G., Bergmann, K., Gibson, P. H., and Perry, R. H. (1978). Correlation of cholinergic abnormalities with senile plaques and mental test scores in senile dementia. *Br. Med. J.*, **2**, 1457–9.

Perry, R. H., Candy, J. M., Perry, E. K., Irving, D., Blessed, G., Fairbairn, A. F., *et al.* (1982). Extensive loss of choline acetyltransferase activity is not reflected by neuronal loss in the nucleus of Meynert in Alzheimer's disease. *Neurosci. Lett.*, **33**, 311–15.

Perry, R. H., Irving, D., Blessed, G., Fairbairn, A., and Perry, E. K. (1990). Senile dementia of Lewy body type. A clinically and neuropathologically distinct form of Lewy body dementia in the elderly. *J. Neurol. Sci.*, **95**, 119–39.

Peskind, E. R., Wingerson, D., Pascualy, M., Thal, L., Veith, R. C., Dorsa, D. M., *et al.* (1995). Oral physostigmine in Alzheimer's disease: effects on norepinephrine and vasopressin in cerebrospinal fluid and plasma. *Biol. Psychiatry*, **38**, 532–8.

Piggott, M. A. and Marshall, E. F. (1996). Neurochemical correlates of pathological and iatrogenic extrapyramidal symptoms. In *Dementia with Lewy bodies: Clinical, pathological, and treatment issues* (ed. R. H. Perry, I. G. McKeith, and E. K. Perry), pp. 449–67. Cambridge: Cambridge University Press.

Piggott, M. A., Perry, E. K., Marshall, E. F., McKeith, I. G., Johnson, M., Melrose, H. L., *et al.* (1998). Nigrostriatal dopaminergic activities in dementia with Lewy bodies in relation to neuroleptic sensitivity: comparison with Parkinson's disease. *Biol. Psychiatry*, **44**, 764–74.

Piggort, M. A., Marshall, E. F., Thomas N., Lloyd, S., Court, J. A., Jaros, E., Burn, D., Johnson, M., Perry, R. H., McKeith , I. G., Ballard, C., Perry, E. K. 1999. Striatal dopaminergic markers in dementia with Lewy bodies, Alzheimer's and Parkinson's disease; rostro-caudal distribution. *Brain* **122**, 1449–68.

Pike, C. J. and Cotman, C. W. (1993). Cultured GABA-immunoreactive neurons are resistant to toxicity induced by beta-amyloid. *Neuroscience*, **56**, 269–74.

Pizzolato, G., Chierichetti, F., Fabbri, M., Cagnin, A., Dam, M., Ferlin, G., *et al.* (1996). Reduced striatal dopamine receptors in Alzheimer's disease: single photon emission tomography study with the D2 tracer [^{123}I]-IBZM. *Neurology*, **47**, 1065–8.

Pollock, B. G., Mulsant, B. H., Sweet, R., Burgio, L. D., Kirshner, M. A., Shuster, K., *et al.* (1997). An open pilot study of citalopram for behavioural disturbances of dementia. Plasma levels and real-time observations. *Am. J. Geriatr. Psychiatry*, **5**, 70–8.

Proctor, A. W., Francis, P. T., Stratmann, G. C., and Bowen, D. M. (1992). Serotonergic pathology is not widespread in Alzheimer patients without prominent aggressive symptoms. *Neurochem. Res.*, **17**, 917–22.

Ragneskog, H., Eriksson, S., Karlsson, I., and Gottfries, C. G. (1996). Long-term treatment of elderly individuals with emotional disturbanes: an open study with citalopram. *Int. Psychogeriatr.*, **8**, 659–68.

Reiner, A., Albin, R. L., Anderson, K. D., D'Amato, C. J., Penney, J. B., and Young, A. B. (1988). Differential loss of striatal projection neurones in Huntington's disease. *Proc. Natl. Acad. Sci. USA*, **85**, 5733–7.

Reynolds, G. P. and Pearson, S. J. (1987). Decreased glutamic acid and increased 5-hydroxytryptamine in Huntington's disease brain. *Neurosci. Lett.*, **78**, 233–8.

Reynolds, G. P., Pearson, S. J., and Heathfield, K. W. G. (1990). Dementia in Huntington's disease is associated with neurochemical deficits in the caudate nucleus, not the cerebral cortex. *Neurosci. Lett.*, **113**, 95–100.

Rinne, J. O., Sahlberg, N., Ruottinen, H., Nagren, K., and Lehikoinen, P. (1998). Striatal uptake of the dopamine reuptake ligand [^{11}C]beta-CFT is reduced in Alzheimer's disease assessed by positron emission tomography. *Neurology*, **50**, 152–6.

Robinson, M. R. and Harrell, L. E. (1997). Cholinergic activity and amyloid precursor protein metabolism. *Brain Res. Rev.*, **25**, 50–69.

Ryoo, H. L., Pierrotti, D., and Joyce, J. N. (1998). Dopamine D3 receptor is decreased and D2 receptor is elevated in the striatum of Parkinson's disease. *Mov. Disorders*, **13**, 788–97.

Sabbagh, M. N., Corey-Bloom, J., Alford, M., Masliah, E., and Thal, L. (1998). Correlation of nicotinic receptor binding with clinical and neurochemical markers in Alzheimer's disease and dementia with Lewy bodies. *Neurobiol. Aging*, **19**, S207.

Samuel, W., Alford, M., Hofstetter, C., and Hansen, L. (1997). Dementia with Lewy bodies versus pure Alzheimer's disease: differences in cognition neuropathology, cholinergic dysfunction and synapse density. *J. Neuropathol. Exp. Neurol.*, **56**, 499–508.

Sax, D. S., O'Donnell, B., and Butters, N. (1983). Computed tomographic, neurologic, and neuropsychological correlates of Huntington's disease. *Int. J. Neurosci.*, **18**, 21–36.

Scatton, B., Javoy-Agid, F., Rouquier, L., Dubois, B., and Agid, Y. (1983). Reduction of cortical dopamine, noradrenaline, serotonin and their metabolites in Parkinson's disease. *Brain Res.*, **275**, 321–8.

Schneider, C., Risser, D., Kirchner, L., Kitzmuller, E., Cairns, N., Prast, H., *et al.* (1997). Similar deficits of central histaminergic system in patients with Down syndrome and Alzheimer disease. *Neurosci. Lett.*, **222**, 183–6.

Schneider, L. S. and Sobin, P. B. (1992). Non-neuroleptic treatment of behavioural symptoms and agitation in Alzheimer's disease and other dementia. *Psychopharmacol. Bull.*, **28**, 71–9.

Schröder, H., de Vos, R. A. I., Jansen, E. N. H., Birtsch, C., Wevers, A., Lobron, C., *et al.* (1995). Gene expression of the nicotinic acetylcholine receptor alpha4 subunit in the frontal cortex in Parkinson's disease patients. *Neurosci. Lett.*, **187**, 173–6.

Schröder, H., Giaobini, E., Struble, R. G., Zilles, K., and Maelicke, A. (1991). Nicotinic cholinoceptive neurons of the frontal cortex are reduced in Alzheimer's disease. *Neurobiol. Aging*, **12**, 259–62.

Schubert, P., Ogata, T., Rudolphi, K., Marchini, C., McRae, A., and Ferroni, S. (1997). Support of homeostatic glial cell signaling: a novel therapeutic approach by propentofylline. *Ann. N. Y. Acad. Sci.*, **826**, 337–47.

Seeman, P., Bzowej, N. H., Guan, H. C., Bergeron, C., Reynolds, G. P., Bird, E. D., *et al.* (1987). Human brain D1 and D2 dopamine receptors in schizophrenia, Alzheimer's, Parkinson's, and Huntington's diseases. *Neuropsychopharmacology*, **1**, 5–15.

Sheline, Y. I., Miller, K., Bardgett, M. E., and Csernansky, J. G. (1998). Higher cerebrospinal fluid MHPG in subjects with dementia of the Alzheimer type. Relationship with cognitive dysfunction. *Am. J. Geriatr. Psychiatry*, **6**, 155–61.

Singh, V. K., Warren, R. P., and Singh, E. A. (1990). Binding of [^{3}H] serotonin to lymphocytes in patients with neuropsychiatric disorders. *Mol. Chem. Neuropathol.*, **13**, 167–73.

Sjogren, M., Minthon, L., Passant, K., and Wallin, A. (1998). Decreased monoamine metabolites in frontotemporal dementia and Alzheimer's disease. *Neurobiol. Aging*, **19**, 379–84.

Soininen, H., Laulumaa, V., Helkala, E. L., Hartikainen, P., and Riekkinen, P. J. (1992). Extrapyramidal signs in Alzheimer's disease: a 3-year follow-up study. *J. Neural Transm. — Parkinson's Disease and Dementia Section*, **4**, 107–19.

Sparks, D. L., Beach, T. G., and Lukas, R. J. (1998). Immunohistochemical localization of nicotinic β2 and α4 receptor subunits in normal human brain and individuals with Lewy body and Alzheimer's disease: Preliminary observations. *Neurosci. Lett.*, **256**, 151–4.

Sparks, D. L. and Markesbery, W. R. (1991). Altered serotonergic and cholinergic synaptic markers in Pick's disease. *Arch. Neurol.*, **48**, 796–9.

Starr, M. S. (1995). Glutamate/dopamine D1/D2 balance in the basal ganglia and its relevance to Parkinson's disease. *Synapse*, **19**, 264–93.

Stern, Y., Liu, X., Albert, M., Brandt, J., Jacobs, D. M., Del Castillo-Castaneda, C., *et al.* (1996). Modelling the influence of extrapyramidal signs on the progression of Alzheimer disease. *Arch. Neurol.*, **53**, 1121–6.

Storey, E. and Beal, M. F. (1993). Neurochemical substrates of rigidity and chorea in Huntington's disease. *Brain*, **116**, 1201–22.

Storey, E., Kowell, N. W., Finn, S. F., Mazurek, M. F., and Beal, M. F. (1992). The cortical lesion of Huntington's disease: Further neurochemical characterisation, and reproduction of some of the histological and neurochemical features by N-methyl-D-aspartate lesions of rat cortex. *Ann. Neurol.*, **32**, 526–34.

Storga, D., Vrecko, K., Birkmayer, J. G., and Reibnegger, G. (1996). Monoaminergic neurotransmitters, their precursors and metabolites in brains of Alzheimer patients. *Neurosci. Lett.*, **203**, 29–32.

Struble, R. G., Cork, L. C., Whitehouse, P. J., and Price, D. L. (1982). Cholinergic innervation in neuritic plaques. *Science*, **216**, 413–15.

Sunderland, T., Esposito, G., Molchan, S. E., Coppola, R., Jones, D. W., Gorey, J., *et al.* (1995). Differential cholinergic regulation in Alzheimer's patients compared to controls following chronic blockade with scopolamine: a SPECT study. *Psychopharmacology*, **121**, 231–41.

Swartz, J. R., Miller, B. L., Lesser, I. M., and Darby, A. L. (1997). Frontotemporal dementia: treatment response to serotonin selective reuptake inhibitors [published erratum appears in *J. Clin. Psychiatry*, 1997 Jun; **58** (6), 275]. *J. Clin. Psychiatry*, **58**, 212–16.

Tejani-Butt, S. M., Yang, J., and Zaffar, H. (1993). Norepinephrine transporter sites are decreased in the locus coeruleus in Alzheimer's disease. *Brain Res.*, **631**, 147–50.

Thorns, V., Mallory, M., Hansen, L., and Masliah, E. (1997). Alterations in glutamate receptor 2/3 subunits and amyloid precursor protein expression during the course of Alzheimer's disease and Lewy body variant. *Acta Neuropathol.*, **94**, 539–48.

Tissingh, G., Booij, J., Bergmans, P., Winogrodzka, A., Janssen, A. G., van Royen, E. A., *et al.* (1998). Iodine-123-N-omega-fluoropropyl-2beta-carbomethoxy-3beta-(4-iod ophenyl)tropane SPECT in healthy controls and early-stage, drug-naive Parkinson's disease. *J. Nucl. Med.*, **39**, 1143–8.

Tissingh, G., Booij, J., Winogrodzka, A., van Royen, E. A., and Wolters, E. C. (1997). IBZM- and CIT-SPECT of the dopaminergic system in parkinsonism. *J. Neural Transm.* (Suppl), **50**, 31–7.

Tohgi, H., Abe, T., Takahashi, S., Kimura, M., Takahashi, J., and Kikuchi, T. (1992). Concentrations of serotonin and its related substances in the cerebrospinal fluid in patients with Alzheimer type dementia. *Neurosci. Lett.*, **141**, 9–12.

Tohgi, H., Abe, T., Takahashi, S., Saheki, M., Kimura, M. 1995. Indoleamine concentrations in celebrospinal fluid from patients with Alzheimer type and Binswanger type dementias before and after administration of citalopram, a synthetic serotonin uptake inhibitor. *J. Neurol. Transm - Parkinson's Disease & Dementia Section* **9**, 121–131.

Torack, R. M., Morris, J. C. 1998. The association of ventral tegmental area histopathology with adult dementia. *Arch. Neurol.* **45**, 497–501.

Tyrrell, P. J., Sawle, G. V., Ibanez, V., Bloomfield, P. M., Leenders, K. L., Frackowiak, R. S., *et al.* (1990). Clinical and positron emission tomographic studies in the 'extrapyramidal syndrome' of dementia of the Alzheimer type. *Arch. Neurol.*, **47**, 1318–23.

Ulas, J., Weihmuller, F. B., Brunner, L. C., Joyce, J. N., Marshall, J. F., and Cotman, C. W. (1994). Selective increase in NMDA-sensitive glutamate binding in the striatum of Parkinson's disease, Alzheimer's disease, and mixed Parkinson's disease/Alzheimer's disease patients: an autoradiographic study. *J. Neurosci.*, **14**, 6317–24.

Ulrich, J., Johannson-Locher, G., Seiler, W. O., and Stahelin, H. B. (1997). Does smoking protect from Alzheimer's disease? Alzheimer-type changes in 301 unselected brains from patients with known smoking history. *Acta Neuropathol.*, **94**, 450–4.

Van Dyck, C. H., Lin, C. H., Robinson, R., Cellar, J., Smith, E. O., Nelson, J. C., *et al.* (1997). The acetylcholine releaser linopridine increases parietal regional cerebral blood flow in Alzheimer's disease. *Psychopharmacology*, **132**, 217–26.

Vonsattel, J.-P. and DiFiglia, M. (1998). Huntington's disease. *J. Neuropathol. Exp. Neurol.*, **57**, 369–84.

Voytko, M. L. (1998). Cognitive functions of the basal forebrain cholinergic system in monkeys: memory or attention? *Behav. Brain Res.*, **75**, 13–25.

Wagster, M. V., Hedreed, J. C., Peyser, C. E., Folstein, S. E., and Ross, C. A. (1994). Selective loss of [3H] kainic acid and [3H] AMPA binding in layer VI frontal cortex in Huntington's disease. *Exp. Neurol.*, **127**, 70–5.

Westlake, T. M., Howlett, A. C., Bonner, T. I., Matsuda, L. A., and Herkenham, M. (1994). Cannabinoid receptor binding and messenger RNA expression in human brain: an in vitro receptor autoradiography and *in situ* hybridization histochemistry study of normal aged and Alzheimer's brains. *Neuroscience*, **63**, 637–52.

Wenning, G. K., Donnemiller, E., Granata, R., Riccabona, G., and Poewe, W. (1998). ^{123}I-beta-CIT and ^{123}I-IBZM-SPECT scanning in levodopa-naive Parkinson's disease. *Mov. Disorders*, **13**, 438–45.

Wilson, J. M., Levey, A. I., Rajput, A., Ang, L., Guttman, M., Shannak, K., *et al.* (1996). Differential changes in neurochemical markers of striatal dopamine nerve terminals in idiopathic Parkinson's disease. *Neurology*, **47**, 718–26.5.

Whitehouse, P. J., Trifiletti, R. R., Jones, B. E., Folstein, S., Price, D. L., Snyder, S. H., *et al.* (1985). Neurotransmitter receptor changes in Huntington's disease: autoradiographic and homogenate studies with special reference to benzodiazepine receptor complexes. *Ann. Neurol.*, **18**, 202–10.

Winkler, J., Thal, L. J., Gage, F. H., and Fisher, L. J. (1998). Cholinergic strategies for Alzheimer's disease. *J. Mol. Med.*, **76**, 555–67.

Wolfe, N., Katz, D. I., Albert, M. L., Almozlino, A., Durso, R., Smith, M. C., *et al.* (1990). Neuropsychological profile linked to low dopamine: in Alzheimer's disease, major depression, and Parkinson's disease. *J. Neurol. Neurosurg. Psychiatry*, **53**, 915–17.

Wu, J. Y., Bird, E. D., Chen, M. S., and Huang, W. M. (1979). Abnormalities of neurotransmitter enzymes in Huntington's chorea. *Neurochem. Res.*, **4**, 575–86.

Wyper, D. J., Brown, D., Patterson, J., Owens, J., Hunter, R., Teasdale, E., *et al.* (1993). Deficits in iodine-labelled 3-quinuclidinyl benzilate binding in relation to cerebral blood flow in patients with Alzheimer's disease. *Eur. J. Nucl. Med.*, **20**, 379–86.

Yates, C. M., Simpson, J., Maloney, A. F., and Gordon, A. (1980). Neurochemical observations in a case of Pick's disease. *J. Neurol. Sci.*, **48**, 257–63.

Young, A. B., Greenamyre, J. T., Hollingsworth, Z., Albin, R., D'Amato, C., Shoulson, I., *et al.* (1988). NMDA receptor losses in the putamen from patients with Huntington's disease. *Science*, **241**, 981–3.

Zilles, K. and Schleicher, A. (1995). Correlative imaging of transmitter receptor distributions in human cortex. In *Autoradiography and correlative imaging* (ed. W. E. Stumpf and H. F. Solomon), pp. 277–307. London: Academic Press Inc.

Zubenko, G. S., Moossy, J., Martinez, A. J., Rao, G., Claassen, D., Rosen, J., *et al.* (1991). Neuropathologic and neurochemical correlates of psychosis in primary dementia. *Arch. Neurol.*, **48** (6), 619–24.

10 Neuropathology

Peter L. Lantos and Nigel J. Cairns

1 Alzheimer's disease

Within the nosological entity of Alzheimer's disease (AD), there is both clinical and pathological heterogeneity. Subgroups include sporadic and familial forms; there are also phenotypic differences according to the gene and location of the genetic defect within a single gene. Occasionally, atypical cases may be seen and Alzheimer's disease may also be found in combination with other diseases, which may contribute to the dementing illness (see chapter 11).

Patients with AD usually die of bronchopneumonia and few abnormalities are found outside the nervous system. The naked eye appearances of the brain range from unremarkable to grossly abnormal. Brain weight is quite often reduced, sometimes below 1000 g. The atrophy is usually diffuse and symmetrical, although the fronto-parietal region and the temporal lobes may be more severely affected than the rest of the brain (Figure 10.1). The neurohistological features of AD are complex and variable. The two hallmark lesions, senile plaques and neurofibrillary tangles, are complemented by granulovacuolar degeneration, Hirano bodies, neuronal loss, abnormalities of neuronal processes and synapses, astrocytic and microglial response, and vascular changes. The white matter may also be affected (for review see Esiri and Morris 1997).

The senile or neuritic plaque is one of the major lesions found in the AD brain and is present to a lesser extent in the ageing brain (Figure 10.2). These structures ranging in size from 50–200 μm (Terry 1985) can be readily demonstrated by silver impregnation methods. The lesion consists of an amyloid core with a corona of argyrophilic axonal and dendritic processes, amyloid fibrils, glial cell processes, and microglial cells. Neuritic processes in the periphery of the SP are frequently dystrophic and contain paired helical filaments (PHFs), which are

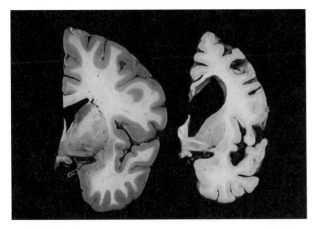

Figure 10.1 On the right, a coronal slice of the hemi-brain of a 47-year-old patient with severe Alzheimer's disease showing atrophy: the lateral ventricle is enlarged with rounding of its angle and several gyri are narrowed and the lateral fissure is widened. On the left, a slice of the right hemi-brain of a normal subject.

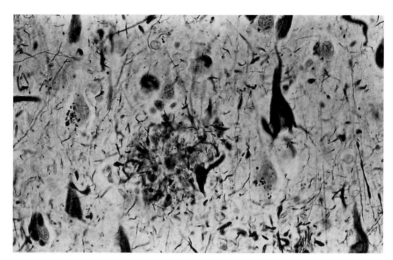

Figure 10.2 Neurofibrillary tangles and a neuritic plaque in the hippocampus. Glees and Marsland silver impregnation.

composed largely of abnormally phosphorylated tau protein (Gonatas *et al.* 1967; Hanger *et al.* 1991). The amyloid is composed of 5–10 nm filaments made up of a 40–43 amino acid (4 kDa) protein which was sequenced by Glenner and Wong (1984), and is now referred to as Aβ protein according to its proposed secondary structure of β-pleated sheets.

Studies using antibodies raised against Aβ protein have revealed the presence of a much more widespread deposition of amyloid than is visualized by traditional staining methods (Majocha *et al.* 1988; Gentleman *et al.* 1989; Armstrong *et al.* 1996) (Figure 10.4; see Plate 5). Aβ immunoreactivity has been detected throughout the central nervous system including the neocortex, hippocampus, thalamus, amygdala, caudate nucleus, putamen, nucleus basalis of Meynert, midbrain, pons, medulla oblongata, the cerebellar cortex, and spinal cord (Joachim *et al.* 1989*b*; Ogomori *et al.* 1989). These deposits take a variety of forms and include subpial, vascular, dyshoric, punctate or granular, diffuse, stellar, ring-with-core, and compact deposits (Ogomori *et al.* 1989). A laminar pattern of Aβ deposits in the neocortex has been described with concentrations in layers II, III, and V (Majocha *et al.* 1988). Aβ deposits have been reported in peripheral tissues such as skin and gut in AD (Joachim *et al.* 1989*a*). The widespread deposition of Aβ protein provides evidence that AD is an Aβ-amyloidosis of the central nervous system.

Aβ protein is a 40–43 residue polypeptide cleavage product of a larger precursor protein, amyloid precursor protein (APP). Although all cells have the potential for producing APP it seems likely that the major source of APP is the neuron. Nonetheless, astrocytes and microglial cells have also been implicated. The hypothesis that Aβ deposition is an early event in the pathogenesis of AD has been given support by the presence of extracellular APP and Aβ in diffuse plaques not associated with any neuritic change, or astrocytic involvement (Yamaguchi *et al.* 1991). However, more condensed Aβ is associated with a neuritic change, reactive astrocytosis, and microglial infiltration and phagocytosis. The Aβ fragment may act as a growth-promoting factor causing neuritic attraction and outgrowth leading to promotion of the SP about an Aβ core. Immunohistochemistry using antibodies that recognize a full-length $A\beta_{1-42}$ or a truncated $A\beta_{1-40}$ has detected most species of Aβ. The predominant species in sporadic AD is $A\beta_{42(43)}$ and this is found in plaques of all morphological types. Diffuse plaques contain only $A\beta_{42(43)}$ (Mann *et al.* 1996*a, b*).

Both diffuse and compact Aβ plaques may be immunolabelled by anti-Aβ and anti-ApoE antibodies (Cairns *et al.* 1997*a*; Armstrong *et al.* 1998*a*). The presence of one or more ε4 alleles leads to both an earlier onset and a more severe Aβ-amyloidosis (Roses 1994).

SPs are also immunohistochemically positive for a number of neuroactive substances. Acetylcholinesterase, a marker of the cholinergic system, can be demonstrated in some of the neuritic fibres of the corona. Several other neurotransmitters have been demonstrated in the SP including substance P, neuropeptide Y, neurotensin, cholecystokinin, 5-hydroxytryptamine (5-HT), and catecholamine (Walker *et al.* 1988; Hauw *et al.* 1991). Ubiquitin, a protein acting as a signal for degradation of abnormal proteins, is also present in SPs and NFTs (Perry *et al.* 1987). The presence of complement proteins and inflammatory cytokines suggest the involvement of inflammatory processes (McGeer and McGeer 1998).

The second histological hallmark of AD is the neurofibrillary tangle (NFT). These are not specific to AD, since they occur in ageing and other neurodegenerative disorders, including Down's syndrome, post-encephalitic parkinsonism, dementia pugilistica, amyotrophic lateral sclerosis-parkinsonism-dementia complex of Guam, subacute sclerosing panencephalitis, dementia with tangles with and without calcification, and in myotonic dystrophy (Kiuchi *et al.* 1991). NFTs also develop in progressive supranuclear palsy and sporadic motor neuron disease, but their ultrastructure and immunocytochemistry differ from those seen in ageing and AD.

In AD, NFTs are not only more numerous than in normal ageing, but they also affect the brain more extensively (Figure 10.2). Like in ageing, they are common in the medial temporal structures, in the hippocampus, amygdala, and parahippocampal gyrus, but also occur throughout the neocortex and the deep grey matter. NFTs are neuronal inclusions composed of abnormal cytoskeletal elements. The shape of neurons in which they develop determines their configuration. NFTs are flame-shaped in pyramidal neurons, whilst in the neurons of the brain stem they assume more complex, globose forms. They can be demonstrated by immunocytochemistry using antibodies against various neurofilament proteins, tau protein, and ubiquitin. Electron microscopy reveals their finer structural details: NFTs are mainly composed of paired helical filaments (Kidd 1963) which in turn are formed by two filaments wound around each other (Figure 10.5). Each filament has a diameter of 10 nm with crossover points at every 80 nm resulting in the typical periodicity of a double helix (Crowther and Wischik 1985). NFTs also contain straight filaments with an average diameter of 15 nm (Crowther 1991). In the adult human brain there are six isoforms of tau and all of these are hyperphosphorylated in AD (Goedert *et al.* 1991; Hanger *et al.* 1991). Specific phosphorylation-dependent anti-tau antibodies may be used to identify the three sites of tau pathology: the NFT, dystrophic neurites of SPs, and neuropil threads (Figure 10.3; see Plate 4). Phosphorylation-

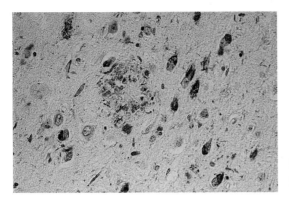

Figure 10.3 Neurofibrillary tangles and a neuritic plaque in the hippocampus. Tau immunohistochemistry.

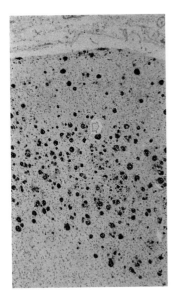

Figure 10.4 Extracellular Aβ deposits are present throughout all layers of the neocortex and have variable morphology. Aβ immunohistochemistry.

dependent antibodies may also be used to distinguish tauopathy in AD from other neurological disorders (Cairns *et al.* 1997*b*).

Neuropil threads or 'curly' fibres and dystrophic neurites have been well documented in silver impregnated preparations developed by Gallyas (1971), but they attracted attention only when it was realized that they could substantially contribute to dementia (Braak *et al.* 1986). These fibres are slender, short structures found in the neuropil of the cortex and in subcortical nuclei.

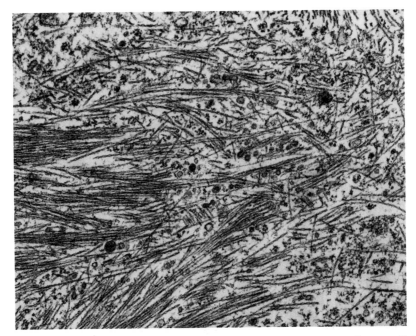

Figure 10.5 A high-power electron micrograph revealing paired helical filaments of a neurofibrillary tangle (kindly provided by the late Professor L. W. Duchen, Institute of Psychiatry, London).

Dystrophic neurites, some of which contribute to the formation of SPs, also appear as somewhat contorted, thread-like structures in these preparations. These abnormal neurites are likely to be a heterogeneous population of dendrites and axons (Tourtellotte and Van Hoesen 1991). Their ultrastructural and immunocytochemical features are strikingly similar to those of NFTs, indicating that they also originate from the altered neuronal cytoskeleton.

Neurofibrillary tangles and SPs have been associated with astrocytosis in AD and ageing brain (Beach *et al.* 1989; Itagakai *et al.* 1989; Cairns *et al.* 1992). In addition to NFTs, SPs, and dystrophic neurites, reactive astrocytosis is associated with degenerating neurons in AD.

Cerebral and leptomengeal blood vessels containing amyloid, when stained with Congo red, appear apple green under polarized light. Pantelakis (1954) called this deposition congophilic angiopathy. Vascular amyloid is now known to be, basically, the same protein, Aβ, as the amyloid found in SPs and other deposits in AD. Occasionally, Aβ appears to extend from the vessel wall into the surrounding cerebral tissue; this is referred to as dyshoric angiopathy.

Although the degenerative process in AD primarily affects the grey matter, the white matter may not be spared. White matter damage, which occurs in the absence of hypertensive vascular degeneration, is thought to be caused by hypoperfusion (Brun and England 1986). However, severe loss of cortical neurons may also contribute to fibre loss and consequent pallor of white matter.

AD is a disease primarily of old age and it is difficult to determine the proportion of genetic cases, as many family members will die before expressing the disease. Familial forms of AD with multiply affected individuals are rare and account for probably fewer than 5% of AD cases (see chapter 11). Mutations in the amyloid precursor protein (APP) gene and two related genes, presenilin 1 (PS1) and presenilin 2 (PS2), account for the majority of early onset autosomal dominant cases of familial AD (Goate *et al.* 1991; Lamb 1997). Although clinical features may differ between families, the neuropathological features are not markedly different between FAD and early onset sporadic cases (Davies 1986). However, prominent cerebellar plaques and Aβ deposition have also been reported in familial cases (Iseki *et al.* 1990; Struble *et al.* 1991; Fukutani *et al.* 1996, 1997). Computerized methods of image analysis have been used to more accurately define the pathological phenotype of AD. Using these techniques, differences in Aβ load have been reported. Mann *et al.* (1996*a, b*) have shown that both APP and PS mutations lead to measurable increases in Aβ load. Also, mutations in the same gene may also produce subtle but measurable changes in the neuropathology.

In those cases with an early onset, below 65 years of age, the duration of illness tends to be shorter, and the density of NFTs and SPs is often greater, than in sporadic, late onset patients. Patients with APP and PS mutations may have combined pathology. Cortical and brain stem Lewy bodies may coexist with AD pathology in APP (Lantos *et al.* 1992) and PS mutation patients. It is now known that the Lewy body and dystrophic neurites of Parkinson's disease and dementia with Lewy bodies contain the protein α-synuclein (Spillantini *et al.* 1997*b*). Familial and sporadic forms of AD may also be found in combination with cerebrovascular disease. Rare sporadic cases of AD have been found in combination with other neurodegenerative disorders including Pick's disease, Creutzfeldt–Jakob disease, motor neuron disease, and progressive supranuclear palsy (Morris 1997).

Even when the neurohistological abnormalities of AD have been established, the neuropathological diagnosis is not always straightforward (Cruz-Sánchez *et al.* 1995). It is important to establish a set of neuropathological criteria. Although several attempts have been made, no universally accepted criteria exist for the neuropathological diagnosis of AD. The most widely used protocol for neuropathological assessment is that developed by the Task Force of the Consortium to Establish a Registry for AD. This takes clinical findings into consideration, and neuropathological criteria for 'definite', 'probable' and 'possible' AD are proposed (Mirra *et al.* 1991). This system is based on a semi-quantitative assessment of plaque scores, while tangles are not formally assessed. The more recent National Institute on Aging and Reagan Institute (NIA-RI) criteria require both semi-quantitative measures of plaque and tangle distribution and additional sampling (Hyman and Trojanowski 1997). A change from previous criteria is the opinion that any Alzheimer lesions should be considered as pathological even when they appear to be incidental. By acknowledging that a spectrum of changes exists within AD, these criteria may prove more successful than previous ones (Hyman and Trojanowski 1997).

2 Dementia in Parkinson's disease and dementia with Lewy bodies

A number of pathological studies have shown that Lewy bodies in the brain stem and cortex may be found in between 10–25% of all dementia cases (Burns *et al.* 1990; Perry *et al.* 1990; McKeith *et al.* 1996). The presentation of progressive cognitive decline with fluctuating cognition, recurrent hallucinations, and parkinsonism with brain stem and cortical Lewy bodies has been defined by an international consensus meeting as dementia with Lewy bodies (McKeith *et al.* 1996) making it the second most common neurodegenerative cause of dementia after Alzheimer's disease (see chapter 13).

Macroscopically there may be mild thickening of the leptomeninges and slight atrophy associated with ageing. Atrophy may be found in patients who have abundant cortical Lewy bodies or coexisting Alzheimer's disease. Occasionally, the frontal lobe may be particularly atrophied with enlargement of the lateral ventricles. The pigmented nuclei, the substantia nigra, and locus coeruleus, appear pale indicating loss of pigment. The thalamus, striatum, and globus pallidus are normal (Daniel 1995).

The Lewy body is the histological hallmark for the diagnosis of idiopathic Parkinson's disease. Lewy bodies are usually spherical intracytoplasmic inclusions 15–30 μm in diameter (Figure 10.6; see Plate 6). They are easily seen in haematoxylin and eosin-stained sections where the central core is characteristically more eosinophilic and with a paler halo. They may be of variable shape and more than one Lewy body can be found in a single neuron. Lewy bodies are argyrophilic and labelled by ubiquitin (Figure 10.8) and neurofilament antibodies. Some Lewy bodies are also labelled by antibodies that recognize a number of different antigens including amyloid precursor protein, tubulin, microtubule-associated proteins, gelsolin-related antigen, and complement proteins (Yamada *et al.* 1992; Esiri and McShane 1997). Purified Lewy bodies obtained from frozen post-mortem brain have been used to show that the major component of the Lewy body is the protein α-synuclein (Figure 10.7), and α-synuclein immunohistochemistry is now the method of choice for detecting these lesions (Spillantini *et al.* 1997*b*). In the electron microscope, Lewy bodies do not appear to have a limiting membrane. The core contains granular material and there is an outer ring of filaments of 8–20 nm in diameter (Galloway *et al.* 1992). In addition to Lewy bodies, pale bodies may also be seen in the substantia nigra in haematoxylin and eosin-stained sections (Dale *et al.* 1992). These pale bodies may represent an intermediate stage of Lewy body formation, but the pathogenesis of the Lewy body is poorly understood.

The substantia nigra is severely affected. In addition to Lewy bodies, pigment-containing macrophages, neuronal loss, α-synuclein immunoreactive dystrophic neurites and astrocytosis may be observed. Neuronal loss in the substantia nigra correlates with the duration of the disease

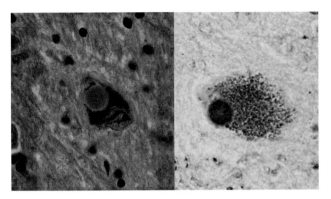

Figure 10.6   On the left, a Lewy body in a pigment-containing neuron in the substantia nigra of dementia with Lewy bodies. The Lewy body is eosinophilic and is circumscribed by a pale halo (haematoxylin and eosin). On the right a Lewy body in a pigmented neuron demonstrated by ubiquitin immunohistochemistry.

(Hughes *et al.* 1992). Lewy bodies and neuronal loss are found in both pigmented and non-pigmented brain stem nuclei, nucleus basalis of Meynert, thalamus, and hypothalamus (Daniel 1995). In the cerebral cortex, Lewy bodies occur in the deeper layers (V and VI) and are found in regular clusters indicating selective vulnerability of cortico-cortical projections (Armstrong *et al.* 1997). The density varies between cortical areas and between patients. Limbic areas including the anterior cingulate and parahippocampal gyri are usually more severely affected than other neocortical areas (Rezaie *et al.* 1996). Dystrophic neurites are frequently seen in the CA2/CA3 subfields of the hippocampus in patients with idiopathic Parkinson's disease and dementia with Lewy bodies (Figure 10.9).

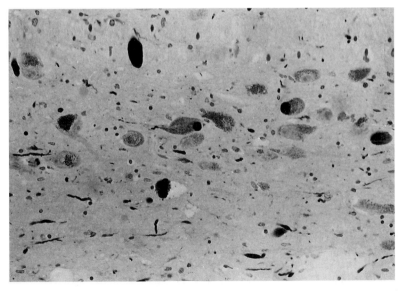

Figure 10.7   Lewy bodies and dystrophic neurites in the midbrain of dementia with Lewy bodies. α-Synuclein immunohistochemistry.

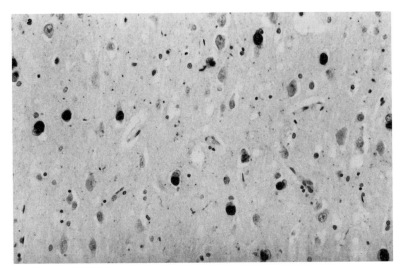

Figure 10.8 Lewy bodies in the cingulate gyrus of the frontal lobe in dementia with Lewy bodies. Ubiquitin immunohistochemistry.

Familial cases of Parkinson's disease are rare and the onset of the disease in these patients is typically at a younger age than sporadic cases. Mutations have been reported in the α-synuclein gene in these familial cases but none has been reported in sporadic cases indicating that mutations are rare causes of Parkinson's disease. The discovery of mutations in this gene and that the gene product, the protein α-synuclein, is a major component of the Lewy body and dystrophic neurites demonstrate the importance of α-synuclein in the pathogenesis of Parkinson's disease and dementia with Lewy bodies.

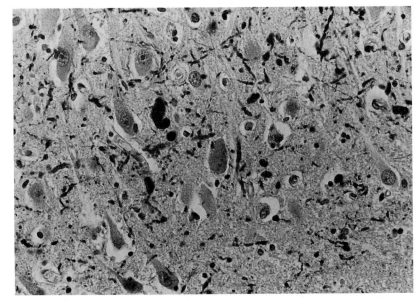

Figure 10.9 Dystrophic neurites in the CA2/CA3 subfields of the hippocampus of dementia with Lewy bodies. Ubiquitin immunohistochemistry.

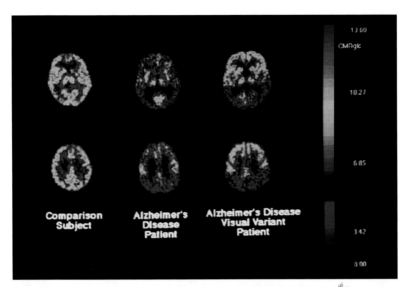

Plate 1 Comparison of glucose metabolism for Alzheimer's disease patients with and without prominent visual symptoms and a healthy control subject. Values of CMRglc reported on the colorimetric scale are in units of milligrams per 100 grams of tissue per minute. Relative to the healthy control subject, the patient with Alzheimer's disease (AD) and no visual symptoms shows the typical pattern of reductions in glucose metabolism in frontal, temporal, and parietal association areas, with preservation of metabolic rates in primary sensory regions. In contrast, compared to the AD patient without visual symptoms, the AD patient with visual symptoms shows a prominent glucose hypometabolism in parietal and occipital areas, including primary visual cortex, along with preservation of metabolism in frontal and temporal regions, which is virtually indistinguishable from that of the healthy control subject. CMRglc = cerebral metabolic rate for glucose. (From Pietrini et al. 1996.)

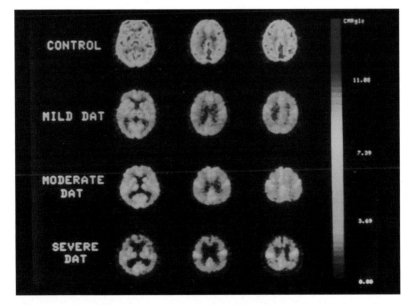

Plate 2 Transverse images at three different levels of brain PET scans in a normal control and in Alzheimer's disease (AD) patients with mild, moderate, and severe dementia, respectively (from top to bottom). rCMRglc values reported on the colorimetric scale are in mg/100 g/min. rCMRglc reductions are present mostly in the association areas and become more severe as AD progresses. Primary neocortical areas are relatively spared, even in the latest stages of the disease.

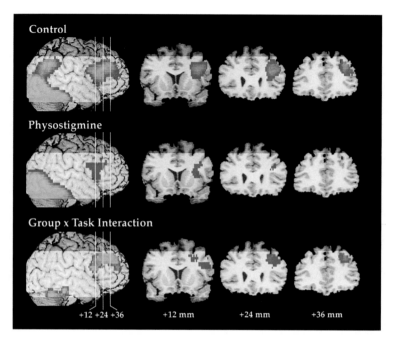

Control

Physostigmine

Group x Task Interaction

+12 +24 +36   +12 mm   +24 mm   +36 mm

Plate 3 Comparison of rCBF for healthy subjects receiving either physostigmine or saline while performing a working memory (WM) task relative to the resting state. For each comparison, the figure shows the result projected onto the right hemisphere and indicates the location for the three coronal sections in frontal cortex, located +12, +24, and +36 mm anterior to the anterior commissure. Z scores that exceeded a threshold of 2.33 (p = 0.01, two-tailed, before correction for multiple comparisons based on spatial extent) and obtained significance after an analysis of spatial extent are shown. Significant rCBF increases during WM task performance relative to rest are shown for the control and physostigmine groups. The group x task interaction shows greater task-related rCBF increases during saline infusion as compared with physostigmine infusion. (From Furey et al. 1997.)

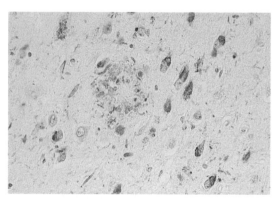

Plate 4 Neurofibrillary tangles and a neuritic plaque in the hippocampus. Tau immunohistochemistry.

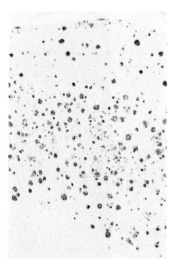

Plate 5 Extracellular Aβ deposits are present throughout all layers of the neocortex and have variable morphology. Aβ immunohistochemistry.

Plate 6   On the left, a Lewy body in a pigment-containing neuron in the substantia nigra of dementia with Lewy bodies. The Lewy body is eosinophilic and is circumscribed by a pale halo (haematoxylin and eosin). On the right a Lewy body in a pigmented neuron demonstrated by ubiquitin immunohistochemistry.

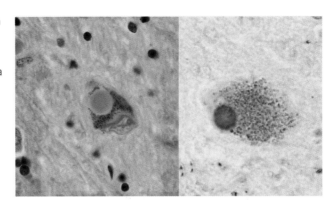

Plate 7   Pick cells or 'ballooned' neurons in the frontal lobe in Pick's disease. αB-crystallin immunohistochemistry.

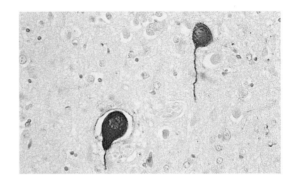

Plate 8   Pick bodies in the granule cells of the dentate gyrus of the hippocampus. Tau immunohistochemistry.

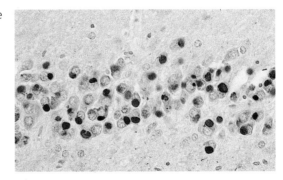

Plate 9   Pick bodies in the frontal lobe. Tau immunohistochemistry.

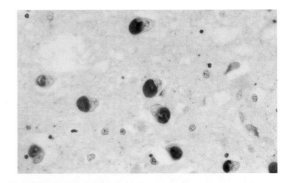

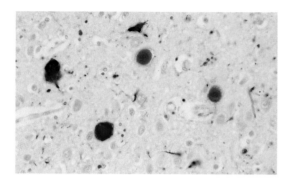

Plate 10 Swollen 'ballooned' neurons in the frontal lobe in corticobasal degeneration. αB-crystallin immunohistochemistry.

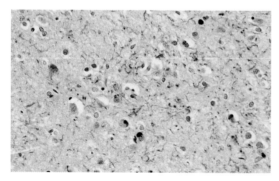

Plate 11 Corticobasal inclusions in the pigmented neurons of the substantia nigra. Tau immunohistochemistry.

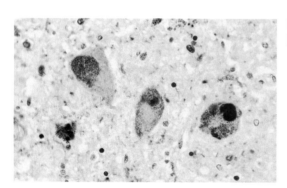

Plate 12 Abnormal astrocytic processes and inclusions in small neurons in the frontal lobe of corticobasal degeneration. Tau immunohistochemistry.

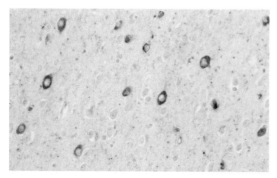

Plate 13 Tau positive neuronal inclusions in the brain of a case of frontotemporal dementia with parkinsonism linked to chromosome 17. Tau immunohistochemistry. (Tissue kindly provided by Professor B. Ghetti.)

Plate 14   Neuronal loss producing a status spongiosus in the superficial layers of the temporal neocortex in frontotemporal dementia with motor neuron disease. Haematoxylin and eosin.

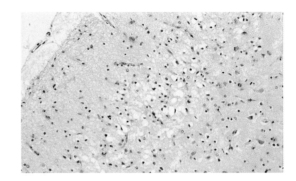

Plate 15   Neuronal inclusions in the granule cells of the dentate gyrus of frontotemporal dementia with motor neuron disease. Ubiquitin immunohistochemistry.

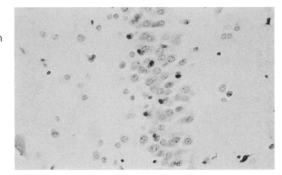

Plate 16   Neuronal loss and vacuolation in the caudate nucleus. Haematoxylin and eosin.

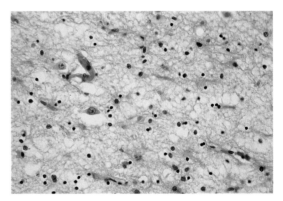

Plate 17   Neurofibrillary tangles in the substantia nigra of progressive supranuclear palsy. Tau immunohistochemistry.

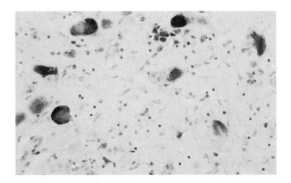

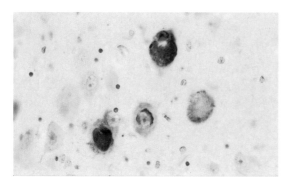

Plate 18 Neurofibrillary tangles in neurons of the raphé nucleus of progressive supranuclear palsy.
Tau immunohistochemistry.

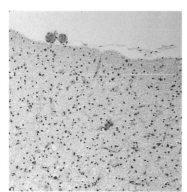

Plate 19 Thorny astrocytes in the caudate nucleus of progressive supranuclear palsy.
Tau immunohistochemistry.

Plate 20 Neuronal loss and vacuolation (status spongiosus) in the frontal lobe (left) and caudate nucleus (right) of Creutzfeldt–Jakob disease. Haematoxylin and eosin.

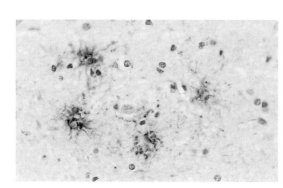

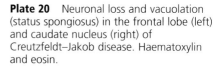

Plate 21 Prion protein deposition in the cerebellum of sporadic CJD on the left and vCJD on the right for comparison. The prion load is much greater in vCJD and is particularly striking in the molecular layer.
Prion protein (12F10) imunohistochemistry.

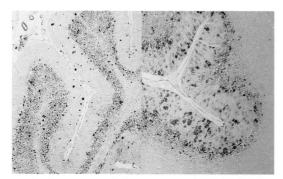

Plate 22 A prion plaque in the brain of vCJD (left) and associated reactive astrocytosis (right). Glial fibrillary acidic protein immunohistochemistry.

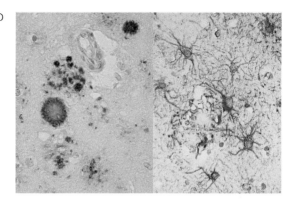

Plate 23 Neuronal loss and vacuolation in the molecular, Purkinje, and granule cell layers of the cerebellum of vCJD.

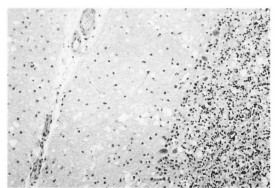

Plate 24 Typical prion protein deposits in the molecular layer of the cerebellum in familial prion disease with a 144 base pair insertion in the prion gene. Prion protein (12F10) imunohistochemistry.

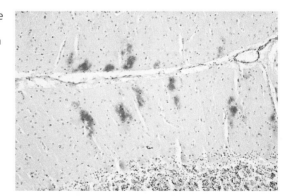

Plate 25 A prion plaque surrounded by vacuoles in kuru. Prion protein (12F10) imunohistochemistry.

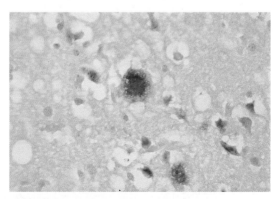

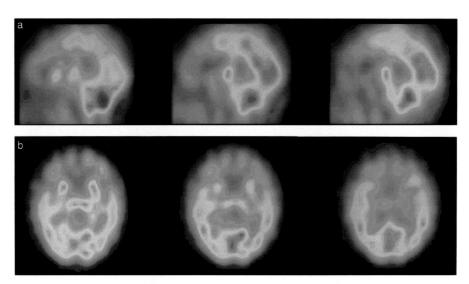

Plate 26 HMPAO-SPECT images from a typical case of frontal variant frontotemporal dementia (dementia of frontal type) showing marked bifrontal hypoperfusion. (a) Three sagittal images; (b) three axial images.

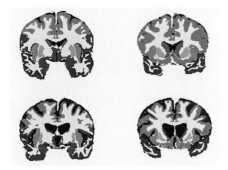

Plate 27 Magnetic resonance image of healthy control (top) and HD patient (bottom). Colours represent areas traced for volumetric analyses; red traces the caudate nucleus.
(Source: Terry L. Jernigan, University of California San Diego. Printed with permission.)

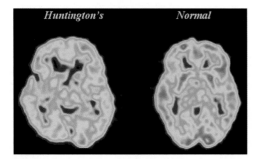

Plate 28 Positron emission tomography (using FDG) of healthy control (right) and HD patient (left). (Source: Mark Guttman, Centre for Addiction and Mental Health. Printed with permission.)

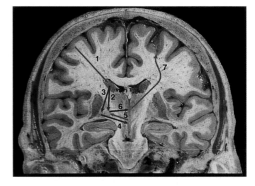

Plate 29 Brain sections including the frontal subcortical circuits. Top: The direct and indirect frontal circuits (red arrows indicate excitatory connections and blue arrows indicate inhibitory connections). (1) Excitatory glutamatergic corticostriatal fibres. (2) Direct inhibitory γ-aminobutyric acid (GABA)/substance P fibres (associated with D1 dopamine receptors) from the striatum to the globus pallidus interna/substantia nigra pars reticulata. (3) Indirect inhibitory GABA/enkephalin fibres (associated with D2 dopamine receptors) from the striatum to the globus pallidus externa. (4) Indirect inhibitory GABA fibres from the globus pallidus externa to the subthalamic nucleus. (5) Indirect excitatory glutamatergic fibres from the subthalamic nucleus to the globus pallidus interna/substantia nigra pars reticulata. (6) Basal ganglia inhibitory outflow via GABA fibres from the globus pallidus interna/substantia nigra pars reticulata to specific thalamic sites. (7) Thalamic excitatory fibres returning to the cortex (shown in contralateral hemisphere for convenience).

Okazaki *et al.* (1961) and Kosaka (1990) first described cortical Lewy bodies associated with dementia with parkinsonism. In some of the patients with an early onset there was little additional pathology. In late onset cases Alzheimer-type pathology is more common and is present in the majority of patients with dementia with Lewy bodies (Gibb *et al.* 1989a). However, there are fewer neurofibrillary tangles than are normally found in Alzheimer's disease. There may be sufficient additional pathology to warrant a combined diagnosis of dementia with Lewy bodies or Parkinson's disease and Alzheimer's disease (Mirra *et al.* 1991). Lewy bodies have also been reported in the brains of patients with mutation of the APP gene (Lantos *et al.* 1992, 1994). In these familial cases the brain stem and cortical Lewy pathology was sufficient to merit the neuropathological diagnosis of dementia with Lewy bodies using established criteria (McKeith *et al.* 1996). Thus, mutations in genes other than the α-synuclein gene may be associated with Lewy body pathology in addition to Alzheimer's disease.

3 Frontotemporal dementias

This is a clinical term, although not only the clinical, but also the neuropathological criteria for frontotemporal dementia have been defined by the Lund-Manchester groups (Brun *et al.* 1994). The underlying pathology may include various neurodegenerative diseases: Pick's disease, corticobasal degeneration, motor neuron disease-associated dementia, frontal lobe degeneration of non-Alzheimer-type, and frontotemporal dementia and parkinsonism linked to chromosome 17 (Jackson and Lowe 1996; Mann 1998; Lantos 1999), see chapter 12 for further details.

3.1 Pick's disease

Pick's disease is an uncommon cause of dementia. In some large pathological studies the disease accounts for about 2% of cases (Boller *et al.* 1989). The age at onset varies between 45 and 65 years and rarely beyond 75 years. Thus, unlike most patients with Alzheimer's disease, patients with Pick's disease have, typically, an early onset dementia. The duration of the disease is on average 5–10 years. Women appear to be slightly more affected than men. The disease has been observed in most geographical zones: 80% of cases are sporadic and less than 20% are familial. However, as the familial cases have come under greater scrutiny, the original diagnosis in some has been revised to take account of recent advances in immunohistochemistry and molecular genetics (see chapter 12).

The brain shows severe atrophy of the frontal or temporal lobe or both and less commonly to the parietal lobe. In classical cases the temporal pole may be particularly affected with relative sparing of the posterior part of the superior temporal gyrus. In the frontal lobes, the inferior aspect including the orbitofrontal region is often severely shrunken. The loss of brain substance may lead to a brain weight below 1000 g. The lateral ventricles may be largely dilated (Figure 10.10).

The diagnostic histological feature is the Pick body (Figure 10.12; see Plate 8). Pick bodies are well-circumscribed, spherical, argyrophilic neuronal intracytoplasmic inclusions. In addition, there are swollen achromatic so-called 'ballooned' neurons or Pick cells (Figure 10.11; see Plate 7), neuronal loss, and astrocytosis. Granulovacuolar degeneration may be seen in the hippocampus. These additional changes are not specific to Pick's disease as they are also found in other neurodegenerative disorders.

Pick bodies are found most abundantly in the granule cells of the dentate gyrus. The predilection for the cells of the dentate gyrus distinguishes Pick's disease from Alzheimer's disease

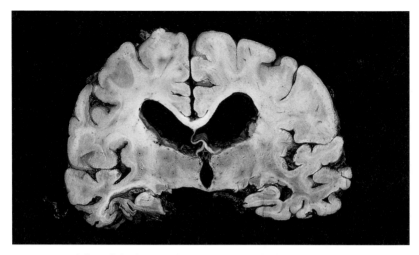

Figure 10.10 A coronal slice of the brain with Pick's disease. The lateral ventricle is dilated and there is increased space in the inferior horns of the lateral ventricle. The medial and inferior parts of the temporal lobe including the hippocampus are markedly shrunken and there is increased space in the lateral fissure. The superior temporal gyrus is relatively well preserved.

where neurofibrillary tangles are rarely found in the granule cells. Pick bodies are found at lower densities in the pyramidal neurons of the frontal and temporal neocortex. The distribution of Pick bodies may be uni- or bilaminar and this difference may reflect the stage of progression of the disease. A prominent band may be seen in layer II and upper layer III and a band in layer IV. These neurons can be contrasted with those in Alzheimer's disease where neurofibrillary tangles are found predominantly in the large pyramidal neurons of layers III and V, the major cortico-cortical projecting neurons. Spatial pattern analysis has shown that Pick bodies appear in regular clusters throughout affected cortical areas (Armstrong *et al.* 1998*b*). Pick bodies may also be found in the amygdala, striatum, thalamus, hypothalamus, brain stem nuclei, and the spinal cord.

Ultrastructurally, Pick bodies consist mainly of bundles of disorganized straight fibrils, which are labelled by anti-tau antibodies (Figure 10.13; see Plate 9), by ubiquitin, and neurofilament antibodies. They have a similar staining pattern to neurofibrillary tangles but recent studies show that the immunohistochemical profile of tau in Pick's disease is different from that in Alzheimer's disease (Delacourte *et al.* 1996).

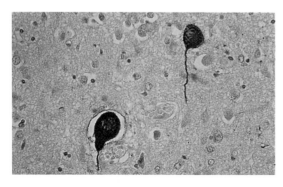

Figure 10.11 Pick cells or 'ballooned' neurons in the frontal lobe in Pick's disease. αB-crystallin immunohistochemistry.

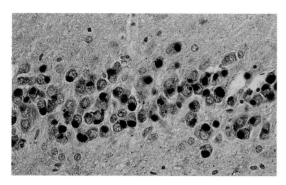

Figure 10.12 Pick bodies in the granule cells of the dentate gyrus of the hippocampus. Tau immunohistochemistry.

Ballooned neurons are readily seen, most often in the deep layers of the cortex in haematoxylin and eosin-stained sections. They are not present in all cases and are usually absent from the most severely affected regions of the cortex. Ballooned neurons have a slightly different immunohistochemical profile from that of Pick bodies. Like Pick bodies, the swollen neurons are labelled by ubiquitin, tau, and neurofilament antibodies, but the staining is usually less intense and more variable within the cytoplasm of ballooned neurons. They are also labelled by the heat-shock protein αB-crystallin (Lowe *et al.* 1997).

The significance of ballooned neurons in the pathogenesis of Pick's disease is unclear. In severely atrophied cortical areas, there may be severe neuronal loss and astrocytosis and an absence of Pick bodies.

Recently, the European Concerted Action against Pick's Disease (1998) proposed that the neuropathological diagnosis should be dependent on the microscopic identification of numerous Pick bodies, swollen cells, neuronal loss, and astrocytosis. The use of specific antibodies allows for the inclusions of different disorders to be distinguished. From a neuropathological viewpoint tau immunohistochemistry will distinguish between the inclusions of Pick's disease from those of frontotemporal dementia with motor neuron disease. The advantage of the European Concerted Action on Pick's Disease criteria over others is that they identify a distinct disease, which will facilitate research into aetiology and pathogenesis.

3.2 Corticobasal degeneration

The clinico-pathological description of corticobasal degeneration was first made by Rebeiz *et al.* in 1967. Males and females are equally affected and the age at onset of sporadic cases is in the

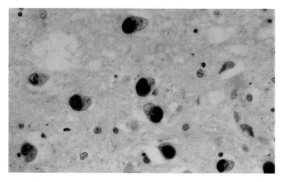

Figure 10.13 Pick bodies in the frontal lobe. Tau immunohistochemistry.

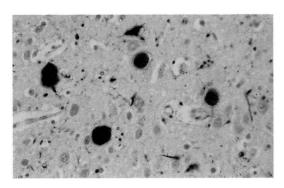

Figure 10.14 Swollen 'ballooned' neurons in the frontal lobe in corticobasal degeneration. αB-crystallin immunohistochemistry.

sixth to eighth decades and duration of illness ranges from 7–10 years. This rare progressive neurodegenerative disorder is characterized pathologically by degeneration of the cortex, basal ganglia, and brain stem. Microscopically, swollen achromatic neurons may be seen as well as glial and neuronal inclusions in the affected areas (Figure 10.14; see Plate 10).

Characteristically, the brain is atrophied asymmetrically in the posterior frontal and parietal lobes; both the pre- and post-central gyri are affected. The cortical atrophy is not usually so pronounced as in Pick's disease. There is dilatation of the lateral ventricles and the striatum may be shrunken. The corticospinal tracts and corpus callosum may appear thinned. The substantia nigra appears pale in the majority of cases but the brain stem atrophy typically found in patients with progressive supranuclear palsy is absent. The loss of neurons may be more severe in the outer cortical laminae and produce a spongy appearance. The white matter underlying the affected areas of cortex may be rarefied and display a reactive astrocytosis. The swollen neurons, also called achromatic or ballooned neurons, are readily seen in haematoxylin and eosin-stained sections where the nuclei are eccentric and the cytoplasm is pale reflecting the loss of basophilic Nissl substance (achromasia). They are found most frequently in cortical laminae III, V, and VI and occasionally in subcortical areas, but may be absent in the most severely affected cortical areas. The swollen neurons are variably labelled by ubiquitin, neurofilament, and tau antibodies; they are best demonstrated by αB-crystallin immunohistochemistry (Lowe *et al.* 1997). Ultrastructurally, swollen neurons contain 10–15 nm filaments and a smaller number of thicker 25–30 nm filaments, granular material, and lipofuscin (Wakabayashi *et al.* 1994).

There is usually severe neuronal loss and accompanying astrocytosis in the substantia nigra. Extracellular pigment may be seen as well as in some macrophages. A characteristic feature is the intraneuronal basophilic corticobasal inclusion: they are argentophilic and fibrillar and are labelled by anti-ubiquitin and anti-tau antibodies (Figure 10.15; see Plate 11) (Wakabayashi *et al.* 1994). Histologically, they resemble the neurofibrillary tangles of progressive supranuclear palsy. Ultrastructurally, the filaments of the inclusions are mainly straight with a diameter of 15 nm (Wakabayashi *et al.* 1994). Similar inclusions may be found in the locus coeruleus and other brain stem nuclei (Gibb *et al.* 1989b). In addition to these corticobasal inclusions, small neuronal inclusions and neuropil threads can be found in the superficial layers of the cortex. These cortical inclusions may be visualized by silver impregnation and with ubiquitin or tau immunohistochemistry (Revesz *et al.* 1995). They can be distinguished from the round well-demarcated Pick bodies of Pick's disease and tau immunohistochemistry may help to distinguish between these two disorders.

A striking feature of corticobasal degeneration is glial pathology in the affected areas (Figure 10.16; see Plate 12). Filamentous argyrophilic structures are seen most commonly in astrocytes and less frequently in oligodendrocytes. The astrocytic inclusions are often dramatic and clusters

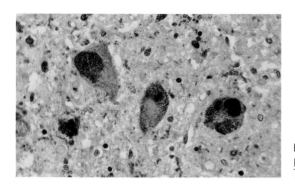

Figure 10.15 Corticobasal inclusions in the pigmented neurons of the substantia nigra. Tau immunohistochemistry.

of astrocytic tangles may form astrocytic plaques (Komori *et al.* 1998). The inclusions in oligo-dendrocytes are argyrophilic coiled bodies. Both the astrocytic and oligodendroglial inclusions in corticobasal degeneration are labelled by ubiquitin and tau antibodies. They are not recognized by antibodies to α-synuclein, the major component of the glial cytoplasmic inclusions (GCIs) of multiple system atrophy (MSA) (Spillantini *et al.* 1998*b*).

3.3 Frontotemporal dementia with parkinsonism linked to chromosome 17

In 1994 frontotemporal dementia in one family was linked to chromosome 17q21-22 (Wilhelmsen *et al.* 1994). This initial discovery resulted in a Consensus Conference on families with the same genetic abnormality (Foster *et al.* 1997).

The clinical symptomatology of FDTP-17 varies not only between kindreds, but also within the same kindred. The disease usually starts insidiously with behavioural or motor manifestations typically in the fifth decade of life, but occasionally earlier in the third or fourth decades or later in the sixth decade. The duration is variable: on average it lasts about 10 years with a range of 3–30 years with a slowly progressive course. The presenting symptoms may include dementia, parkinsonism, non-fluent aphasia, personality changes, or obvious psychosis. The clinical symptomatology (Wilhelmsen and Clark 1998) and the neuropathology (Spillantini *et al.* 1998*a*) of FDTP-17 have been recently reviewed (see chapter 12).

Macroscopically, frontotemporal atrophy with enlargement of the lateral ventricles is the predominant feature with a less obvious tissue loss from the basal ganglia and the substantia nigra. The overall histology shows neuronal loss with vacuolation of the superficial layers of the cortex (status spongiosus) and astrocytosis sometimes extending into the white matter (Figure 10.18; see Plate 14). The caudate nucleus, the putamen, the amygdala, the hippocampus,

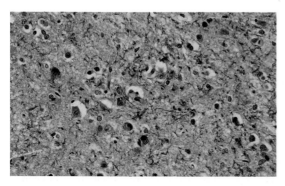

Figure 10.16 Abnormal astrocytic processes and inclusions in small neurons in the frontal lobe of corticobasal degeneration. Tau immunohistochemistry.

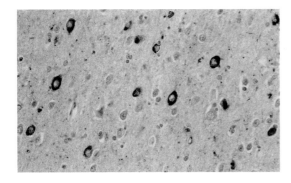

Figure 10.17 Tau positive neuronal inclusions in the brain of a case of frontotemporal dementia with parkinsonism linked to chromosome 17. Tau immunohistochemistry. (Tissue kindly provided by Professor B. Ghetti.)

and the substantia nigra also show neuronal loss and astrocytosis. The amygdala is usually severely affected, while the hippocampus is relatively well preserved. Other histological abnormalities include neuronal and glial inclusions as well as large, swollen achromatic cells. The inclusions are argentophilic and tau positive (Figure 10.17; see Plate 13); these are found in the neocortex, the basal ganglia, the hypothalamus, the brain stem, and the spinal cord. Glial inclusions occur chiefly in oligodendrocytes, but some astrocytes may also be affected.

The distribution, the antigenic profile, and the ultrastructure of the tau positive argyrophilic inclusions have been best characterized in the familial multiple-system tauopathy with presenile dementia (Spillantini *et al.* 1997a, 1998c).

Three recent reports of molecular genetic investigations indicate tau mutations in FDTP-17. The first shows a point mutation of valine to methionine in the coding region of tau (Poorkaj *et al.* 1998), the second a G-A transition in an intron of tau (Spillantini *et al.* 1998a), and the third describes a mixture of exon and intron tau mutations in ten different families (Hutton *et al.* 1998). None of these tau mutations were present in any of the controls. The significance of these findings and recent investigations of molecular genetics are discussed elsewhere in this book (see chapter 8).

3.4 Frontotemporal dementia with motor neuron disease

The disease usually starts in the sixth decade although earlier or later manifestations are known to occur. The duration, with an average course of 2–3 years, is considerably shorter than that of Alzheimer's disease. It is more common in men than in women with a ratio of 2:1. Although most cases are sporadic, familial occurrence is responsible for approximately 15–20%. The familial and sporadic cases do not differ significantly according to sex ratio, age at onset, and disease duration (for review Mann 1998).

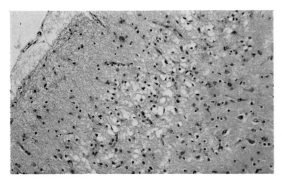

Figure 10.18 Neuronal loss producing a status spongiosus in the superficial layers of the temporal neocortex in frontotemporal dementia with motor neuron disease. Haematoxylin and eosin.

Macroscopically, there is mild-to-moderate cerebral atrophy affecting mainly the anterior frontal, temporal, and parietal lobes. This tissue loss is not as severe as that seen in Alzheimer's disease, Pick's disease, or Creutzfeldt–Jakob disease: the average brain weight of 26 autopsies of Japanese cases was 1240 g (Morita *et al.* 1987). On coronal slices, the lateral ventricles may be enlarged with rounding of the angles while the corpus callosum is thin. The substantia nigra may appear paler than usual.

Histology shows neuronal loss, vacuolar degeneration (status spongiosus), and astrocytosis in the superficial layers of the cortex, and intraneuronal inclusions both in the cortex and in the dentate fascia of the hippocampal formation. The severity of neuronal loss varies, but it can be profound leaving severe status spongiosus in layers II and III of the cortex. Morphometric studies revealed substantial reduction in the number of cortical neurons, particularly those larger than 90 μm in diameter. In addition, there is also an attrition of the dendritic tree: the surviving neurons show reduced dendritic arborization, proximal dendritic varicosities, amputation of the dendrites, and depletion of the dendritic spines (for review see Lantos 1992*a*). The intraneuronal, ubiquitin positive but tau negative and non-argyrophilic inclusions occur in the superficial small cortical neurons in layer II and to a lesser extent in layer III of the cortex, together with abnormal neurites (Lowe *et al.* 1989; Leigh *et al.* 1991) are also seen in the amygdala (Anderson *et al.* 1995). However, neuronal inclusions are most abundant in the dentate gyrus of the hippocampal formation and in the entorhinal cortex (Figure 10.19; see Plate 15) (Okamoto *et al.* 1991). Neuronal loss is accompanied by striking astrocytosis, the distribution of which may be laminar, but occasionally involving the entire thickness of the cortex. In addition, widespread astrocytosis and microglial activation have been demonstrated in the white matter (Cooper *et al.* 1996). The substantia nigra is usually severely affected with neuronal loss and astrocytosis. In addition to these changes, histological abnormalities of motor neuron disease are present including neuronal loss in the anterior horns of the spinal cord and in the motor nuclei of the brain stem. The surviving neurons here contain the typical skein-like and other ubiquitin positive inclusions of motor neuron disease (Ince *et al.* 1998).

However, more recently, a variety of motor neuron disease-associated dementia without the clinical and pathological features of classical motor neuron disease was described and for these cases the term motor neuron disease inclusion dementia was suggested (Jackson *et al.* 1996). Histologically, the intraneuronal inclusions are the same as in motor neuron disease-associated dementia and there are also ubiquitin positive dystrophic neurites, white matter pallor with astrocytosis, and severe neuronal loss with accompanying astrocytosis in the cortex, basal ganglia, and substantia nigra. In a review of three cases of semantic dementia showing the same histological features with ubiquitin positive, but tau negative inclusions, the term ubiquitin body dementia was introduced to describe such cases (Rossor *et al.* 1999). The existence of these cases lends some support to the argument that they are not merely

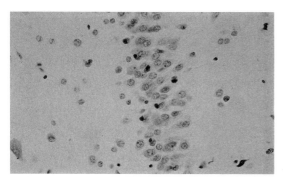

Figure 10.19 Neuronal inclusions in the granule cells of the dentate gyrus of frontotemporal dementia with motor neuron disease. Ubiquitin immunohistochemistry.

phenotypic variations within the spectrum of motor neuron disease, but a separate a clinico-pathological entity.

The occurrence of dementia with motor neuron disease raises the important question of the neuropathological substrate of the patient's mental impairment. The underlying lesions responsible for dementia may include extensive neuronal loss with cortical vacuolation, the severe dendritic damage with synaptic loss, the formation of cortical and hippocampal neuronal inclusions, and the involvement of subcortical structures.

4 Huntington's disease

Huntington's disease is an autosomal dominant neurodegenerative disorder: the mutation was identified in 1993 as an unstable expansion in the length of a cytosine-adenine-guanine (CAG) triplet repeat sequence within the coding region of the gene IT15 (for interesting transcript). This gene is localized on chromosome 4 (4p63) and encodes the protein huntingtin. The genetics of Huntington's disease are discussed elsewhere in this book (see chapters 8 and 15).

Macroscopically, there is evidence of severe cerebral atrophy. In a comparative study of 30 patients with Huntington's disease and 13 controls, a 30% mean reduction in brain weight was found. A striking loss of the cerebral cortex (21–29%), the white matter (29–34%), the caudate nucleus (57%), the putamen (64%), and the thalamus (28%) was observed. The enlargement of the ventricular system ranged from 2.5–13 times of the normal (De la Monte *et al.* 1988). The atrophy of the caudate nucleus is the principal naked-eye diagnostic hallmark lesion of the disease: its convex contour becomes flattened or even concave (Figure 10.20). In addition, there may be atrophy of the globus pallidus and the pars reticularis of the substantia nigra as a result of loss of projections from the corpus striatum. The frontal lobes show atrophy in 80% of the cases. The mean brain weight at post-mortem examination of 163 cases was 1067 g compared to 1350 g in controls (Vonsattel and DiFiglia 1998). The striatal atrophy is bilateral and occurs in 95% of the Huntington brains: severe in 80%, mild in 15%, and hardly notice-

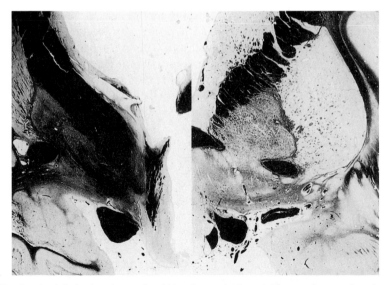

Figure 10.20 On the left the basal ganglia of Huntington's disease. The caudate nucleus is considerably thinned in comparison to the normal brain on the right. Luxol fast blue-Nissl stain.

able in 5% of the brains. The non-striatal regions may also show atrophy of varying severity or are unremarkable. In the advanced stages of the disease, the brain appears to be diffusely smaller than usual.

Histologically, there is neuronal loss of varying severity and astrocytosis in the affected areas of the corpus striatum (Figure 10.21; see Plate 16). The striatal degeneration does not occur in random but follows an ordered topographic distribution. In the caudate nucleus the tail, the body, and the head all show evidence of degeneration in this order of decreasing severity. In the putamen the caudal portion is more affected than the rostral part. As the disease progresses the striatal degeneration spreads both from caudo-rostral and dorso-ventral/medio-lateral directions. The neuronal loss is accompanied by astrocytosis. Surviving neurons may also show degenerative changes: they appear smaller, stain darker, and have an irregular scalloped outline. There is increasing evidence that these neurons undergo apoptosis (Vonsattel and DiFiglia 1998). Based on macroscopical and histological findings of the striatum in three standardized coronal sections, Vonsattel and colleagues (1985) developed a grading system distinguishing five grades from 0–4 of increasing severity.

The cerebral cortex shows atrophy in Grades 3 and 4 of Huntington's disease. Although the question of cortical neuronal loss has been controversial, there is increasing evidence of neuronal fallout in advanced cases of Huntington's disease. These degenerative changes in the cortex and the hippocampus may be at least partly responsible for some of the non-motor symptomatology of Huntington's disease, particularly dementia. Ubiquitin positive neurites, indicating cortical pathology, were also found in the cortex (Cammarata *et al.* 1993; Jackson *et al.* 1995). Intranuclear inclusions, immunostained with antibodies to both ubiquitin and N-terminal huntingtin, are found in Huntington brains and their density correlate with the length of the triplet repeat (Becher *et al.* 1998). Changes in the thalamus, substantia nigra, subthalamic nucleus, and cerebellum have also been reported (for reviews see Vonsattel and DiFiglia 1998; Kowall and Ferrante 1998).

The neuropathology of Huntington's disease is closely associated with pathophysiology, which in turn determines clinical symptomatology. The normal striatum is made of two compartments, the striosome (the so-called patch compartment) and the matrix compartment. In Huntington's disease there is a significant loss of striatal matrix area whereas the total area of patch compartment remains within normal limits (Kowall and Ferrante 1998). Both neuronal cytology and neurochemistry are different in these two compartments. The striosome compartment is rich in the so-called spiny neurons, which contain GABA, encephalin, dynorphin, and substance P. Projection neurons from the striatum are in this class of neurons. The matrix compartment, in contrast, is rich in smooth dendrites, the so-called aspiny neurons which contain acetylcholinesterase, NADPH diaphorase (nitric oxide synthase), somatostatin,

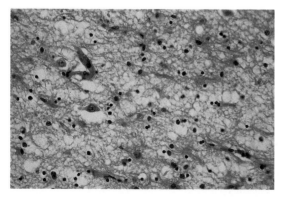

Figure 10.21 Neuronal loss and vacuolation in the caudate nucleus. Haematoxylin and eosin.

neuropeptide Y, and cholecystokinin. Striatal interneurons belong to this class of neurons. The medium-sized spiny projection neurons are affected early and bear the brunt of the disease, whereas the aspiny neurons undergo degeneration at a later stage. NADPH diaphorase containing neurons are relatively well-preserved. This results in an increased GABAergic input to the subthalamic nucleus, reducing its tonic activity on the medial globus pallidus and the pars reticularis component of the substantia nigra. The consequence is reduced inhibitory output of these nuclei to the thalamus which then increases glutamergic stimulation of the cerebral cortex, resulting in chorea (see chapters 9 and 15). Consequently chorea is caused by a diminished striatal inhibition of neurons in the lateral globus pallidus reducing activity of the subthalamic nucleus and releasing thalamic neurons to excite the cortex (Lowe *et al.* 1997; Kowall and Ferrante 1998).

Although the genetic abnormality of Huntington's disease is known, the precise pathogenetic mechanism remains to be elucidated. There is increasing evidence that the impairment of oxidative phosphorylation can produce symptomatology in experimental animals similar to that of Huntington's disease. This reduction in oxidative phosphorylation is also associated with selective neuronal vulnerability. The presence of free radicals and reactive oxygen species could explain some of the pathology of Huntington's disease (Kowall and Ferrante 1998; Vonsattel and DiFiglia 1998).

5 Progressive supranuclear palsy

The clinical and neuropathological features of progressive supranuclear palsy (PSP) was first described by Steele, Richardson, and Olszewski in 1964 (Steele *et al.* 1964). Since this seminal publication cases have been reported from all over the world, and the clinical and neuropathological criteria of PSP have subsequently been defined (Hauw *et al.* 1994; Litvan *et al.* 1996).

The precise incidence of PSP is not known, and only a few epidemiological data are available. The incidence in Western Australia is four cases per 10^6 population per annum (Mastaglia *et al.* 1973), whereas a minimum estimate of prevalence in New Jersey is 1.39 per 100 000 (Golbe *et al.* 1988). The annual incidence rate (new cases per 100 000 population per year) for the age group of 50–99 years was 5 in Olmsted County, Minnesota (Bower *et al.* 1997). There is a male preponderance: 60% of the patients are male and 40% female (Kristensen 1985). In a large series of 202 cases, the average age of onset was 59.6 years, ranging from 12–80 years. The disease most often starts during or after the sixth decade: the age at onset in 71% of patients was between 50–65 years. The duration varies from 1–23 years; the average survival time being 5.7 years (Kristensen 1985). The disease is sporadic, although rare familial cases, indicating autosomal dominant inheritance, have been described (Brown *et al.* 1993; Yebenes *et al.* 1995; Tetrud *et al.* 1996; Gazeley and Macguire 1996). Recently, a dinucleotide repeat polymorphism in a tau intron has been identified: homozygous tau AO allele was found in 95.5% of PSP cases compared to 50% in controls and in Alzheimer's disease (Conrad *et al.* 1997). However, this significant association between tau gene AO homozygosity and PSP has not been confirmed in the Japanese population, suggesting that the role of this dinucleotide repeat in PSP may be different in Caucasian and Japanese populations, or it may not be causal for PSP, but represents a marker for other molecular genetic risk factors within or close to the tau gene on chromosome 17 (Conrad *et al.* 1998).

The neuropathology of PSP has been recently reviewed (Bergeron *et al.* 1998; Hauw *et al.* 1998; Lantos 1999). On gross examination, the brains show variation: they may appear to be normal or may be atrophied. The brain weight may be slightly reduced, but quite often it is within normal limits. On coronal slices the cortex and the white matter are unremarkable. Cortical atrophy, when present, is difficult to assess. Gross pathology is restricted chiefly to the diencephalon, the brain stem, and the cerebellum. The ventricular system, particularly the 3rd and 4th ventricles may be enlarged, but without the overall impression of severe diffuse atrophy, so often encountered in Alzheimer's disease. The midbrain, particularly the superior colliculi, the tegmentum and the periaqueductal grey matter, and the pontine tegmentum are atrophied. The substantia nigra and the locus coeruleus are paler than usual. The subthalamic regions and the inner segment of the globus pallidus may be shrunken and discoloured. The superior cerebellar peduncles and the dentate nucleus of the cerebellum are atrophied (Mann *et al.* 1993; Lantos 1994; Daniel *et al.* 1995).

The principal histological lesions of PSP include neurofibrillary tangles, neuropil threads, neuronal loss, neuroglial pathology, and astrocytosis. The presence of neurofibrillary tangles (NFT) is the single most important feature of PSP. The NFTs of PSP are different from those of Alzheimer's disease in distribution, ultrastructure, antigenic profile, and biochemistry. They are present in the substantia nigra, the subthalamic nucleus, the globus pallidus, the nucleus basalis of Meynert, the pretectal region, the tegmentum of the midbrain, and the pons including the periaqueductal grey matter, the locus coeruleus, the raphé nuclei, and in the nuclei of various cranial nerves. NFTs occur less frequently in the corpus striatum, the red nucleus, the thalamus, and in the inferior olives (Lantos 1994; Daniel *et al.* 1995; Hauw *et al.* 1994; Litvan *et al.* 1996). NFTs as an integral part of PSP, and not representing concomitant ageing changes, are also present in the cerebral cortex (Hauw *et al.* 1990; for review Hauw *et al.* 1998). Depending on the type of neurons in which they occur, two configurations can be distinguished: globose tangles usually in the brain stem and flame-shaped or triangular in the pyramidal cells of the cerebral cortex. More irregular, round or cone-shaped tangles are also seen in smaller neurons. NFTs are easily discernible on routine haematoxylin and eosin-stained sections, but their presence is accentuated in various silver impregnations, including Gallyas, modified Bielschowsky, and Bodian.

Electron microscopy reveals the NFTs to be composed chiefly of straight filaments of indeterminate length and 15 nm in diameter (Tellez-Nagel and Wisniewski 1973) which, in turn, are composed of six or more protofilaments of 2–5 nm (Montpetit *et al.* 1985). In addition to straight filaments, twisted or paired filaments have also been described, and it was suggested that the former represents a stage in the formation of the latter (Tomonaga 1977; Yagashita *et al.* 1979). Immunohistochemically, PSP is characterized by extensive tau pathology, affecting both neuronal and glial cells (Figures 10.22 and 10.23; see Plates 19 and 20). NFTs give positive reactions with antibodies to tau protein (Bancher *et al.* 1987) and to isolated paired helical filaments (Probst *et al.* 1988). Immunoelectron microscopy shows that anti-tau activity is localized predominantly to 15–20 nm straight filaments (Jellinger and Brancher 1992), but it may also be present in diffuse, granular form in the neuronal cytoplasm before it aggregates into filamentous structures. The tau of PSP, however, is different from the biochemical lesion of Alzheimer's disease in that it is composed of a doublet of 64 and 69 kDa on Western blots, whilst the third major band of 55 kDa tau to be present in Alzheimer's disease is missing (for review see Hauw *et al.* 1998). The immunoreactivity of NFTs in PSP to neurofilament proteins and ubiquitin is controversial. Immunostaining with antibodies to ubiquitin and high and medium molecular weight neurofilament subunits gives either negative or weakly positive reaction (for reviews Lantos 1994; Hauw *et al.* 1998). Neuropil threads, demonstrated by the silver impregnation of Gallyas and antibodies to both tau protein and isolated paired helical filaments have been extensively found in the subcortical grey matter (Probst *et al.* 1988), neocortex, and hippocampus (Hauw *et al.* 1990). Ballooned neurons may also be seen in PSP but at a considerably lower density than in corticobasal degeneration (Mori and Oda 1997).

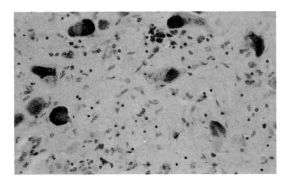

Figure 10.22 Neurofibrillary tangles in the substantia nigra of progressive supranuclear palsy. Tau immunohistochemistry.

There is neuronal loss in various nuclei of the brain stem, the diencephalon, and the cerebellum, including the substantia nigra (Fearnley and Lees 1991), the nucleus basalis of Meynert (Tagliavini *et al.* 1984), in the pedunculopontine nucleus (Hirsch *et al.* 1987), in the pontine reticular formation (Malessa *et al.* 1991), and in the striatum (Oyanagi *et al.* 1988). A recent investigation shows evidence of apoptosis (De la Monte *et al.* 1998).

Glial cells are also extensively involved. In addition to the stereotypic response of astrocytosis, these glial cells also contain tau positive and argyrophilic inclusions, variously referred to as tufts of abnormal fibres, star-like tufts, or glial fibrillary tangles (Figure 10.24; see Plate 19). They are characteristic of PSP and contribute to the neuropathological diagnosis (Matsusaka *et al.* 1998; Komori *et al.* 1998). Thorn-shaped astrocytes, although of somewhat different configuration, are also tau positive. Ultrastructurally these astrocytic inclusions are composed of straight filaments (Nishimura *et al.* 1992). In addition, oligodendrocytes may also contain inclusions, the so-called coiled bodies: these should not be confused with the glial cytoplasmic inclusion of multiple system atrophy (Papp *et al.* 1989) from which they can be distinguished on the basis of different configuration, ultrastructure, and antigenic profile (Lantos 1998).

PSP shows considerable phenotypic variation that makes the diagnosis sometimes difficult. Criteria for the neuropathological diagnosis of PSP, as a result of a series of consensus meetings, have been published (Hauw *et al.* 1994). The diagnosis is based on a semi-quantitative assessment of the distribution of NFTs. The criteria also take into account the presence of neuropil threads and tau positive astrocytes. Based on neuropathological criteria, three types of PSP can be distinguished: typical, atypical, and combined. Typical cases show the pathological features, as originally described, while atypical cases are variants of the histological changes

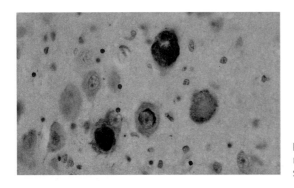

Figure 10.23 Neurofibrillary tangles in neurons of the raphé nucleus of progressive supranuclear palsy. Tau immunohistochemistry.

characteristic of PSP: either the severity or the distribution of the abnormalities, or both, deviate from the typical pattern. In combined cases, in addition to PSP, there is another disease process: this may be another neurodegenerative disorder, for example Alzheimer's disease, or vascular disease (Lantos 1994). Although the atypical forms may present diagnostic difficulties it is important to recognize the clinical and neuropathological heterogeneity of PSP (Gearing *et al.* 1994).

6 Prion diseases

Prion diseases are neurodegenerative disorders affecting man and animals. The previously used, and alternative descriptive term, transmissible spongiform encephalopathy is based on the extensive vacuolation of the grey matter and the transmissibility of disorders. There are four human prion diseases: Creutzfeldt–Jakob disease (CJD), Gerstmann-Sträussler-Scheinker disease (GSSD), fatal familial insomnia (FFI), and kuru. Prion diseases affecting animals include scrapie of sheep and goats, transmissible mink encephalopathy, chronic wasting disease of mule, deer, and elk, bovine spongiform encephalopathy, and feline spongiform encephalopathy. All of the human and veterinary diseases are transmissible. However, of the human diseases, all cases of GSSD and about 10–15% of CJD cases are inherited. Since a review of animal diseases is beyond the scope of this chapter, it will concentrate only on the pathology of the four human disorders.

Human prion diseases can be classified as sporadic (85% of CJD), genetic (GSSD, FFI, and 15% of CJD), and infectious or acquired (kuru, iatrogenic CJD, and the new variant CJD). These neurodegenerative diseases are caused by an unconventional infectious agent the prion, a term introduced by Prusiner 1982 to distinguish these pathogens from viruses and other infectious agents. Prion exists in two isoforms: PrP^C the normal cellular isoform, and PrP^{Sc} the pathogenic isoform. Prion protein, being a neuronal membrane protein, is essential for normal synaptic formation (Collinge *et al.* 1994). It is encoded by a gene on the short arm of chromosome 20 and the dominantly inherited prion diseases are genetically linked to mutations of the PrP gene. The molecular biology and genetics as well as the clinical features of prion diseases are discussed elsewhere in this book (see chapters 8 and 16, respectively).

6.1 Creutzfeldt–Jakob disease

CJD is a rare disease with world-wide distribution. A recent epidemiological study in six European countries (France, Germany, Italy, the Netherlands, Slovakia, and United Kingdom)

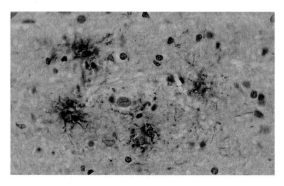

Figure 10.24 Thorny astrocytes in the caudate nucleus of progressive supranuclear palsy. Tau immunohistochemistry.

has shown an overall annual mortality rate of 0.71 cases per million, with a similar incidence rate in all participating countries. According to aetiological subtypes 87% of the cases were sporadic, 8% genetic, and 5% iatrogenic. There were considerable variations from country to country: genetic forms comprised 80% of all cases in Slovakia, whereas iatrogenic cases occurred most frequently in France and the United Kingdom. There was an overall female preponderance with a male to female ratio of 1:1.4. The peak mortality of CJD occurred in the 70–79 years age group with a decline over 80 years of age (Will *et al.* 1998), see chapter 16 for further details.

Post-mortem examination usually reveals terminal bronchopneumonia and otherwise normal internal organs in a wasted body. The brain often shows diffuse or focal atrophy or occasionally may be normal; in several cases the weight may be 1000 g or less. The neurodegenerative process affects the cortical ribbon and the deep grey structures and according to the topographical distribution of the lesions, cortical, corticospinal, cortico-striatal, cortico-striatospinal, and cortico-striatocerebellar forms have been distinguished. The histological features include spongiform change, neuronal loss, astrocytosis, microglial activation, and the deposition of the abnormal form of prion protein (Figures 10.25 and 10.26; see Plates 20 and 21). The spongiform degeneration is characterized by the formation of fine vacuoles of various sizes which may coalesce to form larger vacuoles and microcysts. This microcystic cavitation may lead to status spongiosus and in the most severe cases the cystic cortex collapses to form irregular clefts with obliteration of cortical architecture. Neuronal loss is variable and can be extremely severe and usually is accompanied by astrocytosis. The distribution of these abnormalities is variable and recent investigations have attempted to quantify these changes using computer-based image analysis (for review see Ironside 1998*a*). There is also increasing evidence of microglial activation indicating that microglial cells could produce harmful factors which mediate both astrocytosis and neuronal injury (von Eitzen *et al.* 1998).

Both the clinical symptomatology and the neuropathology of CJD show considerable variation and this phenotypic heterogeneity is determined by the genotype, including the type and the pattern of deposition, of abnormal prion protein. For example, in sporadic CJD amyloid plaques, most frequently found in the cerebellum, occur in approximately 10% of

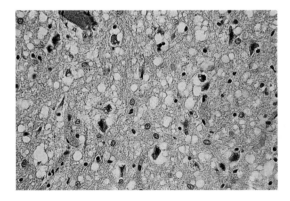
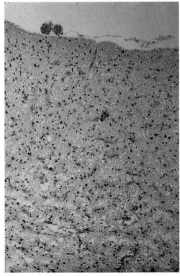

Figure 10.25 Neuronal loss and vacuolation (status spongiosus) in the frontal lobe (left) and caudate nucleus (right) of Creutzfeldt–Jakob disease. Haematoxylin and eosin.

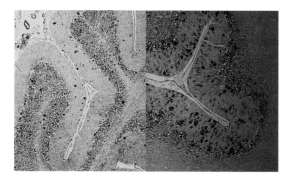

Figure 10.26 Prion protein deposition in the cerebellum of sporadic CJD on the left and vCJD on the right for comparison. The prion load is much greater in vCJD and is particularly striking in the molecular layer. Prion protein (12F10) imunohistochemistry.

those patients who have one or more valine alleles at codon 129 in the prion protein gene (de Silva *et al.* 1994).

6.2 Fatal familial insomnia

This is a dominantly inherited form of prion disease, originally reported in two unrelated families (Lugaresi *et al.* 1986; Medori *et al.* 1992*a, b*). In FFI a D178N mutation occurs on an allele which encodes methionine at position 129. However, if valine is encoded at 129 on the mutated allele, the result will be a familial CJD, with a different clinical and neuropathological phenotype. The disease is characterized clinically by severe and untreatable insomnia, disorders of the autonomic nervous system, endocrine disturbances, and motor signs. Neuropathologically, the lesions are restricted chiefly to the thalamus and there is selective atrophy of the anterior-ventral and medial-dorsal thalamic nuclei. There is neuronal loss and striking astrocytosis while spongiform change is usually mild. The clinical features (Montagna *et al.* 1998), the pathophysiology (Lugaresi *et al.* 1998), and the molecular pathology (Parchi *et al.* 1998) of FFI have all been reviewed.

6.3 Gerstmann-Sträussler-Scheinker disease

GSSD is an extremely rare neurodegenerative disease with an incidence of 2–5 persons per 100 million (Hsiao and Prusiner 1991). Currently there are at least six dominant inherited disorders

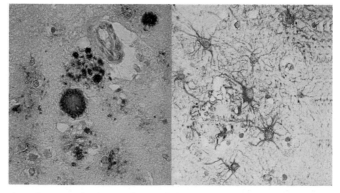

Figure 10.27 A prion plaque in the brain of vCJD (left) and associated reactive astrocytosis (right). Glial fibrillary acidic protein immunohistochemistry.

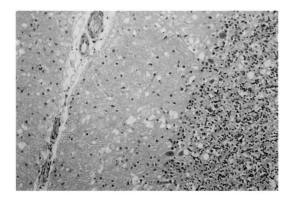

Figure 10.28 Neuronal loss and vacuolation in the molecular, Purkinje, and granule cell layers of the cerebellum of vCJD.

which can be described under this name, all with different neuropathology, different clinical presentation, and linkage to a different mutation of the prion gene (DeArmond and Prusiner 1998). In addition, many other pathogenic point and insertional mutations have been identified in the PrP gene; again, these are associated with different clinical and neuropathological phenotypes (DeArmond and Prusiner 1998; Collinge and Palmer 1997; Prusiner 1998). The disease is characterized by extensive plaque formation and varying degrees of spongiform degeneration, neuronal loss, and astrocytosis. The cerebellum is usually most severely affected. The plaques typically associated with GSSD are multicentric. In one variety of GSSD with the genotype of F198S there is evidence of neurofibrillary tangle formation suggesting an overlap with Alzheimer's disease (Ghetti *et al.* 1989).

The neuropathological manifestations of inherited prion disease can vary, not only in families with different mutations, but also amongst members of the same family with the same mutation. For example, members of a family with an insertional mutation of 144 base pairs in the prion gene showed extremes of pathology ranging from having practically no histological abnormalities to severe and typical changes of neuronal loss, spongiform change, and astrocytosis. However, all members of the family showed deposition of PrP (Figure 10.29; see Plate 24) (Collinge *et al.* 1992; Lantos 1992*b*).

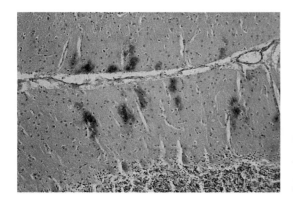

Figure 10.29 Typical prion protein deposits in the molecular layer of the cerebellum in familial prion disease with a 144 base pair insertion in the prion gene. Prion protein (12F10) imunohistochemistry.

6.4 Iatrogenic CJD

Man-to-man infection as iatrogenic transmission via corneal transplants, stereotactic electrodes, dural grafts, and pituitary hormones have been documented. The use of infected stereotactic electrodes was demonstrated in a young man of 17 years and a woman of 23 years who developed CJD after they had been treated by stereotactic surgery for intractable epilepsy. The electrodes used at the operation had been previously implanted into the brain of a 60-year-old woman who had suffered from CJD. The young man died demented aged 19 of CJD, whilst in the case of the woman the clinical diagnosis was supported by EEG (Bernoulli *et al.* 1977). A review of 71 cases with dural graft and 4 cases of corneal transplants has shown that these cases are different from CJD resulting from human growth hormone injections and from the new variant and they are more like sporadic cases. However, the mean age of the dural cases was two decades younger, at 37.7 years, than the sporadic cases and the duration of illness was at 10 months, 5 months shorter than sporadic cases. Clinically, memory loss, disorders of higher cerebral functions, and extrapyramidal signs were fewer, whereas cerebellar abnormalities were more frequent. Genotypic characterization of these cases has revealed that all patients with one exception, receiving corneal or dural grafts who developed CJD and examined for codon 129 polymorphism, were homozygous for methionine or valine (Lang *et al.* 1998).

In 1985, patients who developed and died from CJD following the administration of human growth hormone were reported, both in the United States and in the United Kingdom (for review see Lantos 1992*b*; Collinge and Palmer 1997; Ironside 1998*a*). Of 34 cases of CJD caused by growth hormone, the mean age of onset was 9.6 years, and the mean duration of illness 17 months (Lang *et al.* 1998). The clinical onset was dominated by kuru-like cerebellar syndromes and all presented with dementia (see chapter 16). There are histological differences from classical CJD: the cerebellum tends to be severely involved and plaque formation is usually prominent. In addition to human growth hormone cases, there have been a few cases of CJD among recipients of gonadotrophins for the treatment of infertility (Preece 1991). Again there is evidence for genetic susceptibility to iatrogenic CJD caused by pituitary growth hormone. Initially an excess of codon 129 homozygotes, particularly for valine, has been reported (Collinge *et al.* 1991). A more recent review of 34 cases indicates a 64% homozygosity for methionine (Lang *et al.* 1998).

6.5 Kuru

Kuru, now chiefly of historical interest, occurred mainly in the Fore tribe in the Eastern Highlands of Papua New Guinea and was transmitted by cannibalism. Macroscopically, the cerebral hemispheres may look normal or slightly atrophied, however, the most striking feature is the cerebellar atrophy, particularly the phylogenetically older parts of the vermis and folliculonodular lobe. Histologically, there is loss of Purkinje and granular cells with astrocytosis and fibrillary gliosis throughout the cerebellar cortex and microglial response in the molecular layers. Amyloid plaques are abundant. The cerebral cortex may show slight spongiform degeneration and there is evidence of severe degeneration of the olivo-ponto-cerebellar system (Beck and Daniel 1979). Many neurons in the caudate nucleus and in the putamen contain intracytoplasmic vacuoles. PrP positive plaques are most numerous in the granular layer of the cerebellum but are also found in the Purkinje cell and molecular layer (Figure 10.30; see Plate 25). The neuropathology of kuru has been compared with that of the vCJD on the basis that both types of prion disease are apparently caused by the same route of transmission, i.e. oral ingestion of infected material. These

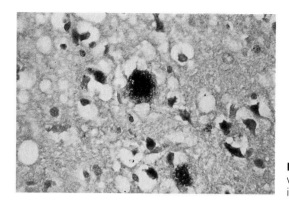

Figure 10.30   A prion plaque surrounded by vacuoles in kuru. Prion protein (12F10) imunohistochemistry.

comparative studies have showed both similarities and differences, both in the general histopathology, as well as in the distribution and type of prion deposits (Lantos *et al.* 1997; Hainfellner *et al.* 1997; McLean *et al.* 1998).

6.6 New variant of Creutzfeldt–Jakob disease

In 1996 ten cases of Creutzfeldt–Jakob disease were reported with unusual clinical and pathological features. The disease developed in a younger age group with a mean age of 26 years (ranging from 16–39 years). The duration of the disease was also longer, with an average of 14 months, than the typical sporadic cases. The vCJD presented with psychiatric symptoms including behavioural and personality changes, depression and sensory symptoms with paraesthesiae, followed by ataxia, and other movement disorders, including myoclonus, chorea, pyramidal, and extrapyramidal signs. Dementia with akinetic mutism, as typical of sporadic disease, developed only in the terminal stages (see chapter 16). Interestingly, none of the patients showed the characteristic electro-encephalogram of sporadic CJD. Moreover, they all were methionine homozygous at codon 129 of the prion protein gene (Will *et al.* 1996). Macroscopically the brains may appear normal, or there may be a tissue loss of up to 10%. There are the usual features of CJD, including spongiform change, neuronal loss, astrocytosis, and amyloid plaques, however, the pattern of pathology is different from sporadic cases. The involvement of the cortex is variable, but the occipital cortex is most severely affected. Although the basal ganglia are not significantly atrophied, the spongiform change is striking, particularly in the caudate nucleus. The thalamus is severely damaged, chiefly the dorsal medial nuclei and the pulvinar. In the hippocampus the spongiform change is not a feature but there are small amyloid plaques. The cerebellar involvement is always striking and there is spongiform change in the molecular layer and considerable, but variable, loss of Purkinje cells and granular neurons. There are also amyloid plaques including florid plaques in which the dense core is surrounded by a halo of vacuoles. There is extensive deposition of prion protein as demonstrated by immunohistochemistry, including plaque formations and more diffuse deposits (Figures 10.27 and 10.29; see Plates 22 and 23). The pericellular and perivascular pattern to be seen in the cerebral and cerebellar cortex are not to be found in sporadic CJD (for review see Ironside 1998*b*). The association of the new variant of CJD with bovine spongiform encephalopathy has been established beyond reasonable doubt (Collinge *et al.* 1996; Bruce *et al.* 1997; Hill *et al.* 1997; and will be reviewed elsewhere in this book).

7 Key points

1   The macroscopic and histological changes associated with early onset dementia are typically more severe than in those cases with a late onset. The naked eye appearance of the brain may vary, however, from the grossly atrophied to the unremarkable.

2   In affected areas of the brain there is neuronal loss and a reactive astrocytosis. In addition, characteristic neuronal and glial inclusions or abnormal aggregates of extracellular protein may be found which may be pathognomonic of a particular neurodegenerative disorder.

3   Standard histological stains reveal frank neurodegeneration but the inclusions and abnormal proteins characteristic of each disease are best demonstrated by immunohistochemistry.

4   The atrophy associated with Alzheimer's disease is generally diffuse and symmetrical. Microscopic examination with silver impregnation reveals intracellular neurofibrillary tangles and extracellular neuritic plaques. Neurofibrillary tangles contain paired helical filaments, which are composed of abnormal accumulations of hyperphosphorylated tau protein. Neuritic plaques contain dystrophic neurites and deposits of β-amyloid. Deposits of β-amyloid of varying morphologies are found within the parenchyma of the brain and commonly in the cerebral vessels, causing amyloid angiopathy. The temporal lobe is usually the most severely affected but all lobes may show Alzheimer-type changes.

5   The substantia nigra is pale, reflecting neuronal loss, in Parkinson's disease and dementia with Lewy bodies. Lewy bodies are found within the substantia nigra and at varying densities in the neocortex. These neuronal inclusions 15–30 μm in diameter are labelled by anti-ubiquitin antibodies but are best demonstrated by α-synuclein immunohistochemistry. Abnormal accumulations of α-synuclein are also found in dystrophic neurites in areas also affected by Lewy bodies.

6   There are five pathological entities associated with frontotemporal dementia. Pick's disease is characterized neuropathologically by frontotemporal atrophy, swollen achromatic neurons, and ubiquitin and tau positive neuronal inclusions called Pick bodies. Corticobasal degeneration has, typically, large swollen achromatic neurons in the cortex and to a lesser extent in the deep grey matter, neuronal inclusions in the substantia nigra and elsewhere in the deep grey matter, and tau positive glial, chiefly astrocytic inclusions in the frontal and parietal lobes. In motor neuron disease-associated dementia, in addition to neuronal loss and astrocytosis in the frontotemporal cortex, there are ubiquitin positive but tau negative neuronal inclusions. Frontotemporal dementia and parkinsonism linked to chromosome 17 (FTDP-17), defined by molecular genetics, is neuropathologically heterogeneous but has tau positive inclusions that overlap morphologically with Pick's disease, corticobasal degeneration, and progressive supranuclear palsy. There is a fifth group, frontal lobe degeneration of non-Alzheimer type, that has neuronal loss and astrocytosis in the context of frontotemporal atrophy but no hallmark lesion.

7   The cerebral hemispheres may be atrophied in Huntington's disease but the most striking macroscopic change is shrinkage of the caudate nucleus and the putamen. Neuronal loss and astrocytosis are associated with abnormal intranuclear inclusions of the protein huntingtin.

8   The neuropathological changes found in progressive supranuclear palsy include tau positive neurofibrillary tangles, neuronal loss, astrocytosis, and tau positive glial inclusions. The distribution, biochemistry, and ultrastructure of these neurofibrillary tangles are different from those in Alzheimer's disease. Although predominantly neocortical structures are affected in supranuclear palsy, the cerebral cortex, particularly if the frontal lobe is also involved.

9   There are four human prion diseases. The Creutzfeldt–Jakob disease (CJD) brain may show diffuse or focal atrophy. The histological features include neuronal loss, status spongiosus, astrocytosis, and abnormal prion deposition in the grey matter. There is often striking prion immunoreactivity in the cerebellum. In fatal familial insomnia the lesions are restricted chiefly to the thalamus. Gerstmann-Sträussler-Scheinker disease (GSSD) is characterized by extensive amyloid plaque formation and varying degrees of spongiform degeneration, neuronal loss, and astrocytosis. Plaques typically associated with GSSD are multicentric. There is neuropathological heterogeneity not only between individuals with the same mutation but also between members of the same family. Transmission of the infectious agent via surgical procedures and pituitary hormone replacement therapy may

produce iatrogenic CJD. A rare form of prion disease is kuru, found mainly in the Fore tribe of Papua New Guinea and spread by cannibalism. The striking feature of kuru is cerebellar atrophy, with numerous prion plaques in the granular layer. Neuropathologically, kuru has been compared with the new variant of Creutzfeldt–Jakob disease (vCJD), as both are likely to have been caused by the ingestion of infected material. There are similarities and differences in the distribution and type of prion deposit between kuru and vCJD but quantitative studies indicate a greater prion load in vCJD than in kuru.

References

Anderson, V. E. R., Cairns, N. J., and Leigh, P. N. (1995). Involvement of the amygdala, dentate and hippocampus in motor neuron disease. *Journal of the Neurological Sciences*, **129**, 75–8.

Armstrong, R. A., Cairns, N. J., Myers, D., Smith, C. U. M., Lantos, P. L., and Rossor, M. N. (1996). A comparison of β-amyloid deposition in the medial temporal lobe in sporadic Alzheimer's disease, Down's syndrome and normal elderly brains. *Neurodegeneration*, **5**, 35–41.

Armstrong, R. A., Cairns, N. J., and Lantos, P. L. (1997). Dementia with Lewy bodies in human patients. *Neuroscience Letters*, **224**, 41–4.

Armstrong, R. A., Cairns, N. J., and Lantos, P. L. (1998*a*). The spatial pattern of β-amyloid (Aβ) deposits in Alzheimer's disease patients is related to apolipoprotein genotype. *Neuroscience Research Communications*, **22**, 99–106.

Armstrong, R. A., Cairns, N. J., and Lantos, P. L. (1998*b*). Clustering of Pick bodies in patients with Pick's disease. *Neuroscience Letters*, **242**, 81–4.

Bancher, C., Lassmann, H., Budka, H., Grundke-Iqbal, I., Iqbal, K., and Wiche, G. (1987). Neurofibrillary tangles in Alzheimer's disease and progressive supranuclear palsy: antigenic similarities and differences. *Acta Neuropathologica*, **74**, 39–46.

Beach, T. G., Walker, R., and McGeer, E. G. (1989). Patterns of gliosis in Alzheimer's disease and aging cerebrum. *Glia*, **2**, 420–36.

Becher, M. W., Kotzuk, J. A., Sharp, A. H., Davies, S. W., Bates, G. P., Price, D. L., *et al.* (1998). Intranuclear neuronal inclusions in Huntington's disease and dentatorubral and pallidoluysian atrophy: correlation between the density of inclusions and IT15 CAG triplet repeat length. *Neurobiology of Diseases*, **4**, 387–97.

Beck, E. and Daniel, P. M. (1979). Kuru and Creutzfeldt–Jakob disease: neuropathological lesions and their significance. *Slow transmissible diseases of the nervous system*, Vol. 1, pp. 253–70. Academic Press, London.

Bergeron, C., Davis, A., and Lang, A. E. (1998). Corticobasal ganglionic degeneration and progressive supranuclear palsy with cognitive decline. *Brain Pathology*, **8**, 355–65.

Bernoulli, C., Siegfried, J., Baumgartner, G., Regli, F., Rabinowicz, T., Gajdusek, D. C., *et al.* (1977). Danger of accidental person-to-person transmission of Creutzfeldt–Jakob disease by surgery. *Lancet*, **i**, 478–9.

Boller, F., Lopez, O. L., and Moossy, J. (1989). Diagnosis of dementia: clinicopathologic correlations. *Neurology*, **39**, 76–9.

Bower, J. H., Maraganore, D. M., McDonnell, S. K., and Rocca, W. A. (1997). Incidence of progressive supranuclear palsy and multiple system atrophy in Olsted County, Minnesota, 1976–1990. *Neurology*, **48**, A299.

Braak, H., Braak, E., Grundke-Iqbal, I., and Iqbal, K. (1986). Occurrence of neuropil thread, in the senile human brain and in Alzheimer's disease: a third location of paired helical filaments outside of neurofibrillary tangles and neuritic plaques. *Neuroscience Letters*, **65**, 351–5.

Brown, J., Lantos, P., Stratton, M., Roques, P., and Rossor, M. (1993). Familial progressive supranuclear palsy. *Journal of Neurology, Neurosurgery and Psychiatry*, **56**, 473–6.

Bruce, M. E., Will, R. G., Ironside, J. W., McConnell, I., Drummond, D., Suttie, A., *et al.* (1997). Transmissions to mice indicate that 'new variant' CJD is caused by the BSE agent. *Nature*, **389**, 498–501.

Brun, A. and Englund, E. (1986). A white matter disorder in dementia of the Alzheimer type: a pathoanatomical study. *Annals of Neurology*, **19**, 253–62.

Brun, A., Englund, B., Gustafson, L., Passant, U., Mann, D. M. A., Neary, D., *et al.* (1994). Clinical and neuropathological criteria for frontotemporal dementia. *Journal of Neurology, Neurosurgery and Psychiatry*, **57**, 416–18.

Burns, A., Luthert, P. J., Levy, R., Jacoby, R., and Lantos, P. L. (1990). Accuracy of clinical diagnosis in Alzheimer's disease. *British Medical Journal*, **301**, 1026.

Cairns, N. J., Chadwick, A., Luthert, P. J., and Lantos, P. L. (1992). Astrocytosis, βA4-protein deposition and paired helical filament formation in Alzheimer's disease. *Journal of the Neurological Sciences*, **112**, 68–75.

Cairns, N. J., Fukutani, Y., Chadwick, A., Barnes, H., Holmes, C., and Lantos, P. L. (1997*a*). Apolipoprotein E, β-amyloid (Aβ), phosphorylated tau and apolipoprotein E genotype in Alzheimer's disease. *Alzheimer's Research*, **3**, 109–14.

Cairns, N. J., Atkinson, P. F., Hanger, D. P., Anderton, B. H., Daniel, S. E., and Lantos, P. L. (1997*b*). Tau protein in the glial cytoplasmic inclusions of multiple system atrophy can be distinguished from abnormal tau in Alzheimer's disease. *Neuroscience Letters*, **230**, 49–52.

Cammarata, S., Caponnetto, C., and Tabaton, M. (1993). Ubiquitin-reative neurites in cerebral cortex of subjects of Huntington's chorea: a pathological correlate of dementia? *Neuroscience Letters*, **156**, 96–8.

Collinge, J., Palmer, M. S., and Dryden, A. J. (1991). Genetic predisposition to iatrogenic Creutzfeldt–Jakob disease. *Lancet*, **337**, 1441–2.

Collinge, J., Brown, J., Hardy, J., Mullan, M., Rossor, M. N., Baker, H., *et al.* (1992). Inherited prion disease with 144 base pair gene insertion. 2. Clinical and pathological features. *Brain*, **115**, 687–710.

Collinge, J. and Palmer, M. S. (1997). Human prion diseases. In *Prion diseases* (ed. J. Collinge and M. S. Palmer), pp. 18–56. Oxford University Press, Oxford.

Collinge, J., Miles, A.-J., Whittington, M. A., Sidle, K. C. L., Smith, C. J., Palmer, M. S., *et al.* (1994). Prion protein is necessary for normal synaptic function. *Nature*, **370**, 295–7.

Collinge, J., Sidle, K. C. L., Meads, J., Ironside, J. W., and Hill, A. F. (1996). Molecular analysis of prion strain variation and the aetiology of 'new variant' CJD. *Nature*, **383**, 685–90.

Conrad, C., Amano, N., Andreadis, A., Xia, Y., Namekataf, K., Oyama, F., *et al.* (1998). Differences in a dinucleotide repeat polymorphism in the tau gene between Caucasian and Japanese populations: implications for progressive supranuclear palsy. *Neuroscience Letters*, **250**, 135–7.

Conrad, C., Andreadis, A., Trojanowski, J. Q., Dickson, D. W., Kang, D., Chen, X., *et al.* (1997). Genetic evidence for the involvement of τ in progressive supranuclear palsy. *Annals of Neurology*, **41**, 277–81.

Cooper, P. N., Siddons, C. A., and Mann, D. M. A. (1996). Patterns of glial cell activity in fronto-temporal dementia (lobar atrophy). *Neuropathology and Applied Neurobiology*, **22**, 17–22.

Crowther, R. A. (1991). Straight and paired helical filaments in Alzheimer's disease have a common structural unit. *Procdings of the National Acadamy of Sciences of the United States of America*, **88**, 2288–92.

Crowther, R. A. and Wischik, C. M. (1985). Image reconstruction of the Alzheimer paired helical filament. *EMBO Journal*, **4**, 3661–5.

Cruz-Sánchez, F. F., Ravid, R., and Cuzner, M. L. (1995). The European Brain Bank Network (EBBN) and the need of standardized neuropathological criteria for brain tissue cataloguing. In *Neuropathological diagnostic criteria for brain banking* (ed. F. F. Cruz-Sánchez, R. Ravid, and M. L. Cuzner), pp. 1–3. IOS Press, Oxford.

Dale, G. E., Probst, A., Luthert, P., Martin, J., Anderton, B. H., and Leigh, P. N. (1992). Relationship between Lewy bodies and pale bodies in Parkinson's disease. *Acta Neuropathologica*, **83**, 525–9.

Daniel, S. E. (1995). Parkinson's disease. In *Neuropathological diagnostic criteria for brain banking* (ed. F. F. Cruz-Sanchez, R. Ravid, and M. L. Cuzner). IOS Press, Oxford.

Daniel, S. E., de Bruin, V. M., and Lees, A. J. (1995). The clinical and pathological spectrum of Steele-Richardson-Olszewski syndrome (progressive supranuclear palsy): a reappraisal. *Brain*, **118**, 759–70.

Davies, P. (1986). The genetics of Alzheimer's disease: a review and a discussion of the implications. *Neurobiology of Aging*, **7**, 459.

DeArmond, S. J. and Prusiner, S. B. (1998). Prion diseases. In *Neuropathology of dementing disorders* (ed. W. R. Markesbery), pp. 340–76. Arnold, London.

Delacourte, A., Robitaille, Y., Sergeant, N., Buée, L., Hof, P. R., Wattez, A., et al. (1996). Specific pathological tau protein variants characterise Pick's disease. *Journal of Neuropathology and Experimental Neurology*, **55**, 159–68.

De la Monte, S. M., Vonsattel, J. P., and Richardson, E. P. (1988). Morphometric demonstration of atrophic changes in the cerebral cortex, white matter, and neostriatum in Huntington's disease. *Journal of Neuropathology and Experimental Neurology*, **47**, 516–25.

De la Monte, S. M., Sohn, Y. K., Ganju, N., and Wands, J. R. (1998). p53 and CD95-associated apoptosis in neurodegenerative diseases. *Laboratory Investigation*, **78**, 401–11.

de Silva, R., Ironside, J. W., McCardle, L., Esmonde, T. G. F., Bell, J. E., Will, R. G., et al. (1994). Neuropathological phenotype and 'prion protein' genotype correlation in sporadic Creutzfeldt–Jakob disease. *Neuroscience Letters*, **179**, 50–2.

Esiri, M. M. and McShane, R. H. (1997). Parkinson's disease and dementia. In *The neuropathology of dementia* (ed. M. M. Esiri and J. H. Morris). Cambridge University Press, Cambridge.

Esiri, M. M. and Morris, J. H. (ed.) (1997). *The neuropathology of dementia*. Cambridge University Press, Cambridge.

European Concerted Action on Pick's Disease (ECAPD) Consortium (1998). Provisional clinical and neuroradiological criteria for the diagnosis of Pick's disease. *European Journal of Neurology*, **5**, 519–20.

Fearnley, J. M. and Lees, A. J. (1991). Ageing and Parkinson's disease: substantia nigra regional selectivity. *Brain*, **114**, 2283–301.

Foster, N. L., Wilhelmsen, K., Sima, A. A. F., Jones, M. Z., D'Amato, C. J., Gilman, S., et al. (1997). Frontotemporal dementia and parkinsonism linked to chromosome 17: a consensus conference. *Annals of Neurology*, **41**, 706–15.

Fukutani, Y., Cairns, N. J., Rossor, M. N., and Lantos, P. L. (1996). Purkinje cell loss and astrocytosis in the cerebellum in familial and sporadic Alzheimer's disease. *Neuroscience Letters*, **214**, 33–6.

Fukutani, Y., Cairns, N. J., Rossor, M. N., and Lantos, P. L. (1997). Cerebellar pathology in sporadic and familial Alzheimer's disease including APP 717(val-ile) mutation cases: a morphometric investigation. *Journal of the Neurological Sciences*, **149**, 177–84.

Galloway, P. G., Mulvihill, P., and Perry, G. (1992). Filaments of Lewy bodies contain insoluble cytoskeletal elements. *American Journal of Pathology*, **47**, 654–63.

Gallyas, F. (1971). Silver staining of Alzheimer's neurofibrillary changes by means of physical development. *Acta Morphologica Academiae Scientiarum Hungaricae*, **19**, 1–8.

Gazeley, S. and Maguire, J. A. (1996). Familial progressive supranuclear palsy. *Clinical Neuropathology*, **15**, 215–20.

Gearing, M., Olson, D. A., Watts, R. L., and Mirra, S. S. (1994). Progressive supranuclear palsy: neuropathologic and clinical heterogeneity. *Neurology*, **44**, 1015–24.

Gentleman, S. M., Bruton, C., Allsop, D., Lewis, S. J., Polak, J. M., and Roberts, G. W. (1989). A demonstration of the advantages of immunostaining in the quantification of amyloid plaque deposits. *Histochemistry*, **92**, 355–8.

Ghetti, B., Tagliavini, F., Masters, C. L., Beyreuther, K., Giaccone, G., Verga, L., et al. (1989). Gerstmann-Sträussler-Scheinker disease. II. Neurofibrillary tangles and plaques with PrP-amyloid coexist in an affected family. *Neurology*, **39**, 1453–61.

Gibb, W. R. G., Luthert, P. J., and Marsden C. D. (1989a). Corticobasal degeneration. *Brain*, **112**, 1171–92.

Gibb, W. R. G., Mountjoy, C. Q., Mann, D. M., and Lees, A. J. (1989b). A pathological study of the association between Lewy body disease and Alzheimer's disease. *Journal of Neurology, Neurosurgery and Psychiatry*, **52**, 701–8.

Glenner, G. G. and Wong, C. W. (1984). Alzheimer's disease and Down's syndrome: sharing of a unique cerebrovascular amyloid fibril. *Biochemical and Biophysical Research Communications*, **122**, 1131–5.

Goate, A., Chartier-Harlin, M. C., Mullan, M., Brown, J., Crawford, F., Fidani, L., et al. (1991). Segregation of a missense mutation in the amyloid precursor protein gene with familial Alzheimer's disease. *Nature*, **349**, 704–6.

Goedert, M., Spillantini, M. G., Cairns, N. J., and Crowther, R. A. (1991). Tau proteins of Alzheimer paired helical filaments: abnormal phosphorylation of all six isoforms. *Neuron*, **8**, 159–68.

Golbe, L. I., Davis, P. H., Schoenberg, B. S., and Duvosin, R. C. (1988). Prevalence and natural history of progressive supranuclear palsy. *Neurology*, **38**, 1031–4.

Gonatas, N. K., Anderson, A., and Vongelista, I. (1967). The contribution of altered synapses in the senile plaque: an electronmicroscopic study in Alzheimer's dementia. *Journal of Neuropathology and Experimental Neurology*, **26**, 25–39.

Hainfellner, J. A., Liberski, P. P., Guiroy, D. C., Cervanáková, L., Brown, P., Gajdusek, D. C., *et al.* (1997). Pathology and immunocytochemistry of kuru brain. *Brain Pathology*, **7**, 547–53.

Hanger, D. P., Brion, J.-P., Gallo, J.-M., Cairns, N. J., Luthert, P. J., and Anderton, B. H. (1991). Tau in Alzheimer's disease and Down's syndrome is insoluble and abnormally phosphorylated. *Biochemical Journal*, **275**, 99–104.

Hauw, J.-J., Verny, M., Delaàre, P., Cervera, Y., and Duyckaerts, C. (1990). Constant neurofibrillary changes in the neocortex in progressive supranuclear palsy. Basic differences with Alzheimer's disease and aging. *Neuroscience Letters*, **119**, 182–6.

Hauw, J.-J., Duyckaerts, C., and Delaère, P. (1991). Alzheimer's disease. In *The pathology of the aging nervous system* (ed. S. Duckett), pp. 113–47. Lea and Febiger, London.

Hauw, J.-J., Daniel, S. E., Horoupian, D. S., Jellinger, K., Lantos, P. L., McKee, A., *et al.* (1994). Preliminary NINDS neuropathologic criteria for Steele-Richardson-Olszewski syndrome (progressive supranuclear palsy). *Neurology*, **44**, 2015–19.

Hauw, J.-J., Verny, M., Ruberg, M., and Duyckaerts, C. (1998). Progressive supranuclear palsy. In *Neuropathology of dementing disorders* (ed. W. R. Markesbery), pp. 219–56. Arnold, London.

Hill, A. F., Desbrulais, M., Joiner, S., Sidle, K. C. L., Gowland, I., Collinge, J., *et al.* (1997). The same prion strain causes vCJD and BSE. *Nature*, **389**, 448–50.

Hirsch, E. C., Graybiel, A. M., Duckyaerts, C., and Javoy-Agid, F. (1987). Neuronal loss in the pedunculopontine tegmental nucleus in Parkinson's disease and in progressive supranuclear palsy. *Proceedings of the National Academy of Sciences of the United States of America*, **84**, 5976–80.

Hsiao, K. and Prusiner, S. B. (1991). Molecular genetics and transgenic model of Gerstmann-Sträussler-Scheinker disease. *Alzheimer Disease and Associated Disorders*, **5**, 155–62.

Hughes, A. J., Daniel, S. E., Kilford, L., and Lees, A. J. (1992). Accuracy of clinical diagnosis of idiopathic Parkinson's disease: a clinico-pathological study of 100 cases. *Journal of Neurology, Neurosurgery and Psychiatry*, **55**, 181–4.

Hutton, M., Lendon, C. L., Rizzu, P., Baker, M., Froelich, S., Houlden, H., *et al.* (1998). Association of missence and 5′-splice-site mutations in tau with the inherited dementia FTDP-17. *Nature*, **393**, 702–5.

Hyman, B. T. and Trojanowski, J. Q. (1997). Editorial on consensus recommendations for the postmortem diagnosis of Alzheimer disease from the National Institute on Aging and the Reagan Institute Working Group on diagnostic criteria for the neuropathological assessment of Alzheimer's disease. *Journal of Neuropathology and Experimental Neurology*, **56**, 1095–7.

Ince, P. G., Lowe, J., and Shaw, P. J. (1998). Amyotrophic lateral sclerosis: current issues in classification, pathogenesis and molecular pathology. *Neuropathology and Applied Neurobiology*, **24**, 104–17.

Ironside, J. W. (1998*a*). Prion diseases in man. *Journal of Pathology*, **186**, 227–34.

Ironside, J. W. (1998*b*). New-variant Creutzfeldt–Jakob disease. *Neuropathology*, **18**, 131–8.

Iseki, E., Matsushita, M., Kosaka, K., Kondo, H., Ishii, T., and Amano, N. (1990). Morphological characteristics of senile plaques in familial Alzheimer's disease. *Acta Neuropathologica*, **80**, 227–32.

Itagakai, S., McGeer, P. L., Akiyama, H., Zhu, S., and Selkoe, D. (1989). Relationship of microglia and astrocytes to amyloid deposits of Alzheimer's disease. *Journal of Neuroimmunology*, **24**, 173–82.

Jackson, M., Gentleman, S., Lennox, G., Ward, L., Gray, T., Randall, K., *et al.* (1995). The cortical neuritic pathology of Huntington's disease. *Neuropathology and Applied Neurobiology*, **21**, 18–26.

Jackson, M., Lennox, G., and Lowe, J. (1996). Motor neurone disease-inclusion dementia. *Neurodegeneration*, **5**, 339–50.

Jackson, M. and Lowe, J. (1996). The new neuropathology of degenerative frontotemporal dementias. *Acta Neuropathologica*, **91**, 127–34.

Jellinger, K. and Brancher, C. (1992). Neuropathology. In *Progressive supranuclear palsy, clinical and research approaches* (ed. I. Litvan and Y. Agid), pp. 44–88. Oxford University Press, New York.

Joachim, C. L., Mori, H., and Selkoe, D. J. (1989*a*). Amyloid β-protein deposition in tissues other than brain in Alzheimer's disease. *Nature*, **341**, 226–30.

Joachim, C. L., Morris, J. H., and Selkoe, D. J. (1989*b*). Diffuse senile plaques occur commonly in the cerebellum in Alzheimer's disease. *American Journal of Pathology*, **135**, 309–19.

Kidd, M. (1963). Paired helical filaments in electron microscopy of Alzheimer's disease. *Nature*, **197**, 192–3.

Kiuchi, A., Otsuka, N., Namba, Y., Nakano, I., and Tomonaga, M. (1991). Presenile appearance of abundant neurofibrillary tangles without senile plaques in the brain in myotonic dystrophy. *Acta Neuropathologica*, **82**, 1–5.

Komori, T., Arai, N., Oda, M., Nakayama, H., Mori, H., Yagishita, S., *et al.* (1998). Astrocytic plaques and tufts of abnormal fibers do not coexist in corticobasal degeneration and progressive supranuclear palsy. (1998). *Acta Neuropathologica*, **96**, 401–8.

Kosaka, K. (1990). Diffuse Lewy body disease in Japan. *Journal of Neurology*, **237**, 197–204.

Kowall, N. W. and Ferrante, R. J. (1998). Huntington's disease. In *Neuropathology of dementing disorders* (ed. W. R. Markesbery), pp. 219–56. Arnold, London.

Kristensen, M. O. (1985). Progressive supranuclear palsy: 20 years later. *Acta Neurologica Scandinavica*, **71**, 177–89.

Lamb, B. T. (1997). Presenilins, amyloid-β and Alzheimer's disease. *Nature*, **3**, 28–9.

Lang, C. J. G., Hechmann, J. G., and Neundörfer, B. (1998). Creutzfeldt–Jakob disease via dural and corneal transplants. *Journal of the Neurological Sciences*, **160**, 128–39.

Lantos, P. L. (1992*a*). Neuropathology of unusual dementias: an overview. In *Baillière's clinical neurology*, Vol. 1, No. 3. Unusual Dementias (ed. M. N. Rossor), pp. 485–516. Baillière Tindall, London.

Lantos, P. L. (1992*b*). From slow virus to prion: a review of transmissible spongiform encephalopathies. *Histopathology*, **20**, 1–11.

Lantos, P. L. (1994). The neuropathology of progressive supranuclear palsy. *Journal of Neural Transmission*, **42**, 137–52.

Lantos, P. L. (1998). The definition of multiple system atrophy: a review of recent developments. *Journal of Neuropathology and Experimental Neurology*, **57**, 1099–111.

Lantos, P. L. (1999). Cracking an enigma: the puzzle of unusual dementias. In *Alzheimer's Disease and Related Disorders*, (ed K. Iqbal, D. F. Swaab, B. Winblad and H. M. Wisniewski) pp. 519–22. John Wiley & Son Ltd, London.

Lantos, P. L., Bhatia, K., Doey, L. J., Al-Sarraj, S., Doshi, R., Beck, J., *et al.* (1997). Is the neuropathology of new variant Creutzfeldt–Jakob disease and kuru similar? *Lancet*, **350**, 187–8.

Lantos, P. L., Luthert, P. J., Hanger, D., Anderton, M., and Rossor, M. (1992). Familial Alzheimer's disease with the amyloid precursor protein position 717 mutation and sporadic Alzheimer's disease have the same cytoskeletal pathology. *Neuroscience Letters*, **137**, 221–4.

Lantos, P. L., Ovenstone, I. M., Johnson, J., Clelland, C. A., Roques, P., and Rossor, M. N. (1994). Lewy bodies in the brain of two members of a family with the 717 (val to ile) mutation of the amyloid precursor protein gene. *Neuroscience Letters*, **172**, 77–9.

Leigh, P. N., Whitwell, H., Garofalo, O., Buller, J., Swash, M., Martin, J. E., *et al.* (1991). Ubiquitin-immunoreactive intraneuronal inclusions in amyotrophic lateral sclerosis. Morphology, distribution, and specificity. *Brain*, **114**, 775–8.

Litvan, I., Hauw, J. J., Bartko, J. J., Lantos, P. L., Daniel, S. E., Horoupian, D. S., *et al.* (1996). Validity and reliability of the preliminary NINDS neuropathologic criteria for progressive supranuclear palsy and related disorders. *Journal of Neuropathology and Experimental Neurology*, **55**, 97–105.

Lowe, J., Aldridge, F., Lennox, G., Doherty, F., Jefferson, D., Landon, M., *et al.* (1989). Inclusion bodies in motor cortex and brainstem of patients with motor neurone disease are detected by immunocytochemical localisation of ubiquitin. *Neuroscience Letters*, **105**, 7–13.

Lowe, J., Lennox, G., and Leigh, P. N. (1997). Disorders of movement and system degenerations. In *Greenfield's neuropathology* (ed. D. I. Graham and P. L. Lantos), pp. 281–366. Arnold, London.

Lugaresi, E., Medori, R., Baruzzi, P. M., Cortelli, P., Lugaresi, A., Tinuper, P., *et al.* (1986). Fatal familial insomnia and dysautonomia with selective degeneration of thalamic nuclei. *New England Journal of Medicine*, **315**, 997–1003.

Lugaresi, E., Tobler, I., Fambetti, P., and Montagna, P. (1998). The pathophysiology of fatal familial insomnia. *Brain Pathology*, **8**, 521–6.

Majocha, R. E., Benes, F. M., Reifel, J. L., Rodenrys, A. M., and Marotta, C. A. (1988). Laminar-specific distribution and infrastructural detail of amyloid in the Alzheimer's disease cortex visualised by computer-enhanced imaging of epitopes recognised by monoclonal antibodies. *Proceedings of the National Academy of Sciences of the United States of America*, **85**, 6182–6.

Malessa, S., Hirsch, E. C., Cervera, P., Javoy-Agid, F., Duyckaerts, C., and Hauw, J.-J. (1991). Progressive supranuclear palsy: loss of choline-acetyltransferase-like immunoreactive neurons in the pontine reticular formation. *Neurology*, **41**, 1593–7.

Mann, D. M. A., Iwatsubo, T., Cairns, N. J., Lantos, P. L., Nochlin, D., Sumi, S. M., *et al.* (1996a). Amyloid β protein (Aβ) deposition in chromosome 14-linked Alzheimer's disease: predominance of A$\beta_{42(43)}$. *Annals of Neurology*, **40**, 149–56.

Mann, D. M. A., Iwatsubo, T., Ihara, Y., Cairns, N. J., Lantos, P. L., Bogdanovic, N., *et al.* (1996b). Predominant deposition of amyloid-$\beta_{42(43)}$ in plaques in cases of Alzheimer's disease and hereditary cerebral haemorrhage associated with mutations in the amyloid precursor protein gene. *American Journal of Pathology*, **148**, 1257–66.

Mann, D., Oliver, R., and Snowden, J. (1993). The topographic distribution of brain atrophy in Huntington's disease and progressive supranuclear palsy. *Acta Neuropathologica*, **85**, 553–9.

Mann, D. M. A. (1998). Dementia of frontal type and dementias with subcortical gliosis. *Brain*, **8**, 325–38.

Mastaglia, F. L., Grainger, K., Kee, F., Sadka, M., and Lefray, R. (1973). Progressive supranuclear palsy (the Steele-Richardson-Olszewski syndrome): clinical and electrophysiological observations in eleven cases. *Proceedings of the Australian Association of Neurology*, **10**, 35–44.

Matsusaka, H., Ikeda, K., Akiyama, H., Arai, T., Inoue, M., and Yagishita, S. (1998). Astrocytic pathology in progressive supranuclear palsy: significance for neuropathological diagnosis. *Acta Neuropathologica*, **96**, 248–52.

McGeer, E. G. and McGeer, P. L. (1998). The importance of inflammatory mechanisms in Alzheimer's disease. *Experimental Gerontology*, **33**, 371–8.

McKeith, I. G., Galasko, G., Kosaka, K., Perry, E. K., and Dickson, D. W. (1996). Consensus guidelines for the clinical and pathologic diagnosis of dementia with Lewy bodies (DLB): report of the consortium on DLB international workshop. *Neurology*, **47**, 1113–24.

McLean, C. A., Ironside, J. W., Alpers, M. P., Brown, P. W., Cervenakova, L., Anderson, R. M., *et al.* (1998). Comparative neuropathology of kuru with the new variant of Creutzfeldt–Jakob disease: evidence for strain of agent predominating over genotype of host. *Brain Pathology*, **8**, 429–37.

Medori, R., Montagna, P., Tritschler, H. J., LeBlanc, A., Cortelli, P., Tinuper, P., *et al.* (1992a). Fatal familial insomnia: a second kindred with mutation of prion protein gene at codon 178. *Neurology*, **42**, 669–70.

Medori, R., Tritschler, H. J., LeBlanc, A., Villare, F., Manetto, V., Chen, H. Y., *et al.* (1992b). Fatal familial insomnia, a prion disease with a mutation at codon 178 of the prion protein gene. *New England Journal of Medicine*, **326**, 444–9.

Mirra, S. S., Heyman, A., McKeel, D., Sumi, S. M., Crain, B. J., Brownlee, L. M., *et al.* (1991). The consortium to establish a registry for Alzheimer's disease (CERAD). Part II. Standardisation of the neuropathologic assessment of Alzheimer's disease. *Neurology*, **41**, 479–86.

Montpetit, V., Clapin, D. F., and Guberman, A. (1985). Substructure of 20nm filaments of progressive supranuclear palsy. *Acta Neuropathologica*, **68**, 311–18.

Montagna, P., Cortelli, P., Avoni, P., Tinuper, P., Plazzi, G., Gallassi, R., *et al.* (1998). Clinical features of fatal familial insomnia: phenotypic variability in relation to a polymorphism at codon 129 of the prion protein gene. *Brain Pathology*, **8**, 515–20.

Mori, H. and Oda, M. (1997). Ballooned neurons in corticobasal degeneration and progressive supranuclear palsy. *Neuropathology*, **17**, 248–52.

Morita, K., Kaiya, H., Ikeda, T., and Namba, M. (1987). Presenile dementia combined with amyotrophy of review of 34 Japanese cases. *Archives of Gerontology and Geriatrics*, **6**, 263–77.

Morris, J. H. (1997). Alzheimer's disease. In *The neuropathy of dementia* (ed. M. M. Esiri and J. H. Morris), pp. 70–121. Cambridge University Press.

Nishimura, M., Namba, Y., Ikeda, K., and Oda, M. (1992). Glial fibrillay tangles with straight tubules in the brains of patients with progressive supranuclear palsy. *Neuroscience Letters*, **143**, 35–8.

Ogomori, K., Kitamoto, T., Tateishi, J., Sato, Y., Suetsugu, M., and Abe, M. (1989). β-protein amyloid is widely distributed in the central nervous system of patients with Alzheimer's disease. *American Journal of Pathology*, **134**, 243–51.

Okamoto, K., Hirai, S., Yamazaki, Y., Sun, X., and Nakazato, Y. (1991). New ubiquitin-positive intraneuronal inclusions in the extra-motor cortices in patients with amyotrophic lateral sclerosis. *Neuroscience Letters*, **129**, 233–6.

Okazaki, H., Lipkin, L. E., and Aronson, S. M. (1961). Diffuse intracytoplasmic ganglionic inclusion (Lewy type) associated with progressive dementia and quadriparesis in flexion. *Journal of Neuropathology and Experimental Neurology*, **20**, 237–44.

Oyanagi, K., Takahashi, H., Wakabayashi, K., and Ikuta, F. (1988). Selective decrease of large neurons in the neostriatum in progressive supranuclear palsy. *Brain Research*, **458**, 218–23.

Pantelakis, S. (1954). Un type particulier d'angiopathie sénile du système nerveux central: l'angiopathie congophile. Topographie et fréquence. *Monatsschrift für Psychiatrie und Neurologie*, **128**, 219–56.

Papp, M. I., Khan, J. E., and Lantos, P. L. (1989). Glial cytoplasmic inclusions in the CNS of patients with multiple system atrophy (striatonigral degeneration, olivopontocerebellar atrophy and Shy-Drager syndrome). *Journal of the Neurological Sciences*, **94**, 79–100.

Parchi, P., Petersen, R. B., Chen, S. G., Autilio-Gambetti, L., Capellari, S., Monari, L., *et al.* (1998). Molecular pathology of fatal familial insomnia. *Brain Pathology*, **8**, 515–20.

Perry, G., Friedman, R., Shaw, G., and Chau, V. (1987). Ubiquitin is detected in neurofibrillary tangles and senile plaque neurites of Alzheimer's disease brains. *Proceedings of the National Academy of Sciences of the United States of America*, **84**, 3033–6.

Perry, R. H., Irving, D., Blessed, G., Fairbairn, A., and Perry, E. K. (1990). Senile dementia of Lewy body type. A clinically and neuropathologically distinct form of Lewy body dementia in the elderly. *Journal of the Neurological Science*, **95**, 119–39.

Poorkaj, P., Bird, T. D., Wijsman, E., Nemens, E., Garruto, R. M., Anderson, L., *et al.* (1998). Tau is a candidate gene for chromosome 17 frontotemporal dementia. *Annals of Neurology*, **43**, 815–25.

Preece, M. A. (1991). Creutzfeldt–Jakob disease following treatment with human pituitary hormones. *Clinical Endocrinology*, **34**, 527–9.

Probst, A., Langui, D., Lautenschlager, C., Ulrich, J., Brion, J.-P., and Anderton, B. H. (1988). Progressive supranuclear palsy: extensive neuropil threads in addition to neurofibrillary tangles. *Acta Neuropathologica*, **77**, 61–8.

Prusiner, S. B. (1982). Novel proteinaceous infectious particles cause scrapie. *Science*, **216**, 136–44.

Prusiner, S. B. (1998). Prions. *Proceedings of the National Academy of Sciences of the Unites States of America*, **95**, 13363–83.

Rebeiz, J. J., Kolodny, E. H., and Richardson, E. P. (1967). Corticodentatonigral degeneration with neuronal achromasia. *Archives of Neurology*, **18**, 20–33.

Revesz, T., Geddes, J. F., and Daniel, S. E. (1995). Corticobasal degeneration. In *Neuropathological diagnostic criteria for brain banking* (ed. F. F. Cruz-Sanchez, R. Ravid, and M. L. Cuzner). IOS Press, Oxford.

Rezaie, P., Cairns, N. J., Chadwick, A., and Lantos, P. L. (1996). Lewy bodies are located preferentially in limbic areas in diffuse Lewy body disease. *Neuroscience Letters*, **212**, 111–14.

Roses, A. D. (1994). Apolipoprotein E affects the rate of Alzheimer's disease expression: β amyloid burden is a secondary consequence dependent on APOE genotype and duration of disease. *Journal of Neuropathology and Experimental Neurology*, **53**, 429–37.

Rossor, M. N., Revesz, T., Lantos, P. L., and Warrington, E. K. (1999). Semantic dementia with ubiquitin inclusion bodies. *Brain*, **123**, 267–76.

Spillantini, M. G., Goedert, M., Crowther, R. A., Murrell, J. R., Farlow, M. R., and Ghetti, B. (1997*a*). Familial multiple system tauopathy with presenile dementia: a disease with abundant neuronal glial tau filaments. *Proceedings of the National Academy of Sciences of the United States of America*, **94**, 4113–18.

Spillantini, M. G., Schmidt, M. L., Lee, V. M.-Y., Trojanowski, J. Q., Jakes, R., and Goedert, M. (1997*b*). α-Synuclein in Lewy bodies. *Nature*, **388**, 839–40.

Spillantini, M. G., Bird, T. D., and Ghetti, B. (1998*a*). Frontotemporal dementia and Parkinsonism linked to chromosome 17: a new group of tauopathies. *Brain Pathology*, **8**, 387–402.

Spillantini, M. G., Crowther, R. A., Jakes, R., Cairns, N. J., Lantos,. P. L., and Goedert, M. (1998*b*). Filamentous α-synuclein inclusions link multiple system atrophy with Parkinson's disease and dementia with Lewy bodies. *Neuroscience Letters*, **251**, 205–8.

Spillantini, M. G., Murrell, J. R., Goedert, M., Farlow, M., Klug, A., and Ghetti, B. (1998*c*). Mutation in the tau gene in familial multiple system tauopathy with presenile dementia. *Proceedings of the National Academy of Sciences of the United States of America*, **95**, 7737–41.

Steele, J. C., Richardson, C., and Olszewski, J. (1964). Progressive supranuclear palsy. *Archives of Neurology*, **10**, 333–59.

Struble, R. G., Polinsky, R. J., Hedreen, J. C., Nee, L. E., Frommelt, P., Feldman, R. G., *et al.* (1991). Hippocampal lesions in dominantly inherited Alzheimer's disease. *Journal of Neuropathology and Experimental Neurology*, **50**, 82–94.

Tagliavini, F., Piller, G., Bouras, C., and Constantinidis, C. (1984). The basal nucleus of Meynert in patients with progressive supranuclear palsy. *Neuroscience Letters*, **44**, 37–42.

Tellez-Nagel, I. and Wisniewski, H. M. (1973). Ultrastructure of neurofibrillay tangles in Steele-Richardson-Olszewski syndrome. *Archives of Neurology*, **29**, 324–7.

Terry, R. D. (1985). Alzheimer's disease. In *Textbook of neuropathology* (ed. R. L. Davis and D. M. Robertson), pp. 824–41. Williams and Wilkins, Baltimore.

Tetrud, J. W., Lawrence, I., Golbe, M. D., Forno, L. S., and Farmer, P. M. (1996). Autopsy-proven progressive supranuclear palsy in two siblings. *Neurology*, **26**, 931–4.

Tomonaga, M. (1977). Ultrastructure of neurofibrillary tangles in progressive supranuclear palsy. *Acta Neuropathologica*, **37**, 177–81.

Tourtellotte, W. G. and Van Hoesen, G. W. (1991). The axonal origin of a subpopulation of dystrophic neurites in Alzheimer's disease. *Neuroscience Letters*, **129**, 11–16.

von Eitzen, U., Egensperger, R., Kosel, S., Grasbon-Frodl, E. M., Imai, Y., Bise, K., *et al.* (1998). Microglia and the development of spongiform change in Creutzfeldt–Jakob disease. *Journal of Neuropathology and Experimental Neurology*, **57**, 246–56.

Vonsattel, J. P. G. and DiFiglia, M. (1998). Huntington disease. *Journal of Neuropathology and Experimental Neurology*, **57**, 369–84.

Vonsattel, J. P. G., Myers, R. H., Stevens, T. J., Ferrante, R. J., Bird, E. D., and Richardson, E. P. (1985). Neuropathological classification of Huntington's disease. *Journal of Neuropathology and Experimental Neurology*, **44**, 559–77.

Wakabayashi, K., Oyanagi, K., and Makifuchi, T. (1994). Corticobasal degeneration: etiopathological significance of the cytoskeletal alterations. *Acta Neuropathologica*, **87**, 545–53.

Walker, L. C., Kitt, C. A., Cork, L. C., Struble, R. G., Delloude, T. L., and Price, D. L. (1988). Multiple transmitter systems contribute neurites to individual senile plaques. *Journal of Neuropathology and Experimental Neurology*, **47**, 138–44.

Wilhelmsen, K. C. and Clarke, L. N. (1998). Chromosome 17-linked dementias. In *Neuropathology of dementing disorders* (ed. W. R. Markesbery), pp. 170–80. Arnold, London.

Wilhelmsen, K. C., Lynch, T., Pavlov, E., Higgins, M., and Nygaard, T. G. (1994). Localization of disinhibition-dementia-parkinsonism-amyotrophy complex to 17q21-22. *American Journal of Human Genetics*, **55**, 1159–65.

Will, R. G., Alperovitch, A., Poser, S., Pocchiari, M., Hofman, A., Mitrova, E., *et al.* (1998). Descriptive epidemiology of Creutzfeldt–Jakob disease in six European countries, 1993–1995. *Annals of Neurology*, **43**, 763–7.

Will, R. G., Ironside, J. W., Zeidler, M., Cousens, S. N., Estibeiro, K., Alperovitch, A., *et al.* (1996). A new variant of Creutzfeldt–Jakob disease in the UK. *Lancet*, **347**, 921–5.

Yagishita, S., Itoh, Y., Amano, N., Nakano, R., and Saitoh, A. (1979). Ultrastructure of neurofibrillary tangles in progressive supranuclear palsy. *Acta Neuropathologica*, **48**, 27–30.

Yamada, T., McGeer, P. L., and McGeer, E. G. (1992). Lewy bodies in Parkinson's disease are recognized by antibodies to complement proteins. *Acta Neuropathologica*, **84**, 100–4.

Yamaguchi, H., Nakazato, Y., Shoji, M., Takamata, M., and Hirai, S. (1991). Ultrastructure of diffuse plaques in senile dementia of the Alzheimer type: comparison with primitive plaques. *Acta Neuropathologica*, **82**, 13–20.

Yebenes, J. G., Sarasa, J. L., Daniel, S. E., and Lees, A. J. (1995). Familial progressive supranuclear palsy: description of pedigree and review of the literature. *Brain*, **118**, 1093–103.

11 Familial and sporadic Alzheimer's disease

A. M. Kennedy, M. N. Rossor, and John R. Hodges

1 Introduction

Ever since the original descriptions of Alzheimer's disease (AD) debate has raged concerning the nosological status of the condition (Alzheimer 1907). For many years a distinction between 'presenile' and 'senile' forms was widely accepted with an arbitrary cut-off at 65 years. More recently, however, a classification based upon age has become less tenable and with the discovery of a range of genetic mutations in familial cases the subdivision of 'familial' versus 'sporadic' has been adopted.

There is now a huge body of literature on the genetics and molecular pathology of AD which is covered in more detail elsewhere in the book (see Chapter 8). In this chapter we describe the clinical, neurological, and cognitive features of familial and sporadic AD and attempt to provide a clinicians guide to the recent molecular advances. Neuropathology is dealt with in Chapter 10 and separate chapters are dedicated to structural and functional imaging (Chapters 6 and 7).

2 The diagnosis of Alzheimer's disease

The question of a precise definition for AD remains unresolved despite many attempts to provide a practical and reliable answer. The gold standard remains pathology and the later parts of this chapter describes specific mutations associated with pathologically confirmed AD. The majority of physicians still rely, however, on clinical criteria for diagnosis. The most widely accepted research criteria were published by the National Institute of Neurological and Communicative Disorders and Stroke and Alzheimer's Disease and Related Disorders Association NINCDS-ADRDA (McKhann *et al.* 1984). These criteria attempt to deal with some of the clinical diagnostic uncertainties by classifying patients into either possible or probable subtypes, reserving the term definite AD only for those which have had post-mortem confirmation. Patients with probable AD have deficits in memory and at least one other cognitive domain sufficient to interfere with social function or employment. The diagnosis rests, therefore, on first establishing dementia, then excluding other possible causes of dementia. With the realization that most cases begin with a phase of pure amnesia before global cognitive deficits set in, plus the development of neuroimaging techniques that show promise of making a positive diagnosis, these criteria are likely to need radical revision in the next few years.

The NINCDS-ADRDA criteria have, however, been extremely useful in unifying criteria for entry into research projects and therapeutic trials (e.g. Burns *et al.* 1990; Kukull *et al.* 1990; Martin *et al.* 1987; Risse *et al.* 1990). Longitudinal follow-up of probable AD cases to post-mortem shows that approximately 80% of cases are correctly classified. Several studies have suggested that the choice of pathological criteria used to corroborate the clinical diagnosis may affect the specificity and sensitivity of the classification (Tierney *et al.* 1988). Neurofibrillary tangle and neuritic plaques, the so-called hallmarks of AD, may also be seen in normal ageing, so the distinction from ageing is quantitative rather than absolute (Wilcock *et al.* 1989). Some workers have suggested that age-related criteria should, therefore, be applied (Khachaturian 1985) and in certain cases tangle formation need not necessarily be present (Braak and Braak 1991).

Despite many attempts, no biological marker has yet emerged which supersedes these clinical criteria and enables precise antemortem diagnosis.

3 The concept of familial Alzheimer's disease

Although references were made to inherited forms of AD during the early 1920s, it was not until the 1930s that detailed descriptions of young onset autosomal dominant pedigrees were reported (e.g. Lowenberg and Waggoner 1934).

These early reports established that AD could rarely occur as an inherited condition, but their importance was not widely appreciated until the 1970s and 80s when gradually many more autosomal dominant pedigrees were described and it became clear that familial AD (FAD) was a rare, but definite, subtype of AD (Bird *et al.* 1989; Cook *et al.* 1979).

Some authors speculated that all cases might be inherited as an autosomal dominant trait, since the apparent lack of family history could be explained by the late onset of the condition together with earlier death from intercurrent disease, precluding disease expression (e.g. Breitner and Folstein 1984; Huff *et al.* 1988).

A number of clinico-epidemiological studies then attempted to estimate the proportion of familial cases and to assess the relative risk of dementia in the relatives of probands. There are many difficulties associated with investigations of this type, the majority of which preceded the molecular revolution, including the selection of cases, diagnostic accuracy, and sampling bias. Most studies showed an increased risk of AD in first degree relatives although this is not a universal finding (see Fitch *et al.* 1988).

Opinions differ and some authorities feel that PS1 mutations account for the majority of young onset pedigrees. The most extensive survey, to date, of an epidemiologically-based series of 101 familial and sporadic cases of early onset AD, applying modern molecular genetic techniques to screen for mutations, showed an overall prevalence for mutations of only 7%: 6% presenilin 1 and 1% presenilin 2 with no cases of APP mutations (Cruts *et al.* 1998). When only those with a clear family history were included in the analyses, the prevalence of mutations rose to 18%. These data suggest that the identified gene mutations are rare and account for less than a fifth of cases with a family history.

4 Molecular studies in familial Alzheimer's disease

By the early 1980s molecular genetic techniques, particularly genetic linkage studies were poised to identify the FAD locus. Shortly before the first reports of genetic linkage, the beta-amyloid peptide (the key constituent of the amyloid protein found in AD plaques) was shown to be derived from a larger precursor protein (the amyloid precursor protein, APP) encoded on the long arm of chromosome 21 (Goldgaber *et al.* 1987; Tanzi *et al.* 1987). APP became an immediate candidate gene when St George Hyslop *et al.* (1987) showed that four early onset FAD families showed genetic linkage to the same region of the long arm of chromosome 21. Others were unable to reproduce these findings (Schellenberg *et al.* 1988; Van Broeckhoven *et al.* 1987). The situation was resolved when a multi-centre study showed that FAD was genetically heterogeneous, and that more than one FAD gene existed (St George Hyslop *et al.* 1990).

4.1 Amyloid precursor protein (APP) gene mutations

As a direct consequence of these observations Goate *et al.* (1991) examined the APP candidate region in one British FAD family (FAD 23) which had strong chromosome 21 linkage (Goate *et al.* 1991). Exons 16 and 17 of APP, which contain the beta-amyloid domain, were directly sequenced and a single point mutation at code 717 resulting in a substitution of isoleucine for valine, was identified. The mutation co-segregated with the affected individuals in this family and was not found in other FAD pedigrees or in 300 controls subjects. Subsequent studies have shown this mutation to be present in only a handful of other FAD families (e.g. Fidani *et al.* 1992; Karlinsky *et al.* 1992; Sorbi *et al.* 1993). Two other point mutations at APP 717 have also been found (Chartier Harlin *et al.* 1991) (VAPPG), (Murrell *et al.* 1991) (VAPPF), both of which lead to an AD phenotype. A double mutation at APP 670/671 locus has been described which leads to an AD phenotype (Mullan *et al.* 1992). Whereas an APP mutation at APP 693 causes predominantly cerebral haemorrhages and amyloid angiopathy (Hendriks *et al.* 1992). Recently APP mutations Val 715 M and I716V have been identified which appears to reduce the total A beta production (Ancolio 1999; Eckman *et al.* 1997). Table 11.1 summarizes the APP pedigrees reported to date.

4.1.1 Is there a distinct APP mutation phenotype?

The APP mutations typically have an age at onset between 45–60 years which is often remarkably constant within a given family. For instance, the mean age at onset in the three UK APP families was similar, with a range between 52–54 years (Kennedy *et al.* 1993*b*). The USA pedigree with APP V717F mutation had a more variable age at onset, with one individual developing cognitive impairment as young as 40 years (Murrell *et al.* 1991). Other genetic factors, such as apolipoprotein E (ApoE) genotype, may account for some of the variability in age at onset within the APP families; individuals with ApoE4 allele having an earlier age at onset (Hardy *et al.* 1993; St George Hyslop *et al.* 1994).

Table 11.1 APP families: age at onset. SD = Standard deviation

Country	Name	Mutation	Age at onset	SD
UK	F23	Val Ile	54.5 yrs	3.5 (n = 11)
	F172	Val Ile	53.9 yrs	6.4 (n = 7)
	F19	Val Gly	52.0 yrs	7.8 (n = 10)
USA	F372	Val Ile	49.4 yrs	6.4 (n = 5)
	Murrell	Val Phe	43.0 yrs	– (n = 7)
Canada	Toronto 3	Val Ile	47.6 yrs	3.0 (n = 11)
Italy	Flo 12	Val Ile	58.0 yrs	4.0 (n = ?)
	Flo 13	Val Ile	50.0 yrs	3.0 (n = ?)
Japan	Osaka	Val Ile ⎫		
	NIIgata 1	Val Ile ⎬	51.5 yrs	4.2 (n = 8)
	NIIgata 2	Val Ile ⎭		

Relatively few studies have described the clinical and neuropsychological features of APP pedigrees in detail. Karlinsky *et al.* (1992) described the Toronto 3 pedigree, an APP V717I family, which had emigrated from the British Isles at the beginning of the 20th century. Memory loss was the initial symptom, but difficulties with calculation, visuospatial function, and language occurred later in the disease. Kennedy *et al.* (1993*b*) reported details of Family 19, a pedigree with a APP V717G mutation. All patients demonstrated prominent memory impairment. Five out of ten individuals had seizures, and all the living affected individuals had myoclonus. Neuropsychological testing showed generalized intellectual impairment with prominent dyscalculia and relative sparing of language (Kennedy *et al.* 1993*b*). In the original APP V717 pedigree myoclonic jerks were present in six cases out of twelve, including all four living individuals (Mullan *et al.* 1993). Post-mortem examinations showed cortical Lewy bodies in addition to typical AD pathology (Lantos *et al.* 1994). A large Swedish family with APP 670–671 mutation showed impairment of memory with prominent depression and other psychiatric symptoms (Axelman *et al.* 1998).

Overall, the clinical features of APP mutation FAD do not reliably distinguish these individuals from sporadic AD or other forms of FAD. The age at onset is probably the most useful pointer.

Mutations in the APP gene adjacent to the putative α-secretase have a different phenotype with prominent amyloid angiopathy. The APP 693 mutation is associated with hereditary cerebral haemorrhage with amyloidosis of the Dutch type (HCHWA-D) in which patients develop cerebral haemorrhage and there is an absence of neuritic pathology. The APP 692 mutation cases (the Flemish mutation) has an intermediary neuropathology (Roks *et al.* 2000).

4.2 Presenilin 1 mutations

After the discovery that the APP mutations accounted for only a small proportion of individuals with FAD (Schellenberg *et al.* 1991), the race to identify other genetic factors continued and two further important genetic factors emerged. First, a genetic risk factor was reported on chromosome 19 which was later shown to be the apolipoprotein E4 locus: the ApoE4 allele being an important risk factor for both sporadic and familial AD (Corder *et al.* 1993; Strittmatter *et al.* 1993). More importantly for younger onset FAD families were the reports that some of these families showed linkage to a locus on chromosome 14 (Mullan *et al.* 1992; Schellenberg *et al.* 1992; St George Hyslop *et al.* 1992; Van Broeckhoven *et al.* 1992). Sherrington *et al.* (1995) completed this work when they reported a novel gene (S182 now referred to as presenilin 1, PS1) located at chromosome 14q24.3. This encoded a seven domain transmembrane protein in which five point mutations were found to co-segregate with early onset FAD pedigrees. During the ensuing five years at least 50 presenilin mutations have been described. The majority are point mutations although two deletions have been reported. Table 11.2 summarizes this literature; the point mutations location and age at onset of these families are shown (Aldudo *et al.* 1998; Aoki *et al.* 1997; Axelman *et al.* 1998; Besancon *et al.* 1998; Campion *et al.* 1995; Crook *et al.* 1997; Cruts *et al.* 1995; Ezquerra *et al.* 1999; Forsell *et al.* 1997; Gomez-Isla *et al.* 1997; Jorgensen *et al.* 1996; Kamino *et al.* 1996; Kowalska *et al.* 1999; Kwok *et al.* 1997; Lendon *et al.* 1997; Lopera *et al.* 1997; Martinez *et al.* 1998; Morelli *et al.* 1998; Palmer *et al.* 1999; Perez-tur *et al.* 1996, 1995; Poorkaj *et al.* 1998; Ramirez-Duenas *et al.* 1998; Reznik-Wolf *et al.* 1996; Sandbrink *et al.* 1996; Sato *et al.* 1999, 1998; Smith *et al.* 1999; Sorbi *et al.* 1995; Taddei *et al.* 1998; Tysoe *et al.* 1998; Wasco 1995; Yasuda *et al.* 1999, 1997).

Table 11.2 A summary of PS1 mutations

Nos	Mutation	Codon	Author	Family code	Age at onset
1	A79V	4	Crutz et al.		53–61–63
2	V82L	4	Campion et al.	gal 508	53 to 58
3	V96F	4	Kamino et al.	OS3	53
4	Y115H	5	Campion et al.	ALZ 025	35 to 37
5	Y115C	5	Kruis et al.		
6	E120K	5	Hutton et al.	F121	32 to 39
7	E120D	5	Poorjah et al.	FV	46
8	E120T	5	Reznik		43 to 48
9	E123K	5	Yasada	ABCD 2	59
10	N135D	5	Crook et al.	USA	34 to 38
11	M139V	5	AD Collab	F148 F206 German 1421	41–39–40
12	M139T	5	Campion et al.	CAE 010	48 to 50
13	M139I	5	Boteva et al.	DUKE AD	
14	I143F	5	Rossor et al.		55
15	I143T	5	Crut et al.	BELGIAN FAMILY A	35
16	M146L	5	Sherrington et al.	OLKA 1 FAD4 TOR 1	43–45–36–35–38
17	M146V	5	AD Collab	Fin 1 MAn 92 NY5201	36–40–37
18	M46 Ile	5	Jorgensen et al.	Danish	44
19	H163Y	6	AD Collab	Swed 2 HR1	47 46
20	H163R	5	Campion et al.	Sal001 LH TK2 for 42 603	42 to 47 47 47
21	S169L	6	Taddei et al.	Perth 4	31
22	S169Pro	6	Ezquerra et al.	Granada	35
23	L171P	6	Ramirez et al.		36 to 40
24	G209V	7	Poorjah et al.	Family L	41
25	I213T	7	Kamino et al.	OS2	45
26	A231T	7	Campion et al.		51
27	A231V	7	Cruts	ALZ 043	45 to 47
28	M233T	7	Kwok et al.	Perth 1	35
29	L235P	7	Campion et al.		32
30	A246E	7	Sherrington et al.		39 53
31	L250S	7	Hutton et al.	F184	50 to 56
32	A260V	8	Rogaev		45
33	C263R	8	Wasco et al.	MGH 12 SAL 511	50
34	L263Phe	8	Forrell et al.		47 to 56
35	P264L	8	Wasco et al.	MGH 6	45 to 50
36	P267S	8	Hutton et al.	F196	32–38
37	R269G	8	Perez Tur et al.	Olka	
38	R269H	8	Gomez Isla et al.	USA	47
39	R278T	8	Kwok et al.	P2	37
40	E280A	8	AD Collab	C1 C2 C3 F771 Col	49–47–47–45–47 46
41	E280G	8	AD Collab	H68 H83	41–43
42	L282R	8	Aldudo et al.		43
43	A285V	8	Aoli et al.	TOH 1	50
44	L286V	8	Sherrington et al.		46–48
45	S290C	SPL	Sato et al.	TK1	47
46	E318G	9	Taddei et al.		47–50s
47	G384A	11	Crut et al.	BELGIAN FAMILY B	35
48	L392V	11	Campion et al.	FADRO1	39 to 52
49	C410Y	11	Campion et al.	ROU011 SNW	40 to 60
50	A426P	12	Poorkaj et al.	HRX 111	
51	P436S	12			
52	P436Q	12		SYD1	20

4.2.1 Is there a presenilin 1 specific phenotype?

Many molecular genetic studies give sparse clinical details, usually concentrating on the age at onset and other demographic and pathological characteristics. It is difficult, therefore, to draw specific conclusions from this literature. Initial reports of PS1 families suggested that the mutations were invariably associated with a very young age at onset, with individuals affected in their early 40s, and a poor prognosis, but as more cases have been discovered (see Table 11.2) it has become apparent that there is a degree of variability with age of onset ranging from 20–60 years. There are quite dramatic differences in the clinical and neuropathological features, even among family members with the identical PS mutations suggesting that further individual or pedigree genetic or epigenetic factors are likely to modulate PS phenotypes strongly (Gomez-Isla *et al.* 1999).

A number of PS1 pedigrees have been described in relative detail. For instance, Kennedy *et al.* (1995) reported a pathologically confirmed UK PS1 family (FAD 148) where three affected individuals were available for prospective assessment. The mean age at onset in this pedigree was 43 years with a mean duration of seven years. All the individuals presented with memory difficulties. Two of the cases developed a deficit in speech production. This hypothesis that the speech deficit might represent a phenotypic characteristic of this pedigree was, however, subsequently disproved since the same clinical characteristic were not found in a further unrelated UK pedigree (F206) which shared an identical presenilin 1 mutation.

Harvey *et al.* (1998) recently reported seven affected members of a further UK kindred with a novel L250S PS1 mutation. All had an early age at onset with prominent myoclonus, depression, and psychosis.

Studies of PS1 pedigrees which have identical point mutations help to determine which phenotypic features are common to the specific mutations or to the PS1 group as a whole. For instance, both Family FAD 4 and Family TOR 1.1 have the M146V PS1 mutation. FAD 4 had a mean age at onset of 45 years, whereas TOR 1.1 had a mean age of onset of 35 years (Bergamini *et al.* 1991; Foncin *et al.* 1985). On the other hand two large Belgian families with extremely similar phenotypes, who were thought until now to have a common ancestor, have been shown to have different PS1 mutations (Martin *et al.* 1991).

The majority of PS1 families have missense mutations although some families have mutations which destroy splice acceptor sites. The clinical features in this pedigree were typical for AD with an age at onset between 44–42 years (Perez-tur *et al.* 1995). This mutation has subsequently been described in other unrelated families (Kwok *et al.* 1997) and interestingly associated with a spastic paraparesis (Crook *et al.* 1998). Neuropathological investigations of a large Finnish pedigree with dementia and paraparesis (Crook *et al.* 1998) revealed numerous, distinct, large, round, and eosinophilic plaques as well as neurofibrillary tangles and amyloid angiopathy throughout the cerebral cortex. An exon 4 splice abnormality has been found in pedigrees of British ancestry including family F160/105 which has an age at onset during the early 30s (De Jonghe *et al.* 1999).

There is no consistent relationship between the distribution of the point mutations the majority of which involve the transmembrane two region or the hydrophilic loop, although some authors have suggested that different clusters have different ages at onset. PS1 mutations appear fully penetrant, although one report has described an individual who carried the mutation who was two standard deviations over the usual age of onset for the family, but had not developed any clinical manifestations of the disease (Rossor *et al.* 1996).

In conclusion, patients with FAD associated with PS1 mutations often, but not always, have a very early age at onset frequently with a relatively short duration. The current literature also indicates that there are other genetic factors that determine age at onset, but unlike APP cases, ApoE status seems not to be important. A spastic paraparesis occurs in some families and myoclonus prominent in others.

4.3 Presenilin 2 mutations

Shortly after the discovery of the PS1 mutations, a related gene was found on chromosome 1. This gene, presenilin 2 (PS2), shows considerable homology to PS1. To date only three disease related missense mutations have been described in this gene. A PS2 mutation occurs in the Volga German pedigrees that originate from Germany and then moved to the Volga region of Southern Russia and subsequently to the USA. For many years the cause of FAD in this genetically distinct group had remained elusive (Levy-Lahad *et al.* 1995; Rogaev *et al.* 1995). One PS2 family is of Italian extraction. In general the age at onset in these families appear older than PS1 families with a range between 50–60 years. Other clinical features pedigrees are similar to PS1 families with a typical amnestic presentation, as well as reports of myoclonus and occasional suggestions of spasticity (Bird *et al.* 1988).

4.4 Other genetic loci

It is clear that other loci remain to be discovered. Recently a number of studies have shown linkage to chromosome 12 in older FAD pedigrees some of which are Amish in origin (Borchelt 1998). Familial British dementia which is associated with spastic paraparesis and amyloid plaques distinct from the β-amyloid of AD and tangles has now been linked to a stop codon mutation in a novel BRI gene on chromosome 13 (Vidal *et al.* 1999; Worster-Drought *et al.* 1944).

5 Sporadic Alzheimer's disease

Most clinical studies concern patients who do not have an autosomal dominant family history of dementia. The assumption has been that these individuals do not have a genetic aetiology and are considered to be 'sporadic' patients. The cognitive, neurological, and neuropsychiatric symptoms reported in sporadic AD will be briefly reviewed in order to compare these with the autosomal dominant familial patients described above. Each section concludes by reflecting whether the feature under discussion distinguishes FAD from sporadic disease. The reader is directed to other chapters for more detailed accounts (e.g. neuropsychological and neuropsychiatric aspects are discussed in Chapters 3 and 4).

6 Cognitive features of sporadic AD

AD, in common with the other dementias, does not begin with non-specific or 'global' impairment in cognitive function, but rather progresses in a relatively predictable pattern through various stages summarized in Table 11.3.

6.1 Memory

When patients present in the early stages of sporadic AD, complaints of memory difficulty are by far the commonest symptom noticed by the patient, and more particularly by their spouse. As

Table 11.3 Stages of cognitive breakdown in typical Alzheimer's disease

	Minimal/ questionable	Mild	Moderate	Severe
Memory				
Working	–	–/+	++	+++
Anterograde episodic	++	+++	+++	+++
Remote	–/+	–/+	++	+++
Semantic	–	–/+	+++	+++
Attention and executive abilities	–/+	++	++	+++
Language (syntax and phonology)	–	–	+	++
Visuospatial and perceptual	–	–/+	++	++
Praxis	–	–	++	++

Key: – absent, + present, –/+ variable.

will be discussed below, there is a growing number of case reports documenting atypical presentations of AD (aphasia, visual agnosia, etc.), but our own experience suggests that these represent only a minority of cases.

Not all aspects of memory are, however, affected equally in early AD. The major impairment is in the domain of anterograde episodic memory. The ability to retain new information, such as a story or word-list, after a period is the most sensitive measure (Locascio *et al.* 1995; Perry and Hodges 2000a; Welsh *et al.* 1992), together with paired associative learning, particularly when subjects are required to acquire cross-modal (pattern and location etc.) associations (Fowler *et al.* 1997; Sahakian *et al.* 1988). The nature of the cognitive deficit underlying this failure of memory is discussed more fully in Chapter 3.

The profound impairment in episodic memory reflects the locus of pathology early in the course of the disease when tangles are found in the transentorhinal cortex, effectively disconnecting the hippocampal complex from heteromodal cortical regions, and then later invade the hippocampal formation proper (Braak and Braak 1995). This early atrophy of hippocampal related structures can now be demonstrated *in vivo* using volumetric MRI techniques (see Chapter 6).

In terms of our ability to understand the very earliest cognitive deficits in AD, patients with sporadic disease provide rather limited opportunities: patients have typically been complaining of memory failure for a number of years and rarely have a pure amnesic syndrome; it is also necessary to follow such patients for years in order to establish that they do indeed have AD pathologically. By contrast, the study of 'at-risk' subjects in families with genetically determined FAD provides the unique opportunity to study the very beginning of the disease. In comparison to the multitude of cognitive studies of sporadic AD, such investigations are in their infancy, but so far it appears that impairment in anterograde episodic memory is also the earliest feature in FAD which may precede other cognitive deficits by a number of years (Fox *et al.* 1998; Harvey *et al.* 1998; Newman *et al.* 1994).

Because patients often become preoccupied with the past, it is commonly believed that such memory is spared in AD. Recent research has shown, however, that most patients early in the course of the disease do, in fact, show impaired performance on tests of autobiographical memory, although the degree of impairment is certainly less than that seen on anterograde memory tests. This loss is temporally-graded with relative sparing of more distant memories; accounting, in part, for the clinical observation above (see Greene and Hodges 1996).

The finding of isolated impairment in episodic memory, often for a number of years, before the onset of other cognitive deficits, in both sporadic and FAD, clearly has profound implications for current diagnostic criteria which require impairment in two or more areas of cognition (Hodges 1998). At present, such cases are referred to as minimal, questionable, or possible AD, and in more recently 'mild cognitive impairment' but follow-up studies of such cases show a very high rate of conversion to full blown dementia (see Perry and Hodges 2000b). Clearly there is need to revise the criteria for the diagnosis of AD to take into account these recent developments.

6.2 Attentional and executive deficits

By the time most patients are diagnosed deficits in attention are usually apparent. Patients are described by carers as distractible, lacking in concentration, slowed up, and easily muddled by tasks which were previously routine, such as setting the washing machine or planning the weekly shopping. At a theoretical level, attentional processes are often characterized in terms of selective, sustained, and divided attention (for review see Perry and Hodges 1999). Although all aspects are impaired at a fairly early stage of the disease, the first component to become impaired appears to be the selective attentional system. In clinical practice the test most sensitive to such deficits is the Stroop Test (Perry and Hodges 1999). The putative neural basis of selective attention involves a network of lateral parietal and anterior midline structures (e.g. the cingulate gyrus) which are known, from FDG-PET studies, to be hypometabolic early in the course of AD (see Chapter 7). Involvement of the basal forebrain cholinergic system may also play an important role in the genesis of attentional dysfunction in AD (see Lawrence and Sahakian 1995).

On tests of divided attention, such as dual-performance tests, in which subjects are required to divide their attention between two simultaneously presented streams of information (e.g. Trail-Making and Digit Span) AD patients also show impairment as the disease progresses (see Perry *et al.* 2000).

Sustained attention, or vigilance, may be defined as the ability to focus attention on a task over an unbroken, but prolonged, period of time and is most frequently measured by the speed and accuracy of detecting infrequent and unpredictable targets among more frequent non-targets. In AD, performance on such tasks declines but only at a later stage of the disease (see Perry and Hodges 1999).

Executive function refers to higher-order cognitive abilities that are called upon to formulate new plans of action, to select and monitor the appropriate sequence of actions. Disorders of executive function have been linked to the dorsolateral prefrontal cortex. Classic tests of executive function include Raven's Progressive Matrices, the Porteus Mazes, the Tower of London Test, Trail-Making (part B), and the Wisconsin Card Sorting Test. Breakdown in executive ability follows behind impairment in episodic memory and before visuospatial problems become prominent (Perry and Hodges 1999).

6.3 Language and knowledge

Patients with AD are also characteristically impaired on tests of semantic memory. Semantic memory refers to our permanent store of representational knowledge including facts, concepts, as well as words and their meaning. Semantic memory is, therefore, central to many other cognitive processes most notably perhaps word production and comprehension.

The task which shows the greatest sensitivity in early AD is category fluency (Garrard *et al.* 1997). Since category fluency is a task which calls upon a range of cognitive abilities — working memory, executive and phonological skills — as well as semantic memory, it is important to note that initial-letter based (or phonological) fluency is usually preserved in AD and that semantic fluency deteriorates at a greater rate than letter fluency as the disease progresses (see Chapter 3).

Naming is also impaired at a fairly early stage in AD. Patients with AD most frequently make semantic and rarely produce either visual or phonological errors (Hodges *et al.* 1991). Moreover, analyses based on a battery of semantic memory tests, all of which test knowledge about the same consistent set of items (e.g. picture naming, word-picture matching, picture sorting, generation of definitions to words), show striking consistency for individual items across tests. In other words, if a patient is unable to name a given item in the battery then he (or she) will almost certainly be unable to generate an adequate definition when presented with the name of the same item (Hodges and Patterson 1995).

Although the main impact of AD falls upon the semantic aspects of language, as the disease progresses there is breakdown of phonological and syntactic abilities (see Croot *et al.* 1999; 2001).

Although reading is well preserved in early AD, breakdown in writing processes is common due to a combination of central (linguistic) and more peripheral (praxic) aspects (see Graham 2001).

6.4 Visuospatial and perceptual deficits

Visuospatial and perceptual symptoms are usually not early features, but rather follow in the wake of episodic memory and attentional deficits (see Perry *et al.* 2000). Occasionally, however, visual symptoms dominate in the so-called visual variant of AD (see below). In more typical cases deficits arise first on complex tasks which require perceptual analysis and spatial planning such as Block Design from the Weschler Intelligence Scale or copying the Rey Complex Figure — although apraxia may also contribute to difficulties copying this figure (see Caine and Hodges 2001).

6.5 Apraxia

Mild apraxia appears common, but rather rarely produces symptoms. For instance, Rapcsak *et al.* (1989) found that all individuals from a cohort of 28 cases with AD were impaired on an apraxia battery. When asked to pantomime the use of objects (e.g. show me how you would brush your teeth?) frequent body part substitution errors were made (the index finger was substituted as the tooth brush.). Tests which were specific to buccofacial apraxia, limb intransitive tasks (e.g. wave good bye) and axial movements were relatively spared. The Florida group have suggested that AD patients exhibit loss of knowledge of tool usage which they term 'conceptual apraxia' (Ochipa *et al.* 1992).

6.6 Insight into cognitive deficits in AD

Patients with AD may lack insight into their cognitive difficulties (so-called anosognosia), although this feature has been overemphasized in the past. A recent meta-analysis of 16 studies (see Markova and Berrios 2000) highlighted the methodological differences in assessment of insight and of dementia, and the not surprising contrast in conclusions between studies.

Nevertheless, certain trends have emerged: most studies suggest that insight is preserved early in the disease and diminishes with progression of the disease although there is marked variability. Analysis of the relationship between disease severity and loss of insight shows mixed results with findings varying between a strong positive correlation (Vasterling *et al.* 1997), a weak association (Michon *et al.* 1994), and a lack of relationship (Reed *et al.* 1993). There appears to be some degree of consensus that AD patients with prominent frontal involvement — as judged by either SPECT hypoperfusion (Starkstein *et al.* 1995) or scores on frontal dysfunction tests (Michon *et al.* 1994) show less insight.

6.7 Atypical presentations of AD

The vast majority of cases with primary progressive aphasia have non-Alzheimer pathology, but there are now a number of well documented AD cases presenting with very severe aphasia, either without other cognitive deficits, or with only mild impairment of non-linguistic function. Galton *et al.* have recently reviewed the topic and described a total of six aphasic cases all with pathologically established AD: two had non-fluent aphasia, which in one was remarkably pure for a number of years; three were fluent with marked anomia and a number of features resembling those seen in semantic dementia (see Chapter 12); and one had a mixed aphasic syndrome (Galton *et al.* 2000).

The other commonly reported variant of AD was highlighted by (Benson *et al.* 1988) under the title of posterior cortical atrophy. A number of subsequent reports have established that within this broad category a number of different presentations may occur. Very occasionally AD may present with progressive visual loss with restriction of fields and a severe apperceptual agnosia. More commonly basic low-level functions (acuity, colour, and shape detection, etc.) are preserved but patients have severe problems with high level visual analysis causing simultagnosia, alexia, and colour agnosia reflecting involvement of the ventral occipito-temporal pathway. The third variant presents with visual disorientation, severe problems with navigation, visual mis-reaching, and apraxia: recently termed the bi-parietal variant of AD to reflect the locus of atrophy (for review see Galton *et al.* 2000).

In addition to these more frequently recognized variants of AD there have been reports of cases presenting with a pure right hemisphere syndrome (Crystal *et al.* 1982) and with a progressive gait disorder resembling that seen in corticobasal degeneration (Rossor *et al.* 1999).

7 Neuropsychiatric features of AD

Non-cognitive symptoms are not only common from an early stage but also cause considerable carer distress (see Chapter 4). Most prominent is apathy, with or without concomitant features of true depression, which has been attributed to anterior cingulate pathology. Around 30–50% have prominent mood change, but relatively few meet criteria for a major depressive episode.

Delusions are commoner than hallucinations with estimates of frequency ranging from 10–70%. Paranoid delusions, often involving theft, are probably the most common type. Misidentification phenomena and the Capras delusion, in which patients believe that a close relative has been replaced by an imposter, may occur. Hallucinations, usually visual, are rare in the early stages but increase in prevalence with disease progression reaching almost 50% in some series (see Chapter 4).

Challenging behaviours including shouting, aggression, agitation disinhibition, and irritability are also common and appear independent of psychosis or depression. Stereotypic ritualized behaviours and changes in eating patterns with a preference for sweet foods that characterize frontotemporal dementia are rare in AD (Bozeat *et al.* 2000).

8 Neurological features in AD

8.1 Extrapyramidal features and Gegenhalten

Parkinsonian features, particularly rigidity and akinesia, occur in around two-thirds of cases (Girling and Berrios 1990). The earliest signs of extrapyramidal disorder are usually abnormal muscular tone, a masking of facial expression and a shuffling gait. Many advanced cases have so-called *Gegenhalten*: a resistance to change in limb position by passive movement, which leads to a variable increases in muscular tension dependent on the manipulating force.

Some authors have suggested that the presence of extrapyramidal signs may signify a subgroup of AD cases (Molsa *et al.* 1984), but others regard parkinsonism solely as a marker of advanced disease (Mayeux *et al.* 1985). Another complicating factor is that most of the studies in this area were conducted before the discovery of dementia with Lewy bodies (DLB see Chapter 13) so that a proportion of the cases classified as AD may in fact have DLB. Some APP pedigrees have cortical Lewy body disease in addition to other cytoskeletal features typical of AD but do not show prominent early extrapyramidal signs.

8.2 Myoclonus

Myoclonus is defined as an involuntary repetitive contraction of a single muscle or muscle group producing sudden and unpredictable muscle contractions which may affect differing muscle groups at differing times. The intensity of the movements range from subtle twitching of the fingers to sudden explosive movements causing significant functional impairment. Myoclonus in AD usually causes twitching of the fingers or toes.

As described above, myoclonus is particularly common in familial young onset cases and has been associated with APP, PS1, and PS2 mutations.

As with extrapyramidal features, some authors have proposed that the presence of myoclonus could be used to define a clinical subgroup of AD cases, which in turn provided further evidence for phenotypic heterogeneity: two large studies (Chui *et al.* 1985; Mayeux *et al.* 1985) observed myoclonus in that less than 10% of AD patients and showed an association between myoclonus, younger age at onset, and a more rapid intellectual decline. Surprisingly, no association with family history was observed in either study.

8.3 Seizures

Seizures occur more commonly in AD than is appreciated, especially in the late stages of both sporadic and FAD. One study showed 8 out of 83 cases with autopsy confirmed AD had a history of seizures, equivalent to a tenfold increase in seizure risk (Hauser *et al.* 1986). A further study followed a cohort of AD cases and an identical number of aged matched controls: 7 out of 44 AD cases developed seizures during 90 months follow-up period, whereas all the controls were seizure free (Romanelli *et al.* 1990). Seizures early in the course of the disease are reported in some FAD families (see above).

9 Studies which compare familial and sporadic phenotypes

Review of the literature from the pre-molecular era of diagnosis reveals a very confusing picture. Some comparisons of patients classified as 'early' or 'late' onset AD showed a clear distinction between these groups with more aphasia and a worse prognosis in the early onset cases (Filley *et al.* 1986; Seltzer and Sherwin 1983). By contrast, a cohort of elderly patients distinguished on the basis of a positive family history showed no difference in age at onset, clinical or imaging features (Duara *et al.* 1993). Likewise, a retrospective analysis using patients from an AD registry found no clinical differences between familial and sporadic cases, although the course of the dementia was thought to be more rapid in the familial group (Luchins *et al.* 1992), another study showed no difference between the neuropsychological profiles in severity matched groups of familial and sporadic cases (Haupt *et al.* 1992). Breitner and Folstein (1984) described more prominent aphasia and apraxia in those with a family history of AD, but the extent of such deficits were not quantified. A more detailed investigation of the neuropsychological features of familial and sporadic AD failed to confirm a significant difference (Swearer *et al.* 1992).

With the ability to identify specific mutations the situation has become somewhat clearer. A recent study comparing three severity matched groups of patients (FAD; FAD with presenilin 1 mutations and sporadic cases) showed that the PS1 FAD group obtained higher scores on graded tests of naming and object perception (Warrington *et al.* 2001). Interestingly some of the same FAD patients were reported earlier to show preserved left hemisphere metabolism compared to a sporadic AD population (Kennedy *et al.* 1993*a*).

10 The role of neuroimaging in AD

In parallel with the growth in neuropsychological studies of AD there has been a burgeoning of the literature on structural and functional neuroimaging. These topics are dealt with more fully elsewhere (see Chapters 6 and 7). In brief, each of the following methods have been advocated in the early diagnosis of AD: temporal orientated computed tomography (CT), volumetric and serial co-registration of magnetic resonance imaging (MRI), single photon emission computed tomography (SPECT), and positron emission tomography (PET). It remains unclear which imaging modality is the most appropriate for the early and accurate detection of particular disease states since the studies, to date, have either been confined very largely to patients with presumed AD, have not been systematically compared with neuropsychological evaluation, or have lacked long-term verification of the pathological diagnosis. Our own experience suggests that neuropsychological evaluation is both more sensitive, and specific, than SPECT changes in early AD. Structural imaging is mandatory in all early onset cases to exclude other rarer causes of dementia (see Chapter 2).

MRI volumetric measurements may detect hippocampal atrophy at an extremely early stage in cases with presenile familial AD (Fox *et al.* 1997), but in the majority of studies of patients with sporadic AD there has been considerable overlap in hippocampal or entorhinal cortical measures between AD cases and matched controls. Such measures might have a role in the confirmation of diagnosis (although the specificity of the changes to AD is questionable) but cannot at present be used for screening or to rule out AD (see Chapter 6). Co-registration of serially acquired MRIs appears at present to be an extremely accurate methods which can detect pathological rates of atrophy in familial AD cases even before the onset of cognitive symptoms, but remains a research tool (Fox *et al.* 1999). Clearly there is a need for further studies which compare a range of diagnostic techniques in a group of patients studied longitudinally with eventual pathological verification of the diagnosis.

11 Conclusions

We have not attempted here to deal with the management of early onset AD cases which requires the dedication of a multidisciplinary team. The needs of patients and there families evolve: at the early stages, sophisticated diagnostic facilities may be needed. Diagnosis of a progressive fatal disorder should always be followed-up with support and practical advice usually best handled by trained nurse counsellors. All families deserve informed advice on genetic issues and disease-modifying therapies. Later the practical management of problematic behaviours will often require the combined input of psychiatry, psychology, and other allied professionals. These aspects are dealt with more fully in Chapters 19 and 20.

12 Key points

1   Autosomal dominant familial Alzheimer's disease is associated with main genetic loci on chromosome 21 (amyloid precursor protein), 14 (presenilin 1), and 1 (presenilin 2).

2   Amyloid precursor protein (APP) mutations FAD affect only 20 families world-wide. No apparent specific phenotype is found in APP mutation FAD apart from an age at onset between 50–55 years.

3   The most common genetic form of FAD is due to mutations in the presenilin 1 gene. Presenilin 2 gene mutations appear to be very rare. Presenilin 1 gene mutations often are associated with a very young age at onset below 40 years of age.

4   The apolipoprotein E4 allele is an established risk factor for familial and sporadic Alzheimer's disease.

5   Studies which compare familial and sporadic cases show no consistent differences apart from age at onset and the presence of myoclonus.

6   Presymptomatic cognitive deficits can be found before the onset of disease in individuals who have FAD mutations.

7   In sporadic AD the most common presentation is impairment in anterograde episodic memory which may precede other cognitive deficits by years and is best detected by measures of delayed recall.

8   Deficits in attentional processes and semantic memory follow the episodic memory impairment.

9   A growing number of atypical cases with progressive aphasia or posterior cortical (visuospatial and perceptual) symptoms have been reported.

10   There is, as yet, no entirely reliable biological or imaging marker of AD. Hippocampal atrophy can be detected by MRI, but is not sensitive or specific.

References

Aldudo, J., Bullido, M. J., Arbizu, T., Oliva, R., and Valdivieso, F. (1998). Identification of a novel mutation (Leu282Arg) of the human presenilin 1 gene in Alzheimer's disease. *Neuroscience Letters*, **240**, 174–6.

Alzheimer, A. (1907). Uber eine eigenartige Erkrankung der Hirnrinde. *Allgemeine Zeitschrift fuer Psychiatrie*, **64**, 146–8.

Ancolio, K. D. C. B. H. (1999). Unusual phenotypic alteration of beta amyloid precursor protein maturation by a new Val 715 Met bAPP 770 mutation responsible for probably early onset AD. *Proceedings of the National Academy of Science USA*, **96**, 4119–21.

Aoki, M., Abe, K., Oda, N., Ikeda, M., Tsuda, T., Kanai, M., *et al.* (1997). A presenilin-1 mutation in a Japanese family with Alzheimer's disease and distinctive abnormalities on cranial MRI. *Neurology*, **48**, 1118–20.

Axelman, K., Basun, H., and Lannfelt, L. (1998). Wide range of disease onset in a family with Alzheimer disease and a His163Tyr mutation in the presenilin-1 gene. *Archives of Neurology*, **55**, 698–702.

Benson, D. F., Davis, R. J., and Snyder, B. D. (1988). Posterior cortical atrophy. *Archives of Neurology*, **45**, 789–93.

Bergamini, L., Pinessi, L., Rainero, I., Brunetti, E., Cerrato, P., Cosentino, L., *et al.* (1991). Familial Alzheimer's disease. Evidences for clinical and genetic heterogeneity. *Acta Neurologica (Napoli)*, **13**, 534–8.

Besancon, R., Lorenzi, A., Cruts, M., Radawiec, S., Sturtz, F., Broussolle, E., *et al.* (1998). Missense mutation in exon 11 (Codon 378) of the presenilin-1 gene in a French family with early-onset Alzheimer's disease and transmission study by mismatch enhanced allele specific amplification. *Human Mutations*, **11**, 481.

Bird, T., Lampe, T., Nemens, E., Miner, G., Sumi, S., and Schellenberg, G. (1988). Familial Alzheimer's Disease in American descendants of the Volga Germans, probable genetic founder effect. *Annals of Neurology*, **23**, 25–31.

Bird, T. D., Sumi, S. M., Nemens, E. J., Nochlin, D., Schellenberg, G., Lampe, T. H., *et al.* (1989). Phenotypic heterogeneity in familial Alzheimer's disease: a study of 24 kindreds. *Annals of Neurology*, **25**, 12–25.

Borchelt, D. R. (1998). Metabolism of presenilin 1: influence of presenilin 1 on amyloid precursor protein processing. *Neurobiology of Aging*, **19**, s15–18.

Bozeat, S., Gregory, C. A., Lambon Ralph, M. A., and Hodges, J. R. (2000). Which neuropsychiatric and behavioural features distinguish frontal and temporal variants of frontotemporal dementia from Alzheimer's disease. *Journal of Neurology, Neurosurgery and Psychiatry*, **69**, 178–86.

Braak, H. and Braak, E. (1991). Neuropathological staging of Alzheimer-related changes. *Acta Neuropathologica*, **82**, 239–59.

Braak, H. and Braak, E. (1995). Staging of Alzheimer's disease related neurofibrillary changes. *Neurobiology of Aging*, **16**, 271–84.

Breitner, J. and Folstein, M. (1984). Familial Alzheimer's disease: a prevalent disorder with specific clinical features. *Psychological Medicine*, **14**, 63–80.

Burns, A., Luthert, P., Levy, R., Jacoby, R., and Lantos, P. (1990). Accuracy of clinical diagnosis of Alzheimer's disease. *British Medical Journal*, **301**, 1026.

Caine, D. and Hodges, J. R. (2001). Evidence for heterogeneity of semantic and spatial deficits in early Alzheimer's disease. *Neuropsychology*, **XXX**, YYY.

Campion, D., Flaman, J. M., Brice, A., Hannequin, D., Dubois, B., Martin, C., *et al.* (1995). Mutations of the presenilin I gene in families with early-onset Alzheimer's disease. *Human Molecular Genetics*, **4**, 2373–2377.

Chartier Harlin, M.-C., Crawford, F., Houlden, H., Warren, A., Hughes, D., Fidani, L., *et al.* (1991). Early onset Alzheimer's disease caused by mutations at codon 717 of the beta amyloid precursor gene. *Nature*, **353**, 844–6.

Chui, H. C., Teng, E. L., Henderson, V. W., and Moy, A. C. (1985). Clinical subtypes of dementia of the Alzheimer type. *Neurology*, **35**, 1544–50.

Cook, R., Ward, B., and Austin, J. (1979). Studies in aging of the brain: Familial Alzheimer's Disease: Relationship to transmissible dementia, aneuploidy and microtubular defect. *Neurology*, **29**, 1402–12.

Corder, E., Saunders, A., Strittmatter, W., Schmechel, D., Gaskell, P., Small, G., *et al.* (1993). Gene dose of Apolipoprotein E Type 4 Allele and the risk of Alzheimer's disease in late onset families. *Science*, **261**, 921–3.

Crook, R., Ellis, R., Shanks, M., Thal, L. J., Perez-Tur, J., Baker, M., *et al.* (1997). Early-onset Alzheimer's disease with a presenilin-1 mutation at the site corresponding to the Volga German presenilin-2 mutation. *Annals of Neurology*, **42**, 124–8.

Crook, R., Verkkoniemi, A., Perez-Tur, J., Mehta, N., Baker, M., Houlden, H., *et al.* (1998). A variant of Alzheimer's disease with spastic paraparesis and unusual plaques due to deletion of exon 9 of presenilin 1. *Nature Medicine*, **4**, 452–5.

Croot, K., Hodges, J. R., and Patterson, K. E. (1999). Evidence for impaired sentence comprehension in early Alzheimer's disease. *Journal of the International Neurological Society*, **5**, 393–404.

Croot, K., Hodges, J. R., Xuereb, J., and Patterson, K. (2000). Phonological and articulatory impairment in Alzheimer's disease: a single case series. *Brain and Language*, **75**, 277–309.

Cruts, M., Backhovens, H., Wang, S. Y., Gassen, G. V., Theuns, J., De Jonghe, C. D., *et al.* (1995). Molecular genetic analysis of familial early-onset Alzheimer's disease linked to chromosome 14q24.3. *Human Molecular Genetics*, **4**, 2363–71.

Cruts, M. van Duijn C. M., Backhoven S. H., Van den Broeck, M., Wehnert, A., Serneels, S., Sherrington, R., Hutton, M, Hardy, J., St. George-Hyslop, P. H., Hofman, A., Van Broeckhoven, C. (1998). Estimation of the genetic contribution of presenile–1 and –2 mutations in a population-based study of presenile Alzheimer Disease, *Human Molecular Genetics*, **43**, 43–51.

Crystal, H. A., Horoupian, D. S., Katzman, R., and Jotkowitz, S. (1982). Biopsy-proved Alzheimer disease presenting as a right parietal lobe syndrome. *Annals of Neurology*, **12**, 186–8.

De Jonghe, C., Cruts, M., Rogaeva, E. A., Tysoe, C., Singleton, A., Vanderstichele, H., *et al.* (1999). Aberrant splicing in the presenilin-1 intron 4 mutation causes presenile Alzheimer's disease by increased Abeta42 secretion. *Human Molecular Genetics*, **8**, 1529–40.

Duara, R., Lopez-Alberola, R. F., Barker, W. W., Loewenstein, D. A., Zatinsky, M., Eisdorfer, C. E., *et al.* (1993). A comparison of familial and sporadic Alzheimer's disease. *Neurology*, **43**, 1377–84.

Eckman, C. B., Mehta, N. D., Crook R., Perez-tur, J., Prihar, G., Pfeiffer, E., *et al.* (1997). A new pathogenic mutation in the APP gene (I716V) increases the relative proportion of A beta 42(43). *Human Molecular Genetics*, **6**, 2087–9.

Ezquerra, M., Carnero, C., Blesa, R., Gelpi, J. L., Ballesta, F., and Oliva, R. (1999). A presenilin 1 mutation (Ser169Pro) associated with early-onset AD and myoclonic seizures. *Neurology*, **52**, 566–70.

Fidani, L., Rooke, K., Chartier Harlin, M.-C., Hughes, D., Tanzi, R., Mullan, M., *et al.* (1992). Screening for mutations in the open reading frame and promoter of the beta amyloid precursor protein gene in familial Alzheimer's disease: identification of a further family with APP 717 Val Ile. *Human Molecular Genetics*, **1**, 165–8.

Filley, C. M., Kelly, J., and Heaton, R. K. (1986). Neuropsychological features of early and late onset Alzheimer's disease. *Archives of Neurology*, **43**, 574–6.

Fitch, N., Becker, R., and Heller, A. (1988). The inheritance of Alzheimer's disease: a new interpretation. *Annals of Neurology*, **23**, 14–19.

Foncin, J., Salmon, D., Supino Viterbo, V., Feldman, R., Macchi, G., Mariotti, P., *et al.* (1985). Demence presenile D'Alzheimer transmise dans une famille etendue. *Revue Neurologique*, **141**, 194–202.

Forsell, C., Froelich, S., Axelman, K., Vestling, M., Cowburn, R. F., Lilius, L., *et al.* (1997). A novel pathogenic mutation (Leu262Phe) found in the presenilin 1 gene in early-onset Alzheimer's disease. *Neuroscience Letters*, **234**, 3–6.

Fowler, K. S., Saling, M. M., Conway, E. L., Semple, J. M., and Louis, W. J. (1997). Computerized neuropsychological tests in the early detection of dementia: prospective findings. *Journal of the International Neuropsychological Society*, **3**, 139–46.

Fox, N. C., Scahill, R. I., Crum, W. R., and Rossor, M. N. (1999). Correlation between rates of brain atrophy and cognitive decline in AD. *Neurology*, **52**, 1687–9.

Fox, N. C., Warrington, E. K., Freeborough, P. A., Hartikainen, P., Kennedy, A. M., Stevens, J. M., *et al.* (1997). Presymptomatic hippocampal atrophy in Alzheimer's disease: A longitudinal MRI study. *Brain*, **119**, 2001–9.

Fox, N. C., Warrington, E. K., Seiffer, A. L., Agnew, S. K., and Rossor, M. N. (1998). Presymptomatic cognitive deficits in individuals at risk of familial Alzheimer's disease: a longitudinal prospective study. *Brain*, **121**, 1631–9.

Galton, C. J., Patterson, K., Xuereb, J. H., and Hodges, J. R. (2000). Atypical and typical presentations of Alzheimer's disease: a clinical, neuropsychological, neuroimaging and pathological study of 13 cases. *Brain*, **123**, 484–98.

Garrard, P., Perry, R., and Hodges, J. R. (1997). Disorders of semantic memory. *Journal of Neurology, Neurosurgery and Psychiatry*, **62**, 431–5.

Girling, D. M. and Berrios, G. E. (1990). Extrapyramidal signs, primitive reflexes and frontal lobe function in senile dementia of the Alzheimer type. *British Journal of Psychiatry*, **157**, 888–93.

Goate, A., Chartier Harlin, M.-C., Mullan, M., Brown, J., Crawford, F., Fidani, L., *et al.* (1991). Segregation of a missense mutation in the amyloid precursor protein gene with familial Alzheimer's disease. *Nature*, **349**, 704–6.

Goldgaber, D., Lerman, M. I., McBride, O. W., Saffiotti, U., and Gajdusek, D. C. (1987). Characterization and chromosomal localization of a cDNA encoding brain amyloid of Alzheimer's Disease. *Science*, **235**, 877–80.

Gomez-Isla, T., Growdon, W. B., McNamara, M. J., Nochlin, D., Bird, T. D., Arango, J. C., *et al.* (1999). The impact of different presenilin 1 andpresenilin 2 mutations on amyloid deposition, neurofibrillary changes and neuronal loss in the familial Alzheimer's disease brain: evidence for other phenotype-modifying factors. *Brain*, **122**, 1709–19.

Gomez-Isla, T., Wasco, W., Pettingell, W. P., Gurubhagavatula, S., Schmidt, S. D., Jondro, P. D., *et al.* (1997). A novel presenilin-1 mutation: increased beta-amyloid and neurofibrillary changes. *Annals of Neurology*, **41**, 809–13.

Graham, N. L. (2000). Dysgraphia in cortical dementia. *Neurocase*, **6**, 365–377.

Greene, J. D. W. and Hodges, J. R. (1996). Identification of famous faces and names in early Alzheimer's disease: Relationship to anterograde episodic and semantic memory impairment. *Brain*, **119**, 111–28.

Hardy, J., Houlden, H., Collinge, J., Kennedy, A., Newman, S., and Rossor, M. (1993). POE genotype and Alzheimer's disease. *Lancet*, **342**, 737–8.

Harvey, R. J., Ellison, D., Hardy, J., Hutton, M., Roques, P. K., Collinge, J., *et al.* (1998). Chromosome 14 familial Alzheimer's disease: the clinical and neuropathological characteristics of a family with a leucine → serine (L250S) substitution at codon 250 of the presenilin 1 gene. *Journal of Neurology, Neurosurgery and Psychiatry*, **64**, 44–9.

Haupt, M., Kurz, A., Pollman, S., and Romerero, B. (1992). Alzheimer's Disease: identical phenotype of familial and non familial cases. *Journal of Neurology*, **239**, 248–50.

Hauser, W., Morris, M., Heston, L., and Anderson, V. (1986). Seizures and myoclonus in patients with Alzheimer's disease. *Neurology*, **36**, 1226–30.

Hendriks, L., Van Duijn, C., Cras, P., Van Hul, P., Harskamp, F., Warren, A., *et al.* (1992). Presenile dementia and cerebral haemorrhage linked to a mutation at codon 692 of the beta amyloid precursor protein gene. *Nature Genetics*, **1**, 218–21.

Hodges, J. R. (1998). The amnestic prodrome in Alzheimer's disease. *Brain*, **121**, 1601–2.

Hodges, J. R. and Patterson, K. (1995). Is semantic memory consistently impaired early in the course of Alzheimer's disease? Neuroanatomical and diagnostic implications. *Neuropsychologia*, **33**, 441–59.

Hodges, J. R., Salmon, D. P., and Butters, N. (1991). The nature of the naming deficit in Alzheimer's and Huntington's disease. *Brain*, **114**, 1547–58.

Huff, F. J., Auerbach, J., Chakravarti, A., and Boller, F. (1988). Risk of dementia in relatives of patients with Alzheimer's Disease. *Neurology*, **38**, 786–90.

Jorgensen, P., Bus, C., Pallisgaard, N., Bryder, M., and Jorgensen, A. L. (1996). Familial Alzheimer's disease co-segregates with a Met146I1e substitution in presenilin-1. *Clinical Genetics*, **50**, 281–6.

Kamino, K., Sato, S., Sakaki, Y., Yoshiiwa, A., Nishiwaki, Y., Takeda, M., *et al.* (1996). Three different mutations of presenilin 1 gene in early-onset Alzheimer's disease families. *Neuroscience Letters*, **208**, 195–8.

Karlinsky, H., Vaula, G., Haines, J., Ridgley, J., Bergeron, C., Mortilla, M., *et al.* (1992). Molecular and prospective phenotypic characterization of a pedigree with Familial Alzheimer's Disease and a missense mutation in codon 717 of the beta amyloid precursor protein gene. *Neurology*, **42**, 1445–53.

Kennedy, A., Agnew, S., Roques, P., Warrington, E. K., Frackowiak, R. S. J., and Rossor, M. (1993*a*). Familial vs Sporadic Alzheimer's disease: A clinical, neuropsychological and PET study. *Neurology*, **43**, 154.

Kennedy, A. M., Newman, S. K., Frackowiak, R. S. J., Cunningham, V. J., Roques, P., Stevens, J., *et al.* (1995). Chromosome 14 linked familial Alzheimer's disease: A clinicopathological study of a single pedigree. *Brain*, **118**, 185–205.

Kennedy, A. M., Newman, S. K., McCaddon, A., Ball, J., Roques, P., Mullan, M., *et al.* (1993*b*). Familial Alzheimer's Disease: A pedigree with a missense mutation in the Amyloid precursor Protein gene (APP 717 valine to glycine). *Brain*, **116**, 309–24.

Khachaturian, Z. S. (1985). Diagnosis of Alzheimer's disease. *Archives of Neurology*, **42**, 1097–105.

Kowalska, A., Forsell, C., Florczak, J., Pruchnik-Wolinska, D., Modestowicz, R., Paprzycki, W., *et al.* (1999). A Polish pedigree with Alzheimer's disease determined by a novel mutation in exon 12 of the presenilin 1 gene: clinical and molecular characterization. *Folia Neuropathologica*, **37**, 57–61.

Kukull, W. A., Larson, E., Reifler, B., Lampe, T., Yerby, M., and Hughes, J. (1990). The validity of 3 clinical diAgnostic criteria for Alzheimer's disease. *Neurology*, **40**, 1364–9.

Kwok, J. B., Taddei, K., Hallupp, M., Fisher, C., Brooks, W. S., Broe, G. A., *et al.* (1997). Two novel (M233T and R278T) presenilin-1 mutations in early-onset Alzheimer's disease pedigrees and preliminary evidence for association of presenilin-1 mutations with a novel phenotype. *NeuroReport*, **8**, 1537–42.

Lantos, P., Ovenstone, I., Johnston, J., Clelland, C., Roques, P., and Rossor, M. N. N. L. (1994). Lewy bodies in the brains of two members of a family with 717 (Val to Ile) mutation of the amyloid precursor protein gene. *Neuroscience Letters*, **172**, 77–9.

Lawrence, A. D. and Sahakian, B. J. (1995). Alzheimer disease, attention, and the cholinogeric system. *Alzheimer Disease and Associated Disorders*, **9**, 43–9.

Lendon, C. L., Martinez, A., Behrens, I. M., Kosik, K. S., Madrigal, L., Norton, J., *et al.* (1997). E280A PS-1 mutation causes Alzheimer's disease but age of onset is not modified by ApoE alleles. *Human Mutations*, **10**, 186–95.

Levy-Lahad, E., Wijsman, E. M., Nemens, E., Anderson, L., Goddard, K. A., Weber, J. L., *et al.* (1995). A familial Alzheimer's disease locus on chromosome 1. *Science*, **269**, 970–3.

Locascio, J. J., Growdon, J. H., and Corkin, S. (1995). Cognitive test performance in detecting, staging, and tracking Alzheimer's disease. *Archives of Neurology*, **52**, 1087–99.

Lopera, F., Ardilla, A., Martinez, A., Madrigal, L., Arango-Viana, J. C., Lemere, C. A., *et al.* (1997). Clinical features of early-onset Alzheimer disease in a large kindred with an E280A presenilin-1 mutation. *Journal of the American Medical Association*, **10**, 793–9.

Lowenberg, K. and Waggoner, R. (1934). Familial Organic Psychosis (Alzheimer's type). *Archives of Neurology and Psychiatry*, **31**, 737–54.

Luchins, D. J., Cohen, D., Hanrahan, P., Eisdorfer, C., Paveza, G., Ashford, J. W., *et al.* (1992). Are there clinical differences between familial and nonfamilial Alzheimer's disease? *American Journal of Psychiatry*, **149**, 1023–7.

Markova, I. S. and Berrios, G. E. (2000). Insight into memory deficits. In *Memory disorders in psychiatric practice* (ed. G. E. Berrios and J. R. Hodges), pp. 204–33. Cambridge: Cambridge University Press.

Martin, E., Wislon, R., Penn, R., Fox, J., Clasen, R., and Savoy, S. (1987). Cortical biopsy results in Alzheimer's disease: Correlation with cognitive deficits. *Neurology*, **37**, 2101–4.

Martin, J. J., Gheuens, J., and Bruyland, M. (1991). Early onset Alzheimer's Disease in two large Belgian families. *Neurology*, **41**, 62–8.

Martinez, M., Campion, D., Brice, A., Hannequin, D., Dubois, B., Didierjean, O., *et al.* (1998). Apolipoprotein E epsilon4 allele and familial aggregation of Alzheimer disease. *Archives of Neurology*, **55**, 810–16.

Mayeux, R., Stern, Y., and Spanton, S. (1985). Heterogeneity in dementia of the Alzheimer type. Evidence of subgroups. *Neurology*, **35**, 453–60.

McKhann, G., Drachman, D., Folstein, M., Katzmann, R., Price, D., and Stadlan, E. M. (1984). Clinical diagnosis of Alzheimer's disease: report of the NINCDS-ADRDA work group under the auspices of department of health and human services task force on Alzheimer's disease. *Neurology*, **34**, 939–44.

Michon, A., Deweer, B., Pillon, B., Agid, Y., and Dubois, B. (1994). Relation of anosognosia to frontal lobe dysfunction in Alzheimer's disease. *Journal of Neurology, Neurosurgery and Psychiatry*, **57**, 805–9.

Molsa, P., Martila, R., and Rinne, U. (1984). Extra pyramidal signs in Alzheimer's disease. *Neurology*, **34**, 1114–16.

Morelli, L., Prat, M. I., Levy, E., Mangone, C. A., and Castano, E. M. (1998). Presenilin 1 Met146Leu variant due to an A → T transversion in an early-onset familial Alzheimer's disease pedigree from Argentina. *Clinical Genetics*, **53**, 469–73.

Mullan, M., Houlden, H., Windelspecht, M., Fidani, L., Lombardi, C., Diaz, P., *et al.* (1992). A locus for familial early onset Alzheimer's disease on the long arm of chromosome 14, proximal to the alpha 1 antichymotrypsin gene. *Nature Genetics*, **2**, 340–2.

Mullan, M., Tsuji, S., Miki, T., Katsuya, T., Naruse, S., Kaneko, K., *et al.* (1993). Clinical comparison of Alzheimer's disease in pedigrees with codon 717 valine to isoleucine mutation in the Amyloid Precursor Protein gene. *Neurobiology of Aging*, **14**, 407–19.

Murrell, J., Farlow, M., Ghetti, B., and Benson, M. (1991). A mutation in the Amyloid Precursor Protein associated with Hereditary Alzheimer's Disease. *Science*, **253**, 97–8.

Newman, S., Warrington, E., Kennedy, A., and Rossor, M. (1994). The earliest cognitive changes in a person with familial Alzheimer's disease: presymptomatic neuropsychological features in a pedigree with familial Alzheimer's disease confined at necropsy *Journal of Neurology Neurosurgery and Psychiatry*, **57**, 967–972.

Ochipa, C., Rothi, L. J. G., and Heilman, K. M. (1992). Conceptual apraxia in Alzheimer's disease. *Brain*, **115**, 1061–71.

Palmer, M. S., Beck, J. A., Campbell, T. A., Humphries, C. B., Roques, P. K., Fox, N. C., *et al.* (1999). Pathogenic presenilin 1 mutations (P436S & I143F) in early-onset Alzheimer's disease in the UK. *Human Mutations*, **13**, 256.

Perez-tur, J., Croxton, R., Wright, K., Phillips, H., Zehr, C., Crook, R., *et al.* (1996). A further presenilin 1 mutation in the exon 8 cluster in familial Alzheimer's disease. *Neurodegeneration*, **5**, 207–12.

Perez-tur, J., Froelich, S., Prihar, G., Crook, R., Baker, M., Duff, K., *et al.* (1995). A mutation in Alzheimer's disease destroying a splice acceptor site in the presenilin-1 gene. *NeuroReport*, **7**, 297–301.

Perry, R. J. and Hodges, J. R. (1999). Attention and executive deficits in Alzheimer's disease: A critical review. *Brain*, **122**, 383–404.

Perry, R. J. and Hodges, J. R. (2000a). Differentiating frontal and temporal variant frontotemporal dementia from Alzheimer's disease. *Neurology*, **54**, 2277–84.

Perry, R. J. and Hodges, J. R. (2000). The fate of patients with questionable (very mild) Alzheimer's disease: longitudinal profiles of individual subjects' decline. *Dementia and Geriatric Cognitive Disorders*, **11**, 342–49.

Perry, R. J., Watson, P., and Hodges, J. R. (2000). The nature and staging of attention dysfunction in early (minimal and mild) Alzheimer's disease: Relationship to episodic and semantic memory impairment. *Neuropsychologia*, **38**, 252–71.

Poorkaj, P., Sharma, V., Anderson, L., Nemens, E., Alonso, M. E., Orr, H., *et al.* (1998). Missense mutations in the chromosome 14 familial Alzheimer's disease presenilin 1 gene. *Human Mutations*, **11**, 216–21.

Ramirez-Duenas, M. G., Rogaeva, E. A., Leal, C. A., Lin, C., Ramirez-Casillas, G. A., Hernandez-Romo, J. A., *et al.* (1998). A novel Leu171Pro mutation in presenilin-1 gene in a Mexican family with early onset Alzheimer disease. *Annals of Genetics*, **41**, 149–53.

Rapcsak, S. Z., Croswell, S. C., and Rubens, A. (1989). Apraxia in Alzheimer's disease. *Neurology*, **39**, 664–8.

Reed, B. R. Jagust, W. J., and Coulter, L. (1993). Anosognosia in Alzheimer's disease: relationships to depression, cognitive function, and cerebral perfusion. *Journal of Clinical and Experimental Neuropsychology*, **15**, 231–44.

Reznik-Wolf, H., Treves, T. A., Davidson, M., Aharon-Peretz, J., St George Hyslop, P. H., Chapman, J., *et al.* (1996). A novel mutation of presenilin 1 in familial Alzheimer's disease in Israel detected by denaturing gradient gel electrophoresis. *Human Genetics*, **98**, 700–2.

Risse, S., Raskind, M., and Nochlin, D. (1990). Neuropathological findings in patients with the clinical diagnoses of probable Alzheimer's disease. *American Journal of Psychiatry*, **147**, 168–72.

Rogaev, E. I., Sherrington, R., Rogaeva, E. M., Levesque, G., Ikeda, M., Liang, Y., *et al.* (1995). Familial Alzheimer's disease in kindreds with missense mutations in a gene on chromosome 1 related to the Alzheimer's disease type 3 gene. *Nature*, **376**, 775–8.

Roks, G., Van Harskamp, F., De Koning, I., Cruts, M., De Jonge, C., Kumar-Singh, S., *et al.* (2000). Presentation of amyloidosis in carriers of the codon 692 mutation in the amyloid precursor protein gene (APP692). *Brain*, **123**, 2130–2140.

Romanelli, M., Morris, J., Ashkin, K., and Cohen, L. (1990). Advanced Alzheimer's disease is a risk factor for late onset seizures. *Archives of Neurology*, **47**, 847–50.

Rossor, M. N., Fox, N. C., Beck, J., Campbell, T. C., and Collinge, J. (1996). Incomplete penetrance of familial Alzheimer's disease in a pedigree with a novel presenilin-1 gene mutation. *Lancet*, **347**, 1560.

Rossor, M. N., Tyrrell, P. J., Warrington, E. K., Thompson, P. D., Marsden, C. D., and Lantos, P. (1999). Progressive frontal gait disturbance with atypical Alzheimer's disease and corticobasal degeneration. *Journal of Neurology, Neurosurgery and Psychiatry*, **67**, 345–52.

Sahakian, B. J., Morris, R. G., Evenden, J. L., Heald, A., Levy, R., Philpot, M., *et al.* (1988). A comparative study of visuospatial memory and learning in Alzheimer-type dementia and Parkinson's disease. *Brain*, **111**, 695–718.

Sandbrink, R., Zhang, D., Schaeffer, S., Masters, C. L., Bauer, J., Forstl, H., *et al.* (1996). Missense mutations of the PS-1/S182 gene in German early-onset Alzheimer's disease patients. *Annals of Neurology*, **40**, 265–6.

Sato, N., Hori, O., Yamaguchi, A., Lambert, J. C., Chartier-Harlin, M. C., Robinson, P. A., *et al.* (1999). A novel presenilin-2 splice variant in human Alzheimer's disease brain tissue. *Journal of Neurochemistry*, **72**, 2498–505.

Sato, S., Kamino, K., Miki, T., Doi, A., Li, K., St George-Hyslop, P. H., *et al.* (1998). Splicing mutation of presenilin-1 gene for early-onset familial Alzheimer's disease. *Human Mutations*, Suppl **1**, S91–4.

Schellenberg, G., Bird, T., Wijsman, E., Moore, D., Boehnke, M., Byrant, E., *et al.* (1988). Absence of linkage of Chromosme 21q21 markers to Familial Alzheimers's disease. *Science*, **241**, 1507–9.

Schellenberg, G. D., Anderson, L., O'dahl, S., Wisjman, E. M., Sadovnick, A. D., Ball, M. J., *et al.* (1991). APP717, APP693, and PRIP gene mutations are rare in Alzheimer disease. *American Journal of Human Genetics*, **49**, 511–17.

Schellenberg, G. D., Bird, T. D., Wijsman, E. M., Orr, H. T., Anderson, L., Nemens, E., *et al.* (1992). Genetic linkage evidence for a famial Alzheimer's disease locus on chromosome 14. *Science*, **258**, 668–71.

Seltzer, B. and Sherwin, I. (1983). A comparison of clinical features in early- and late-onset primary degenerative dementia. *Archives of Neurology*, **40**, 143–6.

Sherrington, R., Rogaev, E. I., Liang, Y., Rogaeva, E. A., Levesque, G., Ikeda, M., *et al.* (1995). Cloning of a gene bearing missense mutations in early-onset familial Alzheimer's disease. *Nature*, **375**, 754–60.

Smith, M. J., Gardner, R. J., Knight, M. A., Forrest, S. M., Beyreuther, K., Storey, E., *et al.* (1999). Early-onset Alzheimer's disease caused by a novel mutation at codon 219 of the presenilin-1 gene. *NeuroReport*, **10**, 503–7.

Sorbi, S., Nacmias, B., Forleo, P., Piacentini, S., Sherrington, R., Rogaev, E., *et al.* (1995). Missense mutation of S182 gene in Italian families with early-onset Alzheimer's disease. *Lancet*, **346**, 439–40.

Sorbi, S., Nacmins, B., Forleo, P., Piacentini, S., and Amaducci, L. (1993). APP717 and Alzheimer's disease in Italy. *Nature Genetics*, **4**, 10.

St George Hyslop, P. H., Tanzi. R. E., Polinsky. R. J., Haines, J. L., Nee. L., Watkins. P. L., *et al.* (1987). The genetic defect causing familial Alzheimer's disease maps on chromosome 21. *Science*, **237**(4791), 885–900.

St George Hyslop, P. H., Haines, J., Farrer, L., Polinsky, R., Van Broeckhoven, C., Goate, A., *et al.* (1990). Genetic studies suggest that Alzheimer's disease is not a single homogeneous disorder. *Nature*, **347**, 194–197.

St George Hyslop, P. H., Haines, J., Rogaev, E., Mortilla, M., Vaula, G., Pericak Vance, M., *et al.* (1992). Genetic evidence for a novel familial Alzheimer's disease locus on chromosome 14. *Nature Genetics*, **2**, 330–4.

St George Hyslop, P. H., McLachan, D. C., Tuda, T., Rogaev, E., Karlinsky, H., Lippa, C. F., *et al.* (1994). Alzheimer's disease and possible gene interaction. *Science*, **263**, 537.

Starkstein, S. E., Vazquez, S., Migliorelli, R., Teson, A., Sabe, L., and Leiguarda, R. (1995). A single-photon emission computed tomographic study of anosognosia in Alzheimer's disease. *Archives of Neurology*, **52**, 415–20.

Strittmatter, W., Saunders, A., Schmechel, D., Pericak Vance, M., Enghild, I., Salvasen, G., *et al.* (1993). Apolipoprotein E; High avidity binding to beta amyloid and increased frequency of type 4 allele in late onset familial Alzheimer disease. *Proceedings of the National Academy of Science USA*, **90**, 1877–81.

Swearer, J., O'Donnell, B., Drachman, D., and Woodward, B. (1992). Neuropsychological features of Familial Alzheimer's disease. *Annals of Neurology*, **32**, 687–94.

Taddei, K., Kwok, J. B., Kril, J. J., Halliday, G. M., Creasey, H., Hallupp, M., *et al.* (1998). Two novel presenilin-1 mutations (Ser169Leu and Pro436Gln) associated with very early onset Alzheimer's disease. *NeuroReport*, **9**, 3335–9.

Tanzi, E., Gusella, J. F., Watkins, P. C., Bruns, G. A. P., St George-Hyslop, P., Van Keuren, M. L., *et al.* (1987). Amyloid B protein gene: cDNA, mRNA distributions, and genetic linkage near the Alzheimer locus. *Science*, **235**, 880–90.

Tierney, M., Fisher, R., Lewis, A., Zorzitto, M. L., Snow, W. G., Reid, D. W., *et al.* (1988). The NINCDS ADRDA Work Group criteria for the clinical diagnosis of probable Alzheimer's disease: a clinopathological study of 57 cases. *Neurology*, **38**, 359–64.

Tysoe, C., Whittaker, J., Xuereb, J., Cairns, N. J., Cruts, M., Van Broeckhoven, C., *et al.* (1998). A presenilin-1 truncating mutation is present in two cases with autopsy- confirmed early-onset Alzheimer disease. *American Journal of Human Genetics*, **62**, 70–6.

Van Broeckhoven, C., Backhovens, H., Cruts, M., De Winter, G., Bruyland, M., Cras, P., *et al.* (1992). Mapping of gene predisposing to early onset Alzheimer's disease to chromosome 14q24.3. *Nature Genetics*, **2**, 334–9.

Van Broeckhoven, C., Genthe, A., Vandeberghe, A., Horsthemke, B., Backhovens, H., Raeymaekers, P., *et al.* (1987). Failure of familial Alzheimer's disease to segregate with the A4 amyloid gene in several European families. *Nature*, **329**, 153–5.

Vasterling, J. J., Seltzer, B., Carpenter, B. D., and Thompson, K. A. (1997). Unawareness of social interaction and emotional control deficits in Alzheimer's disease. *Aging, Neuropsychology and Cognition*, **4**, 280–9.

Vidal, R., Frangione, B., Rostagno, A., Mead, S., Revesz, T., Plant, G., *et al.* (1999). A stop-codon mutation in the BRI gene associated with familial British dementia. *Nature*, **399**, 776–81.

Warrington, E. K., Agnew, S. K., Kennedy, A. M., and Rossor, M. N. (2001). Neuropsychological profiles of familial Alzheimer's disease associated with mutations in the presenilin1 gene. *Journal of Neurology*, **248**, 45–50.

Wasco, W. (1995). Familial Alzheimer's chromosome 14 mutations. *Nature Medicine*, **1**, 848.

Welsh, K. A., Butters, N., Hughes, J. P., and Mohs, R. C. (1992). Detection and staging of dementia in Alzheimer's disease: Use of the neuropsychological measures developed for the Consortium to Establish a Registry for Alzheimer's Disease. *Archives of Neurology*, **49**, 448–52.

Wilcock, G., Hope, R., and Brooks, D. (1989). Recommended minimum data to be collected in research studies on Alzheimer's disease. *Journal of Neurology, Neurosurgery and Psychiatry*, **52**, 693–7000.

Worster-Drought, C., Greenfield, J., and McMenemey, W. (1944). A form of familial presenile demntia with spastic paralysis. *Brain*, **76**, 38–43.

Yasuda, M., Maeda, K., Hashimoto, M., Yamashita, H., Ikejiri, Y., Bird, T. D., *et al.* (1999). A pedigree with a novel presenilin 1 mutation at a residue that is not conserved in presenilin 2. *Archives of Neurology*, **56**, 65–9.

Yasuda, M., Maeda, K., Ikejiri, Y., Kawamata, T., Kuroda, S., and Tanaka, C. (1997). A novel missense mutation in the presenilin-1 gene in a familial Alzheimer's disease pedigree with abundant amyloid angiopathy. *Neuroscience Letters*, **232**, 29–32.

12 Frontotemporal dementia (Pick's disease)

John R. Hodges and Bruce Miller

1 Introduction

The last decade has seen considerable advances in our understanding of the neurodegenerative diseases producing focal cognitive deficits typically involving the frontal and/or temporal lobes (most commonly referred to collectively as either Pick's disease or, more recently, fronto-temporal dementia [FTD]). These advances have come from the fields of neuropsychology, neuropsychiatry, neuroimaging, and molecular genetics. Unfortunately the non-expert's ability to follow these developments has been somewhat marred by the confusing plethora of terms in use. While some labels denote a clinical syndrome without specific histological implications (e.g. progressive aphasia, semantic dementia, or dementia of frontal type), others describe specific neuropathological entities (e.g. Pick's disease, familial tauopathy), hybrid clinicopatho-logical entities (frontotemporal dementia), or even specific familial disorders (e.g. chromosome 17 linked frontotemporal dementia with parkinsonism). While there is a close correspondence between symptoms and the site of pathology, the mapping between other levels is poor, so that it is very difficult to predict the exact pathology (from within the spectrum of Pick and Pick-like diseases). We prefer, therefore, a classification based upon the clinical presentation and distinguish three major clinical syndromes: dementia of frontal type, semantic dementia, and progressive non-fluent aphasia.

The aims of this chapter are to review the evolution of the terms applied to this spectrum of disorders, to describe the key clinical, neuropsychological, and radiological characteristics associated with the major syndromes and to highlight recent developments in the genetics. The molecular pathology and histological changes are dealt with in detail elsewhere in the book (see Chapters 8 and 10, respectively). Issues related to drug therapies and general management are covered in Chapters 19 and 20.

2 Early descriptions by Pick and others

In 1892 Arnold Pick (Girling and Berrios 1994 translation of Pick 1892) reported a 71-year-old man with progressive mental deterioration and unusually severe aphasia who at post-mortem had marked atrophy of the left temporal lobe. Pick wanted to emphasize that progressive brain atrophy can lead to symptoms of local disturbance (in this instance aphasia) through local accentuation of the disease process. He also made specific, and as we will see below highly perceptive, predictions regarding the role of the mid temporal region of the left hemisphere in the representation of word meaning. In subsequent papers (Girling and Berrios 1997 translation of Pick 1904; Girling and Markova 1995 translation of Pick 1901) he described four further patients with left temporal or frontotemporal atrophy again stressing their progressive language disturbance. It was only in his 1906 publication that Pick turned his attention to bilateral frontal atrophy with resultant behavioural disturbance.

The histological abnormalities associated with Pick's disease were described a few years later by Alzheimer (1911) who recognized changes distinct from those found in the form of cerebral degeneration later associated with his name. Alzheimer recognized both argyrophilic intracytoplasmic inclusions (Pick bodies), and diffusely staining ballooned neurons (Pick cells) in association with focal lobar atrophy. Onari and Spatz (1926) were among the first to use the eponym Pick's disease (PD) but Carl Schneider (1927, 1929) is probably most responsible for its introduction. Unfortunately, however, he concentrated on the frontal lobe component of the syndrome and began the neglect of the temporal lobe syndromes associated with focal atrophy which has continued ever since. Many papers appeared in the 1930s and 1940s (for review see Hodges 1994; Tissot *et al.* 1975, 1985).

With the general waning of interest in the cognitive aspects of neurology in the English speaking world, interest in focal dementias faded and some authors went as far as to claim that Alzheimer's and Pick's disease were clinically indistinguishable in life. The focus of interest in English language publications became the neuropathology, and latterly the genetics of the dementias. This resulted in a gradual change in the criteria for Pick's disease which evolved to include the necessity for specific pathological changes (i.e. focal atrophy with Pick cells and/or Pick bodies). In continental Europe, however, there remained a strong interest in the clinical phenomena of the dementias; Pick's disease remained an *in vivo* diagnosis based on a combination of clinical features suggestive of frontal and/or temporal lobe dysfunction and focal lobar atrophy (e.g. Mansvelt 1954; Tissot *et al.* 1975).

3 Rediscovering Pick's disease: from dementia of the frontal type and progressive aphasia to frontotemporal dementia

A renaissance of interest in the focal dementias occurred in the 1980s. Workers from Lund (Brun 1987; Gustafson 1987) reported on a large series of patients with dementia and found that of 158 patients studied prospectively who came to post-mortem, 26 had evidence of frontal lobe degeneration. Since only a small proportion had Pick cells and Pick bodies — the remainder had very similar findings but without specific inclusions (i.e. focal lobar atrophy with severe neuronal loss and spongiosis) — the Lund group preferred to adopt the term 'frontal degeneration of non-Alzheimer type'. At approximately the same time, Neary and co-workers in Manchester (Neary *et al.* 1986), began a series of important clinicopathological studies of patients with presenile dementia. They, likewise, found a high proportion of cases with a progressive frontal lobe syndrome who had neither specific changes of Alzheimer's disease (plaques and tangles) nor specific Pick pathology. They introduced the term 'dementia of frontal type' (DFT). Over the next few years other groups described very similar cases under the labels 'frontal lobe degeneration' (Miller *et al.* 1991) and 'dementia lacking distinct histological features' (Knopman *et al.* 1990).

The other strand of the story concerns the rediscovery of the syndrome of progressive aphasia in association with focal left peri-sylvian or temporal lobe atrophy: In 1982 Mesulam reported six patients with long history of insidiously worsening aphasia in the absence of signs of more generalized cognitive failure one of whom underwent a brain biopsy which revealed non-specific histology without specific markers of either Alzheimer's or Pick's disease. Following Mesulam's seminal paper approximately 100 patients with progressive aphasia were reported over the next 15 years (for review see Garrard and Hodges 1999; Hodges and Patterson 1996; Mesulam and Weintraub 1992; Snowden *et al.* 1996). From this literature it is clear that although the language impairment in patients with progressive aphasia is heterogeneous there are two identifiable and distinct aphasia syndromes: progressive non-fluent aphasia and progressive fluent aphasia. In the later syndrome, speech remains fluent and well articulated but becomes progressively devoid of content words; the language and other non-verbal cognitive deficits observed in these patients reflects a breakdown in semantic memory which has lead many authors to apply the label of 'semantic dementia' (Hodges and Patterson 1996; Hodges *et al.* 1992, 1994; Patterson and Hodges 2000; Saffran and Schwartz 1994; Snowden *et al.* 1989). In non-fluent progressive aphasia speech is faltering and distorted with frequent phonological substitutions and grammatical errors, but the semantic aspects of language remain intact. In both forms of progressive aphasia other non-language based components of cognition remain well preserved, as do activities of daily living.

There are a number of compelling reasons to consider semantic dementia as part of the same disease spectrum as the frontal variant of the disease (DFT). The first is pathological: a meta-analysis of the 14 clinicopathological studies of cases fulfilling criteria for semantic dementia showed that all had either classic Pick's disease (i.e. Pick bodies and/or Pick cells) or non-specific spongiform change of the type found in the majority of cases with the frontal form of lobar atrophy (Hodges *et al.* 1998). Second is the evolution of cognitive and behavioural changes over time; although semantic dementia patients present with progressive anomia and other linguistic deficits, on follow-up the features which characterize DFT emerge (Edwards Lee *et al.* 1997; Hodges *et al.* 1994). Third, is that fact that modern neuroimaging techniques demonstrate subtle involvement of the orbitofrontal cortex in the majority of cases presenting prominent temporal atrophy and semantic dementia (Mummery *et al.* 2000).

The status of patients with the non-fluent form of progressive aphasia within the spectrum of FTD is less certain. Changes in behaviour and personality of the type that typify DFT, and are seen in the later stages of semantic dementia, are rare, but after a number of years, global cognitive decline occurs (Green *et al.* 1990; Hodges and Patterson 1996). In Cambridge, a number of such patients have had classic Alzheimer pathology at post-mortem, albeit with an atypical distribution; that is to say, marked involvement of peri-sylvian language areas but sparing of medial temporal structures (Croot 1997; Greene *et al.* 1996). Review of the published literature reveals that approximately equal numbers of cases with non-fluent aphasia have AD pathology while the remainder have Pick-like pathology but almost invariably without Pick bodies or Pick cells (Mesulam 1982; Mesulam and Weintraub 1992; Weintraub *et al.* 1990).

The final term to be considered is that of frontotemporal dementia (FTD). In 1994 the Lund and Manchester groups introduced the term FTD (Brun *et al.* 1994) and suggested tentative criteria for the diagnosis. The adoption of the term, which has increased enormously with the discovery of tau gene mutations in some families with Pick body negative FTD (see below and Chapter 8), has the advantage of avoiding specific pathological implications. It also brings to attention the fact that patients with the same disease may present with different clinical syndromes and that with time both types of deficit are likely to emerge. It has the disadvantages, however, in blurring levels of description and amalgamating distinct clinical syndromes and, once again, overshadowing the temporal lobe component of the disorder. We now describe the principal clinical variants of FTD which are summarized in Table 12.1.

Table 12.1 A proposed classification of the frontotemporal dementias

Clinical

1 Syndromes based on neuropsychological features and anatomy

Syndrome	Principal symptoms	Site of pathology
Dementia of frontal type	Change in personality and behaviour	Bilateral orbitobasal frontal
Semantic dementia	Fluent anomic aphasia with impaired comprehension and loss of knowledge	Left (or bilateral) temporal pole and infero-lateral cortex
Progressive non-fluent aphasia	Non-fluent, hesitant, distorted speech, with preserved comprehension	Left perisylvian
Progressive prosopagnosia	Impaired face identification followed by loss of person knowledge	Right temporal pole and infero-lateral cortex

2 Familial FTD with parkinsonism
Chromosome 17 linked tauopathy
Chromosome 3 linked Danish variant (one family)
Familial FTD with no known linkage established
(These may present with any of the syndromes listed under 1 (above) and/or with motor neuron disease features)

3 FTD with motor neuron disease
(May present with any of the above clinical syndromes)

Pathological
Pathological classification (after Jackson and Lowe 1996; Spillantini *et al.* 1998a)
Pick's disease proper with tau and ubiquitin positive inclusions (usually non familial)
Familial FTD with characteristic pick-like tau positive inclusions in neurons and glial cells
Motor neuron type with ubiquitin positive inclusions including dentate fascia
Corticobasal degeneration with swollen achromatic neurons containing tau positive inclusions and astrocyte plaques
Microvacuolar degeneration and gliosis but lacking distinctive intraneuronal inclusions

(NB: There is an incomplete correspondence between clinical and pathological syndromes)

Table 12.2 Anatomical divisions of the prefrontal cortex, their hypothesized function, and associated deficits

Brain region	Hypothesized function	Deficit seen with dysfunction
Orbitobasal	Inhibition, social control, eating control	Disinhibition, impulsivity, confabulation, antisocial, stereotypic behaviours, overeating
Dorsolateral	Attention, working memory (area 45), alternate programs, generate words, designs, ideas	Poor attention and focus, working memory deficits, poor organization, planning, poor word/design generation
Medial frontal	Energy, motivation, drive, affect (right > left)?	Apathy, abulia, depression?

4 Dementia of frontal type (frontal variant FTD)

The division of frontal lobe function into three separate areas, each of which has distinctive functions, first proposed by Stuss and Benson (1986), offers a logical way to think about the deficits that develop in patients with frontal variant FTD which for simplicity we shall refer to here as dementia of frontal type (DFT). Table 12.2 lists the anatomical regions of the cortex, describes the functions, and documents the type of deficits that occur in patients when these parts of the brain degenerate.

Patients with DFT are almost invariably lacking in insight (Gregory and Hodges 1996; Gregory *et al.* 1998) and are brought along by relatives or friends who have become aware of the gradual onset of changes in personality and behaviour. The disinhibition and antisocial behaviour, resulting from orbitobasal involvement, occur in approximately one-half of patients and can be the presenting feature (Miller *et al.* 1997). Theft, hit-and-run accidents, and public exposure commonly occur, but violent assaults on others are rare. Poor impulse control places a huge burden on carers, and is the major factor leading to placement in nursing homes. It has been also been suggested that patients with asymmetric right-sided disease are more likely to exhibit socially unacceptable behaviour than those with left-sided involvement (Edwards Lee *et al.* 1997; Miller *et al.* 1993).

Stereotypical or ritualized behaviours (such as insisting on eating the same food at exactly the same time daily or cleaning the house in precisely the same order), the use of a 'catch-phrase', and a change in food preference towards sweet things are also very common and in a recent study were found to be he features that best discriminated DFT from AD (Bozeat *et al.* 2000). Other features of the Kluver-Bucy syndrome (Cummings and Duchen 1981), such as increased sexual activity and hyperorality (a tendency to put any object in the mouth) can develop, but tend to be late.

Apathy is another very common feature and is probably correlated with the severity of medial frontal cingulate involvement. Lack of empathy and a complete lack of concern for others are very distressing and frequent symptoms. Deficits in planning, organization, and other aspects of 'executive' function are likewise universal as the diseases progress and reflect spread of disease to dorso-lateral prefrontal cortex. It should be noted, however, that neither apathy nor dysexecutive symptoms were found in discriminate DFT from AD in a recent large study (Bozeat *et al.* 2000).

One undoubted advance in the area has been the development of standardized carer interviews such as the Neuropsychiatric Inventory (Cummings *et al.* 1994) which appears to differentiate patients with FTD and AD (Levy *et al.* 1996): see Chapter 4. In an attempt to develop a local instrument capable of early diagnosis we identified 15 key symptoms that occurred very commonly in a group of 12 DFT cases and proposed provisional criteria, as shown in Table 12.3 (Gregory and Hodges 1993; 1996.

4.1 Neuropsychological and radiological findings in DFT

Some patients with DFT show clear-cut cognitive deficits at presentation, but since most traditional 'frontal executive' tasks are sensitive to dorso-lateral, rather than orbitobasal frontal, dysfunction, patients may perform perfectly on such tests (Gregory *et al.* 1999). Among the most helpful are the Wisconsin Card Sorting Test and verbal fluency (i.e. the generation of words beginning with a given letter of the alphabet). More recently, quantifiable tasks better able to detect orbitobasal frontal function have been developed. For instance, Rahman *et al.* (1999) have shown that patients with relatively early DFT generally perform very well on the CANTAB battery of computer-based test (including the paired associate learning and delayed matching to sample test which are sensitive to early AD), but show specific deficits at the reversal stage of a discriminate learning test. They also applied a novel test of decision making and risk-taking derived from a popular game show (Rogers *et al.* 1998). The patients with DFT showed marked deficits on this test. Another promising area of development is the application of tests of social judgement initially developed in the field of autism research in which subjects have to judge the mental state of others or to assess the occurrence of socially inappropriate actions or comments, the so-called 'faux pas test' (Stone *et al.* 1998).

Memory is relatively spared in DFT: orientated and recall of recent personal events is good but performance of anterograde memory tests is more variable and patients tend to do poorly on recall (as opposed to recognition) based tasks (Hodges *et al.* 1999*a*). With time, more marked amnesia can develop with non-temporally graded loss of remote memory (Hodges and Gurd 1994).

Table 12.3 Criteria for a diagnosis of dementia of frontal type (suggested by Gregory and Hodges 1993)

A	Presentation with an insidious disorder of personality and behaviour
B	The presence of two or more of the following features:-
	Loss of insight
	Disinhibition
	Restlessness
	Distractibility
	Emotional ability
	Reduced empathy or unconcern for others
	Lack of foresight, poor planning or judgement
	Impulsivity
	Social withdrawal
	Apathy or lack of spontaneity
	Poor self-care
	Reduced verbal output
	Verbal stereotypes or echolalia
	Perseveration
	Features of Kluver-Bucy syndrome (gluttony, pica, sexual hyperactivity)
C	Relative preservation of day-to-day (episodic) memory
D	Psychiatric phenomena may be present (mood disorder, paranoia)
E	Absence of past history of head injury, stroke, chronic alcohol abuse, or major psychiatric illness

A reduction in spontaneous conversation is common, but patients with DFT perform well on tests of involving picture naming, word-picture matching, generation of word definition, and other semantically based tasks such as the Pyramids and Palm Trees Test described below (Hodges *et al.* 1999*a*). The most striking neuropsychological finding is how well subjects perform on tests of visuospatial ability, particularly when the organization aspects are minimized: the Rey Figure Test is often copied poorly due to impulsiveness and poor strategy formation but on subtests of the Visual Object and Space Perception Battery (Warrington and James 1991) subjects can perform perfectly even at an advanced stage of the disease.

Simple cognitive screening tests, such as the Mini-Mental State Examination, are unreliable for the detection and monitoring of patients with DFT who frequently perform normally even when requiring nursing home care (Gregory and Hodges 1996; Gregory *et al.* 1999).

Both functional (single photon emission tomography, SPECT; positron emission tomography, PET) and structural imaging (CT, MRI) may be normal even when the patient exhibits gross behaviour changes (Gregory *et al.* 1999). Functional imaging changes generally precede structural alterations with the appearance of orbitobasal frontal hypoperfusion: an example of typical SPECT scan findings from a patient with DFT are shown in Figure 12.1 (see Plate 26).

5 Semantic dementia (temporal lobe variant FTD)

Warrington (1975) was the first to clearly delineate the syndrome of semantic memory impairment and reported three patients, two of whom were subsequently shown to have Pick's disease at autopsy (Cummings and Duchen 1981; and personal communication). Drawing on the work of Tulving (1972, 1983), Warrington recognized that the progressive anomia in her patients was not simply a linguistic deficit, but reflected a fundamental loss of semantic memory (or knowledge) about the items, which thereby affected naming, word comprehension, and object recognition.

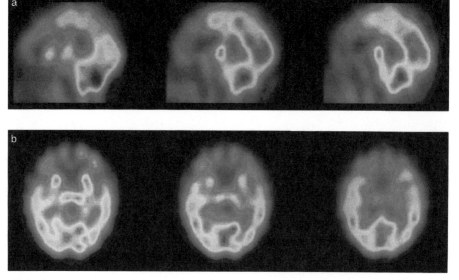

Figure 12.1   (See also Plate 26) HMPAO-SPECT images from a typical case of frontal variant frontotemporal dementia (dementia of frontal type) showing marked bifrontal hypoperfusion. (a) Three sagittal images; (b) three axial images.

Such patients would previously have been described as having a combination of 'amnesic, or sometimes transcortical sensory, aphasia' and 'associative agnosia'. Cases of semantic dementia have also been recognized for many years in Japan as cases of 'Gogi (word meaning) aphasia' (Imura *et al.* 1971; Sasanuma and Mondi 1975; Tanabe *et al.* 1992).

Semantic memory is the term applied to the component of long-term memory which contains the permanent representation of our knowledge about things in the world and their interrelationship, facts and concepts, as well as words and their meaning (Garrard *et al.* 1997; Hodges *et al.* 1998, 1992; Hodges and Patterson 1997).

Patients with semantic dementia typically present complaining of loss of memory for words. They are often painfully aware of their shrinking expressive vocabulary, but are strangely oblivious to their impaired comprehension. Carers note the use of substitute words and phrases such as 'boy' and 'an outdoor thing' and the progressive difficulty understanding less common words. Since the grammatical and phonological structure of language remains intact, these changes are relatively subtle, at least in the early stages.

In contrast to Alzheimer's disease, patients with semantic dementia have good day-to-day (episodic) memory although recent studies show the situation to be more complex that it initially appeared. Orientation is certainly intact and patients are able to relate the details (albeit in a rather empty anomic fashion) of recent life events, but more quantitative assessment shows impaired recall of more distant life events. In other words, they show a reversal of the usual temporal gradient found in Alzheimer's disease and the amnesic syndrome (Graham and Hodges 1997; Hodges and Graham 1998).

Behavioural changes may be slight at presentation but with time features identical to those seen in DFT emerge. The group lead by Miller have also drawn attention to the bizarre behaviours (including irritability, impulsiveness, alterations in dress, limited and fixed ideas, intensification of religious or philosophical thinking, and decreased facial expression) exhibited by patients with predominantly right temporal lobe atrophy (Edwards Lee *et al.* 1997; Miller *et al.* 1997) although this might, in part, reflect the delayed presentation of right-sided cases because of the relative lack of linguistic changes in such cases. The contrasting features of semantic dementia and non-fluent progressive aphasia are summarized in Table 12.4.

5.1 Neuropsychological and radiological findings in semantic dementia

Patients with semantic dementia are globally impaired on tests of semantic memory. This is most apparent on tasks which require a verbal output, such as category fluency tests (in which subjects are asked to produce as many examples as possible defined semantic from categories, such as animals or musical instruments, within one minute), picture naming, and the generation of verbal definitions to words and pictures. The pattern of errors on these tasks reflects a loss of fine grained or attribute knowledge with preservation of broad superordinate information. For instance on naming tasks errors are initially category co-ordinates (elephant for hippopotamus), then with time prototype responses emerge so that all animals are called 'dog', then eventually they are simply called 'animal' (Hodges *et al.* 1994; Lambon Ralph *et al.* 1999). Single-word comprehension is also affected, as judged by tasks such as word-picture matching or 'odd-man-out' synonym tasks (e.g. 'Which of the following is the odd one out; pond, lake, river?'). Non-verbal semantic knowledge is less easy to assess, but the Pyramids and Palm Trees Test (Howard and Patterson 1992) in which the subject is asked to judge the semantic relatedness of pictures almost invariably reveals deficits. The semantic memory battery developed by Hodges and Patterson, based upon the same set of items (in the revised version 64: half natural kinds and half

Table 12.4 Comparison of clinical features of semantic dementia, and progressive non-fluent aphasia

	Semantic dementia	Progressive non-fluent aphasia
Age at onset	Commonly < 65	Commonly < 65
Disease progression	Generally rapid	Slow
Spontaneous speech	Fluent and grammatically correct, but empty of content words	Laboured, telegraphic, with long word finding pauses and frequent phonological and grammatical errors
Paraphasias	Semantic	Phonological

Comprehension:
    Single words
    Syntax
	Impaired
	Intact
		Intact
		Impaired

Repetition	Normal for single words	Phonemic errors
Digit span	Normal	Impaired
Episodic memory	Preserved for recent events	Intact
Frontal 'executive' functions	Intact in early stages	Intact
Visuospatial and perceptual skills	Intact	Intact
Behaviour	Appropriate initially but frontal features invariably appear	Appropriate until very late
General neurological findings	Usually none	Bucco-facial apraxia common
MRI findings	Focal polar and infero-lateral temporal lobe atrophy, often worse on the left	Left perisylvian atrophy

man-made) which are used to assess central representation knowledge via different modalities of input and output including category fluency, picture naming, naming from verbal descriptions, word-picture matching, picture and word sorting, and a probed semantic attribute questionnaire has proven useful in the evaluation of patients with all forms of FTD and Alzheimer's disease (Hodges and Patterson 1995, 1996; Hodges *et al.* 1999*a*, 1996).

In contrast to the profound semantic deficit, other aspects of language competency (phonology and syntax) are strikingly preserved (Hodges *et al.* 1995, 1992). Although able to read and spell words with regular spelling-to-sound correspondence, virtually all cases have difficulty reading — and spelling — irregular words (e.g. reading PINT to rhyme with hint, flint, etc.). This pattern known as surface dyslexia (or dysgraphia) has been attributed to the loss of semantic support that is necessary for the correct pronunciation of irregular words (see Graham *et al.* 2000; Patterson *et al.* 1994). One practical implication of the surface dyslexia is that patients with semantic dementia have great difficulty with National Adult Reading Test (Nelson and Willison 1991), which is based upon irregular words, and is commonly used measure of pre-morbid intellectual ability.

As mentioned above, patients with semantic dementia are characteristically well orientated and have good recall of recent personal events (Graham and Hodges 1997). This distinctive feature is more difficult to detect on formal tests of anterograde memory. Because of their severe semantic deficit, often complicated by additional anomia, patients perform very badly on tests such as logical memory (story recall) from the WMS and word-list learning tests. By contrast, they often score within the normal range on non-verbal memory tests such as recall of the Rey Complex Figure (Hodges *et al.* 1999a). They also show excellent recognition memory when colour pictures are used as the stimuli, although it has been recently demonstrated that they rely heavily upon perceptual information: Graham *et al.* (2000) compared recognition memory for 'known' and 'unknown' items (known items were pictures that subjects were able to name or correctly identify) in two conditions. In one, the item was perceptually identical at study and test (e.g. the same telephone) while in the other condition a different exemplar was presented at study and test (e.g. a different telephone). Patients with semantic dementia showed near perfect recognition memory for both known and unknown items in the former, perceptually identical, condition, but were significantly impaired in the latter (perceptually different) condition. Graham *et al.* concluded that patients with semantic dementia are unusually reliant upon perceptual inputs to medial temporal episodic memory structures whereas normal subjects can use both semantic and perceptually based routes to encode new information. Working (immediate) memory is typically well preserved as illustrated by normal digit span (Hodges *et al.* 1992).

Patients with semantic dementia perform normally on tests of non-verbal problem solving such as Raven's Coloured Progressive Matrices (Hodges *et al.* 1992; Tanaka *et al.* 1998) and, in common with frontal cases, are strikingly good at tests of basic perceptual and spatial ability.

Despite the profound loss of semantic, patients often handle difficult situations surprisingly well in everyday life, at least in their homes. Evidence for apparent preservation of object usage has, however, been based largely upon anecdotal evidence. When investigated systematically a rather different picture emerges. While it is true that patients with even advanced disease are able to use *some* objects for which they have no explicit knowledge — as judged by naming and visually based tests of associative knowledge in which pictures of objects have to be matched with their usual recipient or location — such usage is based upon the visual affordances of the object and mechanical problem solving skills, which are strikingly preserved in semantic dementia (Hodges *et al.* 1999b).

Neuroradiology offers a valuable adjunct to neuropsychological evaluation. Functional changes on HMPAO-SPECT precede visible structural alterations with hypoperfusion of one or both temporal lobes (Garrard and Hodges 1999; Sinnatamby *et al.* 1996). In contrast to DFT, temporal lobe atrophy is much more readily visible. A number of studies have confirmed the anterolateral distribution of changes with severe atrophy involving the polar region, fusiform, and infero-lateral gyri (Mummery *et al.* 1998). An asymmetric pattern is almost invariable with the left temporal lobe much more often involved than the right. The status of the hippocampus and parahippocampal gyrus (containing the entorhinal cortex) is less certain. Despite previous reports of relative sparing of the hippocampus, a recent volumetric analysis of ten cases of semantic dementia has shown asymmetric atrophy of the hippocampus which was actually more marked on the left than in a group of ten Alzheimer disease (AD) patients, matched for disease duration, but equivalent in severity on the right side. The appearance of 'relative' preservation of medial temporal structures is due to the profound atrophy of surrounding structures compared to the hippocampus: the average volume loss of the temporal pole, fusiform, and infero-lateral gyri in semantic dementia was 50%, and in some cases up to 80% compared to 20% loss of hippocampal volume. Whereas in AD the 20% loss of hippocampal volume stands out against the normal polar and infero-lateral structures (Galton *et al.* 2000). The contrasting MRI appearances of AD and semantic dementia are illustrated in Figure 12.2.

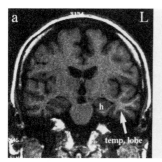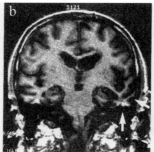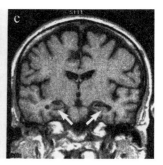

Figure 12.2 Coronal T1-weighted MRI images through the temporal lobes contrasting (a) a normal brain h = hippocampus; (b) a patient with semantic dementia and striking left parahippocampals fusiform and infero-lateral gyri atrophy (arrow), but relative sparing of the hippocampus; (c) a patient with early Alzheimer's disease and bilateral hippocampal atrophy (arrows).

6 Progressive prosopagnosia and loss of knowledge for people with progressive right temporal atrophy

A number of earlier authors had suggested association between right temporal atrophy and selective difficulty with person identification (Tyrrell *et al.* 1990), but the first fully documented cases, VH, was reported by Evans *et al.* (1995). Initially, VH appeared to have the classic features of modality-specific prosopagnosia, i.e. a severe inability to identify familiar people from their face but much better performance on names and voices. With time, however, it became clear that the deficit was one of a loss of knowledge about people affecting all modalities of access to knowledge. She was unable to identify a photograph of Margaret Thatcher or to provide any information when presented with the name yet general semantic and autobiographical memory remained intact (Kitchener and Hodges 1999). MRI showed severe yet selective right anterolateral temporal lobe atrophy. The special role for the right temporal lobe in the representation of knowledge about people has been subsequently confirmed in a number of other cases (Gentileschi *et al.* 1999; Hodges and Graham 1998).

7 Progressive non-fluent aphasia

Patients present with complaints of speech dysfluency and distortion or word finding difficulty. Phonological errors are usually obvious in conversation. Comprehension is relatively well preserved least in the early stages although as the disease progresses there are problems with phoneme discrimination that the patients invariably attribute to poor hearing. Complaints of noise intolerance are common, speech output becomes progressively more sparse, and in the late stages patients may be mute and effectively 'word deaf'.

Memory for day-to-day events is good and patients handle difficult situations well with the skills of everyday life. In our experience, the behavioural changes are usually slight at least for many years. In Cambridge we have followed patients for up to eight years before features of more global dementia emerge.

7.1 Neuropsychological and radiological findings in progressive non-fluent aphasia

The pattern of cognitive deficits presents, in many ways, the mirror image to that found in semantic dementia. Patients perform very well on tests of semantic memory, except on those requiring a spoken output. Although conversational speech is severely disrupted, picture naming is often only mildly impaired and the errors are phonological (efalant for elephant). On tests of fluency, semantic category fluency is less affected than letter fluency. Word-picture matching, synonym tasks, and other semantic tests are usually performed perfectly. On tests of phonological competence (such as repetition of mutisyllabic words, blending word segments and rhyming) they perform poorly. Tests of syntactic comprehension such as the Test for the Reception of Grammar (TROG) (Bishop 1989) in which subjects are asked to match pictures to sentences of increasing complexity, also reveal substantial deficits (Hodges and Patterson 1996). Patients produce phonological errors when repeating multisyllabic words or sentences and show reduced digit span. In common with the other FTD syndromes, however, performance on visuospatial and perceptual function is well preserved.

Much less is know about the radiological changes in non-fluent cases. Structural imaging shows widening of the Sylvian fissure with atrophy of insula, inferior frontal and superior temporal lobes.

8 Genetics of FTD: familial FTD with parkinsonism linked to chromosome 17

It is often fairly difficult to determine if a familial disorder is present. Unlike AD where the presence of progressive memory loss is an excellent marker for disease in previous generations, with FTD the only indications of previous disease can be vaguely described mental disorders, relatives who disappear due to erratic behaviour, alcoholism, or even murder/suicides. Despite this difficulty determining the presence of FTD in previous generations, it is clear that this is often a familial disorder. The UCLA group reported that 40% of all FTD cases showed a familial pattern, with the majority of these familial cases suggesting an autosomal dominant pattern of inheritance (Chow *et al.* 1999). A similar frequency was reported by the Dutch investigators (Stevens *et al.* 1998). It is our impression that patients with semantic dementia have fewer affected relatives than other forms of FTD, although this has not formally been studied. Unlike AD where apolipoprotein E4 is a strong risk factor, in FTD the association between apolipoprotein E4 and dementia is less certain (Geschwind *et al.* 1998). Recent genetic discoveries of tau gene mutations on chromosome 17 have begun to clarify the role of tau in the pathogenesis of dementia.

The story of the chromosome 17 linkage is extraordinary in a number of ways. Families around the world with what has become known as frontotemporal dementia with parkinsonism linked to chromosome 17 (Spillantini *et al.* 1998a) had originally been reported under a range of labels. The link between FTD and chromosome 17 was first reported by (Wilhelmsen *et al.* 1994) in a family with disinhibition–dementia–parkinsonism–amyotrophy–complex (DDPAC) (Wilhelmsen *et al.* 1994). Soon afterwards, linkage was established in a number of other families syndromes not previously connected, including: rapidly progressive autosomal dominant parkinsonism and dementia with pallidoponto-nigral degeneration (Wszolek *et al.* 1992), familial progressive subclinical gliosis (Petersen *et al.* 1995), hereditary dysphasia and dementia (Morris *et al.* 1984), hereditary frontotemporal dementia (Heutink *et al.* 1997), familial multiple system tauopathy with presenile dementia (Spillantini *et al.* 1997), familial presenile dementia with psychosis (Sumi *et al.* 1992), and Pick's disease (Schenk 1958). In 1996 a meeting of representatives from all the groups identifying linkage to chromosome 17 was held in Ann Arbor Michigan (Foster *et al.* 1997). Comparison of clinical and pathological data revealed a great deal of similarity between the families who all shared the characteristics of predominately frontotemporal distribution of pathology with marked behavioural changes. Extrapyramidal dysfunction was present in most. In some families psychotic symptoms were a major feature and a number had amyotrophy. It was recognized then that some of the families shared the common pathology with microtubule-associated protein tau positive inclusions. Progress in the field was then rapid. It was soon discovered that most, if not all, families had tau inclusions with distinctive morphological pattern leading to the coining of the term 'familial tauopathy' and the suggestion that the disease might reflect a mutation in the tau gene known to be located in the 17q21-22 region (Spillantini *et al.* 1998*a*). Within two years of the Ann Arbor meeting, several groups had identified the actual genetic mutation that, as predicted, was in the tau gene (Dumanchin *et al.* 1998; Hutton *et al.* 1998; Spillantini *et al.* 1998*b*). In one large Danish family autosomal dominant FTD linkage has been established to chromosome 3 (Brown *et al.* 1995), the molecular basis in this family remains uncertain.

The discovery of these tau mutations suggests potential mechanisms for why the brain degenerates in patients with FTD. Additionally, progressive supranuclear palsy (PSP) (Conrad *et al.* 1997) and corticobasal degeneration (CBD) (Feany *et al.* 1996; Mori *et al.* 1994) may be linked to FTD through similar abnormalities in tau. Hong *et al.* (1998) found that the cellular inclusions in some families are due to excessive accumulation of tau components, while in other families, mutations in tau lead to abnormal assembly of microtubules. It is still unknown why frontotemporal cortex, basal ganglia, and motor neurons are selectively vulnerable in certain families carrying these mutations.

9 FTD with motor neuron disease

Although motor neuron disease (MND) has traditionally been regarded as a disorder which spares higher cognitive abilities, it has become clear since early reports from Japan (Mitsuyama and Takamiya 1979) that the rate of dementia in MND is significantly greater than expected, and conversely a significant minority of patients with FTD develop features of MND (for review see Bak and Hodges 1999; Caselli *et al.* 1993; Neary *et al.* 1990; Rakowicz and Hodges 1998).

Most patients present with cognitive symptoms, either DFT or progressive aphasia, which then progresses rapidly, followed by the emergence of bulbar features and mild limb amyotrophy, although the reverse sequence can be seen. Up to 10% of patients with MND might show features of dementia and/or aphasia if such features are systematically elicited (Rakowicz and Hodges 1998). There are also suggestions that patients with the MND-dementia/aphasia complex may have disproportionate impairment of verb, compared to noun, knowledge (Bak and Hodges 1997).

The histological features — ubiquitin positive, tau negative, inclusions in cortical regions and the dentate gyrus — which separate MND-associated FTD are described elsewhere in the book although the mapping between clinical syndrome and pathology is incomplete (see Chapter 10).

From a practical perspective, this variant of FTD should be suspected in any cases with rapidly progressive disease or the emergence of bulbar symptoms.

10 The neuropathology of FTD

The neuropathology of FTD has become increasingly complex with the identification of five basic patterns.

(1) Pick's disease proper with tau and ubiquitin positive spherical cortical inclusions best seen in the hippocampal dentate gyrus and frontotemporal cortex.

(2) Familial FTD with characteristic tau positive inclusions in neurons and glial cells.

(3) Motor neuron disease type dementia with ubiquitin positive inclusions in cortical layer II and hippocampal dentate granule cells (see above).

(4) Corticobasal degeneration diagnosed by the presence of tau positive, but ubiquitin negative, inclusions in cortical layer II and the substrate nigra with swollen acromatic neurons and astrocytic plaques.

(5) Microvacular degeneration and gliosis lacking distinctive inclusions. This topic is dealt with more fully elsewhere in the book (see Chapter 10).

While variants 3 and 4 are typically associated with clear-cut clinical syndromes of motor neuron disease associated dementia and corticobasal degeneration, respectively, it is becoming increasingly clear that there is considerable overlap: for instance, patients with classic FTD may have pathological findings more characteristic of corticobasal degeneration and vice versa (Kertesz and Munoz 1998; Mathuranath *et al.* 2000).

There is also continuing controversy regarding whether it is possible to identify cases with Pick bodies in life. The majority of familial cases linked to chromosome 17 have lacked Pick bodies despite having abundant tau positive inclusions, suggesting that classic Pick's disease cases are rarely familial. A multi-centre European initiative has pooled clinical and pathological data on 50 cases with classic Pick's disease (i.e. with Pick bodies) and has proposed criteria that stress the marked asymmetry of atrophy found in many cases and the lack of family history. These criteria are currently being tested prospectively (Rossor 1998).

11 Management

There is no known treatment to delay the progression of FTD although environmental and pharmacological interventions may help considerably (Swartz *et al.* 1997) with behavioural management. FTD patients show a profound serotonergic deficit (see Chapter 9), and we have used selective serotonin reuptake inhibitors with some success in this population (Swartz *et al.* 1997). In particular, irritability, impulsivity, and compulsions often respond to these therapies. In the highly agitated and aggressive FTD patient, selective dopamine blockers such as olanzapine can become necessary. In our experience, anticholinesterase compounds can increase irritability and rarely improve cognitive status. Pharmacological therapies are considered more fully in Chapter 18.

The complete management of patients with FTD and their carers requires a multidisciplinary team with input from clinical psychology, genetics, and specialist nurses. This approach is described in Chapter 19.

12 Key points

1   The term frontotemporal dementia denotes a number of distinct clinical syndromes (dementia of frontal type, semantic dementia, progressive non-fluent aphasia) which reflect the predominant locus of pathology.

2   Dementia of frontal type is characterized by major changes in personality with stereotypical behaviour, change in eating preferences, disinhibition, and loss of empathy being the most common presenting features. These changes reflect orbitobasal involvement.

3   Traditional frontal lobe 'executive' tests are insensitive to orbitobasal pathology, and imaging may be normal initially. Functional brain imaging (SPECT, PET) changes precede atrophy on structural imaging (MRI).

4   Semantic dementia presents with loss of memory for words. Speech is fluent with normal syntax and phonology. Patients show gross impairment on tests of semantic memory (category fluency, picture naming, word-picture and picture-picture matching, word definitions, etc.) with preservation of episodic memory, non-verbal problem solving, visuospatial and perceptual abilities.

5   Structural imaging in semantic dementia shows striking anterolateral temporal lobe atrophy which is typically asymmetric (left > right).

6   A rarer variant of semantic dementia presents with prosopagnosia (inability to recognize faces) with a progressive cross-modality of loss of knowledge about people associated with selective right temporal atrophy.

7   Progressive non-fluent aphasia represents the mirror image of semantic dementia with breakdown of the phonological and syntactic aspects of language associated with left perisylvian brain atrophy.

8   Over a third of cases of FTD have a positive family history. In some cases of familial FTD a tau gene mutation on chromosome 17 has been identified.

9   An association between FTD and motor neuron disease is increasingly recognized with an aggressive course and characteristic histopathology.

10   FTD is associated with a range of different non-Alzheimer histological changes with poor correspondence between clinical syndrome and pathology. Only a minority of cases have classic Pick bodies.

References

Alzheimer, A. (1911). Uber eigenartige Krankheitsfalle des spateren Alters. *Zeitschrift fur die Gesamte Neurologie und Psychiatrie*, **4**, 356–85.

Bak, T. and Hodges, J. R. (1997). Noun-verb dissociation in three patients with motor neuron disease and aphasia. *Brain and Language*, **60**, 38–41.

Bak, T. and Hodges, J. R. (1999). Cognition, language and behaviour in motor neurone disease: evidence of frontotemporal dementia. *Dementia and Geriatric Cognitive Disorders*, **10**, 29–23.

Bishop, D. V. M. (1989). *Test for the Reception of Grammar*: Medical Research Council.

Bozeat, S., Gregory, C. A., Lambon Ralph, M. A., and Hodges, J. R. (2000). Neurobehavioural features distinguish dementia of the frontal type, semantic dementia (frontal and temporal variants of frontotemporal dementia) and Alzheimer's disease. *Journal of Neurology, Neurosurgery and Psychiatry*, **69**, 178–186.

Brown, J., Ashworth, A., Gydesen, S., Sorrensen, A., Rossor, M., Hardy, J., *et al.* (1995). Familial nonspecific dementia maps to chromosome 3. *Human Molecular Genetics*, **4**, 1625–8.

Brun, A. (1987). Frontal lobe degeneration of non-Alzheimer's type. I. Neuropathology. *Archives Gerontology and Geriatrics*, **6**, 209–33.

Brun, A., Englund, B., Gustafson, L., Passant, U., Mann, D. M. A., Neary, D., *et al.* (1994). Consensus statement. Clinical and neuropathological criteria for frontotemporal dementia. Lund and Manchester groups. *Journal of Neurology, Neurosurgery, and Psychiatry*, **57**, 416–18.

Caselli, R. J., Windebank, A. J., Petersen, R. C., Komori, T., Parisi, J. E., Okazaki, H., *et al.* (1993). Rapidly progressive aphasic dementia and motor neuron disease. *Annals of Neurology*, **33**, 200–7.

Chow, T. W., Miller, B. L., Hayashi, V. N., and Geschwind, D. H. (1999). Inheritance of frontotemporal dementia. *Archives of Neurology*, **56**, 817–22.

Conrad, C., Andreadis, A., Trojanowski, J. Q., Dickson, D. W., Kang, D., Chen, X. H., *et al.* (1997). Genetic evidence for the involvement of tau in progressive supranuclear palsy. *Annals of Neurology*, **41**, 277–81.

Croot, K. P. (1997). Phonological disruption in progressive aphaisa and Alzheimer's disease. PhD Thesis, p. 261. Cambridge: University of Cambridge.

Cummings, J. L. and Duchen, L. W. (1981). Kluver-Bucy syndrome in Pick's disease: clinical and pathological correlations. *Neurology*, **31**, 1415–22.

Cummings, J. L., Mega, M., Gray, K., Rosenberg-Thompson, S., Carusi, D. A., and Gornbein, J. (1994). The neuropsychiatric inventory: comprehensive assessment of psychopathology in dementia. *Neurology*, **44**, 2308–14.

Dumanchin, C., Camuzat, A., Campion, D., Verpillat, P., Hannequin, D., Dubois, B., *et al.* (1998). Segregation of a missense mutation in the microtubule-associated protein tau gene with familial frontotemporal dementia and parkinsonism. *Human Molecular Genetics*, **7**, 1825–9.

Edwards Lee, T., Miller, B., Benson, F., Cummings, J. L., Russell, G. L., Boone, K., *et al.* (1997). The temporal variant of frontotemporal dementia. *Brain*, **120**, 1027–40.

Evans, J. J., Heggs, A. J, Antoun, N., and Hodges, J. R. (1995). Progressive prosopagnosia associated with selective right temporal lobe atrophy: a new syndrome? *Brain*, **118**, 1–13.

Feany, M. B., Mattiace, L. A., and Dickson, D. W. (1996). Neuropathologic overlap of progressive supranuclear palsy, Pick's disease and corticobasal degeneration. *Journal of Neuropathology and Experimental Neurology*, **55**, 53–67.

Foster, N. L., Wilhelmsen, K., Sima, A. A. F., Jones, M. Z., DAmato, C. J., Gilman, S., *et al.* (1997). Frontotemporal dementia and parkinsonism linked to chromosome 17: A consensus conference. *Annals of Neurology*, **41**, 706–15.

Galton, C., Gomez-Anson, B., Antoun, N., Scheltens, P., Patterson, K., Graves, M *et al.* (2001). The temporal lobe rating scale: application to Alzheimer's disease and frontotemporal dementia. *Journal of Neurology, Neurosurgery and Psychiatry*, **70**, 157–164.

Garrard, P. and Hodges, J. R. (1999). Semantic Dementia: Implications for the neural basis of language and meaning. *Aphasiology*, **13**, 609–23.

Garrard, P., Perry, R., and Hodges, J. R. (1997). Disorders of semantic memory. *Journal of Neurology, Neurosurgery and Psychiatry*, **62**, 431–5.

Gentileschi, V., Sperber, S., and Spinnler, H. (1999). Progressive defective recognition of familiar people. *Neurocase*, **5**.

Geschwind, D., Karrim, J., Nelson, S. F., and Miller, B. (1998). The apolipoprotein E epsilon 4 allele is not a significant risk factor for frontotemporal dementia. *Annals of Neurology*, **44**, 134–8.

Girling, D. M. and Berrios, G. E. (1994). On the relationship between senile cerebral atrophy and aphasia (translation of Pick, A. Über die Beziehungen der senilen Hirnatrophie zur Aphasie. Prager Medicinische Wochenschrift 1892 17: 165–167. *History of Psychiatry*, **8**, 542–7.

Girling, D. M. and Berrios, G. E. (1997). On the symptomatology of left-sided temporal lobe atrophy (translation of Pick, A. Zur Symptomatologie der linksseitigen Schäfenlappenatrophie. Monatschrift für Psychiatrie und Neurologie 1904 16: 378–388). *History of Psychiatry*, **8**, 149–59.

Girling, D. M. and Markova, I. S. (1995). Senile atrophy as the basis for focal symptoms (translation of Pick, A. Senile Hirnatrophie als Grundlage von Herderescheinungen. Wiener klinische Wochenschrift 1901 14: 403–404). *History of Psychiatry*, **6**, 533–7.

Graham, K. S. and Hodges, J. R. (1997). Differentiating the roles of the hippocampal complex and the neocortex in long-term memory storage; evidence from the study of semantic dementia and Alzheimer's disease. *Neuropsychology*, **11**, 77–89.

Graham, N. L., Patterson, K., and Hodges, J. R. (2000). The impact of semantic memory impairment on spelling: Evidence from semantic dementia. *Neuropsychologia*, **38**, 143–163.

Green, J., Morris, J. C., Sandson, J., McKeel, D. W., and Miller, J. W. (1990). Progressive aphasia: a precursor of global dementia? *Neurology*, **40**, 423–9.

Greene, J. D. W., Patterson, K., Xuereb, J., and Hodges, J. R. (1996). Alzheimer disease and nonfluent progressive aphasia. *Archives of Neurology*, **53**, 1072–8.

Gregory, C. A. and Hodges, J. R. (1993). Dementia of frontal type and the focal lobar atrophies. *International Review of Psychiatry*, **5**, 397–406.

Gregory, C. A. and Hodges, J. R. (1996). Frontotemporal dementia: use of consensus criteria and prevalence of psychiatric features. *Neuropsychiatry, Neuropsychology, and Behavioural Neurology*, **9**, 145–53.

Gregory, C. A., McKenna, P. J. M., and Hodges, J. R. (1998). Dementia of frontal type and simple schizophrenia: two sides of the same coin? *Neurocase*, **4**, 1–6.

Gregory, C. A., Serra-Mestres, J., and Hodges, J. R. (1999). The early diagnosis of the frontal variant of frontotemporal dementia: how sensitive are standard neuroimaging and neuropsychological tests? *Neuropsychiatry, Neuropsychology and Behavioural Neurology*, **12**, 128–35.

Gustafson, L. (1987). Frontal lobe degeneration of non-Alzheimer type. II. Clinical picture and differential diagnosis. *Archives of Gerontology and Geriatrics*, **6**, 209–33.

Heutink, P., Stevens, M., Rizzu, P., Bakker, E., Kros, J. M., Tibben, A., *et al.* (1997). Hereditary frontotemporal dementia is linked to chromosome 17q21-q22: a genetic and clinicopathological study of three Dutch families. *Annals of Neurology*, **41**, 150–9.

Hodges, J. R. (1994). Pick's disease. In *Dementia* (ed. A. Burns and R. Levy), pp. 739–53. London: Chapman and Hall.

Hodges, J. R., Garrard, P., and Patterson, K. (1998). Semantic dementia. In *Pick's disease and Pick complex* (ed. A. Kertesz and D. G. Munoz), pp. 83–104. New York: Wiley-Liss, Inc.

Hodges, J. R. and Graham, K. S. (1998). A reversal of the temporal gradient for famous person knowledge in semantic dementia: Implications for the neural organisation of long-term memory. *Neuropsychologia*, **36**, 803–25.

Hodges, J. R., Graham, N., and Patterson, K. (1995). Charting the progression in semantic dementia: Implications for the organisation of semantic memory. *Memory*, **3**, 463–95.

Hodges, J. R. and Gurd, J. (1994). Remote memory and lexical retrieval in a case of frontal Pick's disease. *Archives of Neurology*, **51**, 821–7.

Hodges, J. R. and Patterson, K. (1995). Is semantic memory consistently impaired early in the course of Alzheimer's disease? Neuroanatomical and diagnostic implications. *Neuropsychologia*, **33**, 441–59.

Hodges, J. R. and Patterson, K. (1996). Nonfluent progressive aphasia and semantic dementia: A comparative neuropsychological study. *Journal of the International Neuropsychological Society*, **2**, 511–24.

Hodges, J. R., Patterson, K., Oxbury, S., and Funnell, E. (1992). Semantic dementia: progressive fluent aphasia with temporal lobe atrophy. *Brain*, **115**, 1783–806.

Hodges, J. R., Patterson, K., and Tyler, L. K. (1994). Loss of semantic memory: Implications for the modularity of mind. *Cognitive Neuropsychology*, **11**, 505–42.

Hodges, J. R., Patterson, K., Ward, R., Garrard, P., Bak, T., Perry, R., *et al.* (1999a). The differentiation of semantic dementia and frontal lobe dementia (temporal and frontal variants of frontotemporal dementia) from early Alzheimer's disease: a comparative neuropsychological study. *Neuropsychology*, **13**, 31–40.

Hodges, J. R. and Patterson, K. E. (1997). Semantic memory disorders. *Trends in Cognitive Science*, **1**, 67–72.

Hodges, J. R., Patterson, K. E., Graham, N., and Dawson, K. (1996). Naming and knowing in dementia of Alzheimer's type. *Brain and Language*, **54**, 302–25.

Hodges, J. R., Spatt, J., and Patterson, K. (1999b). What and How: Evidence for the dissociation of object knowledge and mechanical problem solving skills in the human brain. *Proceedings of the National Academy of Science USA*, **96**, 9444–8.

Hong, M., Zhukareva, V., Vogelsberg-Ragaglia, V., Wszolek, Z., Reed, L., Miller, B. I., *et al.* (1998). Mutation-specific functional impairments in distinct tau isoforms of hereditary FTDP-17. *Science*, **282**, 1914–17.

Howard, D. and Patterson, K. (1992). *Pyramids and Palm Trees: A Test of Semantic Access From Pictures and Words*. Bury St Edmunds, Suffolk: Thames Valley Test Company.

Hutton, M., Lendon, C. L., Rizzu, P., Baker, M., Froelich, S., Houlden, H., *et al.* (1998). Association of missense and 5'-splice-site mutations in tau with the inherited dementia FTDP-17. *Nature*, **18**, 702–5.

Imura, T., Nogami, Y., and Asakawa, K. (1971). Aphasia in Japanese Language. *Nihon University Journal of Medicine*, **13**, 69–90.

Kertesz, A. and Munoz, D. G. (1998). *Pick's disease and Pick complex*. New York: Wiley-Liss, Inc.

Kitchener, E. and Hodges, J. R. (1999). Impaired knowledge of famous people and events and intact autobiographical knowledge in a case of progressive right temporal lobe degeneration: Implications for the organization of remote memory. *Cognitive Neuropsychology*, **16**, 589–607.

Knopman, D. S., Mastri, A. R., Frey, W. H., Sung, J. H., and Rustan, T. (1990). Dementia lacking distinctive histological features: a common non-Alzheimer degenerative disease. *Neurology*, **40**, 251–6.

Lambon Ralph, M., Graham, K. S., Patterson, K., and Hodges, J. R. (1999). Is a picture worth a thousand words? Evidence from concept definitions by patients with semantic dementia. *Brain and Language*, **70**, 309–335.

Levy, M. L., Miller, B. L., Cummings, J. L., Fairbanks, L. A., and Craig, A. (1996). Alzheimer disease and frontotemporal dementias: behavioral distinctions. *Archives of Neurology*, **53**, 687–90.

Mansvelt, J. V. (1954). *Pick's Disease: A syndrome of lobar cerebral atrophy, its clinico-anatomical and histopathological types*. Utrecht: These.

Mathuranath, P. S., Xuereb, J., Bak, T., and Hodges, J. R. (2000). Corticobasal ganglionic degeneration and/or frontotemporal dementia. *Journal of Neurology, Neurosurgery and Psychiatry*, **68**, 304–312.

Mesulam, M. M. (1982). Slowly progressive aphasia without generalised dementia. *Annals of Neurology*, **11**, 592–8.

Mesulam, M. M. and Weintraub, S. (1992). Primary progressive aphasia. In *Heterogeneity of Alzheimer's disease* (ed F. Boller), pp. 43–66. Berlin: Springer–Verlag.

Miller, B. L., Chang, L., Mena, I., Boone, K., and Lesser, I. M. (1993). Progressive right frontotemporal degeneration: clinical, neurpsychological and SPECT characteristics. *Dementia*, **4**, 204–13.

Miller, B. L., Cummings, J. L., Villanueva-Meyer, J., Boone, K., Mehringer, C. M., Lesser, I. M., *et al.* (1991). Frontal lobe degeneration: Clinical, neuropsychological, and SPECT characteristics. *Neurology*, **41**, 1374–82.

Miller, B. L., Darby, A., Benson, D. F., Cummings, J. L., and Miller, M. H. (1997). Aggressive, socially disruptive and antisocial behaviour associated with fronto-temporal dementia. *British Journal of Psychiatry*, **170**, 150–5.

Mitsuyama, Y. and Takamiya, S. (1979). Presenile dementia with motor neurone disease in Japan: A new entity. *Archives of Neurology*, **36**, 592–3.

Mori, H., Nishimura, M., Namba, Y., and Oda, M. (1994). Corticobasal degeneration: a disease with widespread appearance of abnormal tau and neurofibrillary tangles, and its relation to progressive supranuclear palsy. *Acta Neuropathologica (Berlin)*, **88**, 113–21.

Morris, J. C., Cole, M., Banker, B. Q., and Wright, D. (1984). Hereditary dysphasic dementia and the Pick-Alzheimer spectrum. *Annals of Neurology*, **16**, 455–66.

Mummery, C. J., Patterson, K., Price, C. J. Ashburner, J. Frackowiak, R. and Hodges, J. R. (2000). A voxel based morphometry study of semantic dementia: The relation of temporal lobe atrophy to cognitive deficit. *Annals of Neurology*, **47**, 36–45.

Mummery, C. J., Patterson, K., Hodges, J. R., Wise, R. J. S., and Price, C. J. (1998). Functional neuroanatomy of the semantic system: — divisible by what? *Journal of Cognitive Neuroscience*, **10**, 766–77.

Neary, D., Snowden, J. S., Bowen, D. M., Sims, N. R., Mann, D. M. A., Yates, P. O., *et al.* (1986). Cerebral biopsy in the investigation of presenile dementia due to cerebral atrophy. *Journal of Neurology, Neurosurgery and Psychiatry*, **49**, 157–62.

Neary, D., Snowdon, J. S., Mann, D. M. A., Northen, B., Goulding, P. J., and Macdermott, N. (1990). Frontal lobe dementia and motor neuron disease. *Journal of Neurology, Neurosurgery and Psychiatry*, **53**, 23–32.

Nelson, H. and Willison, J. (1991). *The National Adult Reading Test (NART)*. Windsor: NFER-Nelson.

Onari, K. and Spatz, H. (1926). Anatomische Beitrage zur Lehre von der Pickschen umschriebenen Grosshirnrindenatrophie (Piscksche Krankheit). *Zeitschrift fur die Gesamte Neurologie und Psychiatrie*, **101**, 470–511.

Patterson, K., Graham, N., and Hodges, J. R. (1994). The impact of semantic memory loss on phonological representations. *Journal of Cognitive Neuroscience*, **6**, 57–69.

Patterson, K. and Hodges, J. R. (2000) Semantic Dementia: One window on the structure and organisation of semantic memory. In *Revised handbook of neuropsychology: memory disorders* (ed. L. Cermak). Elsevier Science BU, Amsterdam pp. 313–333.

Petersen, R. B., Tabaton, M., Chen, S. G., Monari, L., Richardson, S. L., Lynches, T., *et al.* (1995). Familial progressive subcortical gliosis: Presence of prions and linkage to chromosome 17. *Neurology*, **45**, 1062–7.

Rahman, S., Sahakian, B. J., Hodges, J. R., Rogers, R. D., and Robbins, T. W. (1999). Specific cognitive deficits in early frontal variant frontotemporal dementia. *Brain*, **122**, 1469–93.

Rakowicz, W. and Hodges, J. R. (1998). Dementia and aphasia in motor neurone disease: an under recognised association. *Journal of Neurology, Neurosurgery and Psychiatry*, **65**, 881–9.

Rogers, R. D., Sahakian, B. J., Hodges, J. R., Polkey, C. E., Kennard, C., and Robbins, T. W. (1998). Dissociating executive mechanisms of task control following frontal lobe damage and Parkinson's disease. *Brain*, **121**, 815–42.

Rossor, M. N. (1998). Provisional clinical and neuroradiological criteria for the diagnosis of Pick's disease: European Concerted Action on Pick's Disease (ECAPD) Consortium. *European Journal of Neurology*, **5**, 519–20.

Saffran, E. M. and Schwartz, M. F. (1994). Impairments of sentence comprehension. In *Royal Society meeting on The Acquisition and Dissolution of Language*. London.

Sasanuma, S. and Mondi, H. (1975). The syndrome of Gogi (word meaning) aphasia. *Neurology*, **25**, 627–32.

Schenk, V. W. D. (1958). Re-examination of a family with Pick's disease. *Annals of Human Genetics*, **23**, 325–33.

Schneider, C. (1927). Uber Picksche Krankheit. *Monatschrift fur Psychologie und Neurologie*, **65**, 230–75.

Schneider, C. (1929). Weitere Beitrage zur Lehre von der Pickschen Krankheit. *Zeitschrift fur die Gesamte Neurologie und Psychiatrie*, **120**, 340–84.

Sinnatamby, R., Antoun, N. A., Freer, C. E. L., Miles, K. A., and Hodges, J. R. (1996). Neuroradiological findings in primary progressive aphasia: a comparison of CT, MRI and cerebral perfusion SPECT. *Neuroradiology*, **38**, 232–8.

Snowden, J. S., Goulding, P. J., and Neary, D. (1989). Semantic dementia: A form of circumscribed cerebral atrophy. *Behavioural Neurology*, **2**, 167–82.

Snowden, J. S., Griffiths, H. L., and Neary, D. (1996). Progressive language disorder associated with frontal lobe degeneration. *Neurocase*, **2**, 429–40.

Spillantini, M. G., Bird, T. D., and Ghetti, B. (1998a). Frontotemporal dementia and Parkinsonism linked to chromosome 17: A new group of tauopathies. *Brain Pathology*, **8**, 387–402.

Spillantini, M. G., Goedert, M., Crowther, R. A., Murrell, J. R., Farlow, M. R., and Ghetti, B. (1997). Familial multiple system tauopathy with presenile dementia: a disease with abundant neuronal and glial tau filaments. *Proceedings of the National Academy of Science USA*, **94**, 4113–18.

Spillantini, M. G., Murrell, J. R., Goedert, M., Farlow, M. R., Klug, A., and Ghetti, B. (1998b). Mutation in the tau gene in familial multiple system tauopathy with presenile dementia. *Proceedings of the National Academy of Science USA*, **95**, 7737–41.

Stevens, M., van Duijn, C. M., Kamphorst, W., de Knijff, P., Heutink, P., van Gool, W. A., *et al.* (1998). Familial aggregation in frontotemporal dementia. *Neurology*, **50**, 1541–5.

Stone, V. E., Baron-Cohen, S., and Knight, R. T. (1998). Frontal lobe contributions to theory of mind. *Journal of Cognitive Neuroscience*, **10**, 640–56.

Stuss, D. T. and Benson, D. F. (1986). *The frontal lobes*. New York: Raven Press.

Sumi, S. M., Bird, T. D., Nochlin, D., and Raskind, M. A. (1992). Familial presenile dementia with psychosis associated with cortical neurofibrillary tangles and degeneration of the amygdala. *Neurology*, **42**, 120–7.

Swartz, J. R., Miller, B. L., Lesser, I. M., and Darby, A. L. (1997). Frontotemporal dementia: treatment response to serotonin selective reuptake inhibitors. *Journal of Clinical Psychiatry*, **58**, 212–16.

Tanabe, H., Ikeda, M., Nakagawa, Y., Yamamoto, H., Ikejiri, Y., Kazui, H., *et al.* (1992). Gogi (word meaning) aphasia and semantic memory for words. *Higher Brain Function Research*, **12**, 153–69.

Tanaka, F., Kachi, T., Yamada, T., and Sobue, G. (1998). Auditory and visual event-related potentials and flash visual evoked potentials in Alzheimer's disease: correlations with Mini-Mental State Examination and Raven's Coloured Progressive Matrices. *Journal of the Neurological Sciences*, **156**, 83–8.

Tissot, R., Constantanidis, J., and Richard, J. (1975). *La maladie de Pick*. Paris: Masson.

Tissot, R., Constantinidis, J., and Richard, J. (1985). Pick's disease. In *Handbook of clinical neurology: neurobehavioural disorders*, Vol. 2 (ed. J. A. M. Frederiks), pp. 233–46. Amsterdam: Elsevier Science Publishers.

Tulving, E. (1972). Episodic and semantic memory. In *Organisation of memory* (ed. E. Tulving and W. Donaldson), pp. 381–403. New York and London: Academic Press.

Tulving, E. (1983). *Elements of episodic memory*. Oxford: Clarendon Press.

Tyrrell, P. J., Warrington, E. K., Frackowiak, R. S. J., and Rossor, M. N. (1990). Progressive degeneration of the right temporal lobe studied with positron emission tomography. *Journal of Neurology, Neurosurgery and Psychiatry*, **53**, 1046–50.

Warrington, E. K. (1975). Selective impairment of semantic memory. *Quarterly Journal of Experimental Psychology*, **27**, 635–57.

Warrington, E. K. and James, M. (1991). *The Visual Object and Space Perception Battery*. Bury St Edmunds: Thames Valley Test Company.

Weintraub, S., Rubin, N. P., and Mesulam, M.-M. (1990). Primary progressive aphasia: Longitudinal course, profile, and language features. *Archives of Neurology*, **47**, 1329–35.

Wilhelmsen, K. C., Lynch, T., Pavlou, E., Higgins, M., and Nygaard, T. G. (1994). Localization of disinhibition-dementia-parkinsonism-amyotrophy complex to 17q21–22. *American Journal of Human Genetics*, **55**, 1159–65.

Wszolek, Z. K., Pfeiffer, R. F., Bhatt, M. H., Schelper, R. L., Cordes, M., Snow, B. J., *et al.* (1992). Rapidly progressive autosomal dominant Parkinsonism and dementia with pallido-ponto-nigral degeneration. *Annals of Neurology*, **32**, 312–20.

13 Dementia with Lewy bodies

David P. Salmon, Douglas Galasko, and Lawrence A. Hansen

1 Introduction

Recent clinico-neuropathological studies have shown that 15–25% of patients who manifest a syndrome similar to dementia of the Alzheimer type during life have Lewy bodies diffusely distributed in widespread regions of the neocortex (Kosaka *et al.* 1984; Lennox *et al.* 1989). This cortical Lewy body pathology occurs along with the typical subcortical changes of Parkinson's disease (PD) (i.e. Lewy bodies and cell loss), and in many cases with the typical cortical distribution of senile plaques (but often not neurofibrillary tangles) associated with Alzheimer's disease (AD) (Hansen *et al.* 1990). A variety of designations have been applied to this clinico-neuropathological entity including diffuse Lewy body disease (Dickson *et al.* 1987; Kosaka 1990; Kosaka *et al.* 1984), Lewy body dementia (Gibb *et al.* 1985, 1989), and senile dementia of the Lewy body type (Perry *et al.* 1990a). Recently, the designation dementia with Lewy bodies (DLB) has been proposed as a more descriptive and all encompassing label (McKeith *et al.* 1996b).

The specific subset of patients with DLB who have pathology sufficient to meet standard criteria for AD (e.g. Khachaturian 1985; Mirra *et al.* 1993) and concomitant cortical and subcortical Lewy body pathology are referred to by Hansen and colleagues (Hansen *et al.* 1990) as having the Lewy body variant (LBV) of AD. The term LBV is used to distinguish the condition from diffuse Lewy body disease (DLBD) without concomitant AD and to highlight the extensive pathological, clinical, and genetic overlap the disorder shares with AD (Galasko *et al.* 1994; Katzman *et al.* 1995). Although specific clinical features may distinguish between 'pure' AD and LBV (see Section 3), both are typically characterized by the initial manifestation of insidious and progressive cognitive decline, with memory impairment often the earliest and most prominent feature. In both cases, cognitive deficits become widespread with time and patients inexorably progress to severe dementia. Genetic evidence supporting the notion that LBV is a variant of AD was provided by studies demonstrating that a common risk factor for AD, the e4 allele of apolipoprotein E (ApoE), is over-represented in patients with LBV (29% versus 39.6% in pure AD), but not in patients with pure diffuse Lewy body disease (6%) (Galasko *et al.* 1994; Katzman, *et al.* 1995). In addition, the presence of an e4 allele was found to be strongly associated with neuritic plaques and cerebral amyloid angiopathy in both AD and LBV patients (Olichney *et al.* 1996), and NFT pathology was found to be greater in those LBV patients who were ApoE e4 positive than in those who were e4 negative (Hansen *et al.* 1994).

With the growing realization that the various forms of DLB are most likely the second leading cause of dementia after AD, considerable research on the disorder has been carried out over the past five to ten years. This research has lead to progress in identifying the neuropathological, clinical, and general neuropsychological features associated with DLB. Each of these aspects of the disorder will be discussed in turn.

2 Neuropathology of dementia with Lewy bodies

Studies of the distribution of Lewy body pathology in patients with DLB have shown that these patients have Lewy bodies and cell loss in the substantia nigra and in other pigmented brain stem nuclei (e.g. locus ceruleus and dorsal vagal nucleus) (for reviews see Hansen and Galasko 1992; Ince *et al.* 1998a and chapter 10). The substantia nigra degeneration in DLB patients is reported to be intermediate between that of patients with PD and age-matched normal individuals (Perry *et al.* 1990a). In addition, these patients have diffusely distributed Lewy bodies that appear to have a predilection for cingulate, insula, amygdaloid complex, entorhinal cortex, and transentorhinal cortex, as well as neocortical involvement (usually in deeper layers such as 4, 5, and 6) that is usually most severe in the temporal lobe, somewhat less severe in the parietal and frontal lobes, and least severe in the occipital lobe (Double *et al.* 1996; Ince *et al.* 1998a; Kosaka and Iseki 1996). It should be noted, however, that some Lewy body pathology is observed in the occipital cortex (Pellise *et al.* 1996; Rezaie *et al.* 1996), and that a recent fluoro-deoxyglucose positron emission tomography (PET) study demonstrated hypometabolism in the occipital association cortex and the primary visual cortex in DLB patients (Albin *et al.* 1996).

Both neuropathological (Lippa *et al.* 1994) and neuroimaging studies (Hashimoto *et al.* 1998) indicate that the medial temporal lobe structures, and the hippocampus in particular, are less atrophic in DLB patients than in patients with AD. In the imaging study, this difference in hippocampal volume occurred despite similar degrees of whole brain and amygdala atrophy in the two patient groups. Differences in the histopathological features of hippocampal damage in the two disorders have also been reported with DLB patients having generally less hippocampal pathology than AD patients, but displaying abnormal ubiquinated neurites (i.e. Lewy neurites) in the CA 2/3 region of the hippocampus that are not present in AD (Dickson *et al.* 1991, 1994; Lippa *et al.* 1994). Immunocytochemical and immunoelectron microscopic analyses demonstrated, however, that the neurofibrillary alterations that occur in the granule cells of the dentate gyrus of the hippocampus in patients with AD, LBV, and progressive supranuclear palsy (PSP) are cytoskeletally similar (Wakabayashi *et al.* 1997). Such inclusions were not observed in patients with pure diffuse Lewy body disease.

A recent study by Wakabayashi and colleagues used double immunolabelling with ubiquitin (a Lewy body marker) and SMI32 (a pyramidal cell marker) to demonstrate that cortical cells that contain Lewy bodies are pyramidal cells (Wakabayashi *et al.* 1995). A subsequent study showed that the granular and fragmented appearance of these labelled pyramidal cells in neocortical layers 3 and 5 was apparent in 78% of patients with LBV, but was not found in patients with 'pure' AD. In contrast, Lewy bodies were observed in the pyramidal neurons of layers 5 and 6 in only 44% of the LBV cases. These results suggest that widespread cytoskeletal fragmentation in LBV may be a better explanation for a pathological substrate of dementia than the relatively inconspicuous Lewy body (Smith *et al.* 1995).

The ability to histopathologically identify cortical and subcortical Lewy bodies has been bolstered over the past two years by the recent discovery of the NACP/alpha-synuclein protein in the Lewy body. The synaptic protein NACP (the precursor of non-A beta component of AD) was first purified from plaques in AD brains by Saitoh and colleagues (Ueda *et al.* 1993). Subsequently, this protein (also called alpha-synuclein) was found to be a key constituent of the Lewy body (Spillantini *et al.* 1997), and a mutation of alpha-synuclein was found in a family with Parkinson's disease (PD) (Krugger *et al.* 1998; Polymeropoulous *et al.* 1997). Takeda and colleagues (Takeda *et al.* 1998) recently demonstrated that NACP/alpha-synuclein immunoreactivity is specifically found in cortical and subcortical Lewy bodies, and not in other types of cytoskeletal lesions. These discoveries have led to the development of new, very sensitive histopathological probes for Lewy bodies and Lewy neurites throughout the brain (Irizarry *et al.* 1998; Spillantini *et al.* 1998; Trojanowski and Lee 1998).

As would be expected from the widespread cortical and subcortical pathology that occurs in DLB, a number of neurochemical abnormalities have been identified (for review see Ince *et al.* 1998*a*). As in PD, one of the primary neurochemical changes in DLB is a disruption of dopaminergic input to the striatum due to the loss of pigmented substantia nigra neurons (Perry *et al.* 1990*b*). This loss may be as severe as that in PD (Langlais *et al.* 1993) and most likely mediates the extrapyramidal motor dysfunction that usually accompanies DLB (see chapter 9). Cortical dopamine, in contrast, has been reported to not markedly decrease in DLB (Perry *et al.* 1993); however, neurochemical studies are few and additional research is needed before a strong conclusion can be drawn. In addition to dopaminergic loss, DLB is characterized by a widespread depletion of striatal and neocortical choline acetyltransferase (ChAT) that is greater than that observed in pure AD. Loss of ChAT activity occurs in the striatum due to pathology of intrinsic local circuit neurons and, as suggested by Perry *et al.* (1990*b*) and Langlais *et al.* (1993), this loss may attenuate the manifestation of the severe motor dysfunction that usually occurs with the loss of striatal dopamine in PD. The severe loss of neocortical ChAT activity in DLB is likely to contribute to both the cognitive and neuropsychiatric features (e.g. visual hallucinations; see Section 3) of the disorder.

Several studies have demonstrated that both Lewy body and AD pathology contribute to dementia in patients with DLB. In an initial study, quantitative measures of pathology were compared in patients with LBV (N = 14) and patients with 'pure' AD (N = 12) who were matched for disease duration and who had similar mental status test scores when last evaluated prior to death (Samuel *et al.* 1996). Despite similar levels of dementia, the LBV patients had fewer neurofibrillary tangles (NFT) and plaques than the patients with AD, and were in a lower Braak stage (a semi-quantitative measure of NFT pathology). In addition, the number of NFTs was significantly correlated with level of dementia in the AD patients but not in the LBV patients. The number of neocortical Lewy bodies, on the other hand, was significantly correlated with level of dementia in the LBV patients. In a second study (Samuel *et al.* 1997), the number of neocortical Lewy bodies, Braak stage, the number of neocortical neuritic plaques, and the degree of loss of choline acetyltransferase (ChAT) activity all correlated significantly with dementia severity as measured by the Mini-Mental State Exam (MMSE) and the Blessed Information Memory Concentration (IMC) test in a group of patients with DLB (12 with LBV and 5 with diffuse Lewy body disease). In contrast to patients with AD, however, severity of dementia was not correlated with the number of neocortical NFTs or synaptic density in the patients with DLB. Although measures of AD pathology and level of dementia were not strongly correlated in the LBV patients, a direct comparison of the LBV patients and patients with diffuse Lewy body disease suggests that the AD pathology does contribute to their dementia. Despite comparable numbers of Lewy bodies, the patients with diffuse Lewy body disease were less demented than the LBV patients. In a related study, Hansen *et al.* (1998) demonstrated that synaptophysin concentrations in the mid frontal cortex were significantly lower than normal in patients with AD or LBV, but not in demented patients with 'pure' diffuse Lewy body disease. These results suggest that the loss of mid frontal synapses may contribute to dementia in DLB only when AD pathology is also present. Taken together, these results indicate that neocortical Lewy bodies and ChAT depletion are related to the cognitive deficits that occur in patients with DLB. Furthermore, they suggest that the dementia of patients with LBV is mediated by both Lewy body and AD pathology.

3 Clinical features of dementia with Lewy bodies

Patients who are found at autopsy to have DLB have often been clinically diagnosed with probable or possible AD during life (e.g. Hansen *et al.* 1990). This is not surprising given that DLB often initially produces insidious and progressive cognitive decline without other significant neurological abnormalities. While patients with DLB do not always present with memory impairment as the earliest and most prominent feature, this aspect of cognition is often affected early in the disorder's course. As in AD, the cognitive deficits that occur in DLB are widespread and progressive and have a significant impact on the patient's ability to engage in normal activities of daily living. Both disorders are age-related, usually occurring after the age of 65. However, both DLB and AD have been reported to occur before the age of 50 (Lippa *et al.* 1998).

Despite the similarities in the clinical presentation of the two disorders, retrospective studies indicate that DLB may be clinically distinguishable from AD. Hansen *et al.* (1990), for example, found that patients with LBV differed from patients with 'pure' AD in that a greater proportion had mild parkinsonian or extrapyramidal motor findings (e.g. bradykinesia, rigidity, masked facies; but without a resting tremor). McKeith *et al.* (1992) also found that DLB patients were significantly more likely than 'pure' AD patients to manifest extrapyramidal motor features at some point during the course of the disease, as well as an increased likelihood of fluctuating cognitive impairment, visual or auditory hallucinations, and unexplained falls. In another study, Galasko *et al.* (1996) compared clinical and neuropathological features in 38 autopsy-confirmed DLB (all patients had LBV) and 38 autopsy-confirmed 'pure' AD patients. A significantly higher number of DLB patients than AD patients exhibited rigidity, bradykinesia, masked facies, and parkinsonian gait, and a significantly greater percentage of DLB (32%) than AD (11%) patients reported visual hallucinations. These general findings have now been replicated in numerous studies (Ala *et al.* 1997; Beck 1995; Graham *et al.* 1997; Hely *et al.* 1996; McShane *et al.* 1995; Weiner *et al.* 1996; for reviews see Cercy and Bylsma 1997; Perry *et al.* 1996) and have led to the recent development of clinical criteria for the diagnosis of DLB (McKeith *et al.* 1996*b*).

The primary clinical criteria for DLB that were adopted by the International Consortium on DLB (McKeith *et al.* 1996*b*) include, in addition to dementia, spontaneous motor features of parkinsonism, recurrent and well-formed visual hallucinations, and fluctuating cognition with pronounced variations in attention or alertness (see Table 13.1). Probable DLB is diagnosed if two of these three features are present; possible DLB if only one is present. A recent examination of the performance of these consensus guidelines against autopsy verification of DLB demonstrated 83% sensitivity and 92% specificity. This was comparable to the 78% sensitivity and 87% specificity for AD (using NINCDS-ADRDA criteria) that was obtained in the same study (Ince *et al.* 1998*b*).

A number of additional clinical features of DLB illustrate the importance of being able to accurately differentiate the disorder from AD early in the course of disease. For example, several studies indicate that patients with DLB decline more rapidly than patients with AD (Olichney *et al.* 1998; Armstrong *et al.* 1991). In one of the largest longitudinal studies to date, Olichney *et al.* (1998) found that patients with autopsy-verified LBV (n = 40) declined significantly more rapidly on the MMSE from one year to the next than did patients with autopsy-verified 'pure' AD (n = 153). The average annual rate of decline on the MMSE was 5.6 points per year for the patients with LBV compared to 3.9 points per year for the patients with AD (see Figure 13.1). This more rapid cognitive decline of the LBV patients occurred despite being similar to the patients with AD in terms of initial (i.e. year 1) MMSE score, age, and education.

Table 13.1 Consensus criteria for the clinical diagnosis of probable and possible dementia with Lewy bodies (adapted from McKeith et al. 1996*b*)

1 **Central required feature:**
   Progressive cognitive decline of sufficient magnitude to interfere with normal social or occupational function. Prominent or persistent memory impairment may not necessarily occur in the early stage but is usually evident with progression. Deficits on tests of attention, fronto-subcortical functions and visuospatial abilities may be especially prominent.

2 **Core features (two required for probable DLB and one for possible DLB):**
   A Fluctuating cognition with pronounced variations in attention and alertness
   B Recurrent visual hallucinations that are typically well formed and detailed
   C Spontaneous motor features of parkinsonism

3 **Features supportive of the diagnosis:**
   A Repeated falls
   B Syncope
   C Transient loss of consciousness
   D Neuroleptic sensitivity
   E Systematized delusions
   F Hallucinations in other modalities

4 **Diagnosis of DLB is less likely in the presence of:**
   A Evidence of stroke from focal neurological signs or brain imaging
   B Evidence of any physical illness or other brain disorder sufficient to account for the clinical features

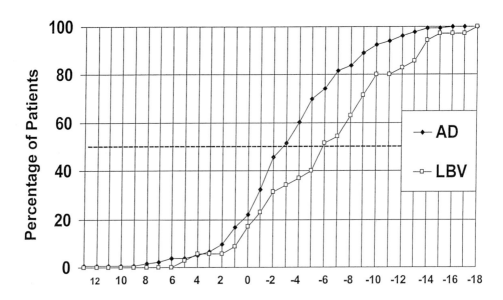

First Year Change of MMSE (points/year)

Figure 13.1   The cumulative percentage of patients with autopsy-confirmed Alzheimer's disease (AD) or the Lewy body variant (LBV) of AD as a function of the amount of change in Mini-Mental State Examination (MMSE) score over a one year interval. Decline is indicated by a negative score. Faster decline in LBV than in AD patients is indicated by a more rapid shift in the distribution towards the negative for the former group. (Adapted from Olichney *et al.* 1998.)

In addition to a more rapid cognitive decline, patients with DLB may develop urinary incontinence earlier in the course of the disease than do AD patients (Del-Ser *et al.* 1996), they appear to be quite susceptible to REM sleep disorder (Boeve *et al.* 1998; Turner *et al.* 1997), they respond poorly to neuroleptic treatment for their psychotic symptoms (for review see McKeith *et al.* 1996*a*), and they may show a better clinical response than AD patients to acetylcholinesterase (AChE) inhibitor treatment of their cognitive deficits (Levy *et al.* 1994). Given the importance of these differences for the prognosis and treatment of the two disorders, it is critical to continue to develop more accurate methods of clinically differentiating between DLB and AD. Better description and understanding of the initial and progressive clinical and neuropsychological manifestations of DLB is a necessary step in this development.

4 Neuropsychological features of dementia with Lewy bodies

Although a number of studies have shown through retrospective review of records that patients with neuropathologically-proven Lewy body disease were demented, very few have provided evidence concerning the specific nature of the cognitive impairment engendered by this disease. Those few early studies that did address this issue reported general memory impairment, constructional and ideomotor apraxia, dysphasia, and dyscalculia (Byrne *et al.* 1989; Gibb *et al.* 1985).

Studies that have retrospectively examined the neuropsychological test performance of patients with autopsy-confirmed DLB in a more detailed manner have focused, for the most part, upon patients with LBV. In one of the first of these studies, Hansen *et al.* (1990) compared the neuropsychological deficits exhibited by nine patients with autopsy-proven LBV and nine age- and education-matched patients with 'pure' AD. Despite equivalent levels of global dementia (as assessed with the Blessed IMC test), patients with LBV exhibited disproportionately severe deficits compared to the AD patients in attention (WAIS-R Digit Span subtest), visuospatial/ constructional ability (WISC-R Block Design subtest, Copy-a-Cross test), verbal concept formation (WAIS-R Similarities subtest), and phonemically-based verbal fluency (i.e. generating words that begin with F, A, or S) (see Figure 13.2). In contrast to these differences, the groups were equivalently impaired on tests of episodic memory (the Buschke-Fuld Selective Reminding Test), confrontation naming (e.g. the Boston Naming Test), semantically-based verbal fluency (i.e. producing exemplars from the categories animals, fruits, and vegetables), and arithmetical ability (WAIS-R Arithmetic subtest).

Galasko *et al.* (1998) recently replicated these findings in much larger cohorts of autopsy-confirmed LBV (N = 50) and AD (N = 95) patients. As in the study by Hansen and colleagues, the LBV and AD patients performed similarly on tests of episodic memory, confrontation naming, and semantic knowledge, but the LBV patients performed significantly worse than the AD patients on tests of visuoconstructive ability, verbal fluency, and abstract reasoning or problem solving. In addition, the patients with LBV exhibited greater psychomotor slowing than the patients with AD. Although attention as measured by the WAIS-R Digit Span subtest was significantly worse in LBV than in AD patients in the Hansen *et al.* (1990) study, this difference was not observed in the more extensive study of Galasko *et al.* (1998). Based upon these results, a logistic regression model was developed by Galasko and colleagues that included performance on phonemic fluency, block design, clock drawing, trail-making (part A), and semantic knowledge tests. The resulting model was highly significant and correctly classified approximately 60% of LBV patients and 88% of AD patients for an overall classification rate of 77%.

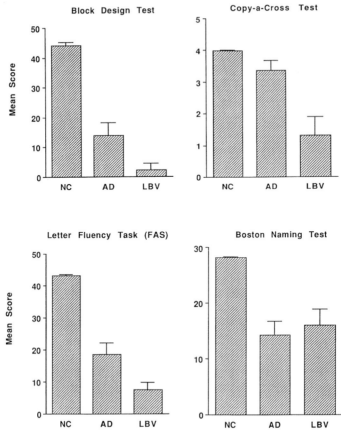

Figure 13.2 The average scores achieved by normal control (NC) subjects, patients with Alzheimer's disease (AD), and patients with the Lewy body variant (LBV) of AD on several neuropsychological tests. Despite equivalent deficits on a test of confrontation naming, the LBV patients were disproportionately impaired compared to the AD patients on tests of visuospatial ability and verbal fluency. (Adapted from Hansen *et al.* 1990.)

The disproportionately severe deficits in visuoconstructive/visuoperceptual abilities, 'executive' functions (e.g. initiation, planning, self-monitoring, self-regulation, volition), verbal fluency (particularly for phonemic categories), and psychomotor speed that were reported for patients with LBV in the studies by Hansen *et al.* (1990) and Galasko *et al.* (1998) have been observed in a number of additional studies with autopsy-confirmed patients (Connor *et al.* 1998; Gnanalingham *et al.* 1996; Wagner and Bachman 1996; Yeatman *et al.* 1994). Furthermore, these differences in the neuropsychological deficits exhibited by LBV and AD patients are robust enough to be detected on relatively brief, standardized tests of mental status (Connor *et al.* 1998). When autopsy-verified LBV (N = 23) and 'pure' AD (N = 23) patients' performances on the subscales of the Mattis Dementia Rating Scale (DRS) were compared, the LBV patients performed significantly worse than those with AD on the Initiation/Perseveration subscale which is heavily weighted towards verbal fluency and other frontal 'executive' functions. In contrast, the AD patients performed significantly worse than those with LBV on the Memory subscale of the test (see Figure 13.3). This latter finding is somewhat different than the equivalent episodic memory impairment exhibited by AD and LBV patients in the studies by Hansen *et al.* (1990)

and Galasko *et al.* (1998), but is similar to the results of other studies that have shown that episodic memory is sometimes less impaired in patients with more general DLB or 'pure' diffuse Lewy body disease than in those with AD (e.g. Salmon *et al.* 1996).

The pattern of neuropsychological deficits exhibited by patients with autopsy-confirmed LBV in the studies described above suggests that LBV and AD patients are, for the most part, equivalently impaired in those cognitive abilities that are most likely to be affected by AD pathology (e.g. episodic memory, language), but LBV patients are more impaired than AD patients in those abilities that are thought to be affected by both AD and cortical and subcortical Lewy body pathology (e.g. verbal fluency, psychomotor speed, visuospatial/constructional ability). Salmon *et al.* (1998) recently completed a longitudinal study of autopsy-confirmed LBV patients to determine if a differential rate of decline was evident in these classes of cognitive abilities. A comparison of the performances of autopsy-confirmed LBV (N = 20) and AD (N = 20) patients on a battery of neuropsychological tests that was administered on two occasions separated by approximately one year revealed that LBV patients exhibit a significantly more rapid decline than patients with 'pure' AD on tests of verbal fluency and visuospatial and constructional abilities, whereas the groups exhibit similar rates of decline in a number of cognitive abilities that are usually affected by AD, including episodic memory, confrontation naming, and semantic knowledge (Salmon *et al.* 1998).

When the results of the studies reviewed above are considered together, they suggest that both AD and Lewy body pathology contribute importantly to the cognitive manifestations of LBV. The Alzheimer-like cognitive deficits of LBV (e.g. impaired long-term memory, confrontation naming, conceptualization, visuospatial apraxia) are most likely mediated to a large extent by the

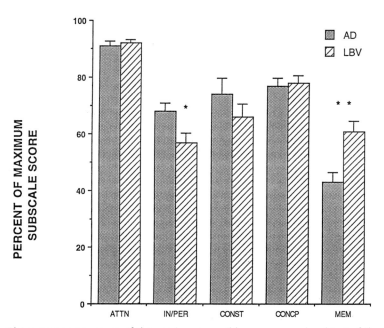

Figure 13.3 The average percentage of the maximum possible score on each subtest of the Mattis Dementia Rating Scale achieved by patients with neuropathologically-confirmed Alzheimer's disease (AD) or the Lewy body variant (LBV) of AD. Patients with LBV scored significantly lower than patients with AD on the Initiation/Perseveration subtest but significantly higher on the Memory subtest. (ATTN = Attention; IN/PER = Initiation/Perseveration; CONST = Construction; CONCP = Conceptualization; MEM = Memory) (Adapted from Connor *et al.* 1998.)

extensive AD pathology that is prominent in medial temporal lobe structures and neocortical association areas. The disproportionately severe deficits exhibited by patients with LBV in those cognitive abilities that have been associated with so-called subcortical dementing disorders such as PD (e.g. psychomotor processing, verbal fluency, 'executive ability, visuospatial functions) may be mediated to a large extent by the subcortical nigral Lewy body pathology that disrupts fronto-striatal circuits that are critical for these cognitive functions (Alexander *et al.* 1986). In addition, their unusual severity may also be a function of the additional cortical Lewy body pathology that occurs in the disorder.

The notion that the specific pattern of cognitive deficits associated with LBV arises from the superimposition of Lewy body and AD pathology receives support from a recently completed study that retrospectively examined the neuropsychological test performance of five patients with diffuse Lewy body disease (DLBD) who had little or no AD pathology (Salmon *et al.* 1996). Despite the lack of AD pathology, these patients were globally demented with deficits in memory, attention, language, 'executive' functions, and psychomotor speed. In addition, these DLBD patients exhibited a strikingly severe deficit in visuospatial/visuoconstructive abilities. The visuoconstructive and psychomotor impairments of the DLBD patients were significantly worse than those of the autopsy-verified 'pure' AD patients, whereas the memory performance of the AD patients was worse than that of the DLBD patients. Thus, cortical and subcortical Lewy body pathology alone can result in a dementia syndrome with particularly severe deficits in psychomotor speed, verbal fluency, executive functions, and visuospatial and visuoconstructive abilities. The notably severe impairments of memory and language that are observed in patients with LBV may occur only when the additional AD pathology is present.

As diagnostic criteria for DLB developed over the years, a number of prospective studies of the neuropsychological features of the disorder were carried out using patients with clinically diagnosed probable DLB. In a series of studies using a microcomputer based testing paradigm (the CANTAB), Sahgal and colleagues found that probable DLB patients performed significantly worse than equally globally demented probable AD patients on tasks that required 'executive' functions such as shifting of attentional set (Sahgal *et al.* 1992), conditional pattern discrimination learning (Galloway *et al.* 1992), or strategy formation (Sahgal *et al.* 1995). In addition, probable DLB patients made more within search and between search errors than AD patients on a spatial working memory task (Sahgal *et al.* 1995).

In two recent studies, Walker *et al.* (1997) and Shimomura *et al.* (1998) independently reported greater visuospatial and visuoconstructive deficits in probable DLB patients than in probable AD patients, even though the AD patients' memory impairment was significantly worse than that of the DLB patients. In a similar study, Rice *et al.* (1996) compared the neuropsychological test performance of patients with clinically diagnosed probable DLB (n = 30) and probable AD (n = 30) and found that despite similar levels of global dementia, language dysfunction, and episodic memory impairment, the probable LBV patients performed worse than the AD patients on measures of visuospatial functioning and verbal fluency. Ballard *et al.* (1996) further showed that the verbal fluency performance of patients with probable DLB declined more rapidly over a one year period than did that of patients with probable AD.

A similar pattern of distinctive neuropsychological features has been identified in studies that have not directly applied clinical criteria for probable DLB, but instead compared the performances of AD patients with and without extrapyramidal motor signs (EPS) that may indicative of DLB. These studies have generally found that those AD patients with EPS are more severely impaired than those without EPS on tests of visuospatial/visuoconstructive ability (e.g. Block Design, Figure Copying), verbal fluency, and 'executive' functions (e.g. Wisconsin Card Sorting Test, Trail-Making Test), whereas the groups are similarly impaired on tests of long-term memory, naming, and verbal comprehension (Girling and Berrios 1990; Merello *et al.* 1994; Richards *et al.* 1993). Furthermore, a longitudinal study demonstrated that AD patients with EPS declined more rapidly than those without EPS on tests of visuospatial praxis and 'executive' abilities, but not on a test of confrontation naming, over a one year period (Soininen *et al.* 1992).

It is interesting to note that the cognitive abilities that appear to be disproportionately impaired in DLB are the same abilities that are mildly impaired in non-demented patients with PD. A number of studies have shown that compared to age-matched normal control subjects PD patients exhibit psychomotor slowing (Brown and Marsden 1991) and have mild deficits in visuospatial abilities (Jacobs *et al.* 1995; Stern *et al.* 1993), verbal fluency (Jacobs *et al.* 1995), and other 'executive' functions that are necessary to perform tasks such as the Wisconsin Card Sorting Test (Brown and Marsden 1988; Lees and Smith 1983), the interference condition of the Stroop Test (Brown and Marsden 1991), dual-processing tasks (Brown and Marsden 1991; Dalrymple-Alford *et al.* 1994), and tasks that require rapid shifts of attention (Filoteo *et al.* 1997).

While there is clearly growing evidence that patients with DLB have disproportionately severe deficits relative to patients with 'pure' AD in visuospatial abilities and some 'executive' functions, the specific neuropsychological processes and neuropathological factors that underlie these deficits remain largely unknown. It is not known, for example, whether the severe visuospatial and visuoconstructive deficits associated with DLB are due to a primary visuoperceptual deficit that might arise from Lewy body pathology in the occipital cortex, to an impaired ability to mentally manipulate information in space that might arise from concomitant AD and Lewy body pathology in parietal lobe cortex, to an inability to plan constructions due to the interruption of fronto-striatal circuits or to AD and Lewy body pathology in the frontal lobe cortex, or to some other factor or combination of factors. Similarly, the specific 'executive' function deficits engendered by DLB have not been systematically examined, nor have they been related to specific pathological features of the disease such as the severity of the nigral pathology that disrupts fronto-striatal circuits or the AD and Lewy body pathology that occurs in the frontal lobe neocortex. Clearly, additional research aimed at identifying these clinico-pathological relationships is warranted.

5 Conclusions

As the brief review presented above attests, the results of a growing number of studies demonstrate that DLB is a clinical and neuropathological entity that can be differentiated from AD on the basis of neuropathological, neurological, and neuropsychological features. Furthermore, the results of these studies show that subcortical and diffusely distributed neocortical Lewy body pathology, without concomitant AD pathology, is associated with global cognitive impairment with particularly severe deficits in visuospatial/visuoconstructional processes, some 'executive' functions, psychomotor abilities, and perhaps attention. In LBV, this pathology is superimposed on the neuropathological changes that typically occur in AD, and the resulting neuropsychological impairment appears to reflect the effects of both. For example, patients with LBV, like AD patients, have deficits in memory and language abilities, most likely due to the severe hippocampal and neocortical damage that occurs in AD. In addition, patients with LBV, like patients with DLBD, have particularly severe deficits in visuospatial abilities, executive functions, attention, and psychomotor processes, which most likely reflects the supplementary effects of Lewy body pathology.

6 Key points

1 Dementia with Lewy Bodies (DLB) may account for 15%-20% of cases of primary degenerative dementia.

2 Many cases have concomittent AD pathology and the distinction between pure DLB and mixed DLB-AD remains unsettled.

3 The principal constituent of Lewy bodies is α synuclein leading to the classification of DLB as an α synucleinopathy.

4 The diagnosis of probable DLB requires a combination of progressive cognitive decline in 2 of the following features: fluctuating cognition, recurrent unprovoked visual hallucinations of motor features of Parkinsonism. Neuroleptic sensitivity is common and may be life threatening.

5 Neuropsychologically DLB may be distinguishable from AD by greater deficits on tests of visuoconstructional, visuoperceptual, attentional and executive abilities, with relative sparing of episodic memory.

6 The rate of progression of DLB appears to be faster than that of AD.

Acknowledgements

Preparation of this chapter was supported by funds from NIA grants AG-05131 and AG-12963 to the University of California, San Diego.

References

Ala, T. A., Yang, K. H., Sung, J. H., and Frey, W. H. (1997). Hallucinations and signs of parkinsonism help distinguish patients with dementia and cortical Lewy bodies from patients with Alzheimer's disease at presentation: A clinicopathological study. *Journal of Neurology, Neurosurgery and Psychiatry*, **62**, 16–21.

Albin, R. L., Minoshima, S., D'Amato, C. J., Frey, K. A., Kuhl, D. A., and Sima, A. A. F. (1996). Fluoro-deoxyglucose positron emission tomography in diffuse Lewy body disease. *Neurology*, **47**, 462–6.

Alexander, G. E., Delong, M. R., and Strick, P. L. (1986). Parallel organization of functionally segregated circuits linking basal ganglia and cortex. *Annual Review of Neuroscience*, **9**, 357–81.

Armstrong, T., Hansen, L., Salmon, D. P., Masliah, E., Pay, M., Kunin, I., *et al.* (1991). Rapid progression of dementia in a patient with the Lewy body variant of Alzheimer's disease. *Neurology*, **41**, 1178–80.

Ballard, C., Patel, A., Oyebode, F., and Wilcock, G. (1996). Cognitive decline in patients with Alzheimer's disease, vascular dementia and senile dementia of the Lewy body type. *Age and Ageing*, **25**, 209–13.

Beck, B. J. (1995). Neuropsychiatric manifestations of diffuse Lewy body disease. *Journal of Geriatric Psychiatry and Neurology*, **8**, 189–96.

Boeve, B. F., Silber, M. H., Ferman, T. J., Kokman, E., Smith, G. E., Ivnik, R. J., *et al.* (1998). REM sleep behavior disorder and degenerative dementia: An association likely reflecting Lewy body disease. *Neurology*, **51**, 363–70.

Brown, R. G. and Marsden, C. D. (1988). An investigation of the phenomenon of 'set' in Parkinson's disease. *Movement Disorders*, **3**, 152–61.

Brown, R. G. and Marsden, C. D. (1991). Dual task performance and processing resources in normal subjects and patients with Parkinson's disease. *Brain*, **114**, 215–31.

Byrne, E. J., Lennox, G., Lowe, J., and Godwin-Austen, R. B. (1989). Diffuse Lewy body disease: Clinical features in 15 cases. *Journal of Neurology, Neurosurgery, and Psychiatry*, **52**, 709–17.

Cercy, S. P. and Bylsma, F. W. (1997). Lewy body and progressive dementia: A critical review and meta-analysis. *Journal of the International Neuropsychological Society*, **3**, 179–94.

Connor, D. J., Salmon, D. P., Sandy, T. J., Galasko, D., Hansen, L. A., and Thal, L. (1998).
Cognitive profiles of autopsy-confirmed Lewy body variant vs. pure Alzheimer's disease.
Archives of Neurology, **55**, 994–1000.

Dalrymple-Alford, J. C., Kalders, A. S., Jones, R. D., and Watson, R. W. (1994). A central executive
deficit in patients with parkinson's disease. *Journal of Neurology, Neurosurgery and Psychiatry*,
57, 360–7.

Del-Ser, T., Munoz, D. G., and Hachinski, V. (1996). Temporal pattern of cognitive decline and
incontinence is different in Alzheimer's disease and diffuse Lewy body disease. *Neurology*, **46**,
682–6.

Dickson, D. W., Davies, P., Mayeux, R., Crystal, H., Horopian, D. S., Thompson, A., *et al.* (1987).
Diffuse Lewy body disease: Neuropathological and biochemical studies of six patients. *Acta
Neuropathologica*, **75**, 8–15.

Dickson, D. W., Ruan, D., Crystal, H., Mark, M. H., Davies, P., Kress, Y., *et al.* (1991).
Hippocampal degeneration differentiates diffuse Lewy body disease (DLBD) from Alzheimer's
disease: Light and electron microscopic immunocytochemistry of CA2–3 neurites specific to
DLBD. *Neurology*, **41**, 1402–9.

Dickson, D. W., Schmidt, M. L., Lee, V. M.-Y., Zhao, M.-L., Yen, S.-H., and Trojanowski, J. Q.
(1994). Immunoreactivity profile of hippocampal CA2/3 neurites in diffuse Lewy body disease.
Acta Neuropathologica, **87**, 269–76.

Double, K. L., Halliday, G. M., McRitchie, D. A., Reid, W. G. J., Hely, M. A., and Morris, J. G. L.
(1996). Regional brain atrophy in idiopathic Parkinson's disease and diffuse Lewy body disease.
Dementia, **7**, 304–13.

Filoteo, J. V., Delis, D. C., Salmon, D. P., Demadura, T., Roman, M. J., and Shults, C. W. (1997).
An examination of the nature of attentional deficits in patients with Parkinson's disease:
Evidence from a spatial orienting task. *Journal of the International Neuropsychological Society*,
3, 337–47.

Galasko, D., Saitoh, T., Xia, Y., Thal, L. J., Katzman, R., Hill, L. R., *et al.* (1994). The
apolipoprotein E e-4 allele is overrepresented in patients with the Lewy body variant of
Alzheimer's disease. *Neurology*, **44**, 1950–1.

Galasko, D., Katzman, R., Salmon, D. P., Thal, L. J., and Hansen, L. (1996). Clinical and
neuropathological findings in Lewy body dementias. *Brain and Cognition*, **31**, 166–75.

Galasko, D., Salmon, D. P., Lineweaver, T., Hansen, L., and Thal, L. J. (1998). Neuropsychological
measures distinguish patients with Lewy body variant from those with Alzheimer's disease.
Neurology, **50**, A181. (Abstract)

Galloway, P. H., Sahgal, A., McKeith, I. G., Lloyd, S., Cook, J. H., Ferrier, I. N., *et al.* (1992).
Visual pattern recognition memory and learning deficits in senile dementias of Alzheimer and
Lewy body types. *Dementia*, **3**, 101–7.

Gibb, W. R. G., Esiri, M. M., and Lees, A. J. (1985). Clinical and pathological features of diffuse
cortical Lewy body disease (Lewy body dementia). *Brain*, **110**, 1131–53.

Gibb, W. R. G., Luthert, P. J., Janota, I., and Lantos, P. L. (1989). Cortical Lewy body dementia:
Clinical features and classification. *Journal of Neurology, Neurosurgery, and Psychiatry*, **52**,
185–92.

Girling, D. M. and Berrios, G. E. (1990). Extrapyramidal signs, primitive reflexes and frontal
lobe function in senile dementia of the Alzheimer type. *British Journal of Psychiatry*, **157**,
888–93.

Gnanalingham, K. K., Byrne, E. J., and Thornton, A. (1996). Clock-face drawing to differentiate
Lewy body and Alzheimer type dementia syndromes. *The Lancet*, **347**, 696–7.

Graham, C., Ballard, C., and Saad, K. (1997). Variables which distinguish patients fulfilling clinical
criteria for dementia with Lewy bodies from those with Alzheimer's disease. *International
Journal of Geriatric Psychiatry*, **12**, 314–18.

Hansen, L. A. and Galasko, D. (1992). Lewy body disease. *Current Opinion in Neurology and
Neurosurgery*, **5**, 889–94.

Hansen, L., Salmon, D., Galasko, D., Masliah, E., Katzman, R., DeTeresa, R., *et al.* (1990).
The Lewy body variant of Alzheimer's disease: A clinical and pathologic entity. *Neurology*, **40**,
1–8.

Hansen, L. A., Galasko, D., Samuel, W., Xia, Y., Chen, X., and Saitoh, T. (1994). Apolipoprotein-E e-4 is associated with increased neurofibrillary pathology in the Lewy body variant of Alzheimer's disease. *Neuroscience Letters*, **182**, 63–5.

Hansen, L. A., Daniel, S. E., Wilcock, G. K., and Love, S. (1998). Frontal cortical synaptophysin in Lewy body diseases: relation to Alzheimer's disease and dementia. *Journal of Neurology, Neurosurgery and Psychiatry*, **64**, 653–6.

Hashimoto, M., Kitagaki, H., Imamura, T., Hirono, N., Shimomura, T., Kazui, H., *et al.* (1998). Medial temporal and whole-brain atrophy in dementia with Lewy bodies. *Neurology*, **51**, 357–62.

Hely, M. A., Reid, W., Halliday, G. M., McRitchie, D. A., Leicester, J., Joffe, R., *et al.* (1996). Diffuse Lewy body disease: clinical features in nine cases without coexistent Alzheimer's disease. *Journal of Neurology, Neurosurgery and Psychiatry*, **60**, 531–8.

Ince, P. G., Jaros, E., Ballard, C., McKeith, I. G., and Perry, R. H. (1998b). Prospective evaluation of consensus diagnosis criteria for dementia with Lewy bodies. *Neuropathology and Applied Neurobiology*, **24**, 138.

Ince, P. G., Perry, E. K., and Morris, C. M. (1998a). Dementia with Lewy bodies: A distinct non-Alzheimer dementia syndrome? *Brain Pathology*, **8**, 299–324.

Irizarry, M. C., Growdon, W., Gomez-Isla, T., Newell, K., George, J. M., Clayton, D. F., *et al.* (1998). Nigral and cortical Lewy bodies and dystrophic nigral neurites in Parkinson's disease and cortical Lewy body disease contain alpha-synuclein immunoreactivity. *Journal of Neuropathology and Experimental Neurology*, **57**, 334–7.

Jacobs, D. M., Marder, K., Cote, L. J., Sano, M., Stern, Y., and Mayeux, R. (1995). Neuropsychological characteristics of preclinical dementia in Parkinson's disease. *Neurology*, **45**, 1691–6.

Katzman, R., Galasko, D., Saitoh, T., Thal, L. J., and Hansen, L. A. (1995). Genetic evidence that the Lewy body variant is indeed a phenotypic variant of Alzheimer's disease. *Brain and Cognition*, **28**, 259–65.

Khachaturian, Z. S. (1985). Diagnosis of Alzheimer's disease. *Archives of Neurology*, **42**, 1097–105.

Kosaka, K. (1990). Diffuse Lewy body disease in Japan. *Journal of Neurology*, **237**, 197–204.

Kosaka, K. and Iseki, E. (1996). Dementia with Lewy bodies. *Current Opinion in Neurology*, **9**, 271–5.

Kosaka, K., Yoshimura, M., Ikeda, K., and Budka, H. (1984). Diffuse type of Lewy body disease: Progressive dementia with abundant cortical Lewy bodies and senile changes of varying degree: A new disease? *Clinical Neuropathology*, **3**, 185–92.

Krugger, R., Kuhn, W., Muller, T., Woitalla, D., Graeber, M., Kosel, S., *et al.* (1998). Ala30Pro mutation in the gene encoding alpha-synuclein in Parkinson's disease. *Nature Genetics*, **18**, 106–8.

Langlais, P. J., Thal, L., Hansen, L., Galasko, D., Alford, M., and Masliah, E. (1993). Neurotransmitters in basal ganglia and cortex of Alzheimer's disease with and without Lewy bodies. *Neurology*, **43**, 1927–34.

Lees, A. J. and Smith, E. (1983). Cognitive deficits in the early stages of Parkinson's disease. *Brain*, **137**, 221–4.

Lennox, G., Lowe, J., Landon, M., Byrne, E. J., Mayer, R. J., and Godwin-Austen, R. B. (1989). Diffuse Lewy body disease: Correlative neuropathology using anti-ubiquitin immunocytochemistry. *Journal of Neurology, Neurosurgery, and Psychiatry*, **52**, 1236–47.

Levy, R., Eagger, S., and Griffiths, M. (1994). Lewy bodies and response to Tacrine in Alzheimer's disease. *The Lancet*, **343**, 176.

Lippa, C. F., Fujiwara, H., Mann, D. M. A., Giasson, B., Baba, M., Schmidt, M. L., *et al.* (1998). Lewy bodies contain altered alpha-synuclein in brains of many familial Alzheimer's disease patients with mutations in presenilin and amyloid precursor protein genes. *American Journal of Pathology*, **153**, 1365–70.

Lippa, C. F., Smith, T. W., and Swearer, J. M. (1994). Alzheimer's disease and Lewy body disease: A comparative clinicopathological study. *Annals of Neurology*, **35**, 81–8.

McKeith, I. G., Perry, R. H., Fairbairn, A. F., Jabeen, S., and Perry, E. K. (1992). Operational criteria for senile dementia of Lewy body type (SDLT). *Psychological Medicine*, **22**, 911–22.

McKeith, I. G., Fairbairn, A., and Harrison, R. (1996*a*). Management of the non-cognitive symptoms of Lewy body dementia. In *Dementia with Lewy bodies* (ed. R. H. Perry, I. G. McKeith, and E. K. Perry). London: Cambridge University Press.

McKeith, I., Galasko, D., Kosaka, K., Perry, E., Dickson, D., Hansen, L., *et al.* (1996*b*). Clinical and pathological diagnosis of dementia with Lewy bodies (DLB): Report of the Consortium on Dementia with Lewy Bodies (CDLB) International Workgroup. *Neurology*, **47**, 1113–24.

McShane, R., Gedling, K., Reading, M., McDonald, B., Esiri, M. M., and Hope, T. (1995). Prospective study of relations between cortical Lewy bodies, poor eyesight, and hallucinations in Alzheimer's disease. *Journal of Neurology, Neurosurgery and Psychiatry*, **59**, 185–8.

Merello, M., Sabe, L., Teson, A., Migliorelli, R., Petracchi, M., Leiguarda, R., *et al.* (1994). Extrapyramidalism in Alzheimer's disease: Prevalence, psychiatric, and neuropsychological correlates. *Journal of Neurology, Neurosurgery, and Psychiatry*, **57**, 1503–9.

Mirra, S. S., Hart, M. N., and Terry, R. D. (1993). Making the diagnosis of Alzheimer's disease. *Archives of Pathology and Laboratory Medicine*, **117**, 132–44.

Olichney, J. M., Hansen, L. A., Galasko, D., Saitoh, T., Hofstetter, C. R., Katzman, R., *et al.* (1996). The apolipoprotein E e-4 allele is associated with increased neuritic plaques and cerebral amyloid angiopathy in Alzheimer's disease and Lewy body variant. *Neurology*, **47**, 190–6.

Olichney, J. M., Galasko, D., Salmon, D. P., Hofstetter, C. R., Hansen, L. A., Katzman, R., *et al.* (1998). Cognitive decline is faster in Lewy body variant than in Alzheimer's disease. *Neurology*, **51**, 351–7.

Pellise, A., Roig, C., Barraquer-Bordas, L., and Ferrer, I. (1996). Abnormal, ubiquinated cortical neurites in patients with diffuse Lewy body disease. *Neuroscience Letters*, **206**, 85–8.

Perry, R. H., Irving, D., Blessed, G., Fairbairn, A., and Perry, E. K. (1990*a*). Senile dementia of the Lewy body type: A clinically and neuropathologically distinct form of Lewy body dementia in the elderly. *Journal of Neurological Sciences*, **95**, 119–39.

Perry, E. K., Marshall, E., Perry, R. H., Irving, D., Smith, C. J., Blessed, G., *et al.* (1990*b*). Cholinergic and dopaminergic activities in senile dementia of Lewy body type. *Alzheimer's Disease and Associated Disorders*, **4**, 87–95.

Perry, E. K., Marshall, E., Thompson, P., McKeith, I. G., Collerton, D., Fairbairn, A. F., *et al.* (1993). Monoaminergic activities in Lewy body dementia: relation to hallucinosis and extrapyramidal features. *Journal of Neural Transmission*, **6**, 167–77.

Perry, R. H., McKeith, I. G., and Perry, E. K. (ed.) (1996). *Dementia with Lewy bodies*. London: Cambridge University Press.

Polymeropoulous, M. H., Lavedant, C., Leroy, E., *et al.* (1997). Mutation in the alpha-synuclein gene identified in families with Parkinson's disease. *Science*, **276**, 2045–7.

Rezaie, P., Cairns, N. J., Chadwick, A., and Lantos, P. L. (1996). Lewy bodies are located preferentially in limbic areas in diffuse Lewy body disease. *Neuroscience Letters*, **212**, 111–14.

Rice, V., Salmon, D., Galasko, D., Connor, D., Thal, L., and Butters, N. (1996). Neuropsychological deficits in patients with clinically diagnosed Lewy body variant of Alzheimer's disease. *Journal of the International Neuropsychological Society*, **2**, 31. (Abstract)

Richards, M., Bell, K., Dooneief, G., Marder, K., Sano, M., Mayeux, R., *et al.* (1993). Patterns of neuropsychological performance in Alzheimer's disease patients with and without extrapyramidal signs. *Neurology*, **43**, 1708–11.

Sahgal, A., Galloway, P. H., McKeith, I. G., Edwardson, J. A., and Lloyd, S. (1992). A comparative study of attentional deficits in senile dementias of Alzheimer and Lewy body types. *Dementia*, **3**, 350–4.

Sahgal, A., McKeith, I. G., Galloway, P. H., Tasker, N., and Steckler, T. (1995). Do differences in visuospatial ability between senile dementias of the Alzheimer and Lewy body types reflect differences solely in mnemonic function? *Journal of Clinical and Experimental Neuropsychology*, **17**, 35–43.

Salmon, D. P., Galasko, D., Hansen, L. A., Masliah, E., Butters, N., Thal, L. J., *et al.* (1996). Neuropsychological deficits associated with diffuse Lewy body disease. *Brain and Cognition*, **31**, 148–65.

Salmon, D. P., Lineweaver, T. T., Galasko, D., and Hansen, L. (1998). Patterns of cognitive decline in patients with autopsy-verified Lewy body variant of Alzheimer's disease. *Journal of the International Neuropsychological Society*, **4**, 228. (Abstract)

Samuel, W., Galasko, D., Masliah, E., and Hansen, L. A. (1996). Neocortical Lewy body counts correlate with dementia in the Lewy body variant of Alzheimer's disease. *Journal of Neuropathology and Experimental Neurology*, **55**, 44–52.

Samuel, W., Alford, M., Hofstetter, R., and Hansen, L. A. (1997). Dementia with Lewy bodies versus pure Alzheimer's disease: Differences in cognition, neuropathology, cholinergic dysfunction and synapse density. *Journal of Neuropathology and Experimental Neurology*, **56**, 499–508.

Shimomura, T., Mori, E., Yamashita, H., Imamura, T., Hirono, N., Hashimoto, M., *et al.* (1998). Cognitive loss in dementia with Lewy bodies and Alzheimer's disease. *Archives of Neurology*, **55**, 1547–52.

Smith, M. C., Mallory, M., Hansen, L. A., Nianfeng, G., and Masliah, E. (1995). Fragmentation of the neuronal cytoskeleton in the Lewy body variant of Alzheimer's disease. *NeuroReport*, **6**, 673–6.

Soininen, H., Helkala, E. L., Laulumaa, V., Soikkeli, R., Hartikainen, P., and Riekkinen, P. J. (1992). Cognitive profile of Alzheimer patients with extrapyramidal signs: A longitudinal study. *Journal of Neural Transmission*, **4**, 241–54.

Spillantini, M. G., Schmidt, M. L., Lee, V., Trojanowski, J. Q., Jakes, R., and Goedert, M. (1997). Alpha-synuclein in Lewy bodies. *Nature*, **388**, 839–40.

Spillantini, M. G., Crowther, R. A., Jakes, R., and Hasegawa, M. (1998). Alpha-synuclein in filamentous inclusions of Lewy bodies from Parkinson's disease and dementia with Lewy bodies. *Proceedings of the National Academy of Sciences USA*, **95**, 6469–73.

Stern, Y., Richards, M., Sano, M., and Mayeux, R. (1993). Comparison of cognitive changes in patients with Alzheimer's and Parkinson's disease. *Archives of Neurology*, **50**, 1040–5.

Takeda, A., Hashimoto, M., Mallory, M., Sundsmo, M., Hansen, L. A., Sisk, A., *et al.* (1998). Abnormal distribution of the non-A beta component of Alzheimer's disease amyloid precursor/alpha-synuclein in Lewy body disease as revealed by proteinase K and formic acid pretreatment. *Laboratory Investigation*, **78**, 1169–77.

Trojanowski, J. Q. and Lee, V. (1998). Aggregation of neurofilament and alpha-synuclein proteins in Lewy bodies. *Archives of Neurology*, **55**, 151–2.

Turner, R. S., Chervin, R. D., Frey, K. A., Minoshima, S., and Kuhl, D. E. (1997). Probable diffuse Lewy body disease presenting as REM sleep behavior disorder. *Neurology*, **49**, 523–7.

Ueda, K., Fukushima, H., Masliah, E., Xia, Y., Iwai, A., Yoshimoto, M., *et al.* (1993). Molecular cloning of cDNA encoding an unrecognized component of amyloid in Alzheimer's disease. *Proceedings of the National Academy of Sciences USA*, **90**, 11282–6.

Wagner, M. T. and Bachman, D. L. (1996). Neuropsychological features of diffuse Lewy body disease. *Archives of Clinical Neuropsychology*, **11**, 175–84.

Wakabayashi, K., Hansen, L. A., and Masliah, E. (1995). Cortical Lewy body-containing neurons are pyramidal cells: Laser confocal imaging of double-immunolabeled sections with anti-ubiquitin and SMI32. *Acta Neuropathologica*, **89**, 404–8.

Wakabayashi, K., Hansen, L. A., Vincent, I., Mallory, M., and Masliah, E. (1997). Neurofibrillary tangles in the dentate granulae cells of patients with Alzheimer's disease, Lewy body disease and progressive supranuclear palsy. *Acta Neuropathologica*, **93**, 7–12.

Walker, Z., Allen, R., Shergill, S., and Katona, C. (1997). Neuropsychological performance in Lewy body dementia and Alzheimer's disease. *British Journal of Psychiatry*, **170**, 156–8.

Weiner, M. F., Risser, R. C., Cullum, C. M., Honig, L., White, C., Speciale, S., *et al.* (1996). Alzheimer's disease and its Lewy body variant: A clinical analysis of postmortem verified cases. *American Journal of Psychiatry*, **153**, 1269–73.

Yeatman, R., McLean, C. A., and Ames, D. (1994). The clinical manifestations of senile dementia of Lewy body type: A case report. *Australian and New Zealand Journal of Psychiatry*, **28**, 512–15.

14 Vascular dementias

John R. Hodges and Naida L. Graham

1 Introduction

Cerebrovascular disease is typically regarded as a condition of the elderly in whom it undoubtedly plays an important, but complex, role in the genesis of cognitive impairment. (For review of this topic readers are recommended to read the many excellent articles in the special issue of *Alzheimer's Disease and Associated Disorders*, Volume 13, supplement 3, December 1999.) Rather surprisingly, in view of the relative rarity of cases in memory clinics (Rockwood *et al.* 1999), epidemiological studies also show that vascular dementias (VaD) contribute significantly in younger cohorts. For instance, in a recent community-based study of two London boroughs by Harvey *et al.* (Chapter 1), VaD was second in prevalence only to Alzheimer's disease (AD) in patients aged under 65. Intuitively it seems likely that rarer causes of VaD are more common in the elderly, although this has not been proven.

Vascular disease is, therefore, an important cause of dementia at all ages. Yet, despite a very considerable literature on the topic (a Medline search revealed 1024 papers published between 1995 and 2000, compared to 12 180 papers on AD), it is remarkably difficult to make definite statements about the clinical, neuropsychiatric, neuropsychological, imaging and other features of VaD. In this chapter we first discuss some of the reasons for the uncertainties that surround the topic. We then describe the three principal clinical syndromes found in patients with VaD, the prevalence of dementia post-stroke, and the role of vascular risk factors. There follows a longer section, which reflects our current research interests, on the neuropsychological differentiation of VaD from AD. Finally, we consider prognosis and management.

1.1 Terminological confusion

The literature contains a plethora of overlapping and confusing terms (including vascular dementia, atherosclerotic dementia and psychosis, vascular cognitive impairment, multi-infarct dementia, lacunar state, cerebral microangiopathy, Binswanger's encephalopathy, leukoaraiosis, subcortical vascular dementia, etc.), some of which relate to clinical syndromes, others to pathological entities, and still others to a syndrome defined on the basis of radiological appearances, and all of which are poorly defined. The important topic of nosology is addressed further below after consideration of other key facts.

1.2 The role of imaging abnormalities

The advent of sophisticated neuroimaging techniques, which one might imagine would have clarified the situation, has caused even more confusion. Up to 60% of patients with clinically 'pure' AD — including some with genetically determined early onset disease (see Chapter 11) — have periventricular and white matter hyperintense lesions particularly visible on T2-

weighted and proton density MRI, which are similar in appearance to those seen, to a greater extent, in patients with VaD (Barber *et al.* 1999; Scheltens *et al.* 1992). These almost certainly reflect the microvascular pathology which occurs together with the classic plaques and tangles in AD (see below). In support of this, studies attempting to show a difference in cognitive profile between patients with and without white matter hyperintensities on MRI have failed to establish a significant difference. Similarly, high signal intensities of this type are seen commonly on T2-weighted MRI in apparently normal asymptomatic middle-aged and elderly individuals. Deciding whether someone has VaD on the basis of their scan is, therefore, more a matter of degree than an absolute distinction between normal and abnormal, and should always be considered in the light of the presenting clinical features. A summary of MRI features suggestive of VaD, based upon a recent international consensus meeting, is shown in Table 14.1 (from Erkinjuntti *et al.* 1999).

1.3 Neuropathology: the gold standard?

Review of the neuropathological literature reveals that the separation of AD from VaD is far from straightforward. As mentioned above, patients with pure AD — even early onset cases — have a high rate of cerebral congophilic angiopathy and non-amyloid small-vessel sclerosis with related microinfarction tissue rarefaction and gliosis occurring in the central, preferentially frontal deep white matter, which some authorities consider contributes significantly to the pathogenesis of the cognitive decline and causes the hyperintensities seen on MRI (see Englund 1998; Kalaria and Ballard 1999). Cases of truly mixed pathology with both classic Alzheimer's type pathology and gross multi-infarct cerebrovascular disease are also common, accounting for up to 20% in many pathological series, although admittedly these series all consist of typical elderly dementia subjects (Gilleard *et al.* 1992; Holmes *et al.* 1999; Jellinger *et al.* 1990; Molsa *et al.* 1985; Todorov *et al.* 1975; Tomlinson *et al.* 1970; Wade *et al.* 1987). It is also increasingly apparent that vascular risk factors heighten the likelihood of developing both AD and vascular pathology (see below). Indeed, we are now entering an era where the distinction between AD and VaD is becoming less clear-cut than it was a decade ago.

Table 14.1 Summary statement of the International Working Group for the Harmonization of Dementia Drug Guidelines regarding imaging in VaD (from Erkinjuntti *et al.* 1999)

1	Not a single feature, but a combination of infarct features, extent and type of white matter lesions, degree and site of atrophy, and host factors constitute correlates of VaD.
2	Infarct features favouring VaD include bilaterality, multiplicity, and location in the dominant hemisphere and in the limbic structures (fronto-limbic or prefrontal-subcortical and medial limbic or medial hippocampal circuits).
3	White matter lesions (WMLs) favouring VaD are extensive WMLs (extending periventricular WMLs and confluent to extending WMLs in the deep white matter) on CT or MRI.
4	It is doubtful that only a single small lesion could support imaging evidence for a diagnosis of VaD. In addition, the heterogeneity of patients with 'strategic infarct dementia' raises questions as to their value as subjects for clinical trials.
5	Absence of cerebrovascular disease related lesions on CT or MRI is evidence against a vascular aetiology.

1.4 Dementia without a stroke history

Related to the above issue is the fact that one-third to one-half of patients with pathological evidence of VaD lack a clinically recognized stroke (Leys *et al.* 1999). Moreover, it remains open to question whether it is necessary to ever suffer an overt, even if subclinical, infarction of brain tissue. The idea that chronic ischaemia may play a part in the genesis of dementia — which was accepted for the first half of the 20th century and then, following the pioneering pathological work of Miller Fisher (1965), Tomlinson *et al.* (1970) and others, was dismissed in favour of the concept of multi-infarct disease — is again finding favour in some quarters as a partial contributor to VaD (Rockwood *et al.* 1999, 2000).

1.5 Many different underlying aetiologies and types of pathology

At its broadest, the term VaD could be applied to patients with a wide range of different underlying aetiologies ranging from cardiac emboli, thrombo-embolic atherosclerotic large vessel disease, microvascular pathology in hypertension, the vasculitidies (SLE, etc.), prothrombotic disorders notably the anti-phospholipid syndrome, and genetic disease such as cerebral autosomal dominant arteriopathy with subcortical infarcts and leucoencephalopathy (CADASIL) or the mitochondrial cytopathies; the rarer causes of genetically determined disease which produce strokes and stroke-like syndromes are covered in Chapters 17 and 18.

The range of mechanisms by which these diseases can damage the brain is also broad and includes at one end of the spectrum lobar haemorrhage and large vessel occlusion, with diffuse microvascular induced damage at the other end. As discussed below, recent pathological evidence suggests that microvascular disease with subcortical white matter damage is the chief substrate of VaD (Englund 1998; Esiri *et al.* 1997).

Table 14.2 NINDS-AIREN criteria for probable VaD (adapted from Roman et al. 1993)

1	Dementia, defined by cognitive decline from a previously higher level of functioning and manifested by impairment of memory and of two or more cognitive domains … severe enough to interfere with activities of daily living and not due to physical effects of stroke alone.
	Exclusion criteria: cases with disturbance of consciousness, delirium, psychosis, severe aphasia, or major sensorimotor impairment precluding neuropsychological testing. Also excluded are systemic disorders or other brain diseases (such as AD) that in and of themselves could account for deficits in memory and cognition.
2	**Cerebrovascular disease** (CVD), defined by the presence of focal signs on neurological examination … consistent with stroke (with or without history of stroke) and evidence of relevant CVD by brain imaging (CT or MRI) including multiple large-vessel infarcts or a single strategically placed infarct …, as well as multiple basal ganglia and white matter lacunes or extensive periventricular white matter lesions or combinations.
3	**A relationship between the above two disorders** manifested or inferred by the presence of one or more of the following: Onset of dementia within three months following a recognized stroke Abrupt deterioration in cognitive functions, or fluctuating, stepwise progression of cognitive deficits Clinical features consistent with the diagnosis of **probable vascular dementia**: Early presence of a gait disturbance History of unsteadiness and frequent, unprovoked falls Early urinary symptoms not explained by urologic disease Pseudobulbar palsy Personality and mood changes, abulia, depression, emotional incontinence, or other subcortical deficits …

1.6 The current concept of vascular dementia: from atherosclerotic dementia to multi-infarct dementia and back again

Not surprisingly, given the above factors, there have until recently been no clear consensus-derived criteria for the diagnosis of VaD. The most widely used diagnostic label, in the modern era, multi-infarct dementia (Hachinski *et al.* 1974) was introduced to emphasize the role of strokes rather than chronic ischaemia, in the genesis of dementia. These authors were influenced by the view of Miller Fisher (1965) and Tomlinson *et al.* (1970) that strokes, most commonly related to extracranial atherosclerotic disease, were the primary cause of dementia and that the dementia was critically related to the volume (> 50 cc) of the infarction. The diagnosis was frequently supported by scores on the Hachinski Ischaemia Scale (HIS) (Hachinski *et al.* 1975) or subsequent modifications (e.g. Loeb and Gandolfo 1983; Small 1985), although the limitations of such scales have been widely appreciated even by Hachinski and colleagues. An extensive critique of the HIS was published by Dening and Berrios (1992) who concluded that 'the HIS deserves a decent burial'. The broader term vascular dementia (Erkinjuntti 1997; Van Gijn 1998) was then gradually introduced to identify intellectual impairment resulting from more diffuse ischaemic (or haemorrhage) damage, with the realization that only a small proportion of patients with dementia in the context of cerebrovascular disease have classic multi-infarct disease. More recently, attempts have been made to establish research guides for VaD — similar to those widely used in studies of AD — which encompass a range of different pathologies: the NINDS-AIREN (National Institute for Neurological Diseases and Stroke Association — Association International pour la Recherché et l'Enseignement en Neurosciences) published criteria for definite, probable, and possible VaD (Roman *et al.* 1993) (see Table 14.2). Another set of guidelines, similar in principal, were proposed by the State of California Alzheimer's Disease Diagnostic and Treatment Centres (ADDTC, Chui *et al.* 1992). The criteria have, so far, been tested rather little against neuropathology. One study concluded that while they appear effective at excluding patients with AD, they failed to diagnose one-third of cases of neuropathologically confirmed VaD (Gold *et al.* 1997). A more recent community based study again confirmed the high specificity (0.95) but low sensitivity (0.43) (Holmes *et al.* 1999). A shortcoming for epidemiological studies is that both the ADDTC and the NINDS-AIREN criteria rely for their diagnosis on neuroimaging which is still not widely available, especially in the community. The criteria appear valuable for the identification of cases of pure VaD for inclusion in research, but many cases with cognitive failure seen in clinical practice in whom vascular factors almost certainly play a major role do not fit the criteria. This is mainly because of the requirements to have 'the presence of focal signs on neurological examination such as hemiparesis, lower facial weakness, Babinski's sign, sensory deficits, hemianopia and dysarthria consistent with stroke' and a clear temporal relationship between the dementia and stroke or a stepwise decline. In the context of a memory clinic very few patients with a suspected vascular aetiology meet these stringent criteria, leading some authors to prefer the term vascular cognitive impairment (for discussion, see Devasenapathy and Hachinski 1997; Rockwood *et al.* 1999); a relevant case vignette is given below. There is also poor agreement between the various diagnostic criteria in current usage (Chui *et al.* 2000). In the absence of prospective clinicopathological validation the issue of which criteria to use remains in a state of flux. In keeping with recent trends, the term vascular dementia will be used in this chapter but with an attempt to distinguish between major syndromes encompassed within the broad rubric.

1.6.1 Case vignette

Ms A, a 65-year-old widow, presented to the memory clinic with a two year history of insidious cognitive decline. Her daughter reported worsening memory with forgetfulness and a decline in activities of daily living — Ms A no longer prepared meals and was unable to use household appliances. Her speech was stereotyped and empty. There was no suggestion of night-time confusion and besides apathy other neuropsychiatric features were absent.

Five years prior to presentation Ms A had three 'mini-strokes'; on each occasion she became dysarthric with facial drooping and limb clumsiness, lasting for a few days. Following these events her memory and other cognitive abilities appeared intact. In addition she suffered from angina, hypertension, and hypercholesterolaemia, all of which were under treatment by a physician.

Examination revealed multiple cognitive deficits: poor attention and executive abilities, markedly impaired episodic memory, mild anomia, and visuospatial dysfunction. Focal neurological signs were absent. MRI showed diffuse periventricular high signal lesions throughout both hemispheres. It seems highly probable that this lady had a subcortical vascular dementia syndrome although she did not fulfil current criteria in that neurological signs were absent and there was no clear relationship between her mini-strokes and the onset of her dementia. She could, of course, have dual pathology but pure AD seems improbable.

2 Clinical vascular dementia syndromes

Patients with dementia in the context of cerebrovascular disease can be divided into three major types, although it should be stressed that individual cases often show features of more than one type and the differences are relative rather than absolute. For summary see Table 14.3.

2.1 Multi-infarct dementia

As mentioned above, there has been considerable shift in the prominence given to dementia arising from recurrent clinically apparent strokes producing so-called multi-infarct dementia (MID). A recent estimate from a large multi-centre Canadian study was that classic MID accounted for only a third of cases of VaD (Rockwood *et al.* 1999). Patients with MID present following recurrent large vessel and lacunar strokes. There is typically a background of thromboembolic disease in the context of hypertension and other evidence of atherosclerotic disease: angina, peripheral vascular disease, etc. The clinical picture depends on the site and number of strokes but patients may show a mixture of cortical and subcortical features, although the latter usually predominate (Ishii *et al.* 1986). The progression is said to be stepwise, with plateaux in the course of the illness, but this feature has probably been overemphasized. Urinary and gait disturbances often occur early in the illness, sometimes before evidence of cognitive impairment.

Table 14.3 A clinical classification of vascular dementia syndromes

1	Multi-infarct dementia

2	Subcortical ischaemic dementia
	    Lacunar state
	    Diffuse leukoaraiosis (Binswanger's encephalopathy)

3	Strategic infarction
	    Medial thalamic infarcts
	    Lateral thalamic — internal capsular infarcts
	    Caudate and pallidal infarction
	    Posterior cerebral artery infarction
	    Left angular gyrus (Gerstmann's) syndrome
	    Basal forebrain infarction

Features of pseudobulbar palsy are said to be characteristic. Fluctuations in cognitive performance and nocturnal confusion are very common and cause difficulty in differentiating VaD from dementia with Lewy bodies. Emotional lability, leading to emotional incontinence and irritability, may be observed. There is often an accentuation of pre-morbid personality, with removal of inhibitions which can lead to disturbances of sexual behaviour. Apathy is also commonly reported and psychotic phenomena may occur.

2.2 Subcortical ischaemic dementia (including lacunar states and leukoaraiosis or Binswanger's encephalopathy)

Patients with long-standing arterial hypertension typically present with a more insidious decline in cognitive function, sometimes punctuated by clear-cut episodes of decline or by lacunar strokes, but rarely major thromboembolic events. Recent studies suggest that such patients constitute the majority of cases with VaD (Leys *et al.* 1999; Rockwood *et al.* 1999, 2000). The small vessel disease is the consequence of the occlusion of small deep perforating arteries caused by fibrinoid degeneration with lipohyalinoisis (Miller Fisher 1965). The difference between the multiple lacunar state and diffuse leukoaraiosis (or Binswanger's disease) is a matter of degree. In the latter, there are confluent changes in the deep white matter with diffuse demyelination predominating in the periventricular and occipital regions. In addition to the dementia, motor symptoms and signs may be present with a mixture of extrapyramidal and pyramidal features, although it should be stressed that many cases with gross white matter changes on MRI in association with hypertension lack focal neurological signs (see case vignette above). The most frequent physical sign is probably a form of gait disturbance which mimics that seen in normal pressure hydrocephalus.

Many patients presenting to memory clinics with cognitive decline in the context of diffuse white matter pathology do not fulfil strict criteria for dementia, in that they show subtle deficits but score above cut-offs on tests such as the Mini-Mental State Examination (MMSE) (Folstein *et al.* 1975). The term vascular cognitive impairment has been proposed by some authors (Devasenapathy and Hachinski 1997; Rockwood *et al.* 1999). It is widely believed that the cognitive syndrome in subcortical vascular dementia is distinct from that seen in AD with a predominance of executive deficits, due to undercutting of the frontal lobes and disconnection of fronto-striatal loops. Clinical experience suggests that such patients are grossly slowed up with poor information retrieval, and problems with tasks that require mental flexibility and shifting of attention (such as on the Wisconsin Card Sorting Test and the Stroop Test). Although forgetful, they are not markedly amnesic and do not show the impairments in semantic memory and visuospatial abilities that occur at an early stage in AD (see Chapter 11). In addition, changes in mood and other neuropsychiatric symptoms appear prominent. As discussed below, however, it has been difficult to substantiate this profile in formal studies contrasting matched groups of patients with VaD and AD.

2.3 Strategic infarction

The concept underlying this term is the idea that a single, discrete lesion of a critical brain region may result in dementia (i.e. impairment in two or more areas of cognition). Of course patients who suffer from a large dominant hemisphere stoke may have marked residual aphasia with concomitant alexia and/or agraphia, and are likely to show some degree of memory or attentional dysfunction if specifically tested, thus qualifying for the label 'dementia'. In general, however, the term 'strategic infarct' has been reserved for cases with small and more cryptic stokes which produce unexpectedly severe cognitive impairment, often without classic focal neurological signs (hemiplegia etc.).

2.3.1 Medial thalamic infarcts

These arise from occlusion of the paramedian thalamic branch of the posterior cerebral artery. The blood supply of thalami and midline structures is complex with marked inter-individual variation, and there is often a single branch of posterior cerebral artery which supplies both medial thalamic regions. Patients present with sudden onset of coma or confusion (due to interruption of components of the reticular activating system traversing the thalamus), followed by persistent amnesia which can be profound and resembles that seen in Korsakoff's syndrome. Apathy is also common. A tell-tale physical sign present in some cases is paralysis of vertical eye movements and/or eyelid apraxia due to infarction of a centre for upgaze at the very top of the brain stem (Crews *et al.* 1996; Graff-Radford *et al.* 1990; Hodges and McCarthy 1993). Functional brain imaging studies in such cases show major reductions in the oxygen metabolism involving the whole cortical mantle, reflecting thalamocortical de-afferentation (Levasseur *et al.* 1992).

2.3.2 Lateral thalamic-internal capsular infarcts

Tatemichi *et al.* (1992*b*) have drawn attention to a group of patients with severe changes in behaviour and memory following infarction of the inferior genu of the internal capsule. In the acute stages patients showed fluctuating alertness, inattention, apathy, and psychomotor retardation. Memory deficits are prominent in the chronic post-stroke state. Functional brain scanning reveals focal cortical hypometabolism in the infero-medial frontal and temporal cortex. These distant effects are thought to reflect interruption of components of the limbic circuitry (the dorsomedial thalamus, cingulate cortex, and orbitomedial frontal cortices) in passage via the inferior capsule.

2.3.3 Caudate and pallidal infarction

Bilateral infarction of the basal ganglia can result in abulia, apathy, and depression in some cases, or alternatively a state of disinhibition, hyperactivity, and inattention (Bhatia and Marsden 1994; Mori *et al.* 1996).

2.3.4 Posterior cerebral artery infarction

Occlusion of the main branch of this artery, by embolus or thrombosis, results in infarction to the following structures:

(a) The hippocampal formation with resultant material-specific memory problems, or if bilateral, severe amnesia.

(b) The medial occipital lobe including the primary visual cortex causing an homonymous hemianopia.

(c) The posterior part of the corpus callosum sometimes causing alexia without agraphia after left-sided strokes.

(d) A variable extent of the inferior temporal lobe producing visual agnosias for objects, colours, or faces according to the side of the lesion (Benson *et al.* 1974; Farah 1990).

2.3.5 Left angular gyrus (Gerstmann's) syndrome

Infarction of a posterior branch of the medial cerebral artery, sparing Wernicke's area in the posterior portion of the superior temporal gyrus, can produce Gerstmann's syndrome. This comprises agraphia, acalculia, left–right disorientation, and finger agnosia, although the syndrome is hardly ever seen in its pure state and most patients have elements of Gerstmann's syndrome plus a degree of aphasia or attentional deficits (Benton 1992; Roeltgen *et al.* 1983).

2.3.6 Basal forebrain infarction

This may complicate surgery for ruptured anterior communicating aneurysm with damage to the small perforating blood vessels in this region. The most consistent abnormality is amnesia, presumably secondary to disruption of the basal forebrain cholinergic system which provides inputs to the hippocampus via the fornix (Rajaram 1997). Change in personality, particularly apathy, is also common. A state of profound abulia may also be seen after infarction in the territory of the anterior bilateral anterior cerebral artery.

3 Dementia after stroke

One way of addressing the vexed issue of the relationship between cerebrovascular pathology and dementia is to look at the long-term outcome of patients who have had a definite stoke. A number of studies have established that the rate of dementia at three months post-stroke is on the order of 20–30%, which represents a ninefold increase in risk above baseline for age (Censori *et al.* 1996; Desmond *et al.* 2000; Kokmen *et al.* 1996; Loeb *et al.* 1992; Pohjasvaara *et al.* 1998; Tatemichi *et al.* 1992a). In the Columbia-Presbyterian Study (Tatemichi *et al.* 1992a) 251 patients aged 60 or older were followed-up at three months with a battery of neuropsychological tasks. Those with deficits involving memory and two other cognitive domains, and some degree of functional handicap, were classified as demented; according to these criteria, 26% were demented three months post-stroke. Interestingly only about half of these cases were thought to be demented purely as a result of vascular disease: 36% had dementia caused by the combined effects of stroke and AD, a diagnosis of which was suggested by their level of pre-stroke abilities, thus emphasizing again the overlap between these two disorders. Another recent large American cohort study of 453 patients revealed almost identical results (Desmond *et al.* 2000). One-fourth of stroke patients are said to develop new onset dementia one year after stroke (Andersen *et al.* 1996). Features associated with an increased risk of dementia include lacunar versus non-lacunar infarcts, dominant versus non-dominant hemisphere involvement (although the latter may reflect the linguistic bias inherent in all cognitive test batteries), prior stroke, advanced age, vascular risk factors, and ApoE status (Desmond *et al.* 2000). In many cases dementia develops insidiously with an AD-like picture and cannot easily be attributed to further stokes or concomitant depression (Tatemichi *et al.* 1994). Interestingly, there is evidence from the Framingham studies that stroke patients have a worse cognitive score on the MMSE prior to their stroke compared to non-stroke cases but the gap widens after the stroke episode (Kase *et al.* 1998).

4 Vascular risk factors and dementia

Although hypertension is the major risk factor for stoke, the relationship between hypertension and dementia (in the absence of stroke) is more complex. Several large studies have shown that raised blood pressure in mid-life is associated with worse cognitive function 20–25 years later (Elias *et al.* 1993; Kilander *et al.* 1998). The effect may be additive with other risk factors such as type 2 diabetes. Cross-sectional studies have produced conflicting evidence with an apparent association between dementia and low systolic pressure in some studies, although all seem agreed that in a younger population high blood pressure has an negative impact (for review see Stewart 1999). There is also a consistent trend for those with type 2 diabetes to be at greater risk of both dementia in general and more specifically vascular-type dementias (Kilander *et al.* 1997; Launer *et al.* 1993). The relationship between hypercholesterolaemia and smoking alone remains unsettled (see Stewart 1999).

Current dogma dictates that vascular risk factors are associated solely with VaD but several studies have now shown that the same factors may substantially increase the risk of AD (for review see Skoog *et al.* 1999). Hypertension, peripheral vascular disease, diabetes mellitus, hyper-cholesterolaemia, and smoking are now considered to be risk factors for AD. As reviewed more fully elsewhere in this book, possession of the apolipoprotein (ApoE) e4 allele has been associated with an increased risk for AD, but there is evidence that it may also be a risk factor for VaD (Bonarek *et al.* 2000; Noguchi *et al.* 1993) and for post-stoke dementia (Slooter *et al.* 1997). Carrying the e4 allele is recognized to be associated with a raised cholesterol level, but the link between ApoE e4 and vascular disease remains obscure. The large Rotterdam community study has suggested an inter-action between ApoE e4 and vascular risk factors in the production of AD with both making a sepa-rate, but additive, contribution such that patients with both hypertension and ApoE e4 are at particularly high risk of developing dementia (Hofman *et al.* 1997). It should be noted, however, that the distinction between AD and VaD in the Rotterdam study is based largely upon clinical assess-ment and not radiological investigations or neuropathology.

5 The neuropsychology of vascular dementia: separating vascular dementia from Alzheimer's disease

Studies of neuropsychological performance in VaD usually involve comparison of VaD with AD patients. Despite a plethora of studies evaluating different aspects of cognition in VaD, no reliable profile of cognitive deficits has emerged, and neuropsychological differentiation of VaD and AD remains problematic. This is because results across studies are often inconsistent. For example, some researchers have found that AD patients are more impaired than those with VaD on confrontation naming (Barr *et al.* 1992; Bayles and Tolmoeda 1983; Lukatela *et al.* 1998; Powell *et al.* 1988; Villardita 1993), while others have found that VaD patients are more impaired (Kontiola *et al.* 1990), and others have found no difference (Almkvist *et al.* 1993; Bentham *et al.* 1997; Laine *et al.* 1997; Loewenstein *et al.* 1991; Starkstein *et al.* 1996). The inconsistencies in the literature arise from several sources, including poor matching across patient groups, deficiencies in diagnostic criteria, and referral bias. These will now be discussed in turn.

Informative comparison across groups requires careful matching of patients. Failure to match AD and VaD groups on demographic variables is one cause of variability in results across studies (see Almkvist *et al.* 1993; Looi and Sachdev 1999; Lukatela *et al.* 1998; Powell *et al.* 1988). Many recent reports have, however, attempted to overcome this failing (see Looi and Sachdev 1999), presumably as a result of it having been highlighted in the literature.

An additional problem is that matching of disease severity across patient groups is not always done (see Bowler *et al.* 1997; Bowler and Hachinski 1997), rendering findings difficult to inter-pret. This is a more challenging problem because there is no ideal method of matching disease severity. Many recent studies have matched groups of VaD and AD patients on the MMSE. This is, however, a potentially flawed method. Consider trying to compare two hypothetical brain dis-eases (X and Y) where X produces profound deficits in memory and Y has its impact predomi-nantly on executive function (or language) and affects memory only late in the course. If you matched groups with disease X and Y using the MMSE, which is heavily weighted towards memory and attention, with virtually no component sensitive to frontal executive dysfunction, this would clearly produce spurious and misleading results. An even more erroneous conclusion could be drawn if comparing disease X with another disease, Z, whose impact was primarily on social cognition, behaviour, and mood, none of which are assessed on the MMSE. These two scenarios are not, however, purely hypothetical because as we shall see below, it has been concluded that VaD does indeed have a differentially severe impact on executive function and produces more neuropsychiatric symptoms.

As recognized by Looi and Sachdev (1999), a more sound approach would be to use indices of function not confounded by the cognitive characteristics of the dementia, or alternatively a more holistic evaluation which takes into account everyday functional ability, as well as neuropsychiatric and cognitive variables. Such studies are underway but have not yet been reported (see Gauthier *et al.* 1999; Roman and Royall 1999).

Inconsistencies in results across studies of VaD also arise from problems with diagnosis. Although several lists of diagnostic criteria for VaD have been published (see above), there is no universally accepted set. Moreover, comparison of criteria has shown that they can lead to different frequencies of diagnosis of VaD, indicating that they are not equivalent (Chui *et al.* 2000; Erkinjuntti *et al.* 1997). This lack of consensus and the resulting variability in classification of patients could account for some of the differences in results across studies. An additional problem with diagnosis is that patients with VaD represent a heterogeneous group. Pooling patients with diverse cerebrovascular pathology will lead to variability in test scores and inconsistent results across studies, as well as failure to recognize distinct patterns of neuropsychological impairments which may be associated with subtypes of VaD (Desmond *et al.* 1999).

An additional problem with diagnosis arises because diagnostic criteria for VaD have been influenced by those developed to identify AD (Bowler and Hachinski 2000; Desmond *et al.* 1999), in which episodic memory impairment is an early and prominent feature. Most diagnostic criteria for VaD require impairment in memory plus one other cognitive domain, e.g. *Diagnostic and Statistical Manual for Mental Disorders*, 4th edition (DSM-IV, American Psychiatric Association 1994), *International Classification of Disease*, 10th edition (ICD-10, World Health Organization 1992, 1993), National Institute of Neurological Disorders and Stroke — Association Internationale pour la Recherché et l'Enseignement en Neurosciences (Roman *et al.* 1993). As a result, the prevalence of episodic memory impairment in VaD may have been overestimated (Bowler and Hachinski 2000; Looi and Sachdev 1999), and patients with VaD but without memory impairment may be excluded from studies. A more serious consequence is that cases of VaD may not be identified early in the course of the illness, and may not, therefore, receive disease-modifying treatment (Bowler and Hachinski 1996, 2000). Bowler and Hachinski (2000) proposed that this problem could be addressed by moving away from the emphasis on episodic memory impairment, and using a criterion requiring impairment in *any* two cognitive domains. It has also been suggested that a requirement for dementia is too stringent, and may preclude early diagnosis and intervention (Bowler and Hachinski 1997). Instead, greater attention should be given to the full spectrum of cognitive impairment, including that which is too mild to fulfil criteria for dementia; it is for this reason that some researchers have adopted the concept of vascular cognitive impairment (see above).

An additional problem arising from the lack of consensus regarding diagnosis of VaD is that studies are open to pitfalls associated with referral bias. Many studies include patients referred to memory/dementia clinics, who are more likely to have (more severe) cognitive impairment than patients referred to vascular/stroke clinics. In addition, it is more probably that subjects referred to memory clinics will have episodic memory impairment than cognitively impaired patients referred to vascular clinics (Bowler and Hachinski 1997; Desmond *et al.* 1999).

In conclusion, the difficulties with accurate diagnosis and with matching patient groups limit the conclusions one can draw regarding neuropsychological deficits in VaD. Nevertheless, review of the literature reveals a number of consistent trends, which are outlined below. These should be interpreted with caution in view of the caveats discussed above.

5.1 Memory

Diagnostic criteria for VaD usually require a deficit in episodic memory (see above), and therefore the observation of this deficit in VaD patients is a self-fulfilling prophecy. Nevertheless, it has often been found that episodic memory impairment is less severe in VaD than in AD. For example, Donnelly and Grohman (1999) found that VaD patients showed significantly worse performance on the memory subscale (only) of the Mattis Dementia Rating Scale. One study compared VaD with Lewy body dementia, and found that the episodic memory impairment was more severe in VaD (Ballard *et al.* 1999).

Looi and Sachdev (1999) reviewed 18 relevant studies employing various tests of verbal learning or recall: virtually all of the more recent studies, using more sophisticated tasks, have shown superior performance in the VaD patients. It should be emphasized, however, that this difference is relative rather than absolute and that some patients with VaD do show severe amnesia of the type seen in AD. On the California Verbal Learning Test (CVLT), VaD patients showed better recall in both spontaneous and cued conditions, particularly after a delay, with fewer intrusions and false positive responses (Lamar *et al.* 1997; Libon *et al.* 1997; Mendez *et al.* 1997; Padovani *et al.* 1995). Similar results were found using a precursor of the CVLT, the Rey Auditory Verbal Learning Test (Carlesimo *et al.* 1993; Gainotti *et al.* 1992). Immediate and delayed recall of stories also tends to be better in VaD than AD (Doody *et al.* 1998; Lafosse *et al.* 1997; Villardita 1993). Note, however, that some studies have shown no difference between VaD and AD patients on tests of verbal learning and recall (e.g. Almkvist *et al.* 1999).

Non-verbal episodic memory has been less extensively studied and results have been somewhat less consistent, but most studies have shown little difference between groups (see Looi and Sachdev 1999). Working (immediate or short-term) memory as assessed by digit span or corsi block tapping span seems to be equivalently impaired in VaD and AD (Almkvist *et al.* 1993, 1999; Gainotti *et al.* 1992; Perez *et al.* 1975).

As discussed elsewhere in this book, breakdown in semantic memory is considered to be one of the hallmarks of AD which is present in most patients fairly early in the course of the disease (see Chapter 11). It is surprising, therefore, that this aspect of memory has been investigated so little in VaD. A pilot study by Bentham *et al.* (1997) comparing ten patients with VaD and ten with AD, matched on the basis of the cognitive component of the CAMDEX, found no differences in performance on a wide range of semantic memory tests (category fluency, picture naming, word-picture matching, generating definitions from words, etc.), although the authors postulated that the deficit in the two groups may reflect different underlying cognitive problems: loss of knowledge in AD versus impaired retrieval of information in VaD. This hypothesis awaits confirmation.

5.2 Executive function

A number of studies have documented superior performance in AD patients on tests of executive function. The most consistently used task has been the Wisconsin Card Sorting Test on which most studies have found greater impairment in VaD (Padovani *et al.* 1995; Tei *et al.* 1997, but for a counter-example see Starkstein *et al.* 1996). Likewise, Villardita (1993) found worse performance on the Porteus mazes test in VaD.

There are hints that attention abilities may also be more compromised in VaD (see Almkvist 1994; Doody *et al.* 1998) but the tests used to draw this conclusion are non-specific such as Digit Symbol Modalities Test and Trail-Making. Compared to the huge literature on attentional function in AD which has employed highly sophisticated tests to assess various aspects of attention (see Perry and Hodges 1999), there are few relevant studies in patients with VaD.

5.3 Language

The results of investigations of naming in VaD have also produced inconsistent results. The most common finding, however, is that VaD patients are anomic; the anomia tends to be more severe than in AD patients (Barr *et al.* 1992; Bayles and Tolmoeda 1983; Lukatela *et al.* 1998; Powell *et al.* 1988; Villardita 1993). This is consistent with Powell *et al.* (1988) results indicating that spontaneous speech in VaD is less empty and more informative than in AD.

One consistent trend to emerge from more recent studies is that initial letter based verbal fluency (sometimes referred to as FAS or the Controlled Oral Word Association Test) is more affected in VaD than AD (Doody *et al.* 1998; Giovannetti Carew *et al.* 1997; Lafosse *et al.* 1997; Lamar *et al.* 1997; Mendez *et al.* 1997; Padovani *et al.* 1995; Starkstein *et al.* 1996). In contrast, category fluency is often found to be equally impaired in the two aetiologies (Bentham *et al.* 1997; Giovannetti Carew *et al.* 1997). Poor verbal fluency is usually thought to reflect frontal/executive dysfunction.

Although it has not been investigated extensively, there is some suggestion that reading and writing are more impaired in VaD (Carey *et al.* 1999; Erkinjuntti *et al.* 1986; Kertesz and Clydesdale 1994). Using the writing subtest from the Western Aphasia Battery, Kertesz and Clydesdale (1994) found that VaD patients were more impaired at writing single dictated letters, and at copying of sentences; moreover, this writing subtest was useful in discriminating between VaD and AD. Powell *et al.* (1988) found that matched groups of VaD and AD patients were equally impaired on narrative writing and writing-to-dictation, but the former group were more impaired on the mechanics of writing. More detailed analyses of a narrative writing task were carried out by Carey *et al.* (1999), who found that in comparison with AD patients, those with VaD made more spelling errors, produced grammatically less complex sentences, and had more difficulty writing in straight horizontal lines. Taken together the results of these studies on writing suggest that both groups showed impairment in linguistic aspects of the writing process, but the VaD patients had greater impairment in handwriting.

Powell *et al.* (1988) compared groups of moderately demented VaD and AD patients, and found differences in their spontaneous speech. The former group showed reduced phrase length and grammatical complexity, as well as abnormal prosody and articulation, yet their speech was less empty and more informative than the AD group. This led the authors to conclude that the mechanics of speech were more affected in the VaD patients, while linguistic aspects were more affected in the AD patients. The reduced information content in the speech of the AD patients is consistent with the finding that they tend to be more anomic than VaD patients.

5.4 Visuospatial and perceptual skills

In their review, Looi and Sachdev (1999) found 11 studies which had compared constructional abilities using tests such as Block Design, Clock Drawing, or copy of the Rey Complex Figure: nine showed no difference between the two groups. Similarly, tests of visuo-perceptual ability in which the potentially confounding effects of praxic deficits were eliminated have also failed to show any consistent difference between AD and VaD.

5.5 Motor performance

In the few studies which have conducted relevant assessments, patients with VaD have been shown to have more difficulty with tests of motor performance (Erkinjuntti *et al.* 1986; Kertesz and Clydesdale 1994); in addition, Kertesz and Clydesdale (1994) found that this was one of the few tests which was useful in discriminating between VaD and AD. Because neither the tests nor the errors have been described in detail, however, it is not possible to specify the nature of the presumably subtle motor impairment. This deficit may account for the VaD patients' relatively greater difficulty with the mechanics of handwriting (see above).

Doody *et al.* (1998) and Almkvist *et al.* (1993) administered speeded tests of finger tapping and fist clenching, and found that patients with VaD performed significantly worse than those with AD, again suggesting some difficulty with motor performance in the VaD groups. In contrast, on higher-order tests of praxis (transitive and intransitive movements performed to command and imitation), there was no difference between the groups (Doody *et al.* 1998).

5.6 Neuropsychiatric features

Patients with VaD are said to show a greater degree of personality and affect change than those with AD with prominent anxiety, agitation, irritability, and emotional incontinence (for full review see Chapter 4). Recent studies have suggested that the degree of apathy and depression is greater in VaD but does not seem to correlate well with the extent of white matter change on MRI (Hargrave *et al.* 2000), although some authors have found an association between frontal white matter hyperintensities and depression scores (Barber *et al.* 1999).

5.7 Summary of the neuropsychological literature

Despite the clinical impression that VaD and AD produce qualitatively quite different patterns of dementia, review of the published literature reveals that it has been hard to find striking differences. In virtually all areas there are contradictory observations. In broad terms, episodic memory appears to be less impaired in VaD, while executive, motor, and possibly attentional, functions are more severely affected. In the language domain there are few differences except that phonological (initial letter) based verbal fluency is more impaired in VaD. The overall pattern is consistent with frontal or subcortical dysfunction.

6 Natural history of vascular dementia

Few good data exist on the prognosis of patients diagnosed with VaD. Chui and Gonthier (1999) recently reported a meta-analysis of the 13 studies (total patient cohort = 470) with survival data reported between 1985 and 1998. All but one used the diagnosis of MID rather than VaD, based largely upon the Hachinski Ischaemic Score. A comparison AD group was included in all but one study. Four of the 13 studies were community based and all concerned elderly rather than young onset cases. In all of the studies survival from either onset of symptoms, or from diagnosis, was poorer in VaD than in AD although the range was wide and the difference usually quite small. On average, patients with MID survived 6.0 years from symptom onset compared to 5.0 for the AD cases. For survival from diagnosis, the figures were 2.6 and 3.4 years for the MID and AD groups, respectively. It should be noted that most patients had fairly advanced dementia at the time of diagnosis and were typically very elderly. These figures should only be extrapolated to younger populations diagnosed at an early stage of disease with great caution.

Nine of the 13 studies included data on cognitive decline giving a total sample size of 175. The rate of change on the MMSE was virtually identical in the AD and MID groups with an average decline of between 2 and 3 points per year. No consistent trends emerged regarding the effects of different variables on rates of decline, but comparison of the studies was difficult because of the different methods used to define progression, variation in the variables included, and differing lengths of follow-up. Of particular note is the fact that the classic 'stepwise' pattern of decline has never been documented in a follow-study, even in patients with MID. The paradoxical findings of a poorer prognosis in VaD compared to AD but an equivalent rate of cognitive decline is probably explicable on the basis of the high rate of subsequent strokes and cardiac events in the VaD group.

7 Treatment and prevention of vascular dementia

The mainstay of treatment in patients with VaD is the prevention of further vascular damage by the meticulous control of risk factors, particularly hypertension. Screening for hypercholesterolaemia, diabetes, and sources of cardiac emboli is essential and patients should receive advice on general life-style issues such as diet and exercise (see Gorelick *et al.* 1999).

Treatment of the cognitive and behavioural symptoms is the same as any other form of dementia and is dealt with elsewhere in this book (see Chapters 19 and 20).

8 Conclusions

Cerebrovascular disease is a common cause of dementia, yet it is poorly understood. Lack of consensus in diagnosis of what is, in fact, a range of pathologies and clinical syndromes has caused confusion, and contributed to difficulty in comparison of results across studies. Nevertheless, progress has been made in the study of VaD. Despite the range of aetiologies, a typical (although not universal) profile of cognitive deficits has emerged, incorporating a mild episodic memory deficit, with more severe impairment in executive functions, and often accompanied by psychiatric problems. In future, large scale studies which combine radiological, neuropsychological, and (ultimately) neuropathological investigations will further our understanding of VaD.

9 Key points

1   Vascular disease is the second commonest cause of dementia in younger as well as older dementia community-based cohorts.

2   A wide range of pathologies contribute including large and small vessel infarction, chronic ischaemia, and haemorrhage.

3   The three principal clinical syndromes are:

   (i) Multi-infarct dementia.

   (ii) Subcortical ischaemic infarction and leukoaraiosis (which includes lacunar states and Binswanger's disease).

   (iii) Strategically sited infarction of critical brain regions such as the medial thalamic nuclei and the basal forebrain.

4   Pathologically and radiologically the separation of VaD from AD is far from straightforward. There is growing evidence that vascular risk factors contribute to the aetiology of AD and microvascular pathology is present in even 'pure' early onset cases of AD; the latter might be the cause of the hyperintensities seen on MRI in many patients with AD.

5   Neuropsychologically, the most consistent findings are better preservation of episodic memory and greater impairment of executive and attention abilities in VaD compared to AD.

6   The prognosis of VaD is probably a little worse than in AD in terms of survival although the rates of cognitive decline are equivalent.

References

Almkvist, O. (1994). Neuropsychological deficits in vascular dementia in relation to Alzheimer's disease: Reviewing evidence for functional similarity or divergence. *Dementia*, **5**, 203–9.

Almkvist, O., Backman, L., Basun, H., and Wahlund, L.-O. (1993). Patterns of neuropsychological performance in Alzheimer's disease and vascular dementia. *Cortex*, **29**, 661–73.

Almkvist, O., Fratiglioni, L., Aguero-Torres, H., Viitanen, M., and Backman L. (1999). Cognitive support at episodic encoding and retrieval: Similar patterns of utilization in community-based samples of Alzheimer's disease and vascular dementia patients. *Journal of Clinical and Experimental Neuropsychology*, **21**, 816–30.

American Psychiatric Association. (1994). *Diagnostic and statistical manual of mental disorders*, 4th edn. Washington, DC: American Psychiatric Association.

Andersen, G., Vestergaard, K., Riis, J. O., and Ingeman Nielsen, M. (1996). Intellectual impairment in the first year following stroke, compared to an age-matched population sample. *Cerebrovascular Disease*, **6**, 363–9.

Ballard, C. G., Ayre, G., O'Brien, J., Sahgal, A., McKeith, I. G., Ince, P. G., *et al.* (1999). Simple standardised neuropsychological assessments aid in the differential diagnosis of dementia with Lewy bodies from Alzheimer's disease and vascular dementia. *Dementia and Geriatric Cognitive Disorders*, **10**, 104–8.

Barber, R., Scheltens, P., Gholkar, A., Ballard, C., McKeith, I., Ince, P., *et al.* (1999). White matter lesions on magnetic resonance imaging in dementia with Lewy bodies, Alzheimer's disease, vascular dementia, and normal aging. *Journal of Neurology, Neurosurgery and Psychiatry*, **67**, 66–72.

Barr, A., Benedict, R., Tune, L., and Brandt, J. (1992). Neuropsychological differentiation of Alzheimer's disease from vascular dementia. *International Journal of Geriatric Psychiatry*, **7**, 621–7.

Bayles, K. A. and Tolmoeda, D. K. (1983). Confrontational naming impairment in dementia. *Brain and Language*, **19**, 98–114.

Benson, D. F., Marsden, C. D., and Meadows, J. C. (1974). The amnesic syndrome of posterior cerebral artery occlusion. *Acta Neurologica Scandinavica*, **50**, 133–45.

Bentham, P. W., Jones, S., and Hodges, J. R. (1997). A comparison of semantic memory in vascular dementia and dementia of Alzheimer's type. *International Journal of Geriatric Psychiatry*, **12**, 575–80.

Benton, A. L. (1992). Gerstmann's syndrome. *Archives of Neurology*, **49**, 445–7.

Bhatia, K. and Marsden, C. (1994). The behavioural and motor consequences of focal lesions of the basal ganglia in man. *Brain*, **117**, 859–76.

Bonarek, M., Barberger-Gateau, P., Letenneur, L., Deschamps, V., Iron, A., Dubroca, B., *et al.* (2000). Relationships between cholesterol, apolipoprotein E polymorphism and dementia: A cross-sectional analysis from the PAQUID study. *Neuroepidemiology*, **19**, 141–8.

Bowler, J. and Hachinski, V. (1996). History of the concept of vascular dementia: Two opposing views on current definitions and criteria for vascular dementia. In *Vascular dementia: current concepts* (ed. I. Prohovnik, J. Wade, S. Knezevic, T. Tatemichi, and T. Erkinjuntti), pp. 1–28. Chichester, England: John Wiley & Sons Ltd.

Bowler, J. V., Eliasziw, M., Steenhuis, R., Munoz, D. G., Fry, R., Merskey, H., *et al.* (1997). Comparative evolution of Alzheimer disease, vascular dementia, and mixed dementia. *Archives of Neurology*, **54**, 697–703.

Bowler, J. V. and Hachinski, V. (1997). Vascular dementia. In *Behavioural neurology and neuropsychology* (ed. T. E. Feinberg and M. J. Farah), pp. 589–603. New York: McGraw Hill.

Bowler, J. V. and Hachinski, V. (2000). Criteria for vascular dementia: Replacing dogma with data. *Archives of Neurology*, **57**, 170–1.

Carey, M. E., Giovannetti, T., and Libon, D. J. (1999). A comparison of written discourse in Alzheimer's disease and subcortical ischemic vascular dementia (abstract). *Archives of Clinical Neuropsychology*, **14**, 45–6.

Carlesimo, G. A., Fadda, L., Bonci, A., and Caltagirone, C. (1993). Differential rates of forgetting from long-term memory in Alzheimer's and multi-infarct dementia. *International Journal of Neuroscience*, **73**, 1–11.

Censori, B., Manara, O., Agostinis, C., Camerlingo, M., Casto, L., Galavotti, B., *et al.* (1996). Dementia after first stroke. *Stroke*, **27**, 1205–10.

Chui, H. and Gonthier, R. (1999). Natural history of vascular dementia. *Alzheimer Disease and Associated Disorders*, **13**, Suppl. 3, S124–30.

Chui, H. C., Mack, W., Jackson, E., Mungas, D., Reed, B. R., Tinklenberg, J., *et al.* (2000). Clinical criteria for the diagnosis of vascular dementia. *Archives of Neurology*, **57**, 191–6.

Chui, H. C., Victoroff, J. I., Margolin, D., Jagust, W., Shankle, R., and Katzman, R. (1992). Criteria for the diagnosis of ischemic vascular dementia proposed by the State of California Alzheimer Disease Diagnostic and Treatment Centers (ADDTC). *Neurology*, **42**, 473–80.

Crews, W. D., Manning, C. A., and Skalabrin, E. (1996). Neuropsychological impairments of executive functions and memory in a case of bilateral paramedian thalamic infarction. *Neurocase*, **2**, 405–12.

Dening, T. R. and Berrios, G. E. (1992). The Hachinski Ischaemic Score: A reevaluation. *International Journal of Geriatric Psychiatry*, **7**, 585–9.

Desmond, D. W., Erkinjuntti, T., Sano, M., Cummings, J. L., Bowler, J. V., Pasquier, F., *et al.* (1999). The cognitive syndrome of vascular dementia: Implications for clinical trials. *Alzheimer Disease and Associated Disorders*, **13**, Suppl. 3, S21–9.

Desmond, D. W., Moroney, J. T., Paik, M. C., Sano, M., Mohr, J. P., Aboumatar, S., *et al.* (2000). Frequency and clinical determinants of dementia after ischemic stroke. *Neurology*, **54**, 1124–31.

Devasenapathy, A. and Hachinski, V. (1997). Vascular cognitive impairment: A new approach. In *Advances in old age psychiatry: chromosomes to community care* (ed. C. Holmes and R. Howard), pp. 79–95. Petersfield, UK: Wrightson Biomedical Publishing Ltd.

Donnelly, K. and Grohman, K. (1999). Can the Mattis Dementia Rating Scale differentiate Alzheimer's disease, vascular dementia, and depression in the elderly? *Brain and Cognition*, **39**, 60–3.

Elias, M. F., Wolf, P. A., D'Agostino, R. B., Cobb, J., and White, L. R. (1993). Untreated blood pressure level is inversely related to cognitive functioning: The Framingham study. *American Journal of Epidemiology*, **138**, 353–64.

Englund, E. (1998). Neuropathology of white matter changes in Alzheimer's disease and vascular dementia. *Dementia and Geriatric Cognitive Disorders*, **9**, Suppl. 1, 6–12.

Erkinjuntti, T. (1997). Vascular dementia: Challenge of clinical diagnosis. *International Psychogeriatrics*, **9**, Suppl. 1, 51–8.

Erkinjuntti, T., Bowler, J. V., DeCarli, C. S., Fazekas, F., Inzitari, D., O'Brien, J. T., *et al.* (1999). Imaging of static brain lesions in vascular dementia: Implications for clinical trials. *Alzheimer Disease and Associated Disorders*, **13**, Suppl. 3, S81–90.

Erkinjuntti, T., Laaksonen, R., Sulkava, R., Syrjalainen, R., and Palo, J. (1986). Neuropsychological differentiation between normal aging, Alzheimer's disease and vascular dementia. *Acta Neurologica Scandinavica*, **74**, 393–403.

Erkinjuntti, T., Ostbye, T., Steenhuis, R., and Hachinski, V. (1997). The effect of different diagnostic criteria on the prevalence of dementia. *New England Journal of Medicine*, **337**, 1667–74.

Esiri, M. M., Wilcock, G. K., and Morris, J. H. (1997). Neuropathological assessment of the lesions of significance in vascular dementia. *Journal of Neurology, Neurosurgery and Psychiatry*, **63**, 749–53.

Farah, M. J. (1990). *Visual agnosia: disorders of object vision and what they tell us about normal vision.* Cambridge, Mass: MIT Press.

Folstein, M. F., Folstein, S. E., and McHugh, P. R. (1975). 'Mini-mental state'. A practical method for grading the cognitive state of patients for the clinician. *Journal of Psychiatric Research*, **12**, 189–98.

Gainotti, G., Parlato, V., Monteleone, D., and Carlomagno, S. (1992). Neuropsychological markers of dementia on visuo-spatial tasks: A comparison between Alzheimer's type and vascular forms of dementia. *Journal of Clinical and Experimental Neuropsychology*, **14**, 239–52.

Gauthier, S., Rockwood, K., Gelinas, I., Sykes, L., Teunisse, S., Orgogozo, J. M., *et al.* (1999). Outcome measures for the study of activities of daily living in vascular dementia. *Alzheimer Disease and Related Disorders*, **13**, Suppl. 3, S143–7.

Gilleard, C. J., Kellett, J. M., Coles, J. A., Millard, P. H., Honavar, M., and Lantos, P. L. (1992). The St. George's dementia bed investigation study: A comparison of clinical and pathological diagnosis. *Acta Psychiatrica Scandinavica*, **85**, 264–9.

Giovannetti Carew, T., Lamar, M., Cloud, B. S., Grossman, M., and Libon, D. J. (1997). Impairment in category fluency in ischemic vascular dementia. *Neuropsychology*, **11**, 400–12.

Gold, G., Giannakopoulos, P., Montes-Paixao, C., Herrman, F. R., Mulligan, R., Michel, J. P., *et al.* (1997). Sensitivity and specificity of newly proposed clinical criteria for possible vascular dementia. *Neurology*, **49**, 690–4.

Gorelick, P. B., Erkinjuntti, T., Hofman, A., Rocca, W. A., Skoog, I., and Winblad, B. (1999). Prevention of vascular dementia. *Alzheimer Disease and Associated Disorders*, **13**, Suppl. 3, S131–9.

Graff-Radford, N. R., Tranel, D., Van Hoesen, G. W., and Brandt, J. P. (1990). Diencephalic amnesia. *Brain*, **113**, 1–25.

Hachinski, V. C., Iliff, L. D., Zilhka, E., du Boulay, G. H., McAllister, V. L., Marshall, J., *et al.* (1975). Cerebral blood flow in dementia. *Archives of Neurology*, **32**, 632–7.

Hachinski, V. D., Lassen, N. A., and Marshall, J. (1974). Multi-infarct dementia. A cause of mental deterioration in the elderly. *Lancet*, **ii**, 207–10.

Hargrave, R., Geck, L. C., Reed, B., and Mungas, D. (2000). Affective behavioural disturbances in Alzheimer's disease and ischaemic vascular disease. *Journal of Neurology, Neurosurgery and Psychiatry*, **68**, 41–6.

Hodges, J. R. and McCarthy, R. A. (1993). Autobiographical amnesia resulting from bilateral paramedian thalamic infarction: A case study in cognitive neurobiology. *Brain*, **116**, 921–40.

Hofman, A., Ott, A., Breteler, M. M. B., Bots, M. L., Slooter, A. J. C., van Harskamp, F., *et al.* (1997). Atherosclerosis, apolipoprotein E, and prevalence of dementia and Alzheimer's disease in the Rotterdam study. *Lancet*, **349**, 151–4.

Holmes, C., Cairns, N., Lantos, P., and Mann, A. (1999). Validity of current clinical criteria for Alzheimer's disease, vascular dementia and dementia with Lewy bodies. *British Journal of Psychiatry*, **174**, 45–50.

Ishii, N., Nishihara, Y., and Imamira, T. (1986). Why do frontal lobe symptoms predominate in vascular dementia with lacunas? *Neurology*, **36**, 340–5.

Jellinger, K., Danielczyk, W., Fischer, P., and Gabriel, E. (1990). Clinico-pathological analysis of dementia disorders in the elderly. *Journal of the Neurological Sciences*, **95**, 239–58.

Kalaria, R. N. and Ballard, C. (1999). Overlap between pathology of Alzheimer disease and vascular dementia. *Alzheimer Disease and Associated Disorders*, **13**, Suppl. 3, S115–23.

Kase, C. S., Wolf, P. A., Kelly-Hayes, M., Kannel, W. B., Beiser, A., and D'Agostino, R. B. (1998). Intellectual decline after stroke. The Framingham study. *Stroke*, **29**, 805–12.

Kertesz, A. and Clydesdale, S. (1994). Neuropsychological deficits in vascular dementia vs. Alzheimer's disease. *Archives of Neurology*, **51**, 1226–31.

Kilander, L., Nyman, H., Boberg, M., Hansson, L., and Lithell, H. (1998). Hypertension is related to cognitive impairment. A 20-year follow-up of 999 men. *Hypertension*, **31**, 780–6.

Kilander, L., Nyman, H., Boberg, M., and Lithell, H. (1997). Cognitive function, vascular risk factors and education. A cross-sectional study based on a cohort of 70-year-old men. *Journal of Internal Medicine*, **242**, 313–21.

Kokmen, E., Whistman, J. P., O'Fallon, W. M., Chu, C. P., and Beard, C. M. (1996). Dementia after ischemic stroke: A population-based study in Rochester, Minnesota (1960–1984). *Neurology*, **19**, 154–9.

Kontiola, P., Laaksonen, R., Sulkava, R., and Erkinjuntti, T. (1990). Pattern of language impairment is different in Alzheimer's disease and multi-infarct dementia. *Brain and Language*, **38**, 364–83.

Lafosse, J. M., Reed, B. R., Mungas, D., Sterling, S. B., Wahbeh, H., and Jagust, W. J. (1997). Fluency and memory differences between ischemic vascular dementia and Alzheimer's disease. *Neuropsychology*, **11**, 514–22.

Laine, M., Vuorinen, E., and Rinne, J. O. (1997). Picture naming deficits in vascular dementia and Alzheimer's disease. *Journal of Clinical and Experimental Neuropsychology*, **19**, 126–40.

Lamar, M., Carew, T. G., Resh, R., Goldberg, E., Podell, K., Cloud, B. S., *et al.* (1997). Perseverative behavior in Alzheimer's disease and subcortical ischemic vascular dementia. *Neuropsychology*, **11**, 523–34.

Launer, L. J., Dinkgreve, M. A. H. M., Jonker, C., Hooijer, C., and Lindeboom, J. (1993). Are age and education independent correlates of the mini-mental state exam performance of community-dwelling elderly? *Journals of Gerontology*, **48**, P271–7.

Levasseur, M., Baron, J. C., Sette, G., Legaultdemare, F., Pappata, S., Mauguiere, F., *et al.* (1992). Brain energy-metabolism in bilateral paramedian thalamic infarcts: A positron emission tomography study. *Brain*, **115**, 795–807.

Leys, D., Erkinjuntti, T., Desmond, D. W., Schmidt, R., Englund, E., Pasquier, F., *et al.* (1999). Vascular dementia: The role of cerebral infarcts. *Alzheimer Disease and Associated Disorders*, **13**, Suppl. 3, S38–48.

Libon, D. J., Bogdanoff, B., Bonavita, J., Skalina, S., Cloud, B. S., Resh, R., *et al.* (1997). Dementia associated with periventricular deep white matter alterations: A subtype of subcortical dementia. *Archives of Clinical Neuropsychology*, **12**, 239–50.

Loeb, C. and Gandolfo, C. (1983). Diagnostic evaluation of degenerative and vascular dementia. *Stroke*, **14**, 399–401.

Loeb, C., Gandolfo, C., Croce, R., and Conti, M. (1992). Dementia associated with lacunar infarction. *Stroke*, **23**, 1225–9.

Loewenstein, D. A., D'Elia, L., Guterman, A., Eisdorfer, C., Wilkie, F., LaRue, A., *et al.* (1991). The occurrence of different intrusive errors in patients with Alzheimer's disease, multiple cerebral infarctions, and major depression. *Brain and Cognition*, **16**, 104–17.

Looi, J. C. L. and Sachdev, P. S. (1999). Differentiation of vascular dementia from AD on neuropsychological tests. *Neurology*, **53**, 670–8.

Lukatela, K., Malloy, P., Jenkins, M., and Cohen, R. (1998). The naming deficit in early Alzheimer's and vascular dementia. *Neuropsychology*, **12**, 565–72.

Mendez, M. F., Cherrier, M. M., and Perryman, K. M. (1997). Differences between Alzheimer's disease and vascular dementia on information processing measures. *Brain and Cognition*, **43**, 301–10.

Miller Fisher, C. (1965). Lacunes: Small deep cerebral infarcts. *Neurology*, **15**, 774–84.

Molsa, P. K., Paljarvi, L., Rinne, J. O., Rinne, U. K., and Sako, E. (1985). Validity of clinical diagnosis in dementia: A prospective clinicopathological study. *Journal of Neurology, Neurosurgery and Psychiatry*, **48**, 1085–90.

Mori, E., Yamashita, H., Takauchi, S., and Kondo, K. (1996). Isolated athymhormia following hypoxic bilateral pallidal lesions. *Behavioural Neurology*, **9**, 17–23.

Noguchi, S., Murakami, K., and Yamada, N. (1993). Apolipoprotein E genotype and Alzheimer's disease. *Lancet*, **342**, 737.

Padovani, A., Di Piero, V., Bragoni, M., Iacoboni, M., Gualdi, G. F., and Lenzi, G. L. (1995). Patterns of neuropsychological impairment in mild dementia: A comparison between Alzheimer's disease and multi-infarct dementia. *Acta Neurological Scandinavica*, **92**, 433–42.

Perez, F. I., Gay, J. R. A., Taylor, R. L., and Rivera, V. M. (1975). Patterns of memory performance in the neurologically impaired aged. *The Canadian Journal of Neurological Sciences*, **2**, 347–55.

Perry, R. J. and Hodges, J. R. (1999). Attentional and executive deficits in Alzheimer's disease: A review. *Brain*, **122**, 383–404.

Pohjasvaara, T., Erkinjuntti, T., Ylikoski, R., Hietanen, M., Vataja, R., and Kaste, M. (1998). Clinical determinants of poststroke dementia. *Stroke*, **29**, 75–81.

Powell, A. L., Cummings, J. L., Hill, M. A., and Benson, D. F. (1988). Speech and language alterations in multi-infarct dementia. *Neurology*, **38**, 717–19.

Rajaram, S. (1997). Basal forebrain amnesia. *Neurocase*, **3**, 405–15.

Rockwood, K., Howard, K., MacKnight, C., and Darvesh, S. (1999). Spectrum of disease in vascular cognitive impairment. *Neuroepidemiology*, **18**, 248–54.

Rockwood, K., Wentzel, C., Hachinski, V., Hogan, D. B., MacKnight, C., and McDowell, I. (2000). Prevalence and outcomes of vascular cognitive impairment. Vascular cognitive impairment investigators of the Canadian Study of Health and Aging. *Neurology*, **54**, 447–51.

Roeltgen, D. P., Sevush, S., and Heilman, K. M. (1983). Pure Gerstmann's syndrome from a focal lesion. *Archives of Neurology*, **40**, 46–7.

Roman, G. C. and Royall, D. R. (1999). Executive control function: A rational basis for the diagnosis of vascular dementia. *Alzheimer Disease and Related Disorders*, **13**, Suppl. 3, S69–80.

Roman, G. C., Tatemichi, T. K., Erkinjuntti, T., Cummings, J. L., Masdeu, J. C., Garcia, J. H., *et al.* (1993). Vascular dementia: Diagnostic criteria for research studies. *Neurology*, **43**, 250–60.

Scheltens, P. H., Barkhof, F., Valk, J., Algra, P. R., Gerritsen van der Hoop, R., Nauta, J., *et al.* (1992). White matter lesions on magnetic resonance imaging in clinically diagnosed Alzheimer's disease. *Brain*, **115**, 735–48.

Skoog, I., Kalaria, R. N., and Breteler, M. B. (1999). Vascular factors and Alzheimer disease. *Alzheimer Disease and Associated Disorders*, **13**, Suppl. 3, S106–14.

Slooter, A. J. C., Tang, M. X., van Duijn, C. M., Stern, Y., Ott, A., Bell, K., *et al.* (1997). Apolipoprotein E epsilon 4 and the risk of dementia with stroke: A population-based investigation. *Journal of the American Medical Association*, **277**, 818–21.

Small, G. W. (1985). Revised ischemic score for diagnosing multi-infarct dementia. *Journal of Clinical Psychiatry*, **46**, 514–17.

Starkstein, S. E., Sabe, L., Vazquez, S., Teson, A., Petracca, G., Chemerinski, E., *et al.* (1996). Neuropsychological, psychiatric, and cerebral blood flow findings in vascular dementia and Alzheimer's disease. *Stroke*, **27**, 408–14.

Stewart, R. (1999). Vascular disease, cognitive impairment and dementia. In *Everything you need to know about old age psychiatry* (ed. R. Howard), pp. 55–71. Petersfield, UK: Wrightson Biomedical Publishing Ltd.

Tatemichi, T. K., Desmond, D. W., Mayeux, R., Paik, M., Stern, Y., Sano, M., *et al.* (1992*a*). Dementia after stroke: Baseline frequency, risks and clinical features in a hospitalised cohort. *Neurology*, **42**, 1185–93.

Tatemichi, T. K., Desmond, D. W., Prohovnik, I., Cross, D. T., Gropen, T. I., Mohr, J. P., *et al.* (1992*b*). Confusion and memory loss from capsular genu infarction: A thalamocortical disconnection syndrome? *Neurology*, **42**, 1966–79.

Tatemichi, T. K., Paik, M., Bagiella, E., Desmond, D. W., Stern, Y., Sano, M., *et al.* (1994). Risk of dementia after stroke in a hospitalised cohort: Results of a longitudinal study. *Neurology*, **44**, 1885–91.

Tei, H., Miyazaki, A., Iwata, M., Osawa, M., Nagata, Y., and Maruyama, S. (1997). Early stage Alzheimer's disease and multiple subcortical infarction with mild cognitive impairment: Neuropsychological comparison using an easily applicable test battery. *Dementia and Geriatric Cognitive Disorders*, **8**, 355–8.

Todorov, A. B., Go, R. C. P., Constantinidis, J., and Elston, R. C. (1975). Specificity of the clinical diagnosis dementia. *Journal of the Neurological Sciences*, **26**, 81–98.

Tomlinson, B., Blessed, G., and Roth, M. (1970). Observations on the brains of demented old people. *Journal of the Neurological Sciences*, **11**, 205–42.

Van Gijn, J. (1998). Leukoaraiosis and vascular dementia. *Neurology*, **51**, Suppl. 3, S3–8.

Villardita, C. (1993). Alzheimer's disease compared with cerebrovascular dementia: Neuropsychological similarities and differences. *Acta Neurologica Scandinavica*, **87**, 299–308.

Wade, J. P. H., Misen, T. R., Hachinski, V. C., Misman, M., Lau, C., and Merskey, H. (1987). The clinical diagnosis of Alzheimer's disease. *Archives of Neurology*, **44**, 24–9.

World Health Organization. (1992). The ICD-10 Classification of Mental and Behavioral Disorders: Clinical Descriptions and Diagnostic Guidelines. Geneva, Switzerland: World Health Organization.

World Health Organization. (1993). The ICD-10 Classification of Mental and Behavioral Disorders: Diagnostic Criteria for Research. Geneva, Switzerland: World Health Organization 1993.

15 Huntington's disease

Jane S. Paulsen and Robert G. Robinson

1 Introduction

Numerous collaborative efforts have been formed in the spirit understanding and conquering Huntington's disease (HD), many of which have resulted in significant changes to our understanding of and care for people with the disease. The goal of this chapter is to summarize what is known about HD and what challenges remain. Several aspects of the disease will be covered, including genetics, pathophysiology, clinical characteristics, treatment, and predictive testing. When possible, manifestions of HD will be addressed in terms of basal ganglia circuitry dysfunction.

2 Genetics of HD

2.1 Gene characteristics

Huntington's disease (HD) is one of the only lethal dominant genetic diseases found in humans. It typically manifests in early-to-middle adulthood, after childbearing years have started, and causes up to 40 years of slow neurodegenerative decline before it eventually kills. HD is characterized by a triad of symptoms including motor disturbance, cognitive impairment, and psychiatric features. The autosomal dominant genetic abnormality consists of expansion of the trinucleotide repeat CAG (i.e. cytosine, adenosine, guanine) in the gene IT-15 on chromosome 4 and encodes the protein huntingtin (The Huntington's Disease Collaborative Research Group 1993; MacDonald and Gusella 1996). The CAG repeat is found in all people, but normally repeats 10–35 times. Repeat sizes of 27 to 35 are at the upper end of normal and sometimes increase into the abnormal range in the next generation; the risk for this has not been quantified. CAG lengths of 36–39 are in the low end of the abnormal range and can result in disease if the individual lives a long life. Repeat lengths greater than 39 will result in manifest HD in a person who lives a normal life span.

2.2 Clinical correlates of the gene: onset age

Although it is not known when HD will become manifest in a given individual, numerous studies have described a significant inverse relationship between CAG repeat length and age of onset (Andrew *et al.* 1997). As shown in Figure 15.1, the length of the CAG repeat explains about 50–60% of the variance in age of onset. Despite having a significant association with onset age, CAG repeat length cannot be used clinically to predict onset in a specific individual. Clearly, the scatterplot of CAG length and onset age (Figure 15.1) shows the futility of making distinct pre-

Age at onset by CAG repeat size

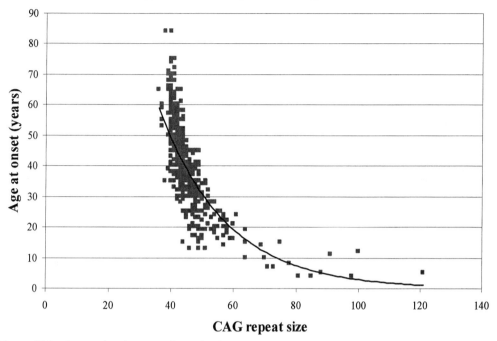

Figure 15.1 Scatterplot showing relationship between age at onset and CAG repeat length.
(Source: Michael Hayden and Ryan Brinkman, University of British Columbia. Printed with permission.)

dictions based solely upon these two variables. For instance, Figure 15.1 shows that people with a CAG of 41 demonstrated onset ages from 33–75.

Clinical implications of genetic knowledge: Amy's story

> Amy is a 25-year-old married attorney employed in a large firm. Amy has always wanted to set up her own small law practice so that she can enjoy flexible hours that would allow her to work and raise a family. Amy had never heard of HD until her dad's diagnosis last year at age 51; he is currently enrolled in a clinical trial to slow the progression of HD.

2.3 Inheritance of the gene

Amy sounds like a rather typical case presenting to any health care professional in any city in the world. Although ten years ago Amy might have had minimal data to help her make life choices, today she has access to information that may influence her decision-making (Nance 1996). Every son or daughter born to a parent with HD has a 50% chance of inheriting the disease. The clinical features of HD usually emerge in early adulthood, although about 10% have onset before age 20 and 25% have onset after age 50 (Myers *et al.* 1985). Although genes with normal repeat sizes almost always undergo stable transmission from parent to child, genes with expanded CAG repeat sizes are inclined to further expand with each generation, particularly in the case of paternal transmission (although expansions occur in maternal transmission as well). As a consequence, children who inherit the abnormal gene often have a larger repeat number than their parent and develop symptoms at a younger age. This is called genetic anticipation and can result in a child having symptomatic HD before their parent.

2.4 Estimating probability of onset

Although it is well established that age of onset cannot be predicted for a specific individual based upon repeat length alone, Brinkman and his colleagues (Brinkman *et al.* 1997) estimated the probability of HD onset by a particular age for a specific CAG size (see Table 15.1). For example, the per cent increase in the number of affected individuals in five year intervals for the CAG repeat length of 46, starting at age 25, is 3%, 3%, 3%, 34%, 43%, and 13%. Thus, a 25-year-old person with a CAG of 46 can expect to have 15 years with a low probability of disease onset followed by 10 years during which onset is likely to occur. Career, family, financial, and recreational decisions might be based upon these probabilities.

2.5 The test

The direct HD gene test is highly sensitive and specific and is considered definitive. Genetic testing for HD is useful in three clinical situations:

(a) To confirm a diagnosis of HD in a person with symptoms of HD, with or without a family history (confirmatory testing).

(b) To inform a healthy individual who wants to know whether (s)he carries the expanded gene (predictive testing).

(c) To determine the risk status of a fetus (prenatal testing).

Table 15.1 Per cent increase in number of affected individuals by five year intervals, based upon age and CAG repeat length[a]

Age range (years)	CAG repeat length											
	39	40	41	42	43	44	45	46	47	48	49	50
25–29								3.1	2.1	2.9	12.9	12.5
30–34								3.1	11.3	8.8	10.5	13.1
35–39						3.4	10.0	3.2	18.7	**33.3**	**16.1**	**24.9**
40–44					11.6	16.3	18.0	**34.3**	28.0	33.8	29.2	34.6
45–49		5.8	6.0		19.2	25.5	37.1	**43.0**	28.5	8.6	18.7	
50–54		5.0	7.5	16.8	18.4	25.7	18.8	13.3	11.4	9.8		
55–59		9.1	16.0	**26.0**	**31.5**	15.9						
60–64		14.1	18.4	**26.2**	7.5	7.2						
65–69		**21.5**	**24.1**	18.4	5.3	4.0						
70–74	10.7	**21.0**	14.2	1.4	1.3							
75–79	**32.2**	12.9	6.3									
85–89		4.8										

Bold percentages indicate range of highest onset chance.
[a] Source: Michael Hayden and Ryan Brinkman, University of British Columbia Centre for Molecular Medicine and Therapeutics, printed with permission.

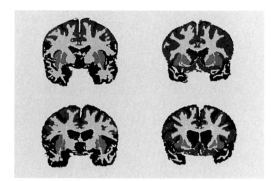

Figure 15.2 (See also Plate 27) Magnetic resonance image of healthy control (top) and HD patient (bottom). Colours represent areas traced for volumetric analyses; red traces the caudate nucleus. (Source: Terry L. Jernigan, University of California San Diego. Printed with permission.)

2.6 Considerations prior to genetic testing

The World Federation of Neurology, the International Huntington Association, and the Huntington's Disease Society of America have published guidelines regarding the ethical conduct of genetic testing that should be followed by all health personnel. In general, testing should be undertaken with extreme caution given the significant impact the genetic information can have on all family members, their relationships, their employment, and their insurance. There are psychosocial risks to genetic testing as well, including adverse effects on the individual's mental health. Codori and her colleagues (1997) followed 160 people undergoing genetic testing for HD and found that those less well adjusted had tested positive, were married, had no children, or were closer to their estimated ages of onset.

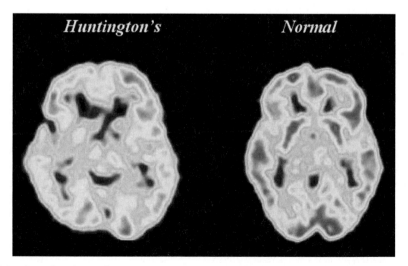

Figure 15.3 (See also Plate 28) Positron emission tomography (using FDG) of healthy control (right) and HD patient (left). (Source: Mark Guttman, Centre for Addiction and Mental Health. Printed with permission.)

3 Pathophysiology

3.1 Neuroimaging

Although not needed for diagnostic purposes since the availability of the gene test, neuro-imaging studies show abnormalities in HD (Figures 15.2 and 15.3; see Plates 29 and 30). Several imaging studies have demonstrated basal ganglia abnormalities, such as caudate volume reduction using magnetic resonance imaging (Starkstein *et al.* 1992) and glucose metabolism (Young *et al.* 1986), and dopamine receptor binding deficiencies in the caudate and putamen (Ginovart *et al.* 1997) using positron emission tomography. A number of these reports have demonstrated significant associations between imaging indices and clinical correlates of the disease including illness duration and functional capacity (Young *et al.* 1986), chorea severity (Kuwert *et al.* 1990), cognitive impairment (Hasselbalch *et al.* 1992), and CAG repeat length (Aylward *et al.* 1997).

3.2 Neuropathology

The pathology of HD is characterized by diffuse brain atrophy with severe neuronal loss and gliosis occurring selectively in the caudate nucleus and putamen with vulnerability in other regions such as deep layers of the cortex (see Vonsattel and DiFiglia 1998 for a review). The earliest changes associated with HD occurred microscopically in the medial paraventricular portion of the caudate nucleus (CN), the tail of the CN, and, to a lesser extent, in the dorsal putamen. Neurodegeneration progresses laterally and basally, and eventually affects most structures in the basal ganglia (Vonsattel and DiFiglia 1998). For more details see Chapter 10.

3.3 Basal ganglia circuitry

There are five recognized, discrete, parallel circuits uniting regions of the frontal lobe (motor, frontal eye, dorsolateral, orbitofrontal, and anterior cingulate areas) with the striatum, globus pallidus, and thalamus in functional systems (Figure 15.4; see Plate 29) (Litvan *et al.* 1998). Each circuit is differentially modulated by two opposing, but parallel pathways: 'direct' and 'indirect'. The motor system has received the most attention and several movement disorders have been successfully 'mapped' onto these circuits. For instance, the chorea associated with HD has been explained by dysfunction in the indirect pathway of the motor circuit (DeLong 1990), which is theorized to connect the putamen to the motor cortex through the external globus pallidus and subthalamic nucleus before reaching the internal globus pallidus/substantia nigra pars reticulata (GPi/SNr) (Alexander and Crutcher 1990). The selective loss of GABA- and enkephalin-containing neurons in the putamen may result in a reduction in the inhibitory signal projected from the GPi/SNr to the thalamus. The thalamus, in turn, projects excessive excitatory signals to the precentral motor strip. Similarly, the rigid akinesia often seen in juvenile or advanced HD has been associated with loss of the GABA- and substance P-containing neurons of the direct pathway (Albin *et al.* 1990). Loss of these neurons removes the inhibitory signal to the GPi/SNr, and leads to increased discharge of the partially deafferented GPi/SNr neurons. The end-result of these changes may be decreased discharge of excitatory signal to the premotor cortex, and a reduction in the amount of movement exhibited by the patient.

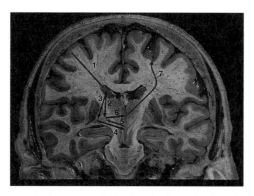

Figure 15.4 (See also Plate 29) Brain sections including the frontal subcortical circuits. Top: The direct and indirect frontal circuits (red arrows indicate excitatory connections and blue arrows indicate inhibitory connections). (1) Excitatory glutamatergic corticostriatal fibres. (2) Direct inhibitory γ-aminobutyric acid (GABA)/substance P fibres (associated with D1 dopamine receptors) from the striatum to the globus pallidus interna/substantia nigra pars reticulata. (3) Indirect inhibitory GABA/enkephalin fibres (associated with D2 dopamine receptors) from the striatum to the globus pallidus externa. (4) Indirect inhibitory GABA fibres from the globus pallidus externa to the subthalamic nucleus. (5) Indirect excitatory glutamatergic fibres from the subthalamic nucleus to the globus pallidus interna/substantia nigra pars reticulata. (6) Basal ganglia inhibitory outflow via GABA fibres from the globus pallidus interna/substantia nigra pars reticulata to specific thalamic sites. (7) Thalamic excitatory fibres returning to the cortex (shown in contralateral hemisphere for convenience).

4 The motor disorder

4.1 Choreoathetosis

Choreoathetosis, or chorea, is the primary involuntary movement disorder associated with HD. Although chorea is the most noticeable feature of the disease, the impairments of voluntary movement are more highly associated with functional disability and are often independent of chorea (Van Vugt *et al.* 1996).

4.2 Diagnosis of HD

Despite the availability of a genetic test, the diagnosis of HD is based upon a neurological evaluation and requires the presence of an unequivocal movement disorder that cannot be explained by other cause(s). Diagnostic criteria may be revised as evidence mounts that behavioural and cognitive changes can manifest before motoric symptoms begin. Some recent reports have described small numbers of individuals with phenotypes similar to HD but who do not have an expanded CAG repeat in IT-15 (Rosenblatt *et al.* 1998).

4.3 Course of motor disorder

The motor disorder of HD changes over time. Early signs often include interrupted pursuit of gaze, an inability to suppress reflexive glances to novel visual stimuli, hypometric saccades, tongue impersistence, impaired rapid alternating movements, and akathisia (Harper 1991; Siemers *et al.* 1996). Epilepsy is rare in adult onset HD, though more common in juvenile onset. Choking is an increasing hazard in HD, as it becomes harder to co-ordinate chewing, swallowing, and breathing. Early chorea may be suppressed or masked by purposeful movements, but as the disease progresses, the choreic movements become larger and less easy to conceal. The severity of the chorea tends to plateau, and in middle stages decline, while rigidity, spasticity, dystonia, and bradykinesia become more prominent (Feigin *et al.* 1995). In later stages, when dystonia often occurs, patients become immobile and bedridden.

5 Collaborative research efforts in HD

A recent international collaborative research assembly, the Huntington Study Group (HSG), was formed in 1993 and consists of over 300 investigators throughout the world. Its primary goal is to develop and test experimental therapeutics aimed at the treatment, and eventual cure, of HD. To date, the HSG has conducted numerous single-site and multiple-site clinical trials. In addition to the support and development of collaborative research, the HSG developed a uniform rating scale for the assessment of HD. The *Unified Huntington's Disease Rating Scale* (UHDRS) (The Huntington Study Group 1996) assesses four components of HD: motor function, cognition, behaviour, and functional abilities. The reliability and internal consistency of the four components of the UHDRS have been evaluated and published (The Huntington Study Group 1996), as has a shortened version of the motor section (Siesling *et al.* 1997).

6 The cognitive disorder

The cognitive disorder in HD is often considered a 'subcortical' syndrome and usually lacks features such as aphasia, amnesia, or agnosia that are associated with dementia of the Alzheimer's type. Although the cortical-subcortical nomenclature has been criticized over the years, it continues to provide an effective means of classifying and understanding the neurodegenerative disorders (see chapter 8).

Zakzanis (1998) recently conducted an effect–size analysis incorporating meta-analytic principles to summarize neuropsychological performances from 760 HD patients and 943 healthy controls. Results indicated that patients with HD are most deficient in delayed recall, memory acquisition, cognitive flexibility, manual dexterity, attention, speed of processing, and verbal skill. Although Zakzanis provides a rank-order list of specific neuropsychological tests in order of HD sensitivity to aid in the interpretation of the quantitative results, she also reports that executive dyscontrol may be an overriding deficit contributing to poorer performance on numerous specific tests. It is well established that among the most prominent cognitive impairments in HD are the so-called 'executive functions'. These fundamental abilities can affect performance in many cognitive areas including reasoning, planning, judgement, decision-making, attention, learning, memory, flexibility, and timing. Cognitive functions have also been shown to be useful predictors of functional capacity (Marder *et al.* 2000).

6.1 Executive dysfunction

Several studies have demonstrated that HD patients are impaired on tests that require executive functions. For instance, HD patients demonstrate impairment on the Wisconsin Card Sorting Test (Paulsen *et al.* 1995*b*) and the Stroop Color Word Test, as well as clinical rating scales of executive dyscontrol (Paulsen *et al.* 2001*a*). In fact, brief tests of executive functions have been suggested as sensitive tools for differential diagnosis. That is, the Serial Sevens item on the Mini-Mental Status Exam (Folstein *et al.* 1975), the Initiation and Perseveration subtest of the Dementia Rating Scale (Mattis 1976), and an abbreviated battery of frontal lobe tests have been demonstrated to be distinctly sensitive to patients with HD (Brandt *et al.* 1988; Rothlind and Brandt 1993; Paulsen *et al.* 1995*a*).

Some recent research has evaluated HD patients' performance on clinically relevant, face-valid tests of judgement and decision-making. Stout and her colleagues (Stout *et al.* 2001) used a simulated gambling task to quantify decision-making deficits in HD patients. The gambling task involved repeatedly choosing from four decks of cards, two with good consequences and two with poor outcome. Findings showed that HD patients made fewer advantageous selections than age- and education-matched healthy controls and dementia-severity-matched patients with Parkinson's disease (PD) (see Figure 15.5). Number of advantageous selections for the HD patients was not associated with overall dementia severity but was significantly correlated with brief measures of conceptualization and memory. It is important to note that several HD patients

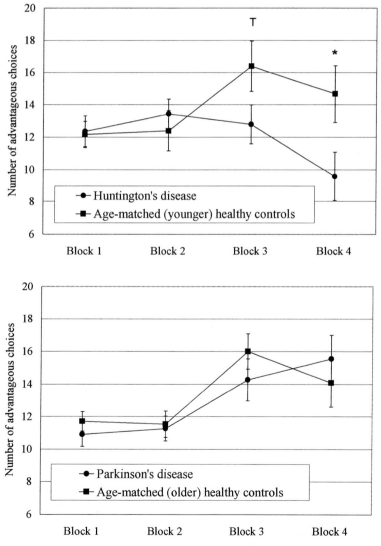

Figure 15.5 Gambling task outcomes for HD, PD, and healthy controls. (Source: Julie Stout, Indiana University. Printed with permission.)

indicated that one or more of the card decks were 'bad' but continued to make selections from the identified 'bad' decks. Findings were similar to results reported in patients with focal ventromedial frontal lobe damage (Bechara *et al.* 1994), indicating that dysfunction at the level of the caudate can result in behavioural disturbances similar to those seen in patients with primary cortical damage.

Another study used an experimental test of Twenty Questions, the well-known parlour game (Stout *et al.* 1996). HD patients were instructed to ask as few yes/no questions as possible to determine which one item in an array, consisting of line drawings of common living and non-living things (see Figure 15.6) (Stout *et al.* 1996), was the preselected target. Compared to age- and education-matched healthy controls, HD patients asked fewer constraint-seeking questions (e.g. 'Is it living/non-living?' or 'Is it in the top half of the page?') and relied upon less-efficient constraint-seeking questions (e.g. 'Is it yellow?') and on questions which eliminated only one item (e.g. 'Does it buzz and sting you?').

Impairments on tasks requiring decision-making may be due to various cognitive decrements, including learning, attention, inhibition, or appreciation for future consequences. Findings can also be interpreted as further evidence that HD patients are less able to benefit from feedback and have difficulty varying output based upon performance (Paulsen *et al.* 1993). Despite evidence of explicit knowledge for the tasks, HD patients were unable to update existing 'programs' based upon new experience and to alter their responses. Numerous wide-ranging consequences of these types of executive deficits are self-evident.

Both HD and Parkinson's disease (PD) patients have subcortical damage within the frontal-subcortical circuits; however, specific areas of damage may explain why HD but not PD is associated with decrements in the simulated gambling task. In HD, loss of the medium spiny neurons occurs more in the caudate nucleus than in the putamen. Behaviour changes similar to those exhibited with damage to the ventromedial frontal lobe damage or damage to other areas of pre-

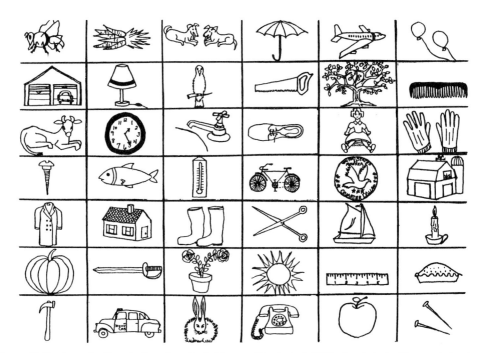

Figure 15.6 Array for Twenty Questions Test. (Source: Stout *et al.* 1996. Reprinted with permission.)

frontal cortex may occur in HD because caudate efferents ultimately affect the prefrontal cortex, which is important in cognitive and personality functions. In contrast, loss of neurons in the substantia nigra pars compacta in PD affects primarily the putamenal efferents, which project more strongly to the premotor regions of the frontal cortex (Alexander 1997), involved more in response selection for executing movement than in cognition and personality.

6.2 Attention and working memory

Early neuropsychological studies using the Wechsler Adult Intelligence Scales (Wechsler 1997) consistently reported that HD patients perform most poorly on subtests requiring attention and working memory (e.g. Arithmetic, Digit Span, Digit Symbol) (e.g. Strauss and Brandt 1986). More recent studies have emphasized dysfunction in unique aspects of attention, including resource allocation, response flexibility, and vigilance (Lange *et al.* 1995; Sprengelmeyer *et al.* 1995). For instance, Lawrence and his colleagues (1996) reported that HD patients are able to maintain attention for a previously learned response set but have difficulty shifting attention to a new set.

The clinical implications of the attentional impairment in HD are significant. Many people with HD perform better when they avoid tasks involving divided attention. Patients and families agree that trying to divide the already-compromised attentional resources can contribute to discomfort and increased safety risks. For instance, driving a car while listening to the radio, talking to the kids in the back seat, or talking on the cell phone is not recommended. To reduce choking risk, the environment should be quiet and calm at mealtimes to emphasize concentration on chewing and swallowing, rather than the TV, doorbell, and conversation.

Recent studies of working memory (Lange *et al.* 1995; Lawrence *et al.* 1996) have also demonstrated that HD patients tend to perseverate on previously correct responses and demonstrate difficulty maintaining attention on updated information in immediate memory. Tests of attention and working memory have been so well established as sensitive to HD that these types of tests are among those incorporated into longitudinal research programs and clinical trials for HD (The Huntington Study Group 1998).

6.3 Learning and memory

Hahn-Barma and colleagues (1998) administered a comprehensive neuropsychological battery of tests to 91 asymptomatic at-risk individuals. CAG repeat lengths were measured to separate those with the HD mutation from those with normal expansion sizes. Performances on learning and memory tests divided those with the gene mutation into two groups, without overlap. The performance of subjects without cognitive deficits was similar to that of healthy normals on all tests. The subjects with cognitive deficits differed from the other groups on several tests, and performances were significantly associated with CAG repeat length. These data suggest that impairments of learning and memory may be early manifestations of disease in people with the HD mutation who do not yet have motor abnormalities.

Deficits in learning and memory are the most frequently reported cognitive complaints from people with HD and their family members. HD patients exhibit verbal learning deficits even in the earliest stages of the illness (Butters *et al.* 1986). The majority of studies have described the memory impairment as a primary encoding and retrieval deficit because recognition memory is often preserved (Kramer *et al.* 1988) (see Chapter 3).

HD patients manifest relatively intact retention over a delay period (Massman *et al.* 1990), indicating no abnormal forgetting or rapid loss of information. When tested on memory for information acquired long ago, they demonstrate no temporal gradient in performance, indicating that memory performance is equivalent for all periods of their lives (Butters and Albert 1982).

Observations that skill learning is intact in patients with medial-temporal and diencephalic damage and deficient in patients with HD led to an explosion of research investigating the existence of multiple, independent memory systems in the brain. It has become well accepted that skill learning is dependent upon the integrity of the basal ganglia. More recently, however, Gabrieli and colleagues (1997) documented dissociable skill learning performances in HD, suggesting separable neural circuits for skill learning. They propose that a striatal memory system may be essential for sequence or open-loop skill learning but not for skills that involve the closed-loop learning of novel visual-response mappings.

In summary, the memory impairment of HD is characterized by a mild encoding deficit, moderately impaired retrieval in the context of relatively intact memory storage when measured with a less-effortful strategy (viz., recognition). Other learning and memory skills that are less dependent on working memory capacity may be relatively intact.

6.4 Primary sensory processing

Several studies have shown olfaction impairments in HD. In the most comprehensive research to date, Nordin and colleagues (1995) assessed absolute detection, intensity discrimination, quality discrimination, short-term recognition memory, and lexical- and picture-based identification for odour, using taste and vision as comparison modalities. Results suggested that although odour-recognition memory is not affected in HD patients, absolute detection, intensity discrimination, quality discrimination, and identification were significantly impaired. Poor detection sensitivity explained performance on several other olfactory tasks where odour identification was the function most impaired. Recently, Moberg and Doty (1997) evaluated olfactory functions in people at-risk for HD. Findings were not significant, and the authors argue that olfaction cannot serve as a indicator of genetic vulnerability in HD.

6.5 Spatial-perceptual skill

Deficits in the ability to copy simple geometric designs, to copy block designs, and to put together puzzles are evident in HD. Although some of these impairments likely reflect motor abnormalities, performance is also impaired on motor-free untimed perceptual tasks (Mohr *et al.* 1991). A consistent and primary spatial impairment has been identified in the perception of personal, or egocentric, space (Brouwers *et al.* 1984). For instance, people with HD experience difficulty with map reading, directional sense, and varying their motor responses following alterations in space. Individuals with HD typically misjudge distances and the relationship of their body to walls, curbs, and other potential obstacles. Although the underlying basis for these impairments is not fully understood, disruptions in corticostriatal circuitry make it difficult to update spatial relations based upon feedback. Cortico-cortico connections to the parietal cortex may also be compromised secondary to disruption of the prefrontal cortex.

6.6 Language

One of the most prominent features of HD is the motor speech impairment, or dysarthria, that is characteristic of the illness. Early speech changes may include insufficient breath support, varying prosody, increased response latencies, and mild misarticulations. As HD progresses, phrase length becomes reduced and pauses in speech output lengthen (Podoll *et al.* 1988).

Performances on tasks of letter and category fluency are impaired early in the disease (Randolph *et al.* 1993), although the integrity of word associations remains relatively intact with little evidence of intrusion or perseveration errors (Randolph 1991). Despite significant impairments in verbal fluency, speed of output, and complexity, syntactic structure remains intact and speech content is usually appropriate (Illes 1989). Although there are some reports in late-stage HD of mild deterioration in semantic knowledge structure (Smith *et al.* 1988), several other studies have shown that errors in confrontation naming are more likely due to visual-perceptual deficits (Hodges *et al.* 1991) and retrieval slowing (Rohrer *et al.* 1999).

Speech output becomes severely impaired as the disease progresses, typically resulting in a profound communication deficit. Assistive devices for language expression are recommended early in the disease to assure that preferences are understood and needs are met in later stages when traditional communication is no longer possible. Computer devices are useful for a brief period, after which motor dyscontrol limits use of a keyboard or joystick. Infrared detectors are often prone to error due to involuntary movements. Alphabet boards and pictures that summarize frequently requested needs are adaptive and can be used throughout the illness. Simple computer response keys and large YES/NO cards are critical in late stages of HD.

Although motor output of speech is the primary impairment, there are several more subtle language impairments associated with HD. Comprehension of conversational speech is limited by its length and complexity. Poor executive control impairs the ability to sequence and organize the information communicated. In addition, there is some evidence that people with HD cannot benefit from affective and propositional prosody (Speedie *et al.* 1990).

6.7 Time perception and production

Recent findings have suggested that people with HD (Woodruff-Pak and Papka 1996), have difficulty with the estimation and production of time. These findings are corroborated clinically; people often complain that their once-punctual spouse becomes frequently late and misestimates how long activities will take.

7 Psychiatric and behavioural symptoms

Research on the incidence of psychiatric symptoms in HD is encumbered by limitations within and across studies (Mendez 1994; Zappacosta *et al.* 1996). Some limitations of the available research:

(a) Affected people are often medicated to minimize abnormal involuntary movements; such treatment may mask psychiatric and behavioural symptoms.

(b) Most available neuropsychiatric assessment tools use conventional psychiatric terminology based upon idiopathic psychiatric illness, which fails to distinctly reflect the symptoms associated with striatal deterioration.

(c) Most research has emphasized the motor and cognitive impairments associated with HD, despite family reports that psychiatric disturbances are most strongly associated with stress, disability, and placement decisions (see also Chapter 4).

Data from 1857 HSG subjects with a diagnosis of definite HD are presented in Table 15.2. Subjects are grouped into disease stages according to ratings obtained on the Total Functional Capacity Scale (Shoulson and Fahn 1979).

Table 15.2 Percentage of HD patients endorsing psychiatric symptoms by TFC stage[a]

Symptom	Stage 1 (n = 432)	Stage 2 (n = 660)	Stage 3 (n = 520)	Stage 4 (n = 221)	Stage 5 (n = 84)
Depression	57.5%	62.9%	59.3%	52.1%	42.2%
Suicide	6.0%	9.7%	10.3%	9.9%	5.5%
Aggression	39.5%	47.7%	51.8%	54.1%	54.4%
Obsessions	13.3%	16.9%	25.5%	28.9%	13.3%
Delusions	2.4%	3.5%	6.1%	9.9%	2.2%
Hallucinations	2.3%	4.2%	6.3%	11.2%	3.3%

[a] Source: The Huntington Study Group. Printed with permission.

7.1 Depression

Depression is one of the most common concerns for individuals and families with HD, occurring in 9–63% of patients (see Chapter 4) (Table 15.2). Recent data from the HSG indicate that depression is most common immediately prior to diagnosis, when neurological soft signs and other subtle abnormalities become evident. Following a definite diagnosis of HD, however, depression is most prevalent in the middle stages of the disease (i.e. Shoulson-Fahn stages 2 and 3) and may diminish in the later stages. Mayberg *et al.* (1992) examined regional brain metabolic activity using positron emission tomography (PET) in patients with and without depression matched for age and duration of involuntary movements. Patients with depression had greater hypometabolism in the inferior frontal cortex and thalamus than non-depressed HD patients or normal, age-comparable controls. Although less well studied, mania episodes occur in 2–12% of HD patients (see Chapter 4).

7.2 Suicide

Suicide is more common in HD than in other neurological disorders with high rates of depression, such as stroke and Parkinson's disease. Most studies have found a four- to sixfold increase of suicide in HD, and some studies have reported it to be 8–20 times higher than the general population (Almqvist *et al.* 1999). Suicidal ideation, as measured by the behavioural rating scale on the UHDRS, is highly prevalent throughout the disease, with 10% of all individuals diagnosed with HD having active ideation.

7.3 Psychosis

Psychosis occurs with increased frequency in HD, with estimates ranging from 3–12% (Folstein 1989; Folstein *et al.* 1979). Psychosis is more common among early adult-onset cases than among those whose disease begins in middle or late adulthood. Psychosis associated with HD is more resistant to treatment than psychosis in schizophrenia (Caine and Shoulson 1983). HSG data suggests that psychosis may increase somewhat as the disease progresses (see Table 15.2).

Table 15.3 Percentage of subjects in each category endorsing psychiatric symptoms (categories estimated by UHDRS neurological examination)[a]

Symptom	Normal (n = 425)	Soft signs (n = 252)	Probable HD (n = 313)	Definite HD (n = 2095)
Depression	45.2%	61.5%	62.9%	58.2%
Suicidal ideation	2.8%	8.4%	11.5%	8.8%
Aggression	23.1%	34.5%	39.0%	47.8%
Obsessions	8.0%	11.5%	17.6%	19.7%
Delusions	0.2%	3.6%	4.5%	4.8%
Hallucinations	0.9%	4.4%	6.1%	5.1%

[a] Source: The Huntington Study Group. Printed with permission.

7.4 Obsessive-compulsiveness

Although true obsessive-compulsive disorder is not often reported in HD (Cummings and Cummingham 1992), obsessive and compulsive behaviours are prevalent (i.e. 13–30%). As shown in the preliminary data in Table 15.3, obsessional thinking often increases with proximity to disease onset and then remains somewhat stable throughout the illness. Obsessional thinking associated with HD is reminiscent of perseveration, such that individuals get 'stuck' on a previous occurrence or need and are unable to shift. For instance, patients often emphasize a time in the past when they felt wronged (e.g. divorce, job loss) and maintain discussion on this topic for several years. Another example of obsessional thinking in HD is when patients get fixated on a specific need, such as needing a cigarette, soda, sweater, or specific kind of juice.

7.5 Irritability, agitation, aggressiveness

A spectrum of behaviours ranging from irritability to intermittent explosive disorders occurs in 19–59% of HD patients (Burns *et al.* 1990; Folstein 1991). One recent study using a standardized scale to rate neuropsychiatric symptoms in 52 HD patients showed that at least 66% were rated by their spouses as having significant irritability and aggressive outbursts (Paulsen *et al.* 2001*a*).

Understanding aggression in HD: Joan's story

Alice, a staff member in a nursing home, was rearranging the night table of Joan, a woman with Huntington's disease. Joan had been busy in the adjoining bathroom while Alice tidied up her room and threw away some dead flowers on the night table. Suddenly, without warning, Joan leaped out of the bathroom and wrestled Alice to the floor. She attacked her with such force that Alice was sent to the hospital. The staff at the nursing home agreed that this was a product of the unpredictable irritability and aggression of Huntington's disease. Joan's family was contacted and asked to find her another, more restrictive, placement.

Unfortunately, this interpretation of aggression in HD is not uncommon. It's often easy to forget to look beyond the diagnosis to the distinct individual, her history, and life course. Oftentimes, it is important to consider the individual person and how the disease has interfered with his or her life. In the story above, the bouquet of flowers was the only gift Joan had received from her son that year. Their removal by Alice was the source of her anger. Her response was certainly exaggerated, but the nursing staff viewed her behaviour quite differently knowing the full story. 'When we see things in a new way, we can intervene in a different way', says Dr Allen Rubin, who shared this story.

Given the frequency of agitation in HD and the significant consequences of this behaviour, a formal survey was developed to investigate staff perspectives of HD care in skilled nursing facilities throughout California. 189 skilled nursing facilities completed a survey addressing the needs and problems involved in caring for people with HD. Well over half of the facilities surveyed reported that they would be hesitant to consider admitting an HD patient. When queried as to the reasons for the difficulty in acceptance, 52% reported it was due to excessive care requirements, 41% to inadequate training, 28% to the behavioural problems associated with HD, and 26% reported it was due to insufficient staffing or funding. Table 15.4 shows what percentage of skilled nursing facilities surveyed rated behaviours as problematic in caring for an individual with HD. The final column represents the overall rank of each behaviour from most problematic (10) to least problematic (1) in providing care for HD. Findings reveal that agitation is the most prominent behaviour problem cited. Irritability, disinhibition, and depression were the next most common behaviour problems cited by the facilities surveyed (Paulsen *et al.* 2001*a*).

7.6 Apathy

Early signs of HD may include withdrawal from activities and friends, decline in personal appearance, lack of behavioural initiation and initiative, decreased spontaneous speech, and constriction of emotional expression. Oftentimes, however, these symptoms are considered merely reflective of depression, and more conclusive evaluations are precluded. Although difficult to distinguish, apathy is defined as diminished motivation not attributable to cognitive impairment, emotional distress, or decreased level of consciousness (Marin 1990). Levy and colleagues (1998) recently examined the relationship of apathy and depression in 34 people with HD and concluded that apathy is common (59%) in HD and is separable from depression (70%). 53% of HD patients had mutually exclusive apathy or depression, and the two symptoms were not correlated ($r = -0.15$, $p = .40$). Apathy was correlated with lower cognitive function, however, repli-

Table 15.4 Ratings by nursing home staff of problematic behaviours in patients with Huntington's disease

Behaviour problem	Percentage	Rank
Agitation	76%	2.0
Irritability	72%	2.9
Disinhibition	59%	3.3
Depression	51%	4.2
Anxiety	50%	4.4
Appetite	54%	5.1
Delusions	43%	5.5
Sleep disorders	50%	5.5
Apathy	32%	6.8
Euphoria	40%	6.9

cating previous research indicating relationships between apathy and dementia (Caine and Shoulson 1983). Although the frequency of complaints from patients and family members about apathy may be low, the prevalence of this behaviour is not. The consequences of apathy are rarely problematic (in contrast to temper outbursts which are less frequent but highly distressing), but effective treatment of apathy (see treatment section later this chapter) is typically appreciated by both patients and family members.

A problem with initiation: Elsie's story

> Elsie did not have a problem with interest and she was not depressed. She still enjoyed and cared about many things in her life. She was very disappointed, however, that she never did anything anymore. She seemed to just sit around the house all day, sometimes never getting up from her easy chair except to use the toilet. After she complained about her inactivity to several others, including her family, it was agreed that the family would try to replace Elsie's lack of initiative with external structure and begin activities for her. This strategy worked very well. Elsie was a good 'follower' and enjoyed all of the activities that her family members encouraged her to attend or participate in. After about six weeks, however, it became evident that the family was experiencing a significant amount of distress having to guide and begin every one of Elsie's activities. First of all, the family was small, so the work load could not be spread out. Secondly, all of the other family members had full-time commitments to work and/or school. They grew tired of providing constant initiation for Elsie and began to neglect her. One day Elsie's daughter came home with an abandoned puppy which had been left at school. At the family's protest, Elsie adopted the puppy. The next time Elsie and her family were seen in support group, the whole family announced that the puppy had become Elsie's external initiator. The puppy initiated play-time, dinner-time, time to go outside to the bathroom, and time to go for a walk. Elsie was no longer inactive!

7.7 Awareness of illness

One of the most frequent behavioural complaints about HD from family members is that the affected individual 'refuses to accept' or 'denies' the disease and its consequences. Ample evidence suggests that the apparent 'denial' represents a neurologically based unawareness or anosognosia (Deckel and Morrison 1996; Snowden *et al.* 1998). One recent study (Deckel and Morrison 1996) administered an 8-item self-rating scale to 19 individuals with HD and 15 consecutive patients referred for neuropsychological assessment with non-HD diagnoses. HD patients showed higher anosognosia than the comparison patients. In addition, performances on the Wisconsin Card Sorting Test and the visual-spatial subtests of the WAIS-R were significantly associated with levels of anosognosia for the HD patients. These findings suggest that unawareness in HD is likely to reflect circuitry dysfunction affecting the frontoparietal lobes and their connections, not merely unwillingness to face the diagnosis.

7.8 Sexual disorders

Although little research has been conducted on sexual disorders (SDs) in HD, one study assessed the frequency and type of SDs in 39 HD patients and their partners (Fedoroff *et al.* 1995). 80% of HD patients and 64% of their partners had one or more SDs by Diagnostic and Statistical Manual of Mental Disorders-III-R (DSM-III-R) criteria. Findings showed that SDs are frequent among HD families and that SDs among HD patients often take the form of increased sexual interest or paraphilias.

7.9 Clinical correlates of psychiatric symptoms in HD

Psychiatric measures have been shown to be independent of illness duration, general cognitive impairment, activities of daily living, chorea severity, and CAG repeat length (Caine and Shoulson 1983; Mayberg *et al.* 1992; Paulsen *et al.* 1996; Zappacosta *et al.* 1996), although a few studies have provided descriptions of typical behaviours for distinct stages of the disease process (e.g. Dewhurst *et al.* 1969) (see Tables 15.2 and 15.3).

Relationships among the various types of behavioural changes in HD have been reported in a few studies. Litvan and her colleagues (1998) compared disorders of the basal ganglia with increased activity (chorea, HD) and decreased activity (akinesia, progressive supranuclear palsy [PSP]). They reported that patients with a hyperactive motor disturbance had more agitation (45%), irritability (38%), and anxiety (34%), whereas patients with progressive supranuclear palsy (PSP) exhibited more apathy (82%). Findings were interpreted in terms of dysfunction of thalamocortical circuitry and suggest that patients with hyperkinesia (i.e. HD) display more hyperactive behaviours secondary to an excitatory subcortical output through the medial and

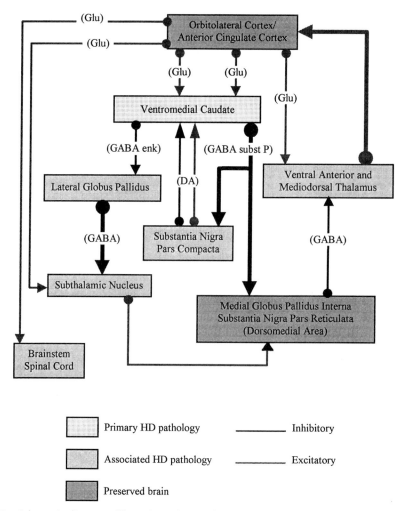

Figure 15.7 Schematic diagram of hypothetical orbitofrontal circuits.

orbitofrontal cortical circuits, while patients with hypokinesia (PSP) display hypoactive behaviours (i.e. apathy). A schematic diagram of the proposed orbitofrontal circuit in HD and the anatomical output areas is shown in Figure 15.7.

Paulsen and her colleagues (2001*a*) recently found a significant association between agitation and irritability, as well as between anxiety and depression, in 50 HD patients. These consistent associations suggest a common pathway for these behavioural changes in both neurodegenerative (i.e. HD and AD) and psychiatric populations.

8 Longitudinal research

Several studies have relied upon the Total Functional Capacity (TFC) scale (Shoulson *et al.* 1989; Marder *et al.* 2000) to quantify disease stages and functional dependence associated with HD. Research has been largely consistent, with most studies demonstrating an average rate of 0.63 ± 0.75 units/year on the TFC (see Feigin *et al.* 1995 for a recent overview). Although controversial, there is some evidence that rate of progression is more rapid in juvenile onset and more gradual in late onset (Kieburtz *et al.* 1994; Penney 1997). Marder and her colleagues reported evidence that better cognitive status at baseline, lower baseline TFC, and longer disease duration were associated with a less rapid rate of decline, whereas depressive symptoms were associated with more rapid functional decline. Longitudinal neuropsychological evaluations suggested that processing speed and executive skills diminish early whereas memory, receptive language and simple attention remain relatively intact throughout the stages of HD (Paulsen *et al.* 1995*a*; Bamford *et al.* 1996). It is important for professionals and family members to educate staff at care facilities regarding the pattern of impaired

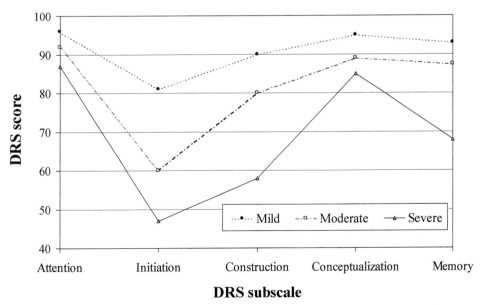

Figure 15.8 DRS subscore performances by HD patients at three stages of disease: mild, moderate, and severe. (Source: Adapted from Paulsen *et al.* 1995*a*.)

and preserved cognitive functions in later stages of HD, when verbal output is severely limited (Paulsen *et al.* 1995*a*) (see Figure 15.8).

9 Presymptomatic HD

9.1 Neurobiological evidence of early changes

There is mounting evidence that atrophy, reduced glucose metabolism, reduced dopamine receptor binding, and neuron loss precede the development of clinical signs and symptoms in HD (see above). Recent studies using indices of quantitative volumetric MRI and PET raclopride binding found that abnormalities in the basal ganglia were associated negatively with the estimated number of years to onset and positively with CAG length in presymptomatic CAG-expanded individuals (Antonini *et al.* 1996; Aylward *et al.* 1996). Lawrence and his colleagues (1998) found a significant relationship between striatal dopamine receptor binding on PET and cognitive performances in 17 presymptomatic individuals with the HD mutation.

9.2 Cognitive-behavioural studies in at-risk individuals

More than 30 studies of individuals at risk for HD have been published since the 1970s. Despite some mixed findings (Strauss and Brandt 1990; Giordani *et al.* 1995), the overall evidence is strong that cognitive and behavioural changes can be detected prior to diagnosis in individuals at-risk for HD (for review see Foroud *et al.* 1995; Hahn-Barma *et al.* 1998; Kirkwood *et al.* 1999). The available studies have varied significantly in terms of study samples and specific cognitive measures utilized, however, limiting comparison across studies. Thus, the magnitude and time-course of early changes in HD are still unclear. Despite these limitations, some recent studies have suggested that inhibitory control mechanisms (i.e. set shifting and fluency) and speed of processing (e.g. Digit Symbol) are among the first to be impaired in at-risk individuals (Lawrence *et al.* 1998).

There are 155 subjects in the HSG database who have been gene-tested who showed no HD symptoms on first testing and have had at least one follow-up evaluation, at an average of 21 months later. 34 of these individuals have been diagnosed with manifest HD at subsequent visits. Initial values and rates of change of cognitive variables among the 121 who did not convert and

Table 15.5 Baseline performance and estimated change rate in presymptomatic HD[a]

Cognitive measure	Non-converters n = 121		Converters n = 34	
	Initial value (SD)	Change rate (SD)	(Initial value (SD)	Change rate (SD)
Verbal Fluency	32.3 (12.1)	1.7 (2.4)	33.9 (13.2)	−0.5 (1.2)
Symbol Digit	48.8 (11.4)	0.1 (2.2)	40.4 (13.6)	−1.8 (1.6)
Stroop Colour	70.8 (14.2)	0.6 (3.0)	62.9 (15.9)	−2.0 (2.5)
Stroop Reading	85.6 (16.2)	0.7 (3.3)	78.7 (17.1)	−2.1 (3.5)
Stroop Interference	40.9 (11.7)	0.5 (2.8)	37.3 (13.8)	−2.2 (0.4)

[a] Source: The Huntington Study Group. Printed with permission.

the 34 who demonstrated HD at follow-up visit(s) (converters) are given below. Rates of change and their standard deviations were estimated from a mixed-model analysis (see Table 15.5). Findings suggest that there are clear differences in cognitive performance change rates between at-risk individuals close to onset and far from onset (or without CAG expansion). Neuropsychological performances in at-risk individuals close to onset declined at a much more rapid rate than in at-risk individuals far from onset and effect sizes of the group differences were robust with every cognitive measure, ranging from 0.8 to 1.9 (see Paulsen *et al.* 2001*b*).

9.3 Neuropsychiatric symptoms in at-risk individuals

Table 15.3 provides a description of the frequency of specific neuropsychiatric symptoms endorsed by HSG subjects via the UHDRS. Groups are defined as follows:

(a) Normal individuals demonstrating no findings on the standardized neurological examination and considered healthy normals.

(b) Soft signs are present on the neurological examination but the pattern, frequency, and/or severity of neurological signs are not consistent with HD.

(c) Probable HD is considered when extrapyramidal and neurological signs are found that are consistent with HD and the examiner is 60–80% confident that the abnormal neurological findings reflect HD.

(d) Definite HD is used to describe neurological findings that are unequivocally HD and the examiner is 99% confident that symptoms represent HD.

10 Potential treatments for HD

At present, treatments for HD are aimed at symptom reduction and maximizing functional capacity. Given the progressive nature of HD, symptoms vary over time such that treatments effective in one stage may be unnecessary, or problematic, in a later stage. Although a brief overview of treatment suggestions is offered here, please see additional references for more thorough treatment recommendations for clinical manifestations of HD (Leroi and Michalon 1998; Rosenblatt *et al.* 1999).

10.1 Chorea

Typically, the chorea associated with HD is not associated with other clinical aspects of the disease, such as depression, functional capacity, or cognitive skill. Hence, the individual with HD rarely presents with complaints of abnormal movements. Treatment for chorea is most often initiated at the request of family members or professionals; it is important to query the purpose of chorea treatment. It is helpful to educate patients and families that pharmacological management of chorea will not decrease falling or improve intelligibility of speech. Assistive devices are often helpful to manage chorea, such as padded beds, reclining chairs, and wrist or ankle weights to diminish the amplitude of chorea.

Some individuals with HD prefer to manage chorea when its high visibility represents a significant source of distress. Three classes of medication are used to suppress chorea in HD: neuroleptics, benzodiazepines, and dopamine-depleting agents. A recent study with risperidone demonstrated improvement of motor disability, psychiatric symptoms, and daily activity levels

Table 15.6 Medications used to suppress chorea[a]

Class	Medication	Starting dose	Maximum dose	Adverse effects
Neuroleptics	Haloperidol	0.5–1 mg/day	6–8 mg/day	Sedation, parkinsonism, dystonia, akathisia, hypotension, constipation, dry mouth, weight gain
	Fluphenazine	0.5–1 mg/day	6–8 mg/day	Same as for haloperidol
	Risperidone	0.5–1 mg/day	6 mg/day	Less parkinsonism than haloperidol
	Thiothixene	1–2 mg/day	10–20 mg/day	Less parkinsonism, more sedation and postural hypotension than haloperidol
	Thioridazine	20 mg/day	200 mg/day	Similar to thiothixene
Benzodiazepines	Clonazepam	0.5 mg/day	4 mg/day	Sedation, ataxia, apathy, withdrawal seizures
	Diazepam	1.25 mg/day	20 mg/day	Same as clonazepam
Dopamine-depleting agents	Reserpine	0.1 mg/day	3 mg/day	Hypotension, sedation, depression
	Tetrabenazine	25 mg/day	100 mg/day	Less hypotension than reserpine

[a] Source: Rosenblatt *et al.* 1999. Reprinted with permission.

(Dallocchio *et al.* 1999), although additional research with larger sample sizes is warranted. Recommendations for suppression of chorea are shown in Table 15.6 (adapted from Rosenblatt *et al.* 1999).

Table 15.7 Medications used to treat depression[a]

Class	Medication	Starting dose	Maximum dose	Adverse effects
SSRIs	Fluoxetine	10–20 mg	60–80 mg	Insomnia, diarrhoea, GI upset, restlessness, weight loss
	Sertraline	25–50 mg	200 mg	Similar to fluoxetine
	Paroxetine	10–20 mg	40–60 mg	Similar to fluoxetine, more sedation
Tricyclics	Nortriptyline	10–25 mg	150–200 mg	Dry mouth, blurry vision, constipation, hypotension, tachycardia, sedation
Other	Nefazodone	50–100 mg	450–600 mg	Sedation, nausea, dry mouth, dizziness, constipation
	Bupropion	100–200 mg	300–450 mg	Seizures, agitation, dry mouth, insomnia, nausea
	Venlafaxine	25–37.5 mg	225 mg	Hypertension, nausea, headache, constipation

[a] Source: Rosenblatt *et al.* 1999. Reprinted with permission.

10.2 Depression

The first line of choice for depression treatment in HD is a selective serotonin reuptake inhibitor (SSRI), such as sertraline, paroxetine, fluoxetine, or fluvoxamine. The SSRIs are particularly useful for HD due to minimal side-effects, once-a-day dosing, safety in the event of overdose, and evidence that other non-specific psychiatric symptoms (i.e. irritability, apathy, obsessiveness) often respond to SSRI treatment. Other, newer antidepressants used with success in HD include bupropion, venlafaxine, and nefazodone. Tricyclic antidepressants (TCAs) (such as nortriptyline, imipramine, or amitriptyline) remain an important option for the treatment of depression in HD, although side-effects are problematic and TCAs are dangerous in overdose. Recommendations for depression treatment are shown in Table 15.7 (adapted from Rosenblatt *et al.* 1999).

10.3 Psychosis

If the patient's depression is accompanied by delusions, hallucinations, or significant agitation, it may be necessary to add an antipsychotic medication to the regimen, preferably in low doses to minimize the risk of sedation, rigidity, or parkinsonism. High-potency agents such as haloperidol or fluphenazine are less sedating but can cause much more parkinsonism. Newer agents such as risperidone, olanzapine, or quetiapine have a lower incidence of side-effects and appear to be just as helpful. Benzodiazepines may be useful in the short-term management of agitation. Any treatment prescribed for the management of acute agitation should be tapered as soon as possible. (For recommendations for the treatment of psychosis, see Rosenblatt *et al.* 1999).

10.4 Obsessiveness

The SSRIs are often used to treat OCD and are effective in ameliorating obsessive symptoms in HD. Higher doses are often required than are necessary for depression treatment (e.g. 40–60 mg of fluoxetine).

10.5 Irritability and temper outbursts

Treatments for irritability often include the SSRIs and may involve mood stabilizers such as carbamazepine. Low-dose neuroleptics may be helpful (particularly the atypical ones), and long-acting benzodiazepines may also be effective. A recent study demonstrated the efficacy of sertraline in abating aggressive behaviour (Ranen *et al.* 1996*a*). The most effective management of irritability and temper outbursts involves a combination of pharmacotherapy, environmental evaluation, and sociopsychological considerations. Calm and routine environments that minimize novelty, noise, and unpredictability are preferred. It is best to determine the behavioural antecedents of aggressiveness; oftentimes, enhanced communication and emotional support can diminish frustration contributing to agitation.

Understanding temper outbursts in HD: Todd's story
The HD clinic at a large university teaching hospital received a phone call from a nursing care facility requesting immediate admission of a patient. According to the facility staff, daily temper outbursts resulted in the staff being unable to care for the HD patient any longer. He was currently in restraints and would remain so until escorted to a locked facility.

Further evaluation was conducted. The nursing facility had been very responsive to Todd's needs. Multiple consultations with family members and specialists had resulted in a personal care program for Todd that emphasized his strengths and allowed him assistance with aspects of disability. For example, Todd was served his meals one hour prior to other residents so that he could receive extra staff assistance with feeding. Wearing a helmet and appropriate wrist and knee pads, Todd joyfully participated in recreational therapy (albeit with frequent falls). Most recently, the staff revised their schedule to better accommodate having two staff available for Todd's daily shower. Upon further discussion, it was revealed that Todd's new shower time was 5:00 am. His 'temper outbursts' began immediately when awakened at 4:45 with two young female staff assisting him to the shower. Following a discussion with Todd, the shower schedule was again revised to allow him to shower in the afternoon with male staff assistance. The daily outbursts abated.

10.6 Apathy

Apathy can be difficult to distinguish from depression, but patients with primary apathy sometimes respond to psychostimulants such as methylphenidate, pemoline, or dextroamphetamine. Since these medications are easily abused and may exacerbate irritability, they should be used with extreme caution. Neuroleptics and benzodiazepines can cause or worsen apathy. It is often appropriate to consider an SSRI for apathy, even when criteria for depression are not met. HD people with apathy benefit from having a highly structured and routine environment. Since they are unable to self-initiate behaviours, they are reliant upon the environment to initiate activity for them. Typically, HD patients respond well to gentle encouragement and routinized schedules.

10.7 Experimental therapeutics

Efforts are underway to develop clinical treatments that could slow HD progression rate in clinically affected individuals and/or delay onset in presymptomatic individuals with the gene mutation (Peyser *et al.* 1995; Ranen *et al.* 1996*b*; The Huntington Study Group 1998; Kremer *et al.* 1999). Some compounds are being tested because of their efficacy in animal excitotoxicity models (Emerich *et al.* 1996). Recent studies have shown that inhibition of caspase-1 can slow the behavioural and pathological course in the HD exon-1 transgenic mouse (Ona *et al.* 1999). In addition, compounds to block glutamine entry into the cell body and drugs to delay aggregation and other aspects of the cellular pathology of HD are in development. Growth factors and surgical transplant of fetal striatal cells are being examined for their utility in replacing cells lost to HD (Peschanski *et al.* 1995; Quinn *et al.* 1996; Shannon and Kordower 1996; Philpott *et al.* 1997; Kopyov *et al.* 1998). This momentum in recent HD research will likely result in a drug to slow disease progression (Shoulson 1998).

11 Summary

Progress in the clinical and pathophysiological aspects of HD has increased exponentially over the past five years. Technological advancements, ongoing multidisciplinary collaboration, and the identification of the genetic basis for HD have resulted in a synergistic gain in knowledge. With the momentum established, effective treatments for HD will become available. In the interim, professionals can minimize distress and facilitate adaptive functioning for individuals with this devastating disease.

12 Key points

1 HD is a neurodegenerative disease characterized by a triad of symptoms including motor distur- bance, cognitive impairment, and psychiatric features.

2 The autosomal dominant gene consists of expansion of the trinucleotide repeat CAG in the gene IT-15 on chromosome 4 and encodes the protein huntingtin.

3 It is not known when HD will become manifest in a given individual, although a significant inverse relationship exists between CAG repeat length and age of onset, with evidence of genetic anticipation greater in paternal inheritance.

4 A simple and accurate genetic test is available and is useful in three clinical situations: to confirm a diagnosis; to inform a healthy person whether (s)he has an expanded gene; or to determine the risk status of a fetus.

5 The neuropathology of HD is characterized by severe loss of medium spiny neurons in the caudate and putamen with vulnerability in other regions. Progression of disease is from dorso- medial to ventrolateral caudate.

6 Early motor abnormalities include interrupted pursuit, hypometric saccades, tongue impersis- tence, impaired rapid alternating movements, and akathisia.

7 A recent effect–size analysis using meta-analytic principles indicated that HD patients are most deficient in learning, motor and cognitive speed, flexibility, and attention. Cognitive functions are more highly associated with functional capacity than motor symptoms.

8 Psychiatric symptoms are the least well-studied aspect of HD, although possibly the most chal- lenging in terms of treatment and the most disruptive in terms of functioning. Agitation, irritabil- ity, and unawareness are among the most prevalent and problematic symptoms reported.

9 There is mounting evidence that behavioural ratings, cognitive performance, brain metabolism, and volumetric MR are abnormal prior to HD diagnosis. Some recent studies suggest that these changes occur up to ten years before diagnosis.

10 Current treatments remain symptomatic ones. However, several experimental therapeutic trials are presently ongoing, and successful delay of onset and slowed progression have been accom- plished in a mouse model of HD.

Acknowledgements

This project was supported by National Institutes of Mental Health Grants MH55331, MH01579, NS35284, MH53592, and MH52879, the Howard Hughes Medical Institute, and the Roy Carver Medical Trust.

References

Albin, R. L., Young, A. B., Penney, J. B., Handelin, B., Balfour, R., Anderson, K. D., *et al.* (1990). Abnormalities of striatal projection neurons and N-methyl-D-aspartate receptors in presymptomatic Huntington's disease. *New England Journal of Medicine*, **332**, 1293–8.

Alexander, G. E. (1997). Anatomy of the basal ganglia and related motor structures. In *Movement disorders: neurological principles and practice* (ed. R. L. Watts and W. C. Koller). McGraw Hill, New York.

Alexander, G. E. and Crutcher, M. D. (1990). Functional architecture of basal ganglia circuits: neural substrates of parallel processing. *Trends in Neurosciences*, **13**, 266–71.

Almqvist, E. W., Bloch, M., Brinkman, R., Crauford, D., and Hayden, M. R. (1999). A worldwide assessment of the frequency of suicide, suicide attempts and psychiatric hospitalizations following predictive testing for Huntington disease. *American Journal of Human Genetics*, **64**, 1293–304.

Andrew, S. E., Goldberg, Y. P., and Hayden, M. R. (1997). Rethinking genotype and phenotype correlations in polyglutamine expansion disorders. *Human Molecular Genetics*, **6**, 2005–10.

Antonini, A., Leenders, K. L., Spiegel, R., Meier, D., Vontobel, P., Weigell-Weber, M., *et al.* (1996). Striatal glucose metabolism and dopamine D2 receptor binding in asymptomatic gene carriers and patients with Huntington's disease. *Brain*, **119**, 2085–95.

Aylward, E. H., Codori, A., Barta, P., Pearlson, G., Harris, G., and Brandt, J. (1996). Basal ganglia volume and proximity to onset in presymptomatic Huntington's disease. *Archives of Neurology*, **53**, 1293–6.

Aylward, E. H., Li, Q., Stine, O. C., Ranen, N., Sherr, M., Barta, P. E., *et al.* (1997). Longitudinal change in basal ganglia volume in patients with Huntington's disease. *Neurology*, **48**, 394–9.

Bamford, K. A., Caine, E. D., Kido, D. K., and Cox, C. (1996). A prospective evaluation of cognitive decline in early Huntington's disease: functional and radiographic correlates. *Neurology*, **45**, 1867–73.

Bechara, A., Damasio, H., Tranel, D., and Anderson, S. (1994). Insensitivity to future consequences following damage to human prefrontal cortex. *Cognition*, **50**, 7–15.

Brandt, J., Folstein, S. E., and Folstein, M. F. (1988). Differential cognitive impairment in Alzheimer's disease and Huntington's disease. *Annals of Neurology*, **23**, 555–61.

Brinkman, R. R., Mezei, M. M., Theilmann, J., Almqvist, E., and Hayden, M. R. (1997). The likelihood of being affected with Huntington's disease by a particular age, for a specific CAG size. *American Journal of Human Genetics*, **60**, 1202–10.

Brouwers, P., Cox, C., Martin, A., Chase, T., and Fedio, P. (1984). Differential perceptual-spatial impairment in Huntington's and Alzheimer's dementias. *Archives of Neurology*, **41**, 1073–6.

Burns, A., Folstein, S., Brandt, J., and Folstein, M. (1990). Clinical assessment of irritability, aggression, and apathy in Huntington's and Alzheimer's disease. *Journal of Nervous and Mental Disease*, **178**, 20–6.

Butters, N. and Albert, M. S. (1982). Processes underlying failures to recall remote events. In *Human, memory, and amnesia* (ed. L. S. Cermak). Erlbaum, Hillsdale, NJ.

Butters, N., Wolfe, J., Graholm, E. and Martone, M. (1986). An assessment of verbal recall, recognition and fluency abilities in Huntington's disease *Cortex.*, **22**, 11–32

Caine, E. D. and Shoulson, I. (1983). Psychiatric syndromes in Huntington's disease. *American Journal of Psychiatry*, **140**, 728–33.

Codori, A.-M., Slavney, P. R., Young, C., Miglioretti, D. L., and Brandt, J. (1997). Predictors of psychological adjustment to genetic testing for Huntington's disease. *Health Psychology*, **16**, 36–50.

Cummings, J. L. and Cummingham, K. (1992). Obsessive-compulsive disorder in Huntington's disease. *Biological Psychiatry*, **31**, 263–70.

Dallocchio, C., Buffa, C., Tinelli, C., and Mazzarello, P. (1999). Effectiveness of risperidone in huntington chorea patients. *Journal of Clinical Psychopharmacology*, **19**, 101–3.

Deckel, A. W. and Morrison, D. (1996). Evidence of a neurologically based 'denial of illness' in patients with Huntington's disease. *Archives of Clinical Neuropsychology*, **11**, 295–302.

DeLong, M. R. (1990). Primate models of movement disorders of basal ganglia origin. *Trends in Neurosciences*, **13**, 281–5.

Dewhurst, K., Oliver, J., Trick, K. L., and McKnight, A. L. (1969). Neuro-psychiatric aspects of Huntington's disease. *Confinia Neurologica*, **31**, 258–68.

Emerich, D. F., Linder, M. D., Winn, S. R., Chen, E. Y., Frydel, B. R., and Kordower, J. H. (1996). Implants of encapsulated human CNTF-producing fibroblasts prevent behavioral deficits and striatal degeneration in a rodent model of Huntington's disease. *Journal of Neuroscience*, **16**, 5168–81.

Fedoroff, J. P., Peyser, C. E., Franz, M. L., and Folstein, S. E. (1995). Sexual disorders in Huntington's disease. *Journal of Neuropsychiatry and Clinical Neurosciences*, **6**, 147–53.

Feigin, A., Kieburtz, K., Bordwell, K., Como, P., Steinberg, K., Sotack, J., *et al.* (1995). Functional decline in Huntington's disease. *Movement Disorders*, **10**, 211–14.

Folstein, M. F., Folstein, S. E., and McHugh, P. R. (1975). Mini-Mental State: a practical method for grading the cognitive state of patients for the clinician. *Journal of Psychiatric Research*, **12**, 189–98.

Folstein, S. E. (1989). *Huntington's disease. A disorder of families*. Johns Hopkins University Press, Baltimore, MD.

Folstein, S. E. (1991). The psychopathology of Huntington's disease. In *Genes, brain, and behavior*, Vol. 69 (ed. P. R. McHugh and V. A. McKusick). Raven Press, New York.

Folstein, S. E., Folstein, M. F., and McHugh, P. R. (1979). Psychiatric syndromes in Huntington's disease. *Advances in Neurology*, **23**, 281–90.

Foroud, T., Siemers, E., Kleindorfer, D., Bill, D. J., Hodes, M. E., Norton, J. A., *et al.* (1995). Cognitive scores in carriers of Huntington's disease gene compared to noncarriers. *Annals of Neurology*, **37**, 657–64.

Gabrieli, J. D., Stebbins, G. T., Singh, J., Willingham, D. B., and Goetz, C. G. (1997). Intact mirror-tracing and impaired rotary-pursuit skill learning in patients with Huntington's disease: evidence for dissociable memory systems in skill learning. *Neuropsychology*, **11**, 272–81.

Ginovart, N., Farde, L., Halldin, C., and Swahn, C. G. (1997). Effect of reserpine-induced depletion of synaptic dopamine on [^{11}C]raclopride binding to D2-dopamine receptors in the monkey brain. *Synapse*, **25**, 321–5.

Giordani, B., Berent, S., Boivin, M. J., Penney, J. B., Lehtinen, S., Markel, D. S., *et al.* (1995). Longitudinal neuropsychological and genetic linkage analysis of persons at risk for Huntington's disease. *Archives of Neurology*, **52**, 59–64.

Hahn-Barma, V., Deweer, B., Durr, A., Feingold, J., Pillon, B., Agid, Y., *et al.* (1998). Are cognitive changes the first symptoms of Huntington's disease? A study of gene carriers. *Journal of Neurology, Neurosurgery, and Psychiatry*, **64**, 172–7.

Harper, P. S. (1991). *Huntington's disease*. W. B. Saunders Co., London.

Hasselbalch, S. G., Oberg, G., Sorensen, S. A., Andersen, A. R., Waldemar, G., Schmidt, J. F., *et al.* (1992). Reduced regional cerebral blood flow in Huntington's disease studied by SPECT. *Journal of Neurology, Neurosurgery and Psychiatry*, **55**, 1018–23.

Hodges, J. R., Salmon, D. P., and Butters, N. (1991). The nature of the naming deficit in Alzheimer's and Huntington's disease. *Brain*, **114**, 1547–58.

Illes, J. (1989). Neurolinguistic features of spontaneous language production dissociate three forms of neurodegenerative disease: Alzheimer's, Huntington's, and Parkinson's. *Brain and Language*, **37**, 628–42.

Kieburtz, K., MacDonald, M., Shih, C., Feigin, A., Steinberg, K., Borfwell, K., *et al.* (1994). Trinucleotide repeat length and progression of illness in Huntington's disease. *Journal of Medical Genetics*, **31**, 872–4.

Kirkwood, S. C., Siemers, E., Stout, J. C., Hodes, M. E., Conneally, P. M., Christian, J. C., *et al.* (1999). Longitudinal cognitive and motor changes among presymptomatic Huntington disease gene carriers. *Archives of Neurology*, **56**, 563–8.

Kopyov, O. V., Jaques, S., Lieberman, A., Duma, C. M., and Eagle, K. S. (1998). Safety of intrastriatal neurotransplantation for Huntington's disease patients. *Experimental Neurology*, **149**, 97–108.

Kramer, J. H., Delis, D. C., Blusewicz, M. J., Brandt, J., Ober, B. A., and Strauss, M. (1988). Verbal memory errors in Alzheimer's and Huntington's dementias. *Developmental Neuropsychology*, **4**, 1–15.

Kremer, B., Clark, C. M., Almqvist, E. W., Raymond, L. A., Graf, P., Jacova, C., *et al.* (1999). Influence of Lamotrigine on progression of early Huntington disease: a randomized clinical trial. *Neurology*, **53**, 1000–1011.

Kuwert, T., Lange, H. W., Langen, K. J., Herzog, H., Aulich, A., and Feinendegen, L. E. (1990). Cortical and subcortical glucose consumption measured by PET in patients with Huntington's disease. *Brain*, **113**, 1405–23.

Lange, K. W., Sahakian, B. J., Quinn, N. P., Marsden, C. D., and Robbins, T. W. (1995). Comparison of executive and visuospatial memory function in Huntington's disease and dementia of Alzheimer type matched for degree of dementia. *Journal of Neurology, Neurosurgery, and Psychiatry*, **58**, 598–606.

Lawrence, A. D., Sahakian, B. J., Hodges, J. R., Rosser, A. E., Lange, K. W., and Robbins, T. W. (1996). Executive and mnemonic functions in early Huntington's disease. *Brain*, **119**, 1633–45.

Lawrence, A. D., Weeks, R. A., Brooks, D. J., Andrews, T. C., Watkins, L. H. A., Harding, A. E., *et al.* (1998). The relationship between striatal dopamine receptor binding and cognitive performance in Huntington's disease. *Brain*, **121**, 1343–55.

Leroi, I. and Michalon, M. (1998). Treatment of the psychiatric manifestations of Huntington's disease: a review of the literature [Review] [65 refs]. *Canadian Journal of Psychiatry*, **43**, 933–40.

Levy, M. L., Cummings, J. L., Fairbanks, L. A., Masterman, D., Miller, B. L., Craig, A. H., *et al.* (1998). Apathy is not depression. *Journal of Neuropsychiatry and Clinical Neurosciences*, **10**, 314–19.

Litvan, I., Paulsen, J. S., Mega, M. S., and Cummings, J. L. (1998). Neuropsychiatric assessment of patients with hyperkinetic and hypokinetic movement disorders. *Archives of Neurology*, **55**, 1313–19.

MacDonald, M. E. and Gusella, J. F. (1996). Huntington's disease: translating a CAG repeat into a pathogenic mechanism. *Current Opinion in Neurobiology*, **6**, 638–43.

Marder, K., Zhao, H., Myers, R. H., Cudkowicz, M., Kayson, E., Kieburtz, K., *et al.* (2000). Rate of functional decline in Huntington's disease. *Neurology*, **54**, 452–458.

Marin, R. S. (1990). Differential diagnosis and classification of apathy. *American Journal of Psychiatry*, **147**, 22–30.

Massman, P. J., Delis, D. C., Butters, N., Levin, B. E., and Salmon, D. P. (1990). Are all subcortical dementia's alike? Verbal learning and memory in Parkinson's and Huntington's disease patients. *Journal of Clinical and Experimental Neuropsychology*, **12**, 729–44.

Mattis, S. (1976). Mental status examination for organic mental syndrome in the elderly patient. In *Geriatric psychiatry* (ed. L. Bellak and T. B. Karasu). Grune & Stratton, New York.

Mayberg, H. S., Starkstein, S. E., Peyser, C. E., Brandt, J., Dannals, R. F., and Folstein, S. E. (1992). Paralimbic frontal lobe hypometabolism in depression associated with Huntington's disease. *Neurology*, **42**, 1791–7.

Mendez, M. F. (1994). Huntington's disease: update and review of neuropsychiatric aspects. *International Journal of Psychiatry in Medicine*, **24**, 189–208.

Moberg, P. J. and Doty, R. L. (1997). Olfactory function in Huntington's disease patients and at-risk offspring. *International Journal of Neuroscience*, **89**, 133–9.

Mohr, E., Brouwers, P., Claus, J. J., Mann, U. M., Fedio, P., and Chase, T. N. (1991). Visuospatial cognition in Huntington's disease. *Movement Disorders*, **6**, 127–32.

Myers, R. H., Sax, D. S., Schoenfeld, M., Bird, E. D., Wolfe, P. A., Vonsattel, J. P., *et al.* (1985). Late onset of Huntington's disease. *Journal of Neurology, Neurosurgery, and Psychiatry*, **48**, 800–4.

Nance, M. A. (1996). Huntington disease — another chapter rewritten [invited editorial]. *American Journal of Human Genetics*, **59**, 1–6.

Nordin, S., Paulsen, J. S., and Murphy, C. (1995). Sensory- and memory-mediated olfactory dysfunction in Huntington's disease. *Journal of the International Neuropsychological Society*, **1**, 271–80.

Ona, V. O., Li, M., Vonsattel, J. P. G., Andrews, L. J., Khan, S. Q., Chung, W. M., *et al.* (1999). Inhibition of caspase-1 slows disease progression in a mouse model of Huntington's disease. *Nature*, **399**, 263–7.

Paulsen, J. S., Butters, N., Sadek, J. R., Johnson, S. A., Salmon, D. P., Swerdlow, N. R., *et al.* (1995a). Distinct cognitive profiles of cortical and subcortical dementia in advanced illness. *Neurology*, **45**, 951–6.

Paulsen, J. S., Butters, N., Salmon, D. P., Heindel, W. C., and Swenson, M. R. (1993). Prism adaptation in Alzheimer's and Huntington's disease. *Neuropsychology*, **7**, 73–81.

Paulsen, J. S., Ready, R. E., Hamilton, J., Mega, M., and Cummings, J. L. (2001a). Neuropsychiatric aspects of Huntington's disease. *Journal of Neurology, Neurosurgery and Psychiatry*.

Paulsen, J. S., Salmon, D. P., Monsch, A. U., Butters, N., and Swenson, M. R. (1995*b*). Discrimination of cortical from subcortical dementias on the basis of memory and problem-solving tests. *Journal of Clinical Psychology*, **51**, 48–58.

Paulsen, J. S., Stout, J. C., Delapena, J., Romero, R., Tawfik-Reedy, Z., Swenson, M. R., *et al.* (1996). Frontal behavioral syndromes in cortical and subcortical dementia. *Assessment*, **3**, 327–37.

Paulsen, J. S., Zhao, H., Stout, J. C., Brinkman, R.R., Ross, C. A., Como, P., *et al.*(2001*b*). Clinical markers of early disease in persons near onset of Huntington's disease. *Neurology*. (in press)

Penney, J. B. Jr. (1997). CAG repeat number governs the development rate of pathology in Huntington's disease. *Annals of Neurology*, **41**, 689–92.

Peschanski, M., Cesaro, P. and Hantraye, P. (1995). Rationale for intrastriatal grafting of striatal neuroblasts in patients with Huntington's disease [Review] [159 refs]. *Neuroscience*, **68**, 273–85.

Peyser, C. E., Folstein, M., Chase, G. A., Starkstein, S., Brandt, J., Cockrell, J. R., *et al.* (1995). Trial of *d-a*-tocopherol in Huntington's disease. *American Journal of Psychiatry*, **152**, 1771–5.

Philpott, L. M., Kopyov, O. V., Lee, A. J., Jaques, S., Duma, C. M., Caine, S., *et al.* (1997). Neuropsychological functioning following fetal striatal transplantation in Huntington's chorea: three case presentations. *Cell Transplantation*, **6**, 203–12.

Podoll, K., Caspary, P., Lange, H. W., and Noth, J. (1988). Language functions in Huntington's disease. *Brain*, **111**, 1475–503.

Quinn, N., Brown, R., Craufurd, D., Goldman, S., Hodges, J., Kieburtz, K., *et al.* (1996). Core assessment program for intracerebral transplantation in Huntington's disease (CAPIT-HD) [Review]. *Movement Disorders*, **11**, 143–50.

Randolph, C. (1991). Implicit, explicit, and semantic memory functions in Alzheimer's disease and Huntington's disease. *Journal of Clinical and Experimental Neuropsychology*, **13**, 479–94.

Randolph, C., Braun, A. R., Goldberg, T. E., and Chase, T. (1993). Semantic fluency in Alzheimer's, Parkinson's, Huntington's disease: dissociation of storage and retrieval failures. *Neuropsychology*, **7**, 82–8.

Ranen, N. G., Lipsey, J. R., Treisman, G., and Ross, C. A. (1996*a*). Sertraline in the treatment of severe aggressiveness in Huntington's disease. *Journal of Neuropsychiatry and Clinical Neurosciences*, **8**, 338–40.

Ranen, N. G., Peyser, C. E., Coyle, J. T., Bylsma, F. W., Sherr, M., Day, L., *et al.* (1996*b*). A controlled trial of idebenone in Huntington's disease. *Movement Disorders*, **11**, 549–54.

Rohrer, D., Salmon, D. P., Wixted, J. T., and Paulsen, J. S. (1999). The disparate effects of Alzheimer's disease and Huntington's disease on semantic memory. *Neuropsychology*, **13**, 381–8.

Rosenblatt, A., Ranen, N. G., Nance, M. A., and Paulsen, J. S. (1999). *A physician's guide to the management of Huntington's disease* (2nd edn). Huntington's Disease Society of America.

Rosenblatt, A., Ranen, N. G., Rubinsztein, D. C., Stine, O. C., Margolis, R. L., Wagster, M. V., *et al.* (1998). Patients with features similar to Huntington's disease, without CAG expansion in huntingtin. *Neurology*, **51**, 215–20.

Rothlind, J. C. and Brandt, J. (1993). A brief assessment of frontal and subcortical functions in dementia. *Journal of Neuropsychiatry and Clinical Neurosciences*, **5**, 73–7.

Shannon, K. M. and Kordower, J. H. (1996). Neural transplantation for Huntington's disease: experimental rationale and recommendations for clinical trials [Review]. *Cell Transplantation*, **5**, 339–52.

Shoulson, I. (1998). Experimental therapeutics of neurodegenerative disorders: unmet needs. *Science*, **282**, 1072–4.

Shoulson, I. and Fahn, S. (1979). Huntington's disease: clinical care and evaluation. *Neurology*, **29**, 1–3.

Shoulson, I., Kurlan, R., Rubin, A. J., Goldblatt, D., Behr, J., Miller, C., *et al.* (1989). Assessment of functional capacity in neurodegenerative movement disorders: Huntington's disease as a prototype. In *Quantification of Neurological Deficit* (ed. T. L. Munsat). Butterworths, Boston, MA.

Siemers, E., Foroud, T., Bill, D. J., Sorbel, J., Norton, J. A. J., Hodes, M. E., *et al.* (1996). Motor changes in presymptomatic Huntington disease gene carriers. *Archives of Neurology*, **53**, 487–92.

Siesling, S., Zwinderman, A. H., Van Vugt, J. P., Keiburtz, K., and Roos, R. A. (1997). A shortened version of the motor section of the Unified Huntington's Disease Rating Scale. *Movement Disorders*, **12**, 229–34.

Smith, S., Butters, N., White, R., Lyon, L., and Granholm, E. (1988). Priming semantic relations in patients with Huntington's disease. *Brain and Language*, **33**, 27–40.

Snowden, J. S., Craufurd, D., Griffiths, H. L., and Neary, D. (1998). Awareness of involuntary movements in Huntington's disease. *Archives of Neurology*, **55**, 801–5.

Speedie, L. J., Brake, N., Folstein, S. E., Bowers, D., and Heilman, K. M. (1990). Comprehension of prosody in Huntington's disease. *Journal of Neurology, Neurosurgery, and Psychiatry*, **53**, 607–10.

Sprengelmeyer, R., Lange, H., and Homberg, V. (1995). The pattern of attentional deficits in Huntington's disease. *Brain*, **118**, 145–52.

Starkstein, S. E., Brandt, J., Bylsma, F. W., Peyser, C. E., Folstein, M., and Folstein, S. E. (1992). Neuropsychological correlates of brain atrophy in Huntington's disease: a magnetic resonance study. *Neuroradiology*, **34**, 487–9.

Stout, J. C., Paulsen, J. S., Tawfik-Reedy, Z., Romero, R. L., Delapena, J. H., Swenson, M. R., *et al.* (1996). The nature of problem-solving deficits in patients with early Huntington's disease. *Journal of the International Neuropsychological Society*, **2**, 35.

Stout, J. C., Rodawalt, W. C., and Siemers, E. R. (2001). Risky decision making in Huntington's disease. *Journal of the International Neurological Society*, **7**, 92–101.

Strauss, M. E. and Brandt, J. (1986). An attempt at presymptomatic identification of Huntington's disease with the WAIS. *Journal of Clinical and Experimental Neuropsychology*, **8**, 210–28.

Strauss, M. E. and Brandt, J. (1990). Are there neuropsychologic manifestations of the gene for Huntington's disease in asymptomatic, at-risk individuals? *Archives of Neurology*, **47**, 905–8.

The Huntington's Disease Collaborative Research Group. (1993). A novel gene containing a trinucleotide repeat that is expanded and unstable on Huntington's disease chromosomes. *Cell*, **72**, 971–83.

The Huntington Study Group. (1996). Unified Huntington's Disease Rating Scale: reliability and consistency. *Movement Disorders*, **11**, 136–42.

The Huntington Study Group. (1998). Safety and tolerability of the free-radical scavenger OPC-14117 in Huntington's disease. *Neurology*, **50**, 1366–73.

Van Vugt, J. P., Van Hilten, B. J., and Roos, R. A. (1996). Hypokinesia in Huntington's disease. *Movement Disorders*, **11**, 384–8.

Vonsattel, J. P. and Difiglia, M. (1998). Huntington's disease [Review]. *Journal of Neuropathology & Experimental Neurology*, **57**, 369–84.

Wechsler, D. (1997). *Wechsler Adult Intelligence Scale*, 3rd edn. The Psychological Corporation, San Antonio.

Woodruff-Park, D. S. and Papka, M. (1996). Huntington's disease and eyeblink classical conditioning: normal learning but abnormal timing. *Journal of the International Neuropsychological Society*, **2**, 323–34.

Young, A. B., Shoulson, I., Penney, J. B., Starosta-Rubinstein, S., Gomez, F., Travers, H., *et al.* (1986). Huntington's disease in Venezuela: neurological features and functional decline. *Neurology*, **36**, 244–9.

Zakzanis, K. K. (1998). The subcortical dementia of Huntington's disease. *Journal of Clinical and Experimental Neuropsychology*, **20**, 565–78.

Zappacosta, B., Monza, D., Meoni, C., Austoni, L., Soliveri, P., Gellera, C., *et al.* (1996). Psychiatric symptoms do not correlate with cognitive decline, motor symptoms, or CAG repeat length in Huntington's disease. *Archives of Neurology*, **53**, 493–7.

16 Transmissible spongiform encephalopathies

Paul Brown

1 Introduction

Unique among the neurodegenerative diseases, the spongiform encephalopathies are transmissible, either experimentally or as a result of cannibalistic, iatrogenic, or zoonotic infections in humans. First described in the 1920s by Creutzfeldt and Jakob, whose names memorialize its most common form, human spongiform encephalopathy is now recognized to include four other distinctive syndromes: kuru, Gerstmann-Sträussler-Scheinker disease, fatal familial insomnia, and the recently described 'new variant' of Creutzfeldt–Jakob disease (vCJD).

Scrapie, an endemic disease of sheep and goats, is reliably recorded to have existed in Europe since the mid-1700s (Brown and Bradley 1998), and has since spread to many other parts of the world; in more recent times, a spongiform encephalopathy (chronic wasting disease) has been recognized to be endemic in some species of deer and elk living in the western United States. The appearance of spongiform encephalopathy in two further animal species is attributable to the consumption of scrapie-infected sheep tissues, either in the form of raw carcasses (by mink), or rendered carcass protein (by cattle). Disease outbreaks in mink have been 'dead-end' epidemics, but the more recent occurrence of disease in cattle has been disastrously 'open-ended', with secondary infections from consumption of recycled cattle carcass protein in domestic cats and zoo ungulates, felines, and primates; and, probably as a result of the consumption of beef products contaminated by nervous system tissue, in humans (Figure 16.1). For details of the molecular pathology and histopathology see chapters 8 and 10, respectively.

2 Kuru

The origins of this disease, limited to an isolated population group in the middle of Papua New Guinea, are shrouded in mystery; however, a plausible explanation is that sometime in the early decades of the 1900s, a chance case of sporadic Creutzfeldt–Jakob disease occurred in the area, and because of the widespread practice of ritual endocannibalism, was propagated in exponential fashion until by mid-century it had reached epidemic proportions, becoming the single most important cause of death and annually decimating the most heavily affected villages. Australian governmental displeasure with the practice of endocannibalism led to its cessation by 1960, and kuru subsequently declined to the point of near disappearance by the 1990s, with continuing single digit annual numbers of cases attributed to ever longer incubation periods (now approaching 40 years) following isolated incidents of cannibalism after mid-century.

Clinically, the illness can be classified as a cerebellar degeneration with a variable amount of associated cerebral dysfunction (Gajdusek 1977). The earliest sign is a very subtle loss of coordi-

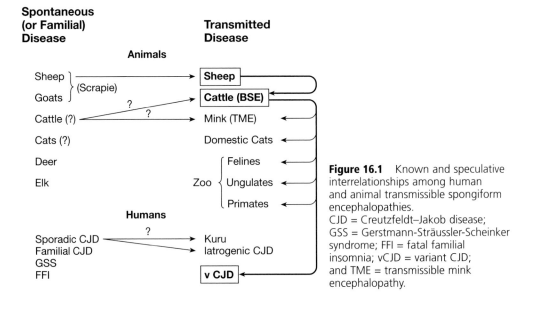

Figure 16.1 Known and speculative interrelationships among human and animal transmissible spongiform encephalopathies. CJD = Creutzfeldt–Jakob disease; GSS = Gerstmann-Sträussler-Scheinker syndrome; FFI = fatal familial insomnia; vCJD = variant CJD; and TME = transmissible mink encephalopathy.

nation apparent only in the performance of a challenging activity, such as crossing a stream on a suspended log. Within a few weeks, this minimal cerebellar dysfunction is extended to postural instability, dysarthria, and generalized 'shivering' tremors. As the ataxia becomes incompatible with an upright posture, the patient enters into a sedentary period characterized by emotional lability, worsening ataxia and tremors, and choreoathetotic and other involuntary movements. In the terminal phase, the patient develops increasing hyperreflexia, dysarthria, and dysphagia. Motor weakness, sensory impairment, and cranial nerve deficits (apart from strabismus) are rarely seen. Death usually occurs from malnutrition and dehydration within 12 months of the appearance of neurological symptoms.

3 Sporadic Creutzfeldt–Jakob disease

Far and away the most common variety of spongiform encephalopathy, sporadic Creutzfeldt–Jakob disease accounts for approximately 90% of all cases, the cause of which remains as perplexing today as when the disease was first described 80 years ago. New cases occur at an annual incidence of about one per million population, the great proportion of which occur in patients between the ages of 55 and 70 years, although verified cases have occurred as early as 16 years, and as late as 84 years (Figure 16.2) (Brown *et al.* 1987; Will *et al.* 1998). Prodromal symptoms, experienced by approximately one-fourth of patients, may occur weeks to months preceding the onset of neurological signs, and include vegetative symptoms such as asthenia, altered sleep and eating patterns, weight loss, and loss of libido. Sometimes, the patient is merely aware of 'not feeling right', or has a sense of impending doom.

In most cases, recognizable neurological disease begins with mental deterioration or cerebellar dysfunction, alone or in combination (Table 16.1) (Brown *et al.* 1994). Family members may notice subtle changes in behaviour such as apathy, self-neglect, depression, or emotional lability, or there may be more obvious episodes of confusion, disorientation, or hallucinations (aggres-

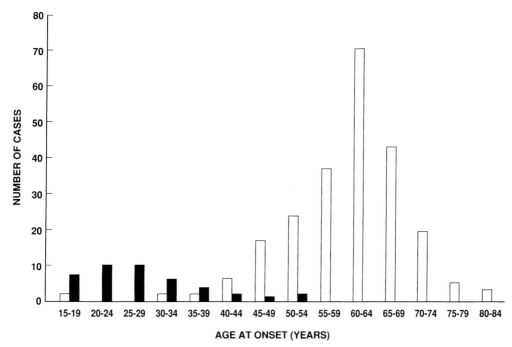

Figure 16.2 Distribution of ages at onset in sporadic (open bars) and new variant (closed bars) Creutzfeldt–Jakob disease. Data on the new variant cases were kindly provided by Dr R. G. Will, CJD Surveillance Unit, Edinburgh, Scotland.

sive, hypersexual, and even violent behaviour is not at all uncommon, but is usually not recounted by the embarrassed spouse). Cerebellar signs typically include gait ataxia, clumsiness, and dysarthria. Often, the clinical presentation also involves the visual system, manifested by diplopia, nystagmus, blurred or distorted vision, altered colour perception, field defects, supranu-clear palsies, or visual agnosias. Headaches and vertigo are infrequent, and sensory symptoms and abnormal movements are rare. Typically, the onset is gradual, occurring over a period of weeks or even months, but in about 15% of patients the onset may occur over a period of a few days, or even with stroke-like suddenness.

As the illness evolves, there is increasing impairment of memory and temporo-spatial orienta-tion, eventually progressing to global dementia, or in some patients, passing directly into a state of mutism. Visual symptoms may evolve into cortical blindness, and increasingly severe ataxia, in conjunction with pyramidal or extrapyramidal deficits in over half of patients, lead to a bed-ridden state. Abnormal movements, especially myoclonic, but often athetotic or choreiform, are eventually observed in most patients. Seizures and lower motor neuron signs are less common and usually late in appearance. The clinical course is typically one of more or less continuous progression, with occasional short periods of stability; however, in the small proportion of patients with long clinical courses, the illness may at first evolve rapidly with a subsequently prolonged period of stability, or as a very slowly progressive memory deficit followed by a rapid terminal dementia and physical deterioration.

Most patients are dead within a year of onset. The mean duration of illness is seven months, but is heavily influenced by the small proportion of long duration cases; thus, the median dura-tion of illness is four months, and the single most frequent duration of illness is only two to three months (Figure 16.3).

Table 16.1 Clinical characteristics of 232 experimentally transmitted cases of sporadic Creutzfeldt–Jakob disease

Symptoms/signs	Percentage of patients with symptoms or signs		
	At onset	On first exam	During course
Mental deterioration	69	85	100
Memory loss	48	66	100
Behavioural abnormalities	29	40	57
Higher cortical functions	16	36	73
Cerebellar	33	56	71
Visual/oculomotor	19	32	42
Vertigo/dizziness	13	15	19
Headache	11	11	18
Sensory	6	7	11
Involuntary movements	4	18	91
Myoclonus	1	9	78
Other (incl. tremor)	3	12	36
Pyramidal	2	15	62
Extrapyramidal	0.5	9	56
Lower motor neuron	0.5	3	12
Pseudobulbar	0.5	1	7
Seizures	0	2	19

4 Iatrogenic Creutzfeldt–Jakob disease

Fortunately rare, but nevertheless responsible for nearly 270 cases since its recognition in the 1970s in a patient receiving a corneal graft and two patients undergoing stereotactic neuroablation therapy, iatrogenic disease has since been principally associated with contaminated pituitary hormones and dura mater grafts (Brown *et al.* 2000).

In 1985, the first case of Creutzfeldt–Jakob disease was reported in a young recipient of cadaveric human growth hormone; the tally has since risen to 139 deaths, almost all in France, England, and the United States, with a few new cases occurring each year after incubation periods that have ranged from less than 5 years to more than 30 years (Table 16.2). However, it is likely that the number of new cases will soon dwindle to zero because of the replacement of natural by recombinant hormone shortly after the first case was discovered in 1985.

The first case of iatrogenic disease due to dura mater grafts was reported in 1988; the total number as of October 2000 was 114 cases, of which 67 have occurred in Japan. Unlike the random contamination of hormones, almost all the infected dura mater grafts were prepared during the early 1980s by a single manufacturer in Germany, who added an effective sterilizing step to the processing protocol in 1987. Currently mandated governmental regulations for the collection and processing of grafts should be adequate to prevent future iatrogenic occurrences from this source.

The incubation period and clinical presentation depend upon the route of introduction of the infectious agent (Table 16.2). When introduced directly into the brain from surgical instru-

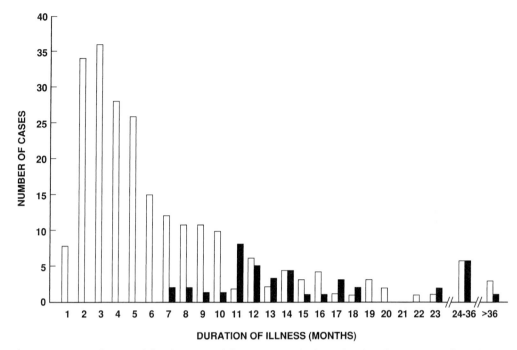

Figure 16.3 Distribution of the durations of illness in sporadic (open bars) and new variant (filled bars) Creutzfeldt–Jakob disease. Data on the new variant cases were kindly provided by Dr R. G. Will, CJD Surveillance Unit, Edinburgh, Scotland.

ments, or via the optic nerve from corneal grafts, the resulting incubation period is usually measured in months (comparable to the incubation period following intracerebral inoculation of experimental animals) and the clinical presentation is indistinguishable from sporadic Creutzfeldt–Jakob disease. When applied to the surface of the brain (dura mater grafts), the incubation period ranges from a few months to more than a decade, and the clinical presentation may resemble sporadic disease, or have a prominent cerebellar or visual onset. When injected by a peripheral route (pituitary hormones), the average incubation period is 15 years (extending up to 30 years), and the clinical presentation is invariably cerebellar in nature. As a

Table 16.2 Summary of iatrogenic cases of transmissible spongiform encephalopathy grouped according to mode of infection, showing different incubation periods and clinical presentations

Mode of infection	Number of patients	Agent entry into brain	Mean incubation period (range)	Clinical presentation
Stereotactic EEG	2	Intra-cerebral	18 months (16, 20)	Dementia/cerebellar
Neurosurgery	5	Intra-cerebral	19 months (12–28)	Visual/dementia/cerebellar
Corneal transplant	3	Optic nerve	16, 18, 320 months	Dementia/cerebellar
Dura mater graft	114	Cerebral surface	6 years (1.5–16)	Cerebellar (visual/dementia)
Growth hormone	139	Hematogenous	12 years (5–30)	Cerebellar
Gonadotrophin	4	Hematogenous	13 years (12–16)	Cerebellar

group, iatrogenic cases have clinical evolutions and durations of illness similar to sporadic Creutzfeldt–Jakob disease.

5 Familial forms of spongiform encephalopathy

A familial form of Creutzfeldt–Jakob disease was recognized in the mid-1920s, only a few years after its original description in sporadic form; then, in the early 1930s, Gerstmann, Sträussler, and Scheinker reported the distinctive familial syndrome that now bears their names; and in 1992, fatal familial insomnia (which had been described six years earlier) was discovered to

Table 16.3 Mutations of the chromosome 20 (PRNP) gene associated with inherited forms of transmissible spongiform encephalopathy

Mutation	Disease phenotype[a]
Octarepeat insertion of 24, 48, 96, 120, 144, 168, 192, or 216 base pairs between codons 51 and 91	CJD, GSS, or atypical dementias
P102L (Pro Leu)	GSS: classical ataxic form
P105L (Pro Leu)	GSS: spastic paraparetic variant
A117V (Ala Val)	GSS: pseudobulbar variant
G131V (Gly Val)	GSS: classical ataxic form
Y145* (Tyr Stop)	Alzheimer-like dementia
D178N (Asp Asn)	CJD (129V on mutant allele)
D178N (Asp Asn)	FFI (129M on mutant allele)
V180I (Val Ile)	CJD
T183A (Thr Ala)	Alzheimer-like dementia
H187R (His Arg)	GSS: classical ataxic form
F198S (Phe Ser)	GSS with neurofibrillary tangles
E200K (Glu Lys)	CJD
D202N (Asp Asn)	GSS with neurofibrillary tangles
V203I (Val Ile)	CJD
R208H (Arg His)	CJD
V210I (Val Ile)	CJD
E211Q (Glu Gln)	CJD
E211Q (Glu Gln)	CJDs
Q212P (Gln Pro)	GSS with Lewy bodies
E217R (Glu Arg)	GSS with neurofibrillary tangles
M232R (Met Arg)	CJD
M232T (Met Thr))	GSS

[a] CJD = Creutzfeldt–Jakob disease; GSS = Gerstmann-Sträussler-Scheinker syndrome; FFI = fatal familial insomnia.

belong to the same group of diseases. All are inherited as autosomal dominant disorders, and all are experimentally transmissible. With the identification of a gene on chromosome 20 that encodes the normal precursor of the pathological amyloid protein deposited in diseased brain tissue, has come the discovery that different mutations in the gene are responsible for the different forms of familial disease (Table 16.3).

It must be clearly appreciated, however, that although genotype–phenotype correlations are satisfying, phenotypic variation is not at all unusual between genotypically identical families, or even among members of the same family, and virtually all well studied families will be found to include at least one member with an illness very similar to classical Creutzfeldt–Jakob disease. Attribution of particular phenotypic features to a given mutation must therefore be made with caution.

5.1 Familial Creutzfeldt–Jakob disease

The first and still most common mutation associated with familial Creutzfeldt–Jakob disease occurs at codon 200. It is responsible for the exceptionally high incidence of disease in the Orava region of rural Slovakia, and among Sephardic Jews (including Libyan-born Israelis) living in many different countries of Europe, North Africa, and the Americas (Lee *et al.* 1999). Except for a slightly earlier average age at onset (55 years), the phenotype is indistinguishable from sporadic disease. Nearby mutations at codons 208 and 210, seen mostly in Italian families, also produce a typical sporadic phenotype (Pocchiari *et al.* 1993). All three mutations are unusual in exhibiting incomplete penetrance, with up to one-half of mutation-positive carriers living to an advanced age, or dying from other diseases.

The second most common mutation associated with familial disease is found at codon 178. It occurs among families of northern European origin, and causes an illness that differs from sporadic disease in having an earlier onset (usually in the fifth decade), and longer duration (1–2 years) (Brown *et al.* 1992). Other mutations have been described in only one or two families of diverse ethnic origins. These include a point mutation at codon 180, and several different insert mutations in the octapeptide repeat region between codons 51 and 91. The point mutation is associated with a typical sporadic phenotype, whereas the insert mutations produce mostly atypical syndromes characterized by a markedly earlier age at onset (third and fourth decades) and much longer duration of illness (5–10 years) than any of the other mutations. Two other point mutations, at codons 145 and 183, are associated with Alzheimer-like clinical courses, and Japanese authors have reported a point mutation at codon 232 in a few patients without known familial disease.

5.2 Gerstmann-Sträussler-Scheinker syndrome

The original family, as well as most of the families discovered later, have a point mutation at codon 102. Onset in the third or fourth decades and a protracted clinical course over several years are common (Piccardo *et al.* 1998; Boellaard *et al.* 1999). Patients typically present with cerebellar dysfunction (ataxia or dysarthria), with dementia appearing later in the course of illness. In some families extrapyramidal or parkinsonian features predominate; others show gaze palsies, deafness, or cortical blindness. Examination frequently reveals loss of deep tendon reflexes in the legs with extensor plantar responses. Myoclonus and periodic electroencephalographic activity are only irregularly present.

Certain distinctive features have been associated with other mutations, notably the occurrence of a pseudobulbar syndrome in patients with a mutation at codon 117, and the presence of Alzheimer-type neurofibrillary tangles in families with mutations at codons 198, 202, and 217. Illnesses associated with point mutations at codons 131 or 187, or with insert mutations, resemble the classical codon 102 syndrome.

5.3 Fatal familial insomnia

The hallmark of this most distinctive member of the spongiform encephalopathy family is a progressive, unremitting insomnia that is associated with dysautonomia, motor signs, and memory loss due to severe thalamic neuronal degeneration (Gambetti *et al.* 1995). Age at onset ranges from 20 to 70 years (average, 50 years), with the duration of illness at least partly dependent upon the genotype of polymorphic codon 129 (6–13 months in homozygotes, 2–4 years in heterozygotes). Autonomic disturbances include sweating, salivation, constipation, impotence, hypertension, tachycardia, tachypnea, and mild fever. Motor signs include dysarthria, dysphagia, diplopia, myoclonus, and seizures, and dystonic attacks. Mental deterioration is usually manifested by severe impairment of vigilance and a selective impairment of memory, with a comparatively good preservation of global intelligence.

The disease has special molecular genetic interest in that the phenotype is associated with the same mutation at codon 178 that produces a Creutzfeldt–Jakob-like illness in other families. The cause of this unique division of phenotypes linked to the same mutation has been traced to the genotype of polymorphic codon 129: when it encodes methionine on the mutant 178 allele the result is fatal familial insomnia; when it encodes valine on the mutant allele the result is Creutzfeldt–Jakob disease (Goldfarb *et al.* 1992). Illustrating the difficulty of defining strict phenotype–genotype correlations is the fact that the same clinicopathological syndrome has been reported in a patient with a codon 200 mutation, and in several patients with sporadic disease.

6 Variant Creutzfeldt–Jakob disease

This most recent variety of human spongiform encephalopathy has now been securely linked to infection by the agent of bovine spongiform encephalopathy, and most likely results from the consumption of beef products that were contaminated by central nervous system tissue. The disease first appeared in 1994 (Will *et al.* 1996) and has since been occurring at a steady state incidence of about 10 to 15 new cases per year; as of March 2001 it had been responsible for nearly 100 deaths in the United Kingdom, three deaths in France and one death in the Republic of Ireland.

Clinically, the most striking feature of variant Creutzfeldt–Jakob disease is the comparative youthfulness of its victims (as young as 14 and averaging 28 years), and thus clearly separate from the major 55–70 year age bracket of sporadic disease (Figure 16.2). In addition, the clinical presentation seen in most patients consists of psychiatric or sensory symptoms, rather than the usual mental and cerebellar onset of sporadic disease. The illness progresses at a comparatively leisurely pace, with an average duration of 14 months, and no case dying in less than 7 months (Figure 16.3), during which most of the features of sporadic disease occur, including dementia and myoclonus. All cases so far tested have been homozygous for methionine at codon 129. Because no single clinical feature (or even combination of features) is peculiar to the new variant, a definitive diagnosis can only be established by the unique neuropathological finding of amyloid plaques surrounded by petals of spongiosis ('daisy plaques').

7 Laboratory diagnosis

Routine laboratory studies of blood and cerebrospinal fluid, useful in the exclusion of alternative diagnostic possibilities, provide no positive clues to the diagnosis of spongiform encephalopathy. In particular, spinal tap opening pressure is normal, and although the fluid may show modestly increased protein concentration (never higher than 100 mg/dl), significant pleo-cytosis is never present. However, three more specialized tests can provide highly significant diagnostic information.

The most time-honoured of these is the electroencephalogram, which in advanced disease typically shows 1–2 cycle/sec triphasic sharp waves superimposed on a depressed background (Figure 16.4) (Steinhoff *et al.* 1996). They are usually asymmetrical in nature, and may or may not occur in synchrony with myoclonic jerks. Less specific but often seen alternative patterns are symmetrical theta and delta waves on an irregularly depressed background, or a 'burst-suppression' slow wave pattern. With serial tracings, the characteristic triphasic sharp wave pattern is seen in up to 80% of patients at some time during the course of illness, with two notable exceptions: periodic patterns have never been seen in the familial form of Creutzfeldt–Jakob disease linked to the codon 178 mutation, or in new variant disease. Also, periodic activity is not entirely restricted to the spongiform encephalopathies; it may be seen in association with tricyclic antidepressant, bismuth, or lithium therapy, and (rarely) in organic neurological disorders, including Alzheimer's disease.

The second useful laboratory examination is an immunological test for the detection of a class of 14–3–3 proteinase inhibitor proteins in cerebrospinal fluid (Hsich *et al.* 1996). Although these proteins are merely a 'seepage' marker of neuronal damage (unrelated to the amyloid protein deposited in brain tissue), they are an excellent surrogate marker of disease, being present in 95% of all patients with spongiform encephalopathy except new variant Creutzfeldt–Jakob disease, in which only about one-half of cases are positive. The overall specificity of the test is also greater than 90%, with the few 'false' positives occurring in patients with encephalitis, hypoxic brain damage, metastatic carcinoma, and metabolic or endocrine encephalopathy (Zerr *et al.* 1998; Saiz *et al.* 1998).

A third laboratory examination, for which data continue to accumulate, is magnetic resonance imaging. A proportion of cases of sporadic Creutzfeldt–Jakob disease have been found to show a symmetric or asymmetric increased signal intensity in the basal ganglia (Pearl and Anderson 1989; Yoon *et al.* 1995; Finkenstaedt *et al.* 1996); whereas cases of new variant disease show a symmetric increased signal intensity in the pulvinar (Figure 16.5) (Sellar *et al.* 1997; Coulthard *et al.* 1999).

In patients with suspected familial disease, molecular analysis of DNA from peripheral blood leukocytes may establish the correct pre-mortem diagnosis by revealing a pathogenic mutation in the amyloid precursor gene. Brain biopsy is not recommended unless the differential diagnosis includes a treatable disease. If new variant disease is suspected, tonsillar biopsy has been pro-posed as a useful diagnostic procedure, as the presence of proteinase-resistant protein in tonsils appears to be specific for this form of disease. It is arguable, however, whether the pre-mortem distinction between two different varieties of the same fatal disease justifies this invasive and painful procedure. The definitive diagnosis is made at autopsy by neuropathological examina-tion, and by immunohistological or Western immunoblot detection of the pathognomonic amyloid protein in brain tissue.

8 Precautions in patient management

Universal precautions should be observed in the general care and management of hospitalized patients. Although the infectious agent of transmissible spongiform encephalopathy can be found in many organs of the body, it does not appear to be present in any external secretion or excre-tion, including tears, saliva, perspiration, urine, and faeces. It is, however, occasionally present in cerebrospinal fluid, and possibly present in blood; therefore, gloves should be worn when han-

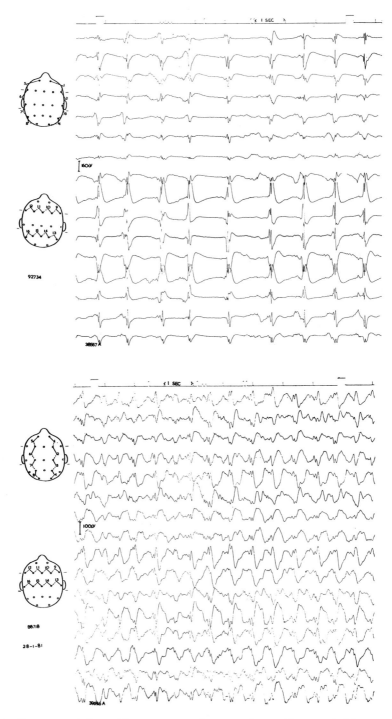

Figure 16.4 Electroencephalographic patterns seen in two patients with transmissible spongiform encephalopathy. Upper tracing shows the nearly pathognomonic 1–2 cycle/sec tri- and multiphasic sharp wave complexes on a very suppressed background; lower tracing shows a suggestive regular slow wave periodicity on a very disorganized background. Tracings were obtained through the courtesy of Dr R. G. Will, CJD Surveillance Unit, Edinburgh, Scotland.

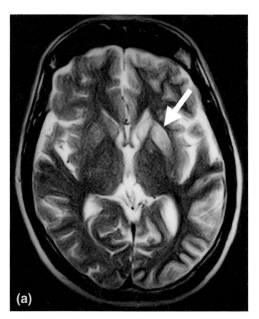 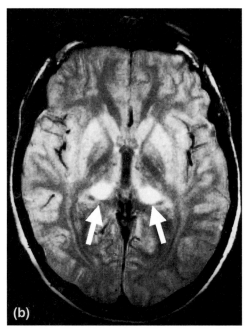

Figure 16.5 Magnetic resonance images of the brain from (A) a patient with sporadic Creutzfeldt–Jakob disease, and (B) a patient with new variant Creutzfeldt–Jakob disease. Arrows indicate areas of signal hyper-intensity in caudate head and putamen (sporadic disease) and pulvinar (new variant disease). Images were kindly supplied by Dr R. G. Will, CJD Surveillance Unit, Edinburgh, Scotland.

dling blood or spinal fluid, or when treating oozing wounds or bed sores. The 'golden rule' is to avoid penetrating injuries from potentially contaminated instruments such as spinal tap needles, venipuncture needles, and scalpel blades. Accidental contamination of intact skin should be treated with the application of fresh undiluted bleach or 1 N sodium hydroxide (one pound of pellets per three gallons of water) to the area for about a minute, followed by thorough washing with soap and water. Disposable instruments and other materials should be used whenever possible; if retained, instruments should be disinfected by immersion in 1 N sodium hydroxide and steam autoclaved for at least 20 minutes at 134°C. Disinfectant procedures are outlined in a recent WHO document (WHO 2000).

9 Prevention and therapy

To date there is neither preventive nor curative treatment for transmissible spongiform encephalopathy, other than the possibility of eliminating familial disease through an acceptance by mutation positive family members either to forebear having children, or to request amniotic fluid mutation screening with a view to therapeutic abortion if the foetus is mutation positive. Future therapies may be directed towards biochemical interruption of the conversion of normal to abnormal protein, or by gene ablation or antisense oligonucleotide therapy to inhibit gene transcription, as studies in mice have shown the absence of a functional gene has no evident detrimental effect on either the health or life-span of genetically altered animals.

9.1 Family concerns

Faced with an incurable and fatal disease, the physician is obliged to exchange the role of healer for that of teacher and comforter. In our experience, the concerns uppermost in the families' minds have to do with therapy, prognosis, symptoms, and the possibility of contagion. We have found it helpful to emphasize the following points in our discussions with families. Although the illness may show periods of stability interspersed with periods of progression, the overall trend is relentless, and invariably fatal; therefore, instead of spending time and money on a fruitless search for non-existent therapies, the family is better advised to devote themselves to ensuring the best and most loving possible care of the patient.

Progression of physical disability is almost always keyed to progression of ataxia and incoordination that eventually lead to immobility. Pain is not a feature of the illness, and muscle twitching and seizures (if they occur) can usually be effectively subdued by medication. Behavioural abnormalities and mood changes are frequent, unpredictable, and often transient. The patient should be assumed to be capable of understanding what is happening around him, even in an unresponsive state of mutism, and may have moments of recognition up to the terminal days of illness. The disease is not contagious, and no special precautions need be taken in the everyday home care of the patient, for example, in the cleaning of eating utensils or bed linens, nor is there any need to avoid casual or even intimate physical contact.

10 Illustrative case reports

This set of 12 clinical histories was presented in the form of a clinicopathological conference to a group of the world's leading experts in transmissible spongiform encephalopathy gathered together at a meeting in Vienna, Austria, in May of 1998. All relevant information available to the patient's neurologist was included in each case history (none of the cases was iatrogenic, because inclusion of the source of infection in the clinical history would have been transparent). In all cases, routine examination of cerebrospinal fluid was normal. Each expert was given a sheet of paper containing a choice of diagnoses that included the categories of sporadic or new variant Creutzfeldt–Jakob disease, familial spongiform encephalopathy (with entries for variety and mutation), and other neurological disorders (two cases). Each clinical history was shown to the audience for one minute, following which the completed sheets were collected, and the diagnoses were evaluated according to the criteria of being appropriate or correct (they did not necessarily coincide). Readers of this chapter are invited to test their own diagnostic skills before reading the neuropathology and diagnostic entries for each case, and may be encouraged to learn that the 'experts' identified the correct diagnosis in only about one-half of the cases.

Case 1

A 63-year-old woman with a history of recurrent depressive episodes experienced the subacute onset of confusion, difficulty speaking, dizzy spells, nocturnal hallucinations, and ataxia. Magnetic resonance imaging showed multiple white matter lesions 'consistent with microvascular ischaemic disease' and moderate bilateral temporal lobe atrophy. Her condition rapidly deteriorated and she developed myoclonic jerking that became almost continuous, associated with periodic triphasic electroencephalographic activity. She became mute and then comatose, dying three months after the onset of illness. Family history was positive only for a non-fatal depressive illness in patient's sister.

(a) **Neuropathology**: spongiform change, neuronal loss, and gliosis throughout cerebral cortex (especially in the occipital lobe) and basal ganglia; similar but milder changes in the thalamus and cerebellum. No plaques were observed. Widespread distribution of proteinase-resistant amyloid protein.

(b) **Diagnosis**: sporadic Creutzfeldt–Jakob disease.

(c) **Comment**: the age is right, the duration is right, and the clinical triad of progressive dementia, ataxia, and myoclonus is supported by the characteristic electroencephalogram. The MRI result remained unexplained at autopsy.

Case 2

A 52-year-old man in previous good health began to experience headaches, stuttering, and occasional 'whispering' speech, followed by weakness and ataxia. Two years later, physical examination revealed a moderately ataxic gait, nystagmus, dysphonia, and mental deterioration with irritability, memory loss, and compromised learning ability. During the next five years, his cerebellar signs slowly worsened, he became increasingly autistic, and he complained of failing vision and hearing. Repeated electroencephalograms showed progressive slowing but no periodic activity. On hospitalization, he was noted to have a global cerebellar syndrome, severe hearing and visual impairment together with oculomotor signs, pyramidal signs, myoclonus, and advanced dementia. He died six years after the onset of illness. Several family members had died with similar illnesses.

(a) **Neuropathology**: marked diffuse gliosis with multicentric and 'kuru type' amyloid plaques, especially abundant in the cerebellar cortex. No spongiosis was observed anywhere in the brain.

(b) **Molecular genetic analysis**: P102L (129MM).

(c) **Diagnosis**: codon 102 Gerstmann-Sträussler-Scheinker disease.

(d) **Comment**: typical clinical evolution, but with an age at onset a little later than the usual case. The absence of spongiform change is unusual, but not unique.

Case 3

A 65-year-old man noted the onset of photophobia and fatigue, with a sense of extreme lassitude, somnolence, and heavy-headedness, and also a tendency to have a swaying gait. On hospitalization two months later, he was found to be apraxic and somnolent, with ataxia, generalized hypertonicity, absent Achilles tendon reflexes, and urinary incontinence. During the next two months, his level of consciousness progressively decreased, he developed a plastic type of rigidity, a bilateral Babinski sign, and generalized myoclonus. An arteriogram was normal, computerized tomography showed mild ventricular dilatation, and the electroencephalogram showed periodic diphasic sharp waves. He died seven months after the onset of symptoms. Family history was negative for neurological disease.

(a) **Neuropathology**: no spongiform change, neuronal loss, gliosis, or plaques. A diffuse reticulosarcoma involved the entire neuroaxis.

(b) **Diagnosis**: primary reticulo-sarcoma of the brain.

(c) **Comment**: no one could have suspected that this case was otherwise than a classic example of Creutzfeldt–Jakob disease. A test for spinal fluid 14–3–3 protein might have been very helpful.

Case 4

A 68-year-old woman experienced the insidious onset of gait imbalance, followed several months later by intermittent episodes of double vision. Hospital examination revealed mild ataxia and decreased cognition. As these symptoms worsened over the next several months, she also complained of progressive hearing loss. Computerized tomography showed cerebellar atrophy. She became unable to walk or speak, and developed extrapyramidal rigidity, dysmetria, resting and intention tremors of all extremities, and myoclonus. Electroencephalographic study was not recorded. She died 20 months after the onset of illness. Family history was positive for degenerative neurological disease characterized principally by cerebellar symptoms in several relatives over three generations: Creutzfeldt–Jakob disease had been considered likely in her sister and son.

(a) **Neuropathology**: modest spongiform change, neuronal loss, and gliosis in the temporal cortex; severe neuronal loss and gliosis in the inferomedial thalamic and inferior olivary nuclei; marked Purkinje cell loss in cerebellum. No plaques were observed.

(b) **Molecular genetic analysis**: D178N (cis-129M).

(c) **Diagnosis**: fatal familial insomnia.

(d) **Comment**: a most atypical clinical course for fatal familial insomnia, as it did not include either insomnia or dysautonomic symptoms. The most appropriate clinical diagnosis would have been the codon 102 variety of Gerstmann-Sträussler-Scheinker disease, by virtue of the cerebellar onset, moderately prolonged illness, and family history.

Case 5

A 71-year-old man experienced the gradual onset of fatigue, uncharacteristic bursts of anger, and difficulty walking. After several months, he also noted a deterioration in both his memory and speech, began having headaches and visual hallucinations, and although suffering from anxiety, became indifferent to the events of daily life. On hospitalization, he was found to have a moderate global dementia that rapidly progressed to a state of mutism, together with an extrapyramidal type of rigidity, myoclonus, and seizures. The electroencephalogram at first showed periodic triphasic sharp waves, and later showed low voltage slow wave activity. He died 12 months after the onset of illness. Family history was negative for neurological disease.

(a) **Neuropathology**: myriad senile plaques and neurofibrillary tangles, without spongiform change or gliosis. Plaques stained positive for β-A4, negative for PrP.

(b) **Diagnosis**: Alzheimer's disease.

(c) **Comment**: an excellent story for sporadic Creutzfeldt–Jakob disease, which was the assumed diagnosis until the surprising results of post-mortem examination. The 14–3–3 spinal fluid protein test, had it been available, might have been a pivotal diagnostic aid.

Case 6

A previously healthy 19-year-old man became increasingly depressed and withdrawn over a period of six months, at which time he noted the onset of unsteadiness and failing memory. Shortly thereafter, he developed hallucinations, choreiform movements, and was found to be frankly ataxic. Two months later he could no longer stand, became bedridden, and finally lapsed into a state of mutism. Two electroencephalograms were normal and a third showed non-specific slow wave activity. He died in coma 13 months after the onset of illness. Family history was negative for neurological disease.

(a) **Neuropathology**: widespread distribution of PrP positive amyloid plaques surrounded by halos of spongiosis ('daisy' plaques), especially pronounced in cerebellum; spongiform change with gliosis in corpus striatum and thalamus.

(b) **Diagnosis**: Variant Creutzfeldt–Jakob disease.

(c) **Comment**: the young age at onset, presenting psychiatric symptoms, prolonged illness, and absence of periodic electroencephalographic activity all point to the correct diagnosis in this case.

Case 7

A previously healthy 26-year-old woman became progressively depressed over a period of several months, and then noted some difficulties with memory, talking, and walking. She was found to be ataxic and dysarthric, with bilateral pyramidal signs, diminished hearing, and horizontal nystagmus. These abnormalities continued slowly to worsen in association with a deteriorating cognition; late in the course of illness, she had increasingly severe dysphagia and rigidity. No abnormal movements were ever observed, and serial electroencephalograms showed only high voltage slow wave activity. She died 22 months after the onset of illness. The patient's mother had died following an operation for cerebellar angioma; otherwise the family history was negative for neurological disease.

(a) **Neuropathology**: massive spongiosis throughout the cerebral cortex, associated with neuronal loss and gliosis; similar but more moderate changes occurred in the caudate and thalamic nuclei, and in the cerebellum. No plaques were observed anywhere in the brain.

(b) **Diagnosis**: sporadic Creutzfeldt–Jakob disease.

(c) **Comment**: every clinical element of this case (except the absence of involuntary movements) pointed to new variant Creutzfeldt–Jakob disease, which would have been the certain pre-mortem diagnosis had the patient become ill after 1994 in the United Kingdom. As it happens, she was a French woman who became ill in 1975.

Case 8

A 64-year-old woman was noted during a two month period to show a personality change, confusion, and insomnia. The insomnia and confusion continued to worsen, and she began to lose weight, hallucinate, and have episodes of disorientation. In hospital, she was found to have a mild cerebellar ataxia, visual hallucinations, and persistent insomnia. A 20 minute electroencephalogram sleep recording showed no specific sleep pattern. She became tachypneic, developed an idiopathic fever, and abruptly lapsed into coma. Myoclonus appeared, and repeated electroencephalograms showed periodic triphasic sharp waves. She died three months after the onset of illness. Family history was positive for neurological disease: a paternal uncle died of a subacute illness diagnosed as a stroke, and a paternal cousin died of an uncategorized illness that was characterized by dementia, ataxia, and myoclonus.

(a) **Neuropathology**: widespread spongiform change, neuronal loss, and gliosis in the cerebral cortex and basal ganglia; severe neuronal loss and gliosis with moderate spongiosis in the mediodorsal thalamic nuclei; minimal spongiosis in the cerebellum. No plaques were observed.

(b) **Molecular genetic analysis**: E200L (cis-129M) mutation in the PRNP gene.

(c) **Diagnosis**: familial codon 200 Creutzfeldt–Jakob disease.

(d) **Comment**: this case was the first published indication that the clinicopathological phenotype of fatal familial insomnia need not be invariably associated with the codon 178 (cis-129M) genotype; and recent reports have extended the mimicry to several cases of sporadic Creutzfeldt–Jakob disease.

Case 9

A pregnant 25-year-old woman noticed difficulty walking disproportionate to her condition, together with some trouble in speaking clearly and swallowing. Her family also noticed a personality change, with unaccountable episodes of crying or laughing, and after delivery, she neglected both her child and her household. On examination, she was found to have significant mental impairment associated with both pyramidal and cerebellar signs (dysarthria, intention tremor, and ataxia). Her illness progressed very gradually over a period of several years, eventually also including an extrapyramidal syndrome, myoclonus, and seizures. At length, fully demented, she became unable to walk, confined to bed, and died ten years after the onset of illness. Repeated electroencephalograms were recorded as normal. Family history was positive for similar dementia/ataxic syndromes.

(a) **Neuropathology** (limited to cerebral biopsy): focal spongiosis and numerous multicentric amyloid plaques, in the absence of neuronal abnormalities or gliosis.

(b) **Molecular genetic analysis**: A117V (cis-129V).

(c) **Diagnosis**: codon 117 Gerstmann-Sträussler-Scheinker disease.

(d) **Comment**: the youthful age, clinical onset with psychiatric symptoms, and absence of periodic electroencephalographic activity would, in the United Kingdom today, raise a pre-mortem suspicion of new variant Creutzfeldt–Jakob disease; however, the duration of illness was exceedingly long, and there was a family history of dementia/ataxic illnesses. The clue here is the presence of a pseudobulbar syndrome (speech and swallowing difficulties, and emotional lability) which is very rare in all forms of spongiform encephalopathy except the codon 117 variety of Gerstmann-Sträussler-Scheinker disease.

Case 10

A 68-year-old woman initially complained of an earache and sense of having saliva 'stuck in her throat'. She then developed a rapidly progressive bulbar syndrome (facial weakness and paresthesia, dysphonia, and dysarthria, with involvement of cranial nerves V, VII, X, and XI), lower limb paresthesias, ataxia, and weakness of the right arm, followed by mutism and coma. The electroencephalogram showed periodic triphasic discharges and she died three months after the onset of illness. Family history was negative for neurological disease.

(a) **Neuropathology**: very slight spongiosis and neuronal loss in the occipital lobe and cerebellum; elsewhere, the brain was entirely normal. Focal occurrence of proteinase-resistant protein (PrP).

(b) **Diagnosis**: sporadic Creutzfeldt–Jakob disease.

(c) **Comment**: not your typical case, but Creutzfeldt–Jakob disease would have at least been included in the differential diagnosis by virtue of age at onset and duration of a multi-system illness with the classical periodic electroencephalogram pattern. The bulbar syndrome is most unusual.

Case 11

A previously healthy 19-year-old woman experienced increasing lethargy, somnulence during the day and insomnia at night, and complained of headaches, pain in the throat, and a trembling of her left hand; her mother also noted a personality change with inappropriate affect and aggressivity. Thereafter, she exhibited progressive unsteadiness and withdrawal, became disoriented, developed bizarre repetitious movements and myoclonus, rigidity, hyperactive reflexes, and a stato-kinetic cerebellar syndrome. Repeated electroencephalograms showed periodic triphasic sharp-wave activity. She died in a state of mutism four months after the onset of illness. Family history was negative for neurological disease.

(a) **Neuropathology** (limited to post-mortem biopsy of temporal cortex): severe spongiform change, neuronal loss, and gliosis; no plaques were observed.

(b) **Diagnosis**: sporadic Creutzfeldt–Jakob disease.

(c) **Comment**: two 'red herrings' complicate the diagnosis in this case: the youthful onset raises a question of new variant disease, and insomnia raises a question of fatal familial insomnia. However, the short clinical course of only four months and typical periodic electroencephalogram argue against new variant disease (the patient died in France in 1982), and the absence of a family history and autonomic symptoms militate against fatal familial insomnia.

Case 12

A 30-year-old mathematician experienced intellectual deterioration and clumsiness that progressed very gradually over a period of many years, leading to repeated failures in less and less challenging jobs, and eventually, to a condition of merely maintaining basic personal hygiene. He remained in this condition for over a decade, then within one week became mute, bedridden, and incontinent. Neurological evaluation at that time revealed a severe global dementia, with mask-like facies, rigidity, tremors, and myoclonus. Computerized tomography showed generalized atrophy, and an electroencephalogram showed a diffuse 3–6 cycle per second slow wave rhythm. He became febrile and died six weeks after hospitalization, 16 years after the onset of his illness. His father and paternal grandfather had died after several year histories of progressive dementia.

(a) **Neuropathology**: severe spongiform change, gliosis, and neuronal loss in the cerebral cortex, corpus striatum, thalami, and cerebellar cortex. No plaques or neurofibrillary tangles were found.

(b) **Molecular genetic analysis**: five octarepeat insert mutation in the PRNP gene.

(c) **Diagnosis**: familial (insert) Creutzfeldt–Jakob disease.

(d) **Comment**: the plausible working diagnosis for this patient was familial Alzheimer's disease; the case illustrates the typically early age at onset and prolonged clinical course in patients with familial Creutzfeldt–Jakob disease associated with insert mutations.

11 Key points

1 Sporadic Creutzfeldt–Jakob disease (CJD) occurs world-wide at an annual frequency of approximately one case per million, chiefly in the 50–75 year age bracket, but with a small number of cases under age 40. The clinical presentation typically consists of mental deterioration and/or cerebellar ataxia, and the average duration of illness is only a few months (but may rarely extend up to ten years).

2 Familial forms of CJD (as well as the allied disorders of Gerstmann-Sträussler-Scheinker disease and fatal familial insomnia) are caused by mutations in the PRNP gene on chromosome 20, and show ages of onset and clinical courses that depend upon the particular mutation, but are usually much younger than sporadic CJD, with symptoms occurring as early as the third or fourth decades of life, and clinical courses that often evolve over years, rather than months.

3 Iatrogenic CJD has so far mainly resulted from treatment with contaminated pituitary hormones or dura mater grafts, and its age at onset depends upon the age at which infection occurred and the route of infection (most direct intra-cerebral infections have incubation periods of about two years, but peripheral infections have unpredictable incubation periods ranging from 5–30 years).

4 Variant CJD, resulting from the consumption of contaminated tissues from cattle dying of bovine spongiform encephalopathy, is distinctive in having a young age at onset (average, 28 years) that probably reflects exposure during the first two decades of life, a psychosensory clinical presentation, and a comparatively long duration of illness (average, 14 months).

References

Boellaard, J., Brown, P., and Tateishi, J. (1999). Gerstmann-Sträussler-Scheinker disease: the dilemma of molecular and clinical correlations. *Clin. Neuropathol.*, **18**, 271–285.

Brown, P. and Bradley, R. (1998). 1755 and all that: a historical primer of transmissible spongiform encephalopathy. *Br. Med. J.*, **317**, 1688–92.

Brown, P., Cathala, F., Raubertas, R. F., Gajdusek, D. C., and Castaigne, P. (1987). The epidemiology of Creutzfeldt–Jakob disease: conclusion of a 15-year investigation in France and review of the world literature. *Neurology*, **37**, 895–904.

Brown, P., Goldfarb, L. G., Kovanen, J., *et al.* (1992). Phenotypic characteristics of familial Creutzfeldt–Jakob disease associated with the codon 178[Asn] mutation. *Ann. Neurol.*, **31**, 282–5.

Brown, P., Gibbs, C. J. Jr, Rodgers-Johnson, P., *et al.* (1994). Human spongiform encephalo-pathy: the National Institutes of Health series of 300 cases of experimentally transmitted disease. *Ann. Neurol.*, **35**, 513–29.

Brown, P., Preece, M., Brandel, J-P, Sato., T, Mc Shane L, Zerr, I *et al.* Iatrogenic Creutzfeldt-Jacob disease at the millenium. *Neurology*, **55**, 1075–1081.

Coulthard, A., Hall, K., English, P. T., *et al.* (1999). Quantitative analysis of MRI signal intensity in new variant CJD. *Br. J. Radiol.*, **72**, 742–8.

Finkenstaedt, M., Szudra, A., Zerr, I., *et al.* (1996). MR imaging of Creutzfeldt-Jakob disease. *Radiology*, **199**, 793–8.

Gajdusek, D. C. (1977). Unconventional viruses and the origin and disappearance of kuru. *Science*, **197**, 943–60.

Gambetti, P., Parchi P., Petersen, R. B., Chen, S. G., and Lugaresi, E. (1995). Fatal familial insomnia and familial Creutzfeldt–Jakob disease: clinical, pathological, and molecular genetic features. *Brain Pathol.*, **5**, 43–51.

Goldfarb, L. G., Petersen, R. B., Tabaton, M., *et al.* (1992). Fatal familial insomnia and familial Creutzfeldt–Jakob disease: disease phenotype determined by a DNA polymorphism. *Science*, **258**, 806–8.

Hsich, G., Kenney, K., Gibbs, C. J. Jr, *et al.* (1996). The 14–3–3 brain protein in cerebrospinal fluid as a marker for spongiform encephalopathies. *N. Eng. J. Med.*, **335**, 924–30.

Lee, H. S., Sambuughin, N., Cervenakova, L., *et al.* (1999). Ancestral origins and worldwide distribution of the PRNP 200K mutation causing familial Creutzfeldt–Jakob disease. *Am. J. Hum. Genet.*, **64**, 1063–70.

Pearl, G. S. and Anderson, R. E. (1989). Creutzfeldt–Jakob disease: high caudate signal on magnetic resonance imaging. *South. Med. J.*, **82**, 1177–80.

Piccardo, P., Dlouhy, S. R., Lievens, P. J. M., *et al.* (1998). Phenotypic variability of Gerstmann-Sträussler-Scheinker disease is associated with prion protein heterogeneity. *J. Neuropathol. Exp. Neurol.*, **57**, 979–88.

Pocchiari, M., Salvatore, M., and Cutruzzolá, F. (1993). A new point mutation of the prion protein gene in Creutzfeldt–Jakob disease. *Ann. Neurol.*, **34**, 802–7.

Saiz, A., Marin, C., Tolosa, E., and Graus, F. (1998). Diagnostic usefulness of the determination of protein 14-3-3 in cerebrospinal fluid in Creutzfeldt–Jakob disease. *Neurologia*, **13**, 324–8 (Article in Spanish).

Sellar, R. J., Will, R. G., and Zeidler, M. (1997). MR imaging of new variant CJD: the pulvinar sign. *Neuroradiology*, **39**, S53 (abstract).

Sano, M., Ernesho, C., Thomas, R. G., *et al.* (1997). A controlled that of seligiline, alpha-tocopheral or both as treatment for Alzheimer's disease *N. Eng. J. Med.* (17) 1216: 220.

Steinhoff, B. J., Racker, S., Herrendorf, G., *et al.* (1996). Accuracy and reliability of periodic sharp wave complexes in Creutzfeldt–Jakob disease. *Arch. Neurol.*, **53**, 162–6.

WHO Infection control guidelines for transmissable spongiform encephalopathies. Report of WHO Constultation, Geneve Switzerland, 23–26 March 1999, WHO/ CDS/ CSR/ APH/ 2000

Will, R. G., Alperovitch, A., Poser, S., *et al.* (1998). Descriptive epidemiology of Creutzfeldt–Jakob disease in six European countries, 1993–1995. *Ann. Neurol.*, **43**, 763–7.

Will, R. G., Ironside J. W., Zeidler M., *et al.* A new variant of Creutzfeldt-Jakob disease in the UK. (1996) *Lancet*, **347**, 921–5.

Yoon, S. S., Chan, S., Chin, S., Lee, K., and Goodman, R. R. (1995). MRI of Creutzfeldt–Jakob disease: asymmetric high signal intensity of the basal ganglia. *Neurology*, **45**, 1932–3.

Zerr, J., Boderuer, M., Gefeller, O., *et al.* (1998). Defection of 14-3-3 protein in the cerebrospinal fluid supports in the diagnosis of Creutzfeldt-Jakob disease *Ann. Neurol.* **1**, 683–4.

17 Inflammatory and infective disorders

Heather C. Wilson and Neil Scolding

1 Introduction

The range and breadth of diseases of the nervous system caused by immunological, infective, or inflammatory disturbances is very large. It includes 'primary' or idiopathic neuroimmune disorders, which may affect any part of the neuraxis (e.g. multiple sclerosis, Guillain-Barré syndrome), and which are very familiar to neurologists. 'Secondary' disorders, where the neurological disturbance reflects involvement of the nervous system in a systemic inflammatory disease, are no less common than idiopathic immune disorders, but most neurologists are rather less familiar and comfortable with them. In this account we can necessarily provide only a brief overview; and our aim is not to be encyclopaedically inclusive, but to rather to follow William Morris's advice, and aim to 'have nothing in … that [we] do not know to be useful or believe to be beautiful'; we therefore offer a summary of those diseases which are either reasonably common, or which illustrate principles of particular interest and relevance. Prion-related disorders are covered elsewhere; Chapters 16 and 18. Where possible, we will point out particular features which might direct the physician (or psychiatrist) towards specific diseases, and approaches to diagnosis. The management of these rare and often life-threatening disorders is beyond the scope of this chapter (see Scolding 1999).

2 Multiple sclerosis

Multiple sclerosis (MS) is an inflammatory disease of the central nervous system of unknown aetiology, characterized by widespread multifocal demyelination within the white matter of the brain and spinal cord. MS commonly presents with episodes of sensory or motor disturbance, incoordination, a characteristic eye movement disorder, internuclear ophthalmoplegia, or with visual symptoms due to optic neuritis. The typical clinical course is one of discrete episodes (relapsing remitting MS) but 50% of these patients develop progressive neurological deficits (secondary progressive MS) within ten years. 10–20% of patients have progressive disease from onset, without clear relapses or remissions (primary progressive MS).

2.1 Cognitive dysfunction

Some degree of cognitive impairment is present in 40% of MS sufferers in the community and 50–60% of hospitalized cases. Particularly severe cognitive deficits are seen in primary progressive disease. Although more usually a feature of advanced disease and correlated with the EDSS score, cognitive dysfunction may be one of the earliest features of MS. Though often subtle, it has an impact on work, social contact, sexual function, and activities of daily living.

The pattern of cognitive deficits seen in MS has been well characterized although (like the physical signs) there is a wide degree of variation between patients. The pattern is characteristic of diseases involving the white matter. In contrast with the changes seen in Alzheimer's disease, deficits are seen in working memory, attention, executive functions, abstracting abilities, learning, and visuo-motor performance, whilst intelligence and language functions are relatively preserved (Rao 1995; Kujula *et al.* 1996).

Deficits in executive function are seen in MS but not all executive skills are affected to the same extent. Memory is the most frequently impaired cognitive function. While primary memory capacity (digit span) is near normal, the storage and processing aspects of working memory are affected, patients performing poorly on tasks requiring spontaneous recall of information, with slowing of information processing speed (auditory more than visual). The changes probably represent both an encoding and a retrieval problem. These deficits may be seen even in patients with clinically isolated lesions (optic neuritis, spinal cord, or brain stem syndromes), a stage when cognitive impairment is subtle or asymptomatic (Pelosi *et al.* 1997); attentional deficits (auditory and visual) may also be identified at this stage.

2.1.1 Natural history of cognitive dysfunction

Some patients develop neuropsychological changes early, others never do. Those who are initially cognitively preserved remain stable over time but those with early mild cognitive deterioration continue to deteriorate in parallel with physical deterioration (Kujula *et al.* 1997). As a rule, deficits tend to be more pronounced in chronic progressive disease, whereas in relapsing remitting MS cognitive impairment remains relatively mild with transient exacerbations during relapses (Foong *et al.* 1998).

2.2 Psychiatric manifestations

Patients with established MS are much more vulnerable to psychiatric illness than the general population (Minden and Schiffer 1990). Transient mood changes, irritability, and anxiety affect two-thirds of patients with MS in the course of a year. There is a lifetime prevalence of major depression of 40–50% (Minden *et al.* 1987). Affective symptoms may begin early in disease, even in patients with clinically isolated lesions. Physical symptoms and signs are almost always present but are often overlooked or misinterpreted. Affective symptoms are commoner during exacerbations and in the chronic progressive group but are not closely correlated to physical disability. Depression and cognitive function are not correlated. There is an increased association with bipolar affective disorder (Minden and Schiffer 1990), and hypomanic episodes can occur, often in association with steroid treatment. Euphoria and eutonia (lack of concern about the disease) are well recognized but rare symptoms occurring in about 10% of patients with established MS and likely to be a clinical expression of executive dysfunction. Lability of mood is seen rarely and may represent a frontal disconnection syndrome caused by pontine, brain stem, or periventricular disease.

2.3 Clinicopathological correlations

Cognitive test performance is related to total cerebral lesion load (Rovaris *et al.* 1998; Rao 1995) and to cerebral atrophy, as estimated by lateral and third ventricle and corpus callosum size. Conversely psychiatric morbidity is not highly correlated to severity of MRI abnormality, with the exception of euphoria and eutonia (Ron 1999). MRI total lesion load is greater in patients with progressive disease than in relapsing remitting MS.

Attempts have been made to relate the location of cerebral white matter lesions to specific patterns of cognitive dysfunction but it is difficult to disentangle the effect of a given lesion when widespread pathology is present. However, short-lived psychoses are associated with increased MRI lesion load around both temporal horns, and frontal lobe lesions have been correlated to amount of perseveration on WCST (Foong *et al.* 1997). Preliminary studies using PET scanning have demonstrated reduced uptake in both frontal lobes and the left temporal lobe in association with reduced verbal fluency and verbal memory deficits in MS.

3 Systemic inflammatory diseases

3.1 Systemic lupus erythematosus (SLE)

SLE, like many autoimmune diseases, occurs perhaps 20 times more commonly in women than in men. Blacks are more commonly affected than whites. Fever and general malaise are accompanied by skin changes — classically, the malar butterfly rash, though various other non-specific manifestations, most typically, photosensitivity, are also described — and a largely symmetrical, non-erosive arthritis affecting large and small joints. Glomerulonephritis, pleurisy and pneumonitis, pericarditis and Libmann-Sachs endocarditis, and haematological disorders — anaemia, thrombocytopoenia, leukocytopoenia, and the generation of circulating anticoagulants — are among the commoner complications. Other laboratory abnormalities include the presence of a variety of autoantibodies (illustrated in Table 17.1).

The diagnosis — particularly for research and therapeutic trial purposes — is now commonly based on the widely accepted revised diagnostic criteria (Table 17.2) suggested by the American College of Rheumatology (Tan *et al.* 1982). The presence of any four (or more) of the listed features, 'serially or simultaneously, during *any interval* of observation' [my italics] are sufficient for the diagnosis, with an estimated specificity and sensitivity of 96%.

Table 17.1 Autoantibodies and their connective tissue disease associations

Immunofluorescence pattern	Antibody	Disease associations
Rim ANA	Anti-native DNA (anti-dsDNA)	SLE (50%)
Homogeneous ANA	Anti-histone	Drug-induced lupus (97%)
NB: low titre (< 1:320) in normals		
Speckled ANA	Anti-Ro (SS-A)	Sjögren's (75%) SLE (30%)
	Anti-La (SS-B)	Sjögren's (60%) SLE (15%)
	Anti-Scl-70	Systemic sclerosis (50%)
	Anti-Sm	SLE (75%)
	Anti-RNP (anti-U1-nRNP)	MCTD (95%) SLE (30%)
Nucleolar ANA	Anti-PM-Scl	? Identifies polymyositis/ scleroderma overlap
Other organelles	Anti-centromere	Systemic sclerosis (85%)

Table 17.2 American College of Rheumatology diagnostic criteria for SLE (Tan *et al.* 1982).

'a person shall be said to have SLE if four or more of the 11 criteria are present, serially or simultaneously, during any interval of observation' (Tan et al. 1982)
Malar flush
Discoid rash
Photosensitivity
Oral ulcers
Arthritis
Serositis (– pleurisy or pericarditis)
Renal disorder (proteinuria > 0.5 g/24 h or cellular casts)
Neurological disorder (seizures, psychosis; other causes excluded)
Haematological disorder (haemolytic anaemia, leukopoenia, or lymphopoenia on two or more occasions, or thrombocytopoenia)
Immunological disorder M LE cells, or anti-dsDNA or anti-Sm or persistent false positive syphilis serology
Anti-nuclear autoantibodies

3.1.1 Neurological complications

Neurological involvement in SLE is not rare, estimates offering an incidence ranging from 25–75% (Futrell *et al.* 1992; Boumpas *et al.* 1995.), 50% representing a reasonable consensus figure. Neurological *presentation*, however, is uncommon, occurring in perhaps 3% of cases (Tola *et al.* 1992). In established SLE, CNS involvement is a poor prognostic sign: a five year survival figure of 55% has been quoted, compared to 75% for patients without neurological features, while epidemiological studies show neurological disease to be second only to renal involvement as the cause of death, excluding iatrogenic causes (Rosner *et al.* 1982).

Cerebral lupus is not a single clinical or pathological entity (Kaell *et al.* 1986). The wide variety of complications reflects two broad pathogenetic mechanisms. Thromboembolic phenomena occur, triggered either by changes in endothelial surfaces, or by disturbances of the coagulation system (including lupus anticoagulant activity). Secondly, there are immunological events more directly affecting the target tissue — neurons or glia — mediated by antibodies, cytokines, lymphocytes, or perhaps particularly nitric oxide (Brundin *et al.* 1998).

Headache (including that associated with dural sinus thrombosis), fits, myelitis, strokes and movement disorders (especially chorea), ataxia and brain stem abnormalities, and cranial and peripheral neuropathies all are seen in the context of SLE. However, in the realm of neurological autoinflammatory disease, SLE has long been recognized particularly to be associated with psychiatric and cognitive disturbances.

3.1.2 Behavioural, cognitive, and neuropsychiatric changes in SLE

While pleomorphism is the rule, three relatively distinct patterns can be discerned:

(a) 'Pure' behavioural or psychiatric illness without clouding of consciousness.

(b) Dementia.

(c) An acute or subacute encephalopathy/encephalitis (organic confusional syndrome or delirium).

Affective disorders, particularly depression, are very widely observed. More pronounced psychotic disease, including schizophrenic syndromes with paranoid or catatonic symptoms, visual and auditory hallucinations, and conversion disorders are also moderately common complications of SLE (Johnson and Richardson 1968), one carefully documented prospective study suggesting a prevalence of 20–25% (Hay 1994). Recurrent, episodic symptoms are common.

Dementia is a commonly accepted complication, though little detailed published information is available. An incidence of cognitive changes in lupus of 55% has been suggested (Denburg *et al.* 1997) but an important and well-validated observation is that cognitive dysfunction in SLE is very often reversible (Hanly *et al.* 1997). This does not apply, however, to multi-infarct dementia, which is also described in lupus (Asherson *et al.* 1989; Briley *et al.* 1989), presumably a consequence of SLE-related cerebro- or cardiovascular complications.

An encephalopathic presentation, with clouding of consciousness with or without headache, often with seizures and usually without focal neurological signs, is also well recognized in SLE. Paranoia, delusions, hallucinations, and excessive restlessness are common. Some have termed this entity *cerebral lupus*, though to avoid confusion with other cerebral manifestations of SLE, perhaps *lupus encephalopathy* is preferable. CSF examination may reveal a raised protein level and a neutrophil or lymphocyte pleocytosis. It is vital in such cases to exclude infectious complications of immune suppressants or steroids, which have become a major cause of death in patients with SLE. Bacterial (including mycobacterial), viral, or fungal meningitis or meningoencephalitis may be seen, and should be sought with vigour.

3.1.3 Diagnosis of neuropsychiatric lupus

The fundamental importance of excluding as a matter of urgency secondary and/or iatrogenic problems — drug-related, metabolic, and especially infectives cannot be overemphasized. Steroids are commonly used in lupus, carrying their own well-described behavioural complications, while immune suppression from these and other agents carries the obvious risk of opportunistic (CNS) infection.

The implications of serological tests have been mentioned above, though an ANA titre more dilute than 1:160 should not be considered significant (Homburger 1995). Lupus anticoagulant activity and anti-cardiolipin antibodies should be sought. Serum anti-ribosomal P antibodies, which can bind to neurons, suggesting a possible direct pathogenetic role, may correlate with the presence of psychiatric disease in lupus (Watanabe *et al.* 1996), and their titre with disease activity. Anti-neuronal antibodies and ANA may be found in CSF (Isshi and Hirohata 1998).

MRI changes are common, though neither specific (Miller *et al.* 1992) nor wholly sensitive — particularly in psychiatric or organic brain disease. The MRI may be normal (West *et al.* 1995), which is hardly surprising since the brain in such cases can be neuropathologically normal (Devinsky *et al.* 1988). Neither MR spectroscopy (Davie *et al.* 1995), nor PET scanning (Sailer *et al.* 1997) appears helpful in the diagnosis. SPECT scanning may show perfusion defects which, while also lacking specificity (the same appearances are seen in vasculitis, for example), may be useful in monitoring disease activity (Kodama *et al.* 1995). Cerebral angiography is often abnormal (Weingarten *et al.* 1997), and also may be important in excluding cerebral venous thrombosis. CSF oligoclonal band analysis is positive in up to 50% patients with CNS lupus and, interestingly, these changes can resolve with successful immunotherapy (West *et al.* 1995). A skin biopsy can be extremely helpful in suspected lupus (West *et al.* 1995).

3.2 Cerebral vasculitis

The vasculitides are an heterogeneous group of disorders which share certain pathological features, in particular intramural inflammation and necrotic changes within the walls of blood vessels. They are classified according to pathological features and vessel size (Table 17.3). CNS vasculitis can occur secondary to any of the systemic vasculitides (Moore and Calabrese 1994; Sigal 1987); additionally, primary isolated vasculitis of the CNS is recognized, where little or no inflammation is apparent systemically. In both, neurological features arise from inflammation and necrosis of the vasculature — principally, through infarction. The cause of the pathological process remains largely a matter of speculation, with much experimental work concentrating on the possible roles of antibody attack of the vasculature, immune complex deposition, and direct and indirect effects of *anti-neutrophil cytoplasmic antibodies* — ANCA-related vasculitis (Jennette *et al.* 1994).

3.2.1 The clinical features of CNS vasculitis

Focal or multifocal infarction, or diffuse ischaemia, affecting any part of the brain, explain the protean manifestations, wide variation in disease activity, course and severity, and the absence of a typical clinical picture (Kissel 1989; Moore 1994; Moore and Calabrese 1994). However, three broad clinical categories of presentation may be delineated (Scolding *et al.* 1997):

(a) Resembling atypical multiple sclerosis ('MS-plus') — with a relapsing–remitting course, and features such as optic neuropathy and brain stem episodes, but also those less common in multiple sclerosis — seizures, severe and persisting headaches, encephalopathic episodes, or hemispheric stroke-like episodes.

(b) Acute or subacute encephalopathy, with headache with an acute confusional state, progressing to drowsiness and coma.

(c) Intracranial mass lesion — with headache, drowsiness, focal signs, and (often) raised intracranial pressure.

This grouping carries neither pathological nor therapeutic implications, but is intended merely to help improve recognition of cerebral vasculitis. Systemic features — fever and night sweats, livedo reticulares, or oligoarthropathy — may be present even in so-called isolated CNS vasculitis.

3.2.2 Neuropsychiatric features

Most studies mention the existence of behavioural features (Kissel 1989; Nishino *et al.* 1993), but there have been few systematic studies of psychiatric complications of cerebral vasculitis, while information concerning cognitive deficits is still more sparse. This is perhaps the more

Table 17.3 Classification of vasculitis

Dominant vessel involved	Primary	Secondary
Large arteries	Giant cell arteritis Takayasu's arteritis	Aortitis with rheumatoid disease; infection (e.g. syphilis)
Medium arteries	Classical polyarteritis nodosa Kawasaki disease	Infection (e.g. hepatitis B)
Small vessels and medium arteries	Wegener's granulomatosis Churg-Strauss syndrome Microscopic polyangiitis	Vasculitis with rheumatoid disease, SLE, Sjögren's syndrome, drugs, infection (e.g. HIV)
Small vessels	Henoch-Schönlein purpura Essential cryoglobulinaemia Cutaneous leukocytoclastic vasculitis	Drugs (e.g. sulfonamides) Infection (e.g. hepatitis C)

unexpected since literature reviews quote the very high incidence of 30–55% for confusion, 'possible psychiatric disorder', 'mental impairment', or 'mental change' (Younger *et al.* 1988), without exploring the nature of these disturbances, or providing detailed descriptions of the clinical psychopathology. Mild depression is said to be very common, hallucinations are not rare. We have seen severe amnestic deficits only partially responding to otherwise successful immunotherapy.

3.2.3 Differential diagnosis

Numerous disorders may cause a combination of headache, encephalopathy, strokes, seizures, and focal deficits or acute or subacute onset, and must therefore be considered in the differential diagnosis of cerebral vasculitis (Table 17.4).

3.2.4 Confirming cerebral vasculitis

No single simple investigation is universally useful in confirming cerebral vasculitis (Moore 1994; Moore and Calabrese 1994; Scolding *et al.* 1997). Serological markers, including ANCA, are important (Hankey 1991; Moore 1994). Spinal fluid examination is, like ESR testing, often abnormal, but lacks specificity, with changes in cell count and/or protein in 65–80% of cases. CSF oligoclonal immunoglobulin band analysis in cerebral vasculitis showed various (and varying) abnormalities in 3/7 cases (Scolding *et al.* 1997). Magnetic resonance imaging may disclose non-specific ischaemic areas, periventricular white matter lesions, haemorrhagic lesions, and parenchymal or meningeal enhancing areas — but may be normal (Greenan *et al.* 1992; Stone *et al.* 1994). Contrast angiography may show segmental (often multifocal) narrowing and areas of localized dilatation or beading, often with areas of occlusion, rarely also with aneurysms (Koo and Massey 1988), though these changes are also non-specific (Hankey 1991). The false negative rate for angiography is between 30–80% (Hankey 1991; Vollmer *et al.* 1993), with a 10% risk of transient neurological deficit, and permanent deficit in 1% (Hellmann *et al.* 1992). Indium-labelled white cell nuclear scanning and examination of the ocular vasculature may be useful (Scolding *et al.* 1997).

Table 17.4 Some systemic disorders which may mimic cerebral vasculitis

Infective endocarditis	Fibromuscular dysplasia
Atrial myxoma	Fabry's disease
Multiple cholesterol emboli	Moyamoya disease
Thrombotic thrombocytopoenic purpura	Amyloid angiopathy
Cerebral sinus thrombosis	CADASIL
Köhlmeyer-Degos disease	Marfan's syndrome
Susac's syndrome	Pseudoxanthoma elasticum
Mitochondrial disease	Homocysteinuria
Infections, including Lyme disease, AIDS	Ehlers-Danlos syndrome
Sarcoidosis	Radiation vasculopathy
Lupus and anti-phospholipid disease	
Behçet's syndrome	

Histopathological confirmation, biopsying an (MRI-)abnormal area of brain where possible, or by 'blind' biopsy, incorporating meninges, and non-dominant temporal white and grey matter (Moore 1989), is important. Biopsy may reveal an underlying process not otherwise suspected with profound therapeutic implications, such as infective or neoplastic (principally lymphomatous) vasculopathies, but is not a trivial procedure, carrying a risk of serious morbidity estimated at 0.5–2% (Barza and Pauker 1980).

A vasculitic process having been confirmed, the specific defining characteristics of the primary and secondary vasculitides (Table 17.3) must be painstakingly sought (Sigal 1987).

3.3 Sarcoidosis

Sarcoidosis is a multisystem granulomatous disease of unknown aetiology which has a propensity to affect the lungs and, in approximately 5% of patients, the nervous system (Zajicek *et al.* 1999). Optic and other cranial neuropathies (especially involving the facial nerve), often due to meningeal infiltration, and brain stem and spinal cord disease are the commoner manifestations.

Cognitive and neuropsychiatric abnormalities are reported in approximately 10% of patients with neurosarcoid, but in the majority of these patients, depression of questionable relationship to direct CNS involvement is postulated (Wirnsberger *et al.* 1998; Drent *et al.* 1998. More pronounced psychotic or dementing neuropsychiatric disease is considerably less common, though recent studies are lacking. There are isolated cases reports of serious cognitive or psychiatric manifestations of neurosarcoidosis (see O'Brien *et al.* 1994; Bona *et al.* 1998).

Serum ACE may be elevated, as may that in the cerebrospinal fluid; more general abnormalities of protein or cell count are present in over 80% of cases at presentation in the British series (Zajicek *et al.* 1999), and oligoclonal bands may be present (McLean *et al.* 1995a). Whole body Gallium scanning remains a useful indicator of systemic disease. Cranial MRI may show multiple white matter lesions or meningeal enhancement (Lawrence *et al.* 1974). The diagnosis is confirmed where possible by biopsy, either of cerebral or meningeal tissue, or of lung or conjunctiva where appropriate.

3.4 Behçet's disease

Behçet's disease is a chronic relapsing multisystem inflammatory disorder whose clinical manifestations vary. The classical triad of recurrent uveitis with oral and genital aphthous ulceration remains clinically useful, though formal diagnostic criteria have since been proposed and generally adopted (Rigby *et al.* 1995). Recurrent oral ulceration (at least three times in one 12 month period) is an absolute criterion, with any two of:

(i) Recurrent genital ulceration.

(ii) Uveitis (anterior or posterior) or retinal vasculitis.

(iii) Skin lesions, including erythema nodosum, or acneiform nodules, pseudofolliculitis or papulopustular lesions.

(iv) A positive pathergy test.

In total, approximately one-third of patients with Behçet's disease develop some form of neurological involvement (O'Duffy 1994), although some studies have suggested a rate of 5% may be more accurate (part of this discrepancy may be due to the variable inclusion of headache as a specific complication — this, when isolated, does not carry serious long-term implications) (Akman *et al.* 1996).

Cerebral venous sinus thrombosis is one of the principal and more specific serious complications (Wechsler *et al.* 1992); others include sterile meningoencephalitis, encephalopathy, brain stem syndromes, cranial neuropathies, and cortical sensory and motor deficits. Investigation may reveal an active CSF with or without oligoclonal IgA and IgM, but not IgG, bands (McLean *et al.* 1995*b*). Evoked potentials may be diagnostically useful (Stigsby *et al.* 1994). Non-specific MRI abnormalities occur (Wechsler *et al.* 1993).

Psychiatric manifestations have not been widely reported in large scale studies, but some studies have suggested an incidence of between 10–38% (Mousa *et al.* 1986; Farah *et al.* 1998). It is suggested that the most serious central nervous system (CNS) manifestation in Behçet's disease is a slowly progressive dementia, which may respond to methotrexate treatment (Hirohata *et al.* 1998).

3.5 Coeliac disease

Coeliac disease (non-tropical sprue) is an immunologically-mediated disorder resulting from intolerance to dietary gluten, a protein present in wheat and many other cereals (Maki and Collin 1997). Affected individuals develop weight loss with steatorrhoea and/or diarrhoea, with clinical evidence of malabsorption. In common with other enteropathies, neurological sequelae of a predictable nature may complicate coeliac disease as a direct consequence of malabsorption. Depression is common in coeliac patients; it may respond to treatment with pyridoxine and is accompanied by reduced central monoamine metabolism (Hallert *et al.* 1983).

CNS complications apparently unrelated to deficiency states may also occur in perhaps 10% of patients (Finelli *et al.* 1980). Rarely, vasculitis is responsible (Mumford *et al.* 1996; Rush *et al.* 1986), but the cause of the most commonly-described and distinctive CNS association, cerebellar, or spino-cerebellar degeneration remains unresolved. The clinical picture may also include brain stem eye movement disorders, myoclonus, and epilepsy.

Major psychiatric complications are well-described as a significant cause of morbidity, and have been studied in detail (Hallert and Derefeldt 1982). Dementia is also recorded, though few details are offered (Hallert and Astrom 1983). A fatal outcome is not uncommon (Kinney *et al.* 1982).

3.6 The thyroid gland

Hyperthyroidism and myxoedema both carry neurological complications generally considered direct consequences of abnormal thyroxine levels: anxiety, tremor, occasionally chorea, etc., in thyrotoxicosis, and lethargy (even progressing to coma), myopathy, and dementia in hypothyroidism. The latter, with its attendant psychiatric disturbances ('myxoedema madness') responds to (judicious) thyroxine hormone replacement (Cook and Boyle 1986). By contrast, the ophthalmoplegia of Grave's disease is thought to be immunologically driven, and an encephalopathy of apparently immunological, not endocrine, origin is also described (Leonard *et al.* 1984).

Hashimoto's encephalopathy exhibits female:male ratio of up to 9:1. It is suggested that two main types of presentation can be delineated (Kothbauer *et al.* 1996). Stroke-like episodes, with or without mild cognitive impairment, focal or generalized seizures, and episodes of encephalopathy, are seen, with a relapsing–remitting course. The second group exhibits a more diffuse progressive disease, almost invariably with progressive dementia and often with psychotic features. These patients may also suffer seizures, myoclonus, and/or tremor and ataxia, but most, in contrast to the first group, have no focal neurological deficits (Kothbauer *et al.* 1996).

Imaging by CT or even MR is often normal (Shaw *et al.* 1991; Barker *et al.* 1996), as is angiography, though isotope brain scanning may show patchy uptake. Spinal fluid examination may reveal a raised protein level but typically a normal cell count. Most cases are clinically and biochemically euthyroid at presentation, but hypo- and hyperthyroid cases are reported (Shaw *et al.* 1991; Barker *et al.* 1996).

Very high titres of anti-thyroid antibodies are found, usually anti-microsomal. Speculative pathogenetic roles include cross-reactivity with neural antigens, or precipitating vasculitis through immune complex formation (Barker *et al.* 1996). An association of Hashimoto's thyroiditis with vasculitis in other tissues has also been reported (Barker *et al.* 1996; Nicholson *et al.* 1984).

4 Infectious diseases

4.1 Human immunodeficiency virus-1 (HIV-1) infection

The late stages of HIV infection are frequently complicated by a dementing process known as the *AIDS dementia complex* or *HIV-1 associated cognitive/motor complex*. 20–30% of AIDS patients eventually develop dementia, half within two years of an AIDS diagnosis, and dementia is the AIDS defining illness in 3%. The condition is classified into two groups according to the severity of clinical manifestations and their impact upon the patient's life. The severe group comprises *HIV-1 associated dementia* (previously referred to as subacute encephalitis, HIV encephalopathy, or AIDS related dementia) and *HIV-1 associated myelopathy* (formerly within the HIV encephalopathy group), the distinguishing factor being the relative prominence of symptoms due to vacuolar myelopathy over cognitive dysfunction. Both are AIDS-defining conditions. The mild form, known as *HIV-1 associated minor cognitive/motor disorder* (formerly HIV-1 associated neuro-cognitive disorder or HIV associated neuro-behavioural abnormalities), is not an AIDS-defining illness (Working group of AAN AIDS task force 1991).

Neuropathological features are widespread reactive astrocytosis, diffuse myelin pallor (due to oedema from leakage of serum proteins, not myelin loss), macrophage infiltration, microglial nodules, and multinucleated giant cells. Neuronal damage is manifest as dendritic pruning, simplification of synaptic contacts, and neuron loss (Lipton and Gendelman 1995).

The clinical picture is one of subcortical dementia with slowness and imprecision of cognition and motor control. Early signs include difficulty with concentration and mental agility and mild forgetfulness. Apathy, lethargy, loss of sexual drive, blunted affect, social withdrawal, irritability, emotional lability, inflexibility to change, and defects in abstract reasoning are common features. Speed of information processing, motor functioning, visuospatial skills, and verbal responses are also slowed (Working group of AAN AIDS task force 1991). Cognitive decline is progressive and eventually leads to a severe global dementia. Motor abnormalities are initially asymptomatic with slowing of rapid movements of the eyes and extremities apparent on examination. Early symptoms such as unsteadiness of gait, limb incoordination, leg weakness, and tremor progress to a spastic, ataxic quadriparesis with the emergence of primitive reflexes.

The majority of neurological complications of AIDS develop during the later stages of infection (Table 17.5). CNS involvement may present as focal or diffuse disease. The common causes of focal disease are toxoplasmosis, primary CNS lymphoma, progressive multifocal leuko encephalopathy (PML), and cryptococcus or TB meningitis. AIDS dementia complex is the

Table 17.5 Late onset, diffuse cognitive impairment in HIV

Alertness preserved	Alertness impaired
AIDS dementia complex	Toxic complications of drugs
CMV encephalitis	Metabolic disease from dysfunction of other organs
Encephalitic form of toxoplasmosis	Sepsis or DIC
Reactive depression	

major cause of diffuse CNS impairment in HIV infection, but must be distinguished from other causes more amenable to treatment; pre-morbid alcohol and substance use, head trauma, or psychiatric illness must be taken into account (Price 1996).

4.1.1 Course and prognosis

AIDS dementia complex is usually progressive but can remain static or fluctuate with treatment and with the patient's general condition. Prognosis is poor, primarily because of the severe underlying immunosuppression. Established disease has a six month cumulative mortality rate of 67% (Neaton *et al.* 1994).

4.1.2 Pathogenesis

HIV invades the CNS early and persists until death without serious CNS illness in the majority of cases. Induction of AIDS dementia complex may depend upon the capacity of the host immune defence to suppress viral replication within the brain, or upon qualitative differences in the infecting virus strain. Macrophages and microglia are the predominantly infected cell type but it is neuronal injury which underlies the cognitive and motor dysfunction seen in AIDS dementia complex. Neuronal damage occurs via a complex network of cytokines, excitotoxins, and free radical mechanisms triggered by HIV-1-infected or immune-stimulated macrophages, microglia, and astrocytes. The final common pathway to neuronal apoptosis involves over-stimulation of neuronal NMDA receptors and an increase in intra-neuronal Ca^{2+} (Price 1996; Lipton 1997).

Although the severity of systemic illness is correlated with viral load in the blood, the degree of neurological or cognitive involvement is not related to the amount of viral RNA or DNA in the CNS (Johnson *et al.* 1996). Severe deficiency in cell-mediated immunity is the most important determinant of neurological disease, clinical dementia being predominantly seen in late AIDS and correlated to very low CD4 counts (Brew *et al.* 1996). Neither are the neuropathological findings tightly correlated with the degree of cognitive dysfunction. Typical changes are present in up to 80% of post-mortem examinations of AIDS patients but are not present in HIV positive subjects without AIDS (Kibayashi *et al.* 1996). Their incidence is similar in early and late AIDS and in demented and non-demented subjects. However, selective susceptibility and loss of specific neuron populations at certain sites may be associated with cognitive dysfunction. Increasing caudate atrophy on MRI is correlated with worsening of some aspects of neuropsychological function, especially motor domains.

4.1.3 Investigation

Atrophy, particularly of the basal ganglia, is seen on MRI, often with a diffuse or fluffy, multifocal increase in T2 and proton density signal in the white matter and basal ganglia. On MR spectroscopy an increase in brain choline, a component of lipid membranes, precedes the onset of dementia and may reflect an increase in glial cell number or neuronal membrane damage. N-acetyl aspartate falls in severe AIDS dementia, confirming the neuronal loss seen histologically.

CSF analysis is non-specific, showing a mild pleocytosis or slightly elevated protein, β-microglobulin and neopterin levels. Antibodies directed against the HIV-1 envelope proteins gp120 and gp160 are more prevalent in the CSF of patients with dementia than without and may serve as a marker of progression (Lipton 1997).

4.2 Lyme disease

Lyme disease is a multisystem illness caused by infection with tick-borne spirochaetes of the *Borrelia burgdorferi* group. It is prevalent in certain parts of North America, Europe, and Asia, the clinical spectrum of disease varying between these geographical areas, reflecting differences in the virulence and organotropism of local *Borrelia* sub-species and in host response (Halperin 1998).

4.2.1 Clinical features

There are two characteristic skin rashes, erythema chronicum migrans (ECM) occurring early in infection and acrodermatitis chronica atrophica, a chronic late manifestation. Rheumatological involvement may produce a relapsing, migratory, large joint oligo-articular arthropathy or may mimic juvenile rheumatoid arthritis. Carditis can cause conduction defects.

A wide variety of neurological presentations has been described, affecting both the peripheral and central nervous systems (Haass 1998). PNS disease includes mononeuritis multiplex and a classical picture of lymphocytic meningitis with cranial neuritis, often affecting both facial nerves, and a painful, patchy polyradiculoneuritis associated with an aseptic meningitis.

The most commonly discussed CNS manifestation is a form of chronic mild confusional state known as Lyme encephalopathy, originally described in patients with unequivocal systemic manifestations of active Lyme disease. This is a subtle syndrome of memory, mood, and sleep disturbance. Patients complain of memory impairment, difficulty concentrating, irritability, emotional lability, fatigue, and sleep disturbance. In some, the disorder is undoubtedly due to subacute CNS infection with a prominent inflammatory response (Halperin *et al.* 1989); in others it is due to parenchymal dysfunction without apparent CNS infection caused by the indirect toxic and metabolic effects of systemic infection, perhaps involving lymphokine-mediated mechanisms (Kaplan *et al.* 1992). In yet other sero-negative, treatment-refractory, patients with primarily neuropsychiatric symptoms, subjective memory loss is probably of psychological origin (Halperin *et al.* 1990; Krupp *et al.* 1989).

There are numerous anecdotal reports of a variety of neuropsychiatric disorders associated with Lyme disease (Reik *et al.* 1985). Severe cognitive impairment and psychosis can be caused by leukoencephalopathy or cerebral vasculitis, and a rare but severe encephalomyelitis producing spasticity, ataxia, and occasionally seizures or significant cognitive impairment affects 0.1% of patients. Suggestions of a common link between Lyme disease and dementia are probably unfounded given the frequency of dementia in the general population and the worsening of symptoms with intercurrent infection in such patients.

4.2.2 Pathophysiology

In the CNS there is perivascular lymphocytic vasculitis with multifocal encephalitis and periventricular demyelination. Limited tissue damage caused directly by the organism is greatly amplified by a local lymphokine-mediated inflammatory response.

4.2.3 Diagnosis

ECM is so specific that patients should be treated immediately on clinical grounds alone. Culture of serum or CSF is difficult as the organism is fastidious and replicates slowly. A two-step sero-diagnostic test for anti-*Borrelia* antibodies (ELISA confirmed with Western blot) is reasonably specific but as many as 25% of patients with CNS borreliosis have negative serology. A more sensitive and specific marker of exposure is IgG or IgM production against *Borrelia* outer surface proteins, OspA and OspC. Most patients with CNS borreliosis have an elevated CSF protein but CSF culture is positive in only 10% and PCR for *Borrelia* DNA is also unreliable. Evidence of intrathecal synthesis of specific anti-*Borrelia* antibodies is a highly specific index of CNS infection (Halperin *et al.* 1989), the only significant false positive results being those seen with neuro-syphilis. Overall sensitivity is less perfect; in patients with indolent, less inflammatory CNS dysfunction only 50% have detectable intrathecal antibodies. Intrathecal IgM OspA reactivity may prove to be an earlier, more sensitive, and specific marker for CNS infection.

4.3 Whipple's disease

Whipple's disease is an uncommon multisystem disorder characterized by arthropathy, respiratory symptoms, anaemia, fever, erythema nodosum, and severe wasting in addition to steatorrhoea and abdominal distension (Fleming *et al.* 1988). The causative organism, *Tropheryma whippelii*, was identified only relatively recently (Relman *et al.* 1992; Wilson *et al.* 1991). Approximately 10% of patients have neurological involvement; 5% are said to present in this way (Brown *et al.* 1990), and a wide variety of features may be seen (Table 17.6).

However, it is reported that commoner than all the above are psychiatric or behavioural difficulties: of 84 reported patients, cognitive changes were recorded in 71%, with episodes of encephalopathy in 50%, and psychiatric abnormalities in 44% (Louis *et al.* 1996). Dementia is

Table 17.6 The neurological features of Whipple's disease (Louis *et al.* 1996)

Supranuclear gaze palsy	51%
Pyramidal signs	37%
Hypothalamic features — somnolence, polydipsia, increased appetite, hypogonadism	31%
Myoclonus	25%
Oculo-masticatory myorhythmia	20%
Cranial neuropathies	25%
Fits	23%
'Eye disease' — keratitis, uveitis, papilloedema, ptosis	23%
Ataxia	20%

not uncommon, usually in the context of other features, though presentation with progressive dementia, accompanied neither by neurological abnormalities nor systemic signs is well described; importantly, successful reversal of cognitive impairment with antibiotic treatment may be seen (Ryser *et al.* 1984), though an unfavourable outcome (despite appropriate treatment) is also possible (Durand *et al.* 1997). Psychosis, responding to treatment (with sulfamethoxazole and trimethoprim) is also reported (Verhagen *et al.* 1996).

4.3.1 Diagnosis and management

Diagnosis can be extremely difficult. Up to 20% of cases of cerebral Whipple's disease occur in the absence of gastrointestinal or indeed other systemic symptoms (Adams *et al.* 1987; Louis *et al.* 1996; Wroe *et al.* 1991). CT and MRI scanning may be normal, although the latter in other cases reveals abnormalities which are essentially non-specific — multiple high signal intensity areas on T2-weighted images, often near the hypothalamus. Enhancing mass lesions warranting biopsy have also been reported (Wroe *et al.* 1991).

Spinal fluid examination reveals an elevated protein and/or raised cell count in approximately 50% of cases (Louis *et al.* 1996); widely varying ratios of monocytes and polymorphonucleocytes are reported. Pathognomic PAS-positive bacilli are identified in the CSF in 29% of samples (Louis *et al.* 1996; Feurle *et al.* 1979); repeat spinal fluid examination may be necessary before organisms are identified. Approximately 30% of reported cases have a normal or noninformative small bowel biopsy (Feurle *et al.* 1979; Finelli *et al.* 1977), though electron microscopy is a vital part of this investigation — none of the 14 non-diagnostic small bowel biopsies in one series had undergone electron microscopy (Louis *et al.* 1996). Lymph node biopsy can also be extremely useful. Polymerase chain reaction analysis of blood, lymph node, spinal fluid, small bowel tissue, or brain (Lynch *et al.* 1997) is increasingly used as a diagnostic test (Cohen *et al.* 1996).

5 Key points

1   A wide variety of immunological, inflammatory, and infective conditions can cause early onset dementia or other neuropsychiatric disorders.

2   These include both primary neurological diseases, such as multiple sclerosis, and systemic disorders, such as vasculitis and systemic lupus erythematosus.

3   In the latter diseases, presentation with cognitive or neuro-behavioural abnormalities in the absence of systemic features, while not common, is well-described.

4   In many of these conditions, the cognitive abnormalities may be reversed, or their progression halted, by appropriate and timely antimicrobial, immunosuppressant, or immunomodulatory therapy.

5   In young patients with rapidly progressive or relapsing–remitting cognitive decline, these disorders should be carefully excluded.

6   This search should include historical enquiry and physical examination for clues suggesting systemic infection or inflammation, including risk factors for HIV infection, tick bites, skin rashes, arthralgia, fever, night sweats.

7   MRI may give some indication, albeit non-specific, of a non-degenerative aetiology — but may also be normal.

8   Other investigations should include extensive autoimmune and infective serology, including ANCA, ANA, and anti-thyroid antibodies, chest X-ray and spinal fluid analysis, SPECT, and possibly labelled leukocyte scanning.

References

Adams, M., Rhyner, P. A., Day, J., DeArmond, S., and Smuckler, E. A. (1987). Whipple's disease confined to the central nervous system. *Ann. Neurol.*, **21**, 104–8.

Akman, D. G., Baykan, K. B., Serdaroglu, P., Gurvit, H., Yurdakul, S., Yazici, H., *et al.* (1996). Seven-year follow-up of neurologic involvement in Behcet syndrome. *Arch. Neurol.*, **53**, 691–4.

Asherson, R. A., Khamashta, M. A., Gil, A., Vazquez, J. J., Chan, O., Baguley, E., *et al.* (1989). Cerebrovascular disease and antiphospholipid antibodies in systemic lupus erythematosus, lupus-like disease, and the primary antiphospholipid syndrome [see comments]. *Am. J. Med.*, **86**, 391–9.

Barker, R., Zajicek, J., and Wilkinson, I. (1996). Thyrotoxic Hashimoto's encephalopathy. *J. Neurol. Neurosurg. Psychiatry*, **60**, 234.

Barza, M. and Pauker, S. G. (1980). The decision to biopsy, treat, or wait in suspected herpes encephalitis. *Ann. Intern. Med.*, **92**, 641–9.

Bona, J. R., Fackler, S. M., Fendley, M. J., and Nemeroff, C. B. (1998). Neurosarcoidosis as a cause of refractory psychosis: a complicated case report. *Am. J. Psychiatry*, **155**, 1106–8.

Boumpas, D. T., Austin, H. A., I. I. I., Fessler, B. J., Balow, J. E., Klippel, J. H., and Lockshin, M. D. (1995). Systemic lupus erythematosus: Emerging concepts. Part 1: Renal, neuropsychiatric, cardiovascular, pulmonary, and hematologic disease. *Ann. Intern. Med.*, **122**, 940–50.

Brew, B. J., Dunbar, N., Pemberton, L., and Kaldor, J. (1996). Predictive markers of AIDS dementia complex: CD4 count and CSF concentrations of beta2microgulin and neopterin. *J. Infect. Dis.*, **174**, 294–8.

Briley, D. P., Coull, B. M., and Goodnight-SH, J. (1989). Neurological disease associated with antiphospholipid antibodies. *Ann. Neurol.*, **25**, 221–7.

Brown, A. P., Lane, J. C., Murayama, S., and Vollmer, D. G. (1990). Whipple's disease presenting with isolated neurological symptoms. Case report. *J. Neurosurg.*, **73**, 623–7.

Brundin, L., Svenungsson, E., Morcos, E., Andersson, M., Olsson, T., Lundberg, I., *et al.* (1998). Central nervous system nitric oxide formation in cerebral systemic lupus erythematosus. *Ann. Neurol.*, **44**, 704–6.

Cohen, L., Berthet, K., Dauga, C., Thivart, L., and Pierrot, D. C. (1996). Polymerase chain reaction of cerebrospinal fluid to diagnose Whipple's disease [letter]. *Lancet*, **347**, 329.

Cook, D. M. and Boyle, P. J. (1986). Rapid reversal of myxedema madness with triiodothyronine. *Ann. Intern. Med.*, **104**, 893–4.

Davie, C. A., Feinstein, A., Kartsounis, L. D., Barker, G. J., McHugh, N. J., Walport, M. J., *et al.* (1995). Proton magnetic resonance spectroscopy of systemic lupus erythematosus involving the central nervous system. *J. Neurol.*, **242**, 522–8.

Denburg, S. D., Carbotte, R. M., and Denburg, J. A. (1997). Psychological aspects of systemic lupus erythematosus: cognitive function, mood, and self-report. *J. Rheumatol.*, **24**, 998–1003.

Devinsky, O., Petito, C. K., and Alonso, D. R. (1988). Clinical and neuropathological findings in systemic lupus erythematosus: the role of vasculitis, heart emboli, and thrombotic thrombocytopenic purpura. *Ann. Neurol.*, **23**, 380–4.

Drent, M., Wirnsberger, R. M., Breteler, M. H., Kock, L. M., de, V. J., and Wouters, E. F. (1998). Quality of life and depressive symptoms in patients suffering from sarcoidosis. *Sarcoidosis Vasc. Diffuse. Lung Dis.*, **15**, 59–66.

Durand, D. V., Lecomte, C., Cathebras, P., Rousset, H., and Godeau, P. (1997). Whipple disease. Clinical review of 52 cases. The SNFMI Research Group on Whipple Disease. Societe Nationale Francaise de Medecine Interne. *Medicine (Baltimore)*, **76**, 170–84.

Farah, S., Al, S. A., Montaser, A., Hussein, J. M., Malaviya, A. N., Mukhtar, M., *et al.* (1998). Behcet's syndrome: a report of 41 patients with emphasis on neurological manifestations. *J. Neurol. Neurosurg. Psychiatry*, **64**, 382–4.

Feurle, G. E., Volk, B., and Waldherr, R. (1979). Cerebral Whipple's disease with negative jejunal histology. *N. Engl. J. Med.*, **300**, 907–8.

Finelli, P. F., McEntee, W. J., Ambler, M., and Kestenbaum, D. (1980). Adult celiac disease presenting as cerebellar syndrome. *Neurology*, **30**, 245–9.

Finelli, P. F., McEntee, W. J., Lessell, S., Morgan, T. F., and Copetto, J. (1977). Whipple's disease with predominantly neuroophthalmic manifestations. *Ann. Neurol.*, **1**, 247–52.

Fleming, J. L., Wiesner, R. H., and Shorter, R. G. (1988). Whipple's disease: clinical, biochemical, and histopathologic features and assessment of treatment in 29 patients. *Mayo Clin. Proc.*, **63**, 539–51.

Foong, J., Rozewicz, L., Quaghebeur, G., Davie, C. A., Kartsounis, L. D., Thompson, A. J., *et al.* (1997). Executive function in multiple sclerosis: the role of frontal lobe pathology. *Brain*, **120**, 15–26.

Foong, J., Rozewicz, L., Quaghebeur, G., Thompson, A. J., Miller, D. H., and Ron, M. A. (1998). Neuropsychological deficits in multiple sclerosis. *J. Neurol. Neurosurg. Psychiatry*, **64**, 529–32.

Futrell, N., Schultz, L. R., and Millikan, C. (1992). Central nervous system disease in patients with systemic lupus erythematosus. *Neurology*, **42**, 1649–57.

Greenan, T. J., Grossman, R. I., and Goldberg, H. I. (1992). Cerebral vasculitis: MR imaging and angiographic correlation. *Radiology*, **182**, 65–72.

Haass, A. (1998). Lyme neuroborreliosis. *Curr. Opin. Neurol.*, **11**, 253–8.

Hallert, C. and Astrom, J. (1983). Intellectual ability of adults after lifelong intestinal malabsorption due to coeliac disease. *J. Neurol. Neurosurg. Psychiatry*, **46**, 87–9.

Hallert, C., Astrom, J., and Walan, A. (1983). Reversal of psychopathology in adult coeliac disease with the aid of pyridoxine (vitamin B6). *Scand. J. Gastroenterol.*, **18**, 299–304.

Hallert, C. and Derefeldt, T. (1982). Psychic disturbances in adult coeliac disease. I. Clinical observations. *Scand. J. Gastroenterol.*, **17**, 17–19.

Halperin, J. J. (1998). Nervous system Lyme disease. *J. Neurol. Sci.*, **153**, 182–91.

Halperin, J. J., Krupp, L. B., Golightly, M. G., and Volkman, D. J. (1990). Lyme borreliosis associated encephalopathy. *Neurology*, **40**, 1340–3.

Halperin, J. J., Luft, B. J., Anand, A. K., Roque, C. T., Alvarez, O., Volkman, D. J., *et al.* (1989). Lyme neuroborreliosis: central nervous system manifestations. *Neurology*, **39**, 753–9.

Hankey, G. (1991). Isolated angiitis/angiopathy of the CNS. Prospective diagnostic and therapeutic experience. *Cerebrovasc. Dis.*, **1**, 2–15.

Hanly, J. G., Cassell, K., and Fisk, J. D. (1997). Cognitive function in systemic lupus erythematosus: results of a 5-year prospective study. *Arthritis Rheum.*, **40**, 1542–3.

Hay, E. M. (1994). Psychiatric disorder and cognitive impairment in SLE. *Lupus*, **3**, 145–8.

Hellmann, D. B., Roubenoff, R., Healy, R. A., and Wang, H. (1992). Central nervous system angiography: Safety and predictors of a positive result in 125 consecutive patients evaluated for possible vasculitis. *J. Rheumatol.*, **19**, 568–72.

Hirohata, S., Suda, H., and Hashimoto, T. (1998). Low-dose weekly methotrexate for progressive neuropsychiatric manifestations in Behcet's disease. *J. Neurol. Sci.*, **159**, 181–5.

Homburger, H. A. (1995). Cascade testing for autoantibodies in connective tissue diseases. *Mayo Clin. Proc.*, **70**, 183–4.

Isshi, K. and Hirohata, S. (1998). Differential roles of the anti-ribosomal P antibody and antineuronal antibody in the pathogenesis of central nervous system involvement in systemic lupus erythematosus. *Arthritis Rheum.*, **41**, 1819–27.

Jennette, J. C., Falk, R. J., and Milling, D. M. (1994). Pathogenesis of vasculitis. *Semin. Neurol.*, **14**, 291–9.

Johnson, R. T., Glass, J. D., McArthur, J. C., and Chesebro, B. W. (1996). Quantitation of human immunodeficiency virus in rains of demented and nondemented patients with acquired immunodeficiency syndrome. *Ann. Neurol.*, **39**, 392–5.

Johnson, R. T. and Richardson, E. P. (1968). The neurological manifestations of systemic lupus erythematosus. *Medicine (Baltimore)*, **47**, 337–69.

Kaell, A. T., Shetty, M., Lee, B. C., and Lockshin, M. D. (1986). The diversity of neurologic events in systemic lupus erythematosus. Prospective clinical and computed tomographic classification of 82 events in 71 patients. *Arch. Neurol.*, **43**, 273–6.

Kaplan, R. F., Meadows, M. E., Vincent, L. C., Logigian, E. L., and Steere, A. C. (1992). Memory impairment and depression in patients with Lyme encephalopathy. *Neurology*, **42**, 1263–7.

Kibayashi, K., Mastri, A. R., and Hirsch, C. S. (1996). Neuropathology of human immunodeficiency virus infection at different disease stages. *Hum. Pathol.*, **27**, 637–42.

Kinney, H. C., Burger, P. C., Hurwitz, B. J., Hijmans, J. C., and Grant, J. P. (1982). Degeneration of the central nervous system associated with celiac disease. *J. Neurol. Sci.*, **53**, 9–22.

Kissel, J. T. (1989). Neurologic manifestations of vasculitis. *Neurol. Clin.*, **7**, 655–73.

Kodama, K., Okada, S., Hino, T., Takabayashi, K., Nawata, Y., Uchida, Y., *et al.* (1995). Single photon emission computed tomography in systemic lupus erythematosus with psychiatric symptoms. *J. Neurol. Neurosurg. Psychiatry*, **58**, 307–11.

Koo, E. H. and Massey, E. W. (1988). Granulomatous angiitis of the central nervous system: Protean manifestations and response to treatment. *J. Neurol. Neurosurg. Psychiatry*, **51**, 1126–33.

Kothbauer, M. I., Sturzenegger, M., Komor, J., Baumgartner, R., and Hess, C. W. (1996). Encephalopathy associated with Hashimoto thyroiditis: diagnosis and treatment. *J. Neurol.*, **243**, 585–93.

Krupp, L. B., LaRocca, N. G., Luft, B. J., and Halperin, J. J. (1989). Comparison of neurologic and psychologic findings in patients with Lyme disease and chronic fatigue syndrome. *Neurology*, **39**, 144.

Kujula, P., Portin, R., and Ruutiainen, J. (1996). Language functions in incipient cognitive decline in multiple sclerosis. *J. Neurol. Sci.*, **141**, 79–86.

Kujula, P., Portin, R., and Ruutiainen, J. (1997). The progress of cognitive decline in multiple sclerosis: a controlled 3 year follow up. *Brain*, **120**, 289–97.

Lawrence, W. P., El, G. T., Pool-WH, J., and Apter, L. (1974). Radiological manifestations of neurosarcoidosis: report of three cases and review of literature. *Clin. Radiol.*, **25**, 343–8.

Leonard, T. J., Graham, E. M., Stanford, M. R., and Sanders, M. D. (1984). Graves' disease presenting with bilateral acute painful proptosis, ptosis, ophthalmoplegia, and visual loss. *Lancet*, **2**, 431–3.

Lipton, S. A. (1997). Neuropathogenesis of acquired immunodeficiency syndrome dementia. *Curr. Opin. Neurol.*, **10**, 247–53.

Lipton, S. A. and Gendelman, H. E. (1995). Dementia associated with the acquired immunodeficiency syndrome. *N. Engl. J. Med.*, **332**, 934–40.

Louis, E. D., Lynch, T., Kaufmann, P., Fahn, S., and Odel, J. (1996). Diagnostic guidelines in central nervous system Whipple's disease. *Ann. Neurol.*, **40**, 561–8.

Lynch, T., Odel, J., Fredericks, D. N., Louis, E. D., Forman, S., Rotterdam, H., *et al.* (1997). Polymerase chain reaction-based detection of Tropheryma whippelii in central nervous system Whipple's disease. *Ann. Neurol.*, **42**, 120–4.

Maki, M. and Collin, P. (1997). Coeliac disease. *Lancet*, **349**, 1755–9.

McLean, B. N., Miller, D., and Thompson, E. J. (1995a). Oligoclonal banding of IgG in CSF, blood-brain barrier function, and MRI findings in patients with sarcoidosis, systemic lupus erythematosus, and Behcet's disease involving the nervous system. *J. Neurol. Neurosurg. Psychiatry*, **58**, 548–54.

McLean, B. N., Miller, D., and Thompson, E. J. (1995b). Oligoclonal banding of IgG in CSF, blood-brain barrier function, and MRI findings in patients with sarcoidosis, systemic lupus erythematosus, and Behcet's disease involving the nervous system. *J. Neurol. Neurosurg. Psychiatry*, **58**, 548–54.

Miller, D. H., Buchanan, N., Barker, G., Morrissey, S. P., Kendall, B. E., Rudge, P., *et al.* (1992). Gadolinium-enhanced magnetic resonance imaging of the central nervous system in systemic lupus erythematosus. *J. Neurol.*, **239**, 460–4.

Minden, S. L., Orar, J., and Reich, P. (1987). Depression in multiple sclerosis. *Gen. Hosp. Psychiatry*, **9**, 426–34.

Minden, S. L. and Schiffer, R. B. (1990). Affective disorders in multiple sclerosis. *Arch. Neurol.*, **47**, 98–104.

Moore, P. M. (1989). Diagnosis and management of isolated angiitis of the central nervous system. *Neurology*, **39**, 167–73.

Moore, P. M. (1994). Vasculitis of the central nervous system. *Semin. Neurol.*, **14**, 307–12.

Moore, P. M. and Calabrese, L. H. (1994). Neurologic manifestations of systemic vasculitides. *Semin. Neurol.*, **14**, 300–6.

Mousa, A. R., Marafie, A. A., Rifai, K. M., Dajani, A. I., and Mukhtar, M. M. (1986). Behcet's disease in Kuwait, Arabia. A report of 29 cases and a review. *Scand. J. Rheumatol.*, **15**, 310–32.

Mumford, C. J., Fletcher, N. A., Ironside, J. W., and Warlow, C. P. (1996). Progressive ataxia, focal seizures, and malabsorption syndrome in a 41 year old woman [clinical conference]. *J. Neurol. Neurosurg. Psychiatry*, **60**, 225–30.

Neaton, J., Wentworth, D., Rhane, F., Hogan, C., and Abrams, D. L. D. (1994). Methods of studying interventions: considerations in choice of a clinical endpoint for AIDS clinical trials. *Stat. Med.*, **13**, 2107–25.

Nicholson, G. C., Gutteridge, D. H., Carroll, W. M., and Armstrong, B. K. (1984). Autoimmune thyroid disease and giant cell arteritis: a review, case report and epidemiological study. *Aust. N. Z. J. Med.*, **14**, 487–90.

Nishino, H., Rubino, F. A., DeRemee, R. A., Swanson, J. W., and Parisi, J. E. (1993). Neurological involvement in Wegener's granulomatosis: an analysis of 324 consecutive patients at the Mayo Clinic. *Ann. Neurol.*, **33**, 4–9.

O'Brien, G. M., Baughman, R. P., Broderick, J. P., Arnold, L., and Lower, E. E. (1994). Paranoid psychosis due to neurosarcoidosis. *Sarcoidosis*, **11**, 34–6.

O'Duffy, J. D. (1994). Behcet's disease. *Curr. Opin. Rheumatol.*, **6**, 39–43.

Pelosi, L., Geesken, J. M., Holly, M., Hayward, M., and Blumhardt, L. D. (1997). Working memory impairment in early multiple sclerosis: evidence from an event-related potential study of patients with clinically isolated myelopathy. *Brain*, **120**, 2039–58.

Price, R. W. (1996). Neurological complications of HIV infection. *Lancet*, **348**, 445–51.

Rao, S. M. (1995). Neuropsychology of multiple sclerosis. *Curr. Opin. Neurol.*, **8**, 216–20.

Reik, L., Smith, L., Khan, A., and Nelson, W. (1985). Demyelinating encephalopathy in Lyme disease. *Neurology*, **35**, 267–9.

Relman, D. A., Schmidt, T. M., MacDermott, R. P., and Falkow, S. (1992). Identification of the uncultured bacillus of Whipple's disease. *N. Engl. J. Med.*, **327**, 293–301.

Rigby, A. S., Chamberlain, M. A., and Bhakta, B. (1995). Behcet's disease. *Baillieres Clin. Rheumatol.*, **9**, 375–95.

Ron, M. A. (1999). Editorial: Multiple sclerosis and the mind. *J. Neurol. Neurosurg. Psychiatry*, **55**, 1–3.

Rosner, S., Ginzler, E. M., Diamond, H. S., Weiner, M., Schlesinger, M., Fries, J. F., *et al.* (1982). A multicenter study of outcome in systemic lupus erythematosus. II. Causes of death. *Arthritis Rheum.*, **25**, 612–17.

Rovaris, J. M., Filippi, M., Falautano, M., Minicucci, L., Rocca, M. A., Martinelli, V., *et al.* (1998). Correlation between MR abnormalities and patterns of cognitive impairment in multiple sclerosis. *Neurology*, **50**, 1601–8.

Rush, P. J., Inman, R., Bernstein, M., Carlen, P., and Resch, L. (1986). Isolated vasculitis of the central nervous system in a patient with celiac disease. *Am. J. Med.*, **81**, 1092–4.

Ryser, R. J., Locksley, R. M., Eng, S. C., Dobbins, W. O., Schoenknecht, F. D., and Rubin, C. E. (1984). Reversal of dementia associated with Whipple's disease by trimethoprim-sulfamethoxazole, drugs that penetrate the blood-brain barrier. *Gastroenterology*, **86**, 745–52.

Sailer, M., Burchert, W., Ehrenheim, C., Smid, H. G. O. M., Haas, J., Wildhagen, K., *et al.* (1997). Positron emission tomography and magnetic resonance imaging for cerebral involvement in patients with systemic lupus erythematosus. *J. Neurol.*, **244**, 186–93.

Scolding, N. J., Jayne, D. R., Zajicek, J. P., Meyer, P. A. R., Wraight, E. P., and Lockwood, C. M. (1997). The syndrome of cerebral vasculitis: recognition, diagnosis and management. *Q. J. Med.*, **90**, 61–73.

Scolding, N. J. (1999). *Immunological and inflammatory disorders of the central nervous system.* Butterworth Heinemann.

Shaw, P. J., Walls, T. J., Newman, P. K., Cleland, P. G., and Cartlidge, N. E. (1991). Hashimoto's encephalopathy: a steroid-responsive disorder associated with high anti-thyroid antibody titers–report of 5 cases. *Neurology*, **41**, 228–33.

Sigal, L. H. (1987). The neurologic presentation of vasculitic and rheumatologic syndromes. A review. *Medicine (Baltimore)*, **66**, 157–80.

Stigsby, B., Bohlega, S., Al, K. M., Al, D. A., and El, R. K. (1994). Evoked potential findings in Behcet's disease. Brain-stem auditory, visual, and somatosensory evoked potentials in 44 patients. *Electroencephalogr. Clin. Neurophysiol.*, **92**, 273–81.

Stone, J. H., Pomper, M. G., Roubenoff, R., Miller, T. J., and Hellmann, D. B. (1994). Sensitivities of noninvasive tests for central nervous system vasculitis: A comparison of lumbar puncture, computed tomography, and magnetic resonance imaging. *J. Rheumatol.*, **21**, 1277–82.

Tan, E. M., Cohen, A. S., Fries, J. F., *et al.* (1982). The 1982 revised criteria for the classification of systemic lupus erythematosus. *Arthritis Rheum.*, **25**, 1271–7.

Tola, M. R., Granieri, E., Caniatti, L., Paolino, E., Monetti, C., Dovigo, L., *et al.* (1992). Systemic lupus erythematosus presenting with neurological disorders. *J. Neurol.*, **239**, 61–4.

Verhagen, W. I., Huygen, P. L., Dalman, J. E., and Schuurmans, M. M. (1996). Whipple's disease and the central nervous system. A case report and a review of the literature. *Clin. Neurol. Neurosurg.*, **98**, 299–304.

Vollmer, T. L., Guarnaccia, J., Harrington, W., Pacia, S. V., and Petroff, O. A. C. (1993). Idiopathic granulomatous angiitis of the central nervous system: Diagnostic challenges. *Arch. Neurol.*, **50**, 925–30.

Watanabe, T., Sato, T., Uchiumi, T., and Arakawa, M. (1996). Neuropsychiatric manifestations in patients with systemic lupus erythematosus: Diagnostic and predictive value of longitudinal examination of anti-ribosomal P antibody. *Lupus*, **5**, 178–83.

Wechsler, B., Dell'lsola, B., Vidailhet, M., Dormont, D., Piette, J. C., Bletry, O., *et al.* (1993). MRI in 31 patients with Behcet's disease and neurological involvement: prospective study with clinical correlation. *J. Neurol. Neurosurg. Psychiatry*, **56**, 793–8.

Wechsler, B., Vidailhet, M., Piette, J. C., Bousser, M. G., Dell, I. B., Bletry, O., *et al.* (1992). Cerebral venous thrombosis in Behcet's disease: clinical study and long-term follow-up of 25 cases. *Neurology*, **42**, 614–18.

Weingarten, K., Filippi, C., Barbut, D., and Zimmerman, R. D. (1997). The neuroimaging features of the cardiolipin antibody syndrome. *Clin. Imaging*, **21**, 6–12.

West, S. G., Emlen, W., Wener, M. H., and Kotzin, B. L. (1995). Neuropsychiatric lupus erythematosus: a 10-year prospective study on the value of diagnostic tests. *Am. J. Med.*, **99**, 153–63.

Wilson, K. H., Blitchington, R., Frothingham, R., and Wilson, J. A. (1991). Phylogeny of the Whipple's-disease-associated bacterium. *Lancet*, **338**, 474–5.

Wirnsberger, R. M., De, V. J., Breteler, M. H., Van, H. G., Wouters, E. F., and Drent, M. (1998). Evaluation of quality of life in sarcoidosis patients. *Respir. Med.*, **92**, 750–6.

Working group of AAN AIDS task force. (1991). Nomenclature and research case definitions for neurologic manifestations of human immunodeficiency virus type 1 (HIV-1) infection. *Neurology*, **41**, 778–85.

Wroe, S. J., Pires, M., Harding, B., Youl, B. D., and Shorvon, S. (1991). Whipple's disease confined to the CNS presenting with multiple intracerebral mass lesions. *J. Neurol. Neurosurg. Psychiatry*, **54**, 989–92.

Younger, D. S., Hays, A. P., Brust, J. C., and Rowland, L. P. (1988). Granulomatous angiitis of the brain. An inflammatory reaction of diverse etiology. *Arch. Neurol.*, **45**, 514–18.

Zajicek, J. P., Scolding, N. J., Foster, O., Rovaris, M., Evanson, J., Moseley, I., *et al.* (1999). Central nervous system sarcoidosis — diagnosis and management based oin a large series. *Q. J. Med.*, **92**, 103–17.

18 Dementia in young adults

P. K. Panegyres

1 Introduction

Of all the problems facing the clinician none is more challenging than the young person with a dementing illness. This problem confronts us with a sense of helplessness as the implications for patient and family become realized. This chapter deals with the clinical approach and management of these patients and specifically deals with the genetic, metabolic, and endocrine disorders that present as a dementing illness in young people.

The care of dementia in young people is relatively under-resourced in most countries and in the future more funds need to be provided for management of this group of individuals and their complex problems. In order to address this problem in Western Australia we have established a new

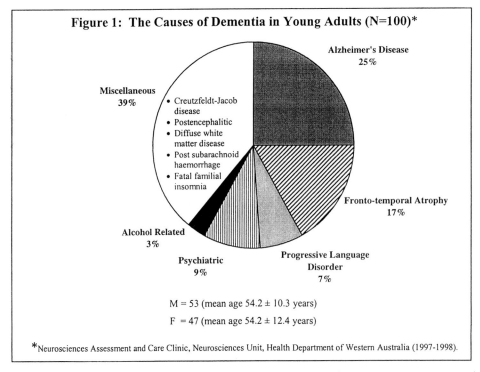

Figure 1: The Causes of Dementia in Young Adults (N=100)*

Alzheimer's Disease 25%

Miscellaneous 39%
- Creutzfeldt-Jacob disease
- Postencephalitic
- Diffuse white matter disease
- Post subarachnoid haemorrhage
- Fatal familial insomnia

Fronto-temporal Atrophy 17%

Alcohol Related 3%

Psychiatric 9%

Progressive Language Disorder 7%

M = 53 (mean age 54.2 ± 10.3 years)

F = 47 (mean age 54.2 ± 12.4 years)

*Neurosciences Assessment and Care Clinic, Neurosciences Unit, Health Department of Western Australia (1997-1998).

Figure 18.1 The causes of dementia in young adults (N = 100). M = 53 (mean age 54.2 ± 10.3 years). F = 47 (mean age 54.2 ± 12.4 years). Neurosciences Assessment and Care Clinic, Neurosciences Unit, Health Department of Western Australia (1997–1998).

service for the management of young patients with dementia. Figure 18.1 has the diagnostic classification from our experience. Alzheimer's disease, frontal lobe atrophy, and lobar atrophies are the most likely causes along with psychiatric disorders and a miscellaneous group. A more extensive discussion of the epidemiology of dementia in young adults is found in Chapter 1.

The purpose of the assessment of a young person with dementia is to determine if the dementia is a primary condition, secondary to some other brain disease or systemic illness, and to identify potentially reversible conditions.

2 Investigations

Blood investigations are performed in all patients and unfortunately they are usually within normal limits. These are the full blood picture and erythrocyte sedimentation rate; urea, creatinine, and electrolytes; liver function tests; calcium; thyroid function tests; vitamin B12 and red blood cell folate; and syphilis serology. Blood is collected in lithium heparin and EDTA tubes for DNA storage in all cases for future research after informed consent for DNA collection has been obtained and ethics committee approval received. At present we see no role for apolipoprotein E (ApoE) genotype analysis in sporadic cases of early onset dementia. We do not use it as a predictive test. We also do not routinely screen our sporadic early onset dementia patients for mutations in the presenilin 1 and 2 genes or in the amyloid precursor gene (APP). Table 18.1 summarizes genetic factors operational to the pathogenesis of Alzheimer's disease. If there is a strong family history of early onset autosomal dominant Alzheimer's disease we use guidelines for gene testing as recommended for Huntington's disease (World Federation of Neurology 1989).

If chromosome 17 autosomal dominant frontal lobe atrophy is a possibility then DNA should be sent to an appropriate laboratory with expertise in the testing for mutations in the tau gene (Hutton *et al.* 1998).

It is likely that new familial syndromes of cerebral atrophy due to novel gene mutations will be recognized in the future and we recommend that young patients with dementia be carefully assessed and DNA stored for research purposes.

There may be an increasing role for a CSF examination of proteins in the diagnosis of dementia (Table 18.2). In Alzheimer's disease there may be reduced levels of $A\beta$ peptide and increased

Table 18.1 Genetic factors in Alzheimer's disease and other causes of dementia in young adults

Alzheimer's disease
- Pathogenic loci
  Presenilin 1
  Presenilin 2
  Amyloid precursor protein gene

- Risk loci
  ApoE e4
  Alpha 2-macroglobulin
  Lipoprotein related polypeptide receptor
  Bleomycin hydrolase gene
  Butyrylcholinesterase K variant

Other dementing diseases
- Prion protein gene
- Tau protein gene in frontal lobe atrophies

Table 18.2 Proteins in blood and CSF that may be useful in the diagnosis of dementia

Blood	S100	CJD
CSF	Aβ	AD
	Tau	AD
	14-3-3	CJD

levels of tau protein (Andreason *et al.* 1998; Hock *et al.* 1998). In Creutzfeldt–Jacob disease the 14-3-3 protein in CSF may be diagnostically useful (Hsich *et al.* 1996). The serum S100 test may also help in the diagnosis of Creutzfeldt–Jacob disease (Otto *et al.* 1998). Further clinical validation of these tests is required.

A cerebral CT scan is considered mandatory in all patients with early onset dementia looking for evidence of cerebral atrophy, white matter disease, or other disease processes such as a brain tumour which may masquerade as a dementing illness. Magnetic resonance imaging (MRI) helps to confirm lobar atrophy in the frontal and temporal lobes which may be difficult to determine using CT scanning alone. MRI is useful in demonstrating white matter changes which would raise the possibility of small vessel disease and arteriosclerotic encephalopathy or a disorder of white matter such as a leukodystrophy. Cerebral perfusion imaging with single photon emission computed tomography (SPECT) may help in the distinction of frontal lobe atrophy from Alzheimer's disease.

An EEG is performed looking for evidence of diffuse periodic sharp waves that suggests a prion disease or slow waves changes that might confirm differential involvement of the frontal or temporal lobes that may reflect a lobar atrophy

Special investigations are necessary if a lysosomal or peroxisomal disorder are considered and these will be discussed below.

3 Specific disease groups

3.1 Alzheimer's disease

Dementia of the Alzheimer type does occur in young adults mostly as a sporadic disorder. In these patients an initial amnesic syndrome might evolve into aphasia and apraxia. In the age range of 35–55 years and in the presence of family history mutations in presenilin 1 and 2 genes should be considered (Giannakopoulos *et al.* 1996). Mutations in presenilin 1 accounting for between 50–60% of mutations in early onset Alzheimer's disease. Mutations in the amyloid precursor protein gene (APP) are responsible for a smaller number. An accelerated dementia with myoclonus may be found in mutational Alzheimer's disease. Further information on the clinical and molecular genetic features of familial Alzheimer's disease are found in Chapter 11.

3.2 Frontotemporal dementia and progressive aphasia

Frontotemporal dementia (FTD) is the second most common cause of dementia in young adults in our experience and may be characterized by change in personality, altered behaviour, reduced speech production, and abnormal stereotype motor behaviour (Neary *et al.* 1988; Lund and Manchester Groups 1994; Neary *et al.* 1998).

The family history should be sought as mutations in the tau gene on chromosome 17 have recently been identified as a cause of familial frontal lobe atrophy (Hutton *et al.* 1998). Patients with frontal lobe atrophy may develop a parkinsonian syndrome. Frontal lobe atrophies are discussed in Chapter 12.

3.3 Progressive language disorders due to lobar atrophy

Some patients who present with a progressive linguistic disorder due to lobar atrophy of the temporal lobes, causing progressive fluent aphasia (semantic dementia) or with progressive non-fluent aphasia (Snowden *et al.* 1992). The key distinguishing features, which are described in Chapter 12, are that patients with non-fluent aphasia have relative preservation of comprehension, while patients with semantic dementia are fluent with impaired understanding of language and its content (Hodges *et al.* 1992). Evaluation of these patients requires both neuropsychological and linguistic assessment. These are essential to exclude abnormalities in other cognitive functions. These patients should be followed long-term as they may evolve into a generalized dementing illness.

3.4 Prion diseases

Prion diseases, such as Creutzfeldt–Jacob disease (CJD), are usually sporadic and may present with early onset dementia leading to death with a mean disease duration of about eight months (Richardson and Masters 1995). However prolonged survival is recognized and may relate to a polymorphism in methionine/valine polymorphism at codon 129 of the prion protein gene (Gambetti *et al.* 1995). Fatal familial insomnia (FFI) and Gerstmann-Sträussler-Scheinker (GSS) syndrome occur in a familial clustering in an autosomal dominant pattern (Ghetti *et al.* 1995). There may often be an overlap in the clinical manifestations of these disorders and in GSS patients may develop a dementing illness before ataxia. In CJD ataxia may develop before dementia. Severe disabling somnolence associated with ataxia and extrapyramidal features raises the possibility of FFI. There is phenotypic variability in the clinical features in all families with prion mutations (Brown 1992). For further details see Chapter 16.

3.5 Wilson's disease

Wilson's disease (familial hepatolenticular degeneration) is an autosomal recessive condition characterized by liver cirrhosis and neuronal degeneration in the corpus striatum. It is a result of a mutation in the copper transporting P-type ATPase on chromosome 13 (Bull *et al.* 1993). In the early stages an extrapyramidal syndrome with tremor, rigidity, and bradykinesia may develop. The tremor may be a coarse action tremor or have features of an intention tremor as found in cerebellar disorders. Dysarthria and dysphagia evolving to anarthria may be seen if untreated and recognized as the bulbar extrapyramidal syndrome. Often the mouth may be permanently open due to a dystonia of the facial muscles with drooling and these patients may have a persistent grimace. The neurological disorder may progress to altered behaviour and psychosis, cognitive decline, and dementia (Dening and Berrios 1989; Akil *et al.* 1991). A variety of neuropsychological phenomena have been observed (Medalia *et al.* 1988). Neurological examination may reveal slow saccadic eye movements, cerebellar ataxia, generalized muscle rigidity, action myoclonus, chorea, and dystonia in advanced untreated patients. If neurological signs are evident Kayser-Fleischer rings will be identified in the cornea and represent copper deposition in Descement's membrane (the deepest layer of the cornea). A slit lamp examination may be necessary in dark-eyed people. Clinical evidence of hepatic cirrhosis may be identified with splenomegaly, jaundice, and features of hypersplenism.

The diagnosis is established by the demonstration of:

(a) Reduced serum ceruloplasmin level.

(b) Reduced serum copper concentrations.

(c) Elevated 24 hour urine copper excretion.

(d) The identification of Kayser-Fleischer rings.

In patients difficult to diagnose a liver biopsy demonstrating an elevated liver copper content may be necessary. Liver enzymes may be elevated. In some centres DNA testing for mutations in the ATPase transporter may be performed. The cerebral CT scan may show hypodensities in the putamen and the MRI may reveal low signal lesions on T1-weighted images and high signal on T2 in the globus pallidus; however the findings may be variable (Starosta-Rubinstein *et al.* 1987; Mochizuki *et al.* 1997).

Chelation therapy with D-penicillamine has been successfully used in the past but serious side-effects such as lupus-like syndromes have limited its usage. In some centres triethylene tetramine (trientene) or zinc acetate are the agents of first choice. The dementia of Wilson's disease may be reversible if treatment is started early (Roselli *et al.* 1987).

3.6 Inherited disorders of metabolism

3.6.1 The organelle dementias

Inherited disorders of metabolism are rare causes of dementia. They must be especially searched for in patients under the age of 40 years. These are difficult disorders for the clinician and the following represents an approach to these conditions.

These disorders are most conveniently classified as disorders of intracellular organelles: lysosomes, peroxisomes, and mitochondria. To the uninitiated they present a bewildering complexity of biochemical pathways and enzymes to which the advances of molecular genetics aid the confusion. This section attempts to simplify the clinician's approach to this complex group of conditions and presents only those disorders that present with dementia in adulthood.

The clinician must consider these diagnoses when multiple neuronal systems are involved. Seizures, myoclonus, retinal involvement in the context of dementia would suggest grey matter involvement and a lysosomal storage disorder should be seriously considered. Corticospinal tract signs, cerebellar dysfunction, optic nerve involvement, and sensory findings are best explained by white matter involvement, and a leukodystrophy or peroxisomal disorder a possibility. Mitochondrial disorders may have a myopathy, peripheral neuropathy, external ophthalmoplegia, myoclonus, optic neuropathy, ataxia, seizures, and strokes.

3.6.2 Lysosomal storage disorders

Lysosomal storage disorders are characterized by the accumulation of material in lysosomes which is harmful to cells. These may be classified according to the nature of the stored substances: glycolipids, glycoproteins, and glycosaminoglycans (Table 18.3). These stored substances causing enlargement of neurons detectable at light and electron microscopy. Examination of extracerebral tissue may therefore be helpful in diagnosis. Enzyme assay, metabolite measurement, DNA analysis, and electron microscopy may all be required to establish the diagnosis (Lake 1997).

Table 18.3 Lysosomal and peroxisomal storage disorders causing dementia in adulthood

- **Glycolipid disorders**
  Gm2 gangliosidosis
  Krabbe's globoid cell leukodystrophy
  Niemann-Pick disease — I and II
  Metachromatic leukodystrophy
  Gaucher's disease
  Mucosulphatidosis

- **Glycosaminoglycan disorders (mucolipidoses)**
  Neuraminidase/β galactosidase deficiency
  Alpha mannosidosis

- **Lipopigment disorders (neuronal ceroid lipofuscinosis)**
  Kufs' disease (adult Batten's disease)

- **Adrenoleukodystrophy**
  Adolescent form
  Adrenomyeloneuropathy
  Adult form

3.6.3 Glycolipid storage disorders

The glycolipid storage disorders are autosomal recessive inherited disorders and dementia is often a feature in early adult life. Hexosaminidase A deficiency is the cause of Gm2 gangliosidosis and dementia may be associated with neurogenic muscle atrophy, ataxia, dystonia (Hurowitz *et al.* 1993; Navon *et al.* 1986). Hexosaminidase A may be assayed in white blood cells (WBC), serum, cultured fibroblasts, tears, or other tissues. In some patients the enzyme assay may be normal and neurons from an intestinal biopsy reveals membranous cytoplasmic bodies (MCB). These patients may have activator protein deficiency (Navon 1991). Hexosaminidase is composed of two subunits — alpha on chromosome 15 and beta on chromosome 5 (Kolter and Sandhoff 1998).

3.6.4 Krabbe's globoid cell leukodystrophy

Krabbe's globoid cell leukodystrophy is due to excess storage of galactocerebroside as a result of inactivity of galactocerebroside — galactosidase (Kolter and Sandhoff 1998). Progressive spasticity leading to a significant gait disorder may occur; there might be an associated demyelinating polyneuropathy. Dementia and visual disturbance are found (Kolodny *et al.* 1991; Lyon *et al.* 1991). The diagnosis is established by the measurement of the enzyme in WBC or fibroblasts. Ultrastructure of peripheral nerve and skin reveal curved tubular profiles. A mutation on chromosome 14q 31 has been reported (Cannizzaro *et al.* 1994).

3.6.5 Niemann-Pick disease

Niemann-Pick disease is classified into two main groups:

    I Sphingomyelinase deficiency

    II Non-sphingomyelinase deficiency — cholesterol homeostasis protein gene abnormality

The enzyme may be measured in WBC and fibroblasts and is normal in type II (Kolter and Sandhoff 1998). In patients with type II there is abnormal cholesterol esterification in cultured fibroblasts (Carstea *et al.* 1997; Vanier and Suzuki 1998). Bone marrow examination identifies vacuolated lymphocytes and rectal biopsy will show abnormal neuronal storage, with involvement of smooth muscle and endothelial cells, and foamy cells in the lamina propria in type I (Long *et al.* 1977). These abnormalities are not found in type II. Cryostat sections searching for PAS positive material and electron microscopy of neurons may be the clues to type II. Type I Niemann-Pick is further subdivided into type A — the neurovisceral form, and type B — the visceral form. Hepatosplenomegaly is found with dementia, spasticity, and seizures. Cherry red spots may be found in the macula (Long *et al.* 1977). Type II is also subclassified into type C — the neurovisceral form and D — a pure visceral type. Patients with Niemann-Pick IIC may develop neurological signs in the fifth decade (Vanier *et al.* 1988). Splenomegaly may be found with dementia. Loss of vertical eye movements is often a feature (Neville *et al.* 1973). Dystonia, spasticity, and seizures are also seen. Neurofibrillary tangles have been identified in the brains of patients dying from Niemann-Pick IIC (Suzuki *et al.* 1995).

3.6.6 Metachromatic leukodystrophy (MLD)

Metachromatic leukodystrophy (MLD) is mostly caused by a deficiency of arylsulfatase A (Bauman *et al.* 1991). Arylsulfatase B and C are normal. Occasionally this enzyme activity is normal and the disease is a result of activator protein deficiency due to a mutation in the saposin B domain of the prosaposin gene (Gieselmann *et al.* 1994). Cerebroside sulfate accumulates giving brown metachromasia in sural nerve biopsies stained with the toluidine blue. Caution must be exercised in the diagnosis of MLD as 10–20% of healthy asymptomatic individuals will have low arylsulfatase deficiency without disease. In fact, pseudodeficiency is more likely to be detected than MLD and the clinical phenotype must be properly established (Gieselmann *et al.* 1991). Multiple sulfatase deficiency is the cause of mucosulfatidosis which is discussed below. Patients with MLD may develop psychosis and dementia (Bosch and Hart 1978). A motor syndrome with pyramidal features is often found and a demyelinating polyneuropathy with slow conduction velocities is revealed in most cases (Macfaul *et al.* 1982). MRI shows widespread symmetrical demyelination (Waltz *et al.* 1987). The enzyme may be determined in urine, WBC, fibroblasts, or tissue samples. Metachromatic deposits should be searched for in urine sediment and neutrophils might show Alder granulation. Ultrastructural studies of peripheral nerve shows prismatic, lamellar, tuffstone, and zebra-like inclusions within Schwann cells and macrophages (Kraus-Ruppert *et al.* 1972). Bone marrow transplantation may retard the progression of the peripheral nervous system manifestations (Krivit *et al.* 1995).

3.6.7 Mucosulfatidosis

Mucosulfatidosis has the features of both MLD and a mucopolysaccharidosis. It is due to a deficiency of at least two arylsulfatases A and B and characterized by abnormal storage of mucopolysaccharides in the form of glycosaminoglycans, gangliosides, and ceramide (Kolter and Sandhoff 1998). It is also referred to as multiple sulfatase deficiency or the Austin variant of metachromatic leukodystrophy (Burch *et al.* 1986). Clinically these patients develop dementia with skeletal abnormalities on X-ray and may have ichthyosis, corneal clouding, and retinitis pigmentosa (Guerra *et al.* 1990). In addition to cerebral atrophy the meninges may be thickened. There is increased urinary excretion of glycosaminoglycans and the urine sediment contains metachromatic granules. The activity of arylsulfatase A and B are absent in WBC and fibroblasts (Tanaka *et al.* 1987). Alder granulation must be present in neutrophils to establish the diagnosis and granulation might also be identified in eosinophils. Metachromatic deposits are seen in peripheral nerve biopsies and ultrastructure shows zebra bodies, lamellated inclusions, membrane sound vacuoles in capillary endothelial cells. Sulfatide inclusions are seen in macrophages (Guerra *et al.* 1990). The biochemical defect results in a post-translational error in the hydrolysis of sulfate esters. No mutations have been described to date.

3.6.8 Gaucher's disease

Gaucher's disease is a result of a deficiency in glucocerebrosidase leading to accumulation of glucocerebroside in spleen, liver, and brain (Patrick 1965). There are multiple forms with two types occurring in adults:

    I Non-neuronopathic

    II Neuronopathic (Norrbottnian type)

Type I is characterized by splenomegaly which may be massive (Zevin *et al.* 1993). Patients with type II often have dementia, myoclonic epilepsy, spasticity, supranuclear gaze palsy, and cerebellar ataxia (Miller *et al.* 1973; King 1975; Winkelman *et al.* 1983). In some patients with Gaucher's disease glucocerebrosidase may be normal and they have deficiency of saposin C (Schnabel *et al.* 1991). Mutations for this protein are found on chromosome 10q21, whereas glucocerebrosidase is on chromosome 1q21 (Dahl *et al.* 1993). The enzyme may be assayed in WBC and fibroblasts; enzyme deficiency is accompanied by increased activity of the enzyme chitotriosidase. Bone marrow examination shows PAS positive enlarged Gaucher's cells — the cytoplasm of which have a striated appearance. Electron microscopy demonstrates elongated tubular inclusions of cerebroside. Gaucher's disease is important to recognize as bone marrow transplantation (Erikson *et al.* 1990) and intravenous enzyme replacement (Zimran *et al.* 1994) may help in the non-neuronopathic form.

3.6.9 Neuronal ceroid lipofuscinosis

Neuronal ceroid lipofuscinosis is a common cause of neurodegenerative disorder in children but very rare in adults where it is known as Kufs' disease (adult Batten's disease) (Goebel and Sharp 1998). It is characterized by the accumulation of autofluorescent lipopigment in neurons with features of ceroid and lipofuscin. In adults autosomal dominant and recessive forms have been discovered and are further classified: type A with progressive myoclonic epilepsy, dementia, and ataxia; and type B with behavioural change, dementia, motor disturbance, and facial dyskinesia (Berkovic *et al.* 1988). Visual problems are not found in either type. Despite advances in the identification of mutations in lysosomal enzymes in infantile and late-infantile forms, no mutation or enzyme abnormalities have yet been identified in the adult form.

Skin and skeletal muscle biopsy may be necessary to observe the autofluorescent pigment and electron microscopy may show a variety of inclusions: curvilinear bodies, fingerprint bodies, rectilinear profiles, and granular osmiophilic deposits (GROD) (Martin *et al.* 1987). Rectal biopsy is not useful in adults because of the normal deposition of lipofuscin in heavy amounts in adults (Gelot *et al.* 1998). Vacuolated lymphocytes are not identified; skin and other biopsies may occasionally be unrewarding.

3.6.10 Mucopolysaccharidoses

Mucopolysaccharidoses are characterized by the accumulation of glycosaminoglycans and usually occur in children; some may survive into adulthood. Neuraminidase/β-galactosidase deficiency is also known as galactosialidosis or mucolipidosis I and may have its onset in early adulthood (Miyatake *et al.* 1979). It is a secondary to absence of a protective protein required for the aggregation of β-galactosidase monomers essential for the activation of neurominidase. The gene localization for this protein is on chromosome 20q13-1 (Galjaard *et al.* 1987). This condition is most common in Japanese where coarse facial features may be accompanied by dementia, myoclonus, ataxia, angiokeratoma, cherry red spots of the macula, and dysostosis multiplex. There is no hepatosplenomegaly. Vacuolated lymphocytes in peripheral blood and foamy cells in bone marrow help to establish the diagnosis. Urine excretion of sialyloligosaccharides is increased and metabolic studies on cultured fibroblasts may be necessary.

3.6.11 Mannosidosis

Mannosidosis may occur in adults and dementia is associated with coarse facial features, gingival hyperplasia, recurrent bacterial infections, and dysostosis multiplex (Ockerman 1967). Deafness, hepatosplenomegaly, and corneal spacities may be found. It is due to a deficiency of lysosomal alpha mannosidase and urine excretion of tetramannosides (Nebes and Schmidt 1994). Cytoplasmic vacuolation in lymphocytes and in bone marrow cells is found. There is no mucopolysacchariduria.

3.6.12 Peroxisomal disorders and adrenoleukodystrophy

Peroxisomes are found in all nucleated cells and synthesize plasmalogens necessary for myelin formation and stability. Peroxisomes are also involved in cholesterol biosynthesis, the βoxidation of fatty acids, and bile acid metabolism. Adrenoleukodystrophy is the major peroxisomal storage disorder that may present in adulthood (Table 18.3) (Powers and Moser 1998). Zellweger syndrome and infantile Refsum disease occur in the neonatal period.

Adrenoleukodystrophy (ALD) is due to a mutation of an ATP binding cassette transporter, an integral component of the peroxisomal membrane, which leads to a reduced capacity to form coenzyme A derivatives of very long chain fatty acids (VLCFA). This gene is located on the X chromosome at position Xq28, a number of mutations have been described and there is no clear genotype–phenotype relationship (Mosser *et al.* 1994). Several subtypes exist: childhood, adolescent, adult cerebral, adrenomyeloneuropathy, Addison's disease only, presymptomatic, and asymptomatic. Manifesting female carriers exist (Moser 1997). The adolescent form has its onset between the ages of 11–21 years and dementia may occur with visual and hearing changes in association with seizures. There may be rapid progression with a progressive pyramidal,

Table 18.4 Case summary: adrenoleukodystrophy

53M **(At death)** **A88/89**	48 years	– Personality change
		 – ↓ Speech output
		 – Abulia
		 – Abusive
		 – Sexually aggressive
		 – ↓ Hygeine
		 – Progressed to:
		   Disorientation
		   Hallucinations
		   Memory loss
		   Incontinence
		   Attempted suicide

	52 years	– Combative – Bilateral extensor plantar responses – CT scan widespread low attenuation in white matter
	53 years	– Death from pulmonary embolism
Neuropathology: Microscopy: EM:		Widespread destruction white matter temporal, frontal parietal lobes Myelin loss Perivascular cuffing mononuclear cells Curvilinear inclusions with electron lucent centre and electron dense membranes diagnostic of ALD

extrapyramidal, and cerebellar syndrome with evolution into a vegetative state. Most of these patients have preceding adrenal insufficiency with increased pigmentation, hypotension, diarrhoea, and vomiting. Not all patients experience adrenal insufficiency.

Adrenomyeloneuropathy (AMN) usually presents as an insidious spastic paraplegia between the ages of 20–30 years — the upper limbs are usually spared. Adrenal insufficiency may precede the onset of AMN. Some patients with AMN might develop a rapidly progressive inflammatory cerebral disease after many years which may have features of a dementing illness.

The adult form of ALD is rare and is a recognized cause of dementia in which schizophrenia-like symptoms may develop (Panegyres *et al.* 1989). These patients may not have adrenal insufficiency and usually do not have AMN. CT and MRI usually identifies changes of demyelination predominantly in the parieto-occipital region with increasing contrast of the advancing margin. Occasionally Addison's disease may occur without any other features. Presentation as a purely progressive cerebellar disorder resembling olivopontocerebellar degeneration is recognized. A case history of a patient presenting with dementia in adulthood is shown (Table 18.4, Figure 18.2).

The diagnosis of ALD is based on the elevation of VLCFA esters in plasma, cultured fibroblasts, and affected tissues. Ultrastructure reveals needle-like trilaminar bodies 7 nm long and 10 nm wide which contain the VLCFA in macrophages in peripheral nerve, conjunction, skin, and rectum (Ceuterick-de Groote and Martin 1998). Confirmation of the diagnosis requires biochemical studies and, in some centres, DNA analysis searching for the mutation. Diagnosis

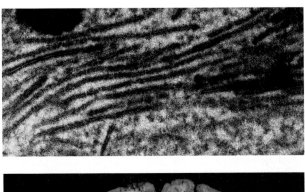

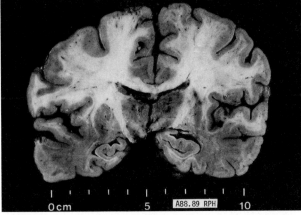

Figure 18.2 The lower figure reveals extensive white matter destruction in the temporal lobes. The upper figure shows the ultrastructural curvilinear inclusions within macrophages which are characteristic of ALD (A88/89; × 192 000).

on the basis of electron microscopy alone may lead to error as the inclusions are not specific for this condition.

Treatment with Lorenzo's oil (glyceryl trierucate/glyceryl trioleate 4:1) and bone marrow transplantation, if performed early, might help to retard the neurological progression before symptoms develop (Odone and Odone 1989; Krivit *et al.* 1995).

A very rare leukodystrophy known as Alexander's disease is found in adults and characterized by dementia, seizures, and spasticity (Soffer and Horoupian 1979). There may be dysphasia and psychiatric disturbances. Little is known about the biochemical and molecular defect of this condition. Pathologically it is characterized by demyelination and rarefaction of white matter with extensive axon loss. Prominent Rosenthal fibres are a distinguishing feature.

3.7 Mitochondrial disorders

Mitochondria are small intracellular organelles about the size of a bacterial cell in which the energy generated by the metabolism of sugars and fats is transformed into ATP by oxidative phosphorylation. Mitochondria contain their own DNA in a circular form composed of 16 569 nucleotides which has been completely sequenced. This DNA encodes information for the following mitochondrial functions: transfer RNA (tRNA), ribosomal RNA (rRNA), and the proteins (cytochrome oxidase, cytochrome *b*, a subunit of ATP synthetase, subunits of NADH–coenzyme Q reductase, and an ATPase). The other proteins originate from nuclear genes. Mitochondria do not have DNA repair enzymes and are therefore predisposed to mutations. A number of mitochondrial disorders are associated with the development of dementia in adults (Table 18.5). There is a wide spectrum of genotype–phenotype correlations (Graeber and Muller 1998).

3.7.1 Leigh's disease

Leigh's disease is a mitochondrial disorder which mostly occurs in children and is also known as subacute necrotising encephalomyelopathy. It is recognized as occurring in adults where dementia may be associated with optic atrophy and cerebellar ataxia (Kalimo *et al.* 1979). It is associated with deficiencies of the pyruvate dehydrogenase and cytochrome oxidase complexes of oxidative phosphorylation (Vazquez-Memije *et al.* 1996). Mitochondrial DNA point mutations at nucleotide 8993 (T → G or T → C) have been described (Rahman *et al.* 1996). The patients may have dystonia. Imaging reveals basal ganglia lucencies or calcifications on CT and MRI shows a high T2-weighted signal in the basal ganglia. Mutations in the ATPase to gene have also been described.

3.7.2 Myoclonic epilepsy and ragged red fibres (MERRF)

Myoclonic epilepsy and ragged red fibres (MERRF) may occur after the second decade of life and myoclonic seizures with ataxia are found. Generalized tonic/clonic seizures and dementia

Table 18.5 Mitochondrial disorders associated with dementia

• Subacute necrotizing encephalomyelopathy (adult Leigh's disease)
• Myoclonic epilepsy ragged red fibres (MERRF)
• Mitochondrial myopathy encephalopathy — lactic acidosis stroke-like episodes (MELAS)

may develop. Short stature, hearing loss, optic atrophy, myopathy, and neuropathy are sometimes identified. There is cytochrome oxidase deficiency on muscle biopsy and electron microscopy might show characteristic mitochondrial inclusions. Point mutations are usually found within the tRNA-Lys gene or tRNA-Leu gene. The most common MERRF mutation is 8344 (A → G) in tRNA-Lys gene but mutations in other genes have been found (Silvestri *et al.* 1993).

3.7.3 Mitochondrial myopathy, encephalopathy, lactic acidosis, and stroke-like episodes (MELAS)

Mitochondrial myopathy, encephalopathy, lactic acidosis, and stroke-like episodes (MELAS) has a wide phenotype of which stroke syndromes and encephalopathy predominate. Dementia may occur and probably a consequence of brain infarction and cerebral white matter disease. A wide phenotype is recognized and includes diabetes mellitus, sensorineural hearing impairment, epilepsy, ophthalmoplegia, hypertrophic cardiomyopathy, and ataxia. Basal ganglia calcification is often found. MELAS is most often a result of a point mutation in the tRNA-Leu gene at nucleotide 3243 (A → G) (Majamaa *et al.* 1998). The muscle biopsy often shows abnormal mitochondrial inclusions and ragged red fibres may be identified by light microscopy.

3.8 Trinucleotide CAG repeat disorders

Inherited neurodegenerative disorders caused by CAG trinucleotide repeat expansions represent an important advance in the understanding of neurodegenerative disease. Huntington's disease is one of the most well studied examples of this group of conditions in which dementia may occur with chorea and psychiatric disturbance — Chapter 15 is devoted to this condition. This section deals with those other CAG repeat disorders in which dementia may be found (Table 18.6).

3.8.1 Spinocerebellar ataxias (SCA)

The spinocerebellar ataxias (SCA) are autosomal dominant disorders caused by CAG repeat expansions in novel genes or in previously discovered genes. At present there are seven SCAs: SCA1–3 involving CAG repeats in new genes and proteins called the ataxins 1–3; SCA4 and 5 which are still being characterized; SCA6 in the Ca^{2+} channel on chromosome 19; and SCA7 involving ataxin 7 (Nance 1997). Dementia is recognized in SCA1–3 and 7 (Geschwind *et al.* 1997; David *et al.* 1997). If dementia develops it is usually a late finding in the context of the features of spinocerebellar ataxia. Chorea, other extrapyramidal features, oculomotor abnormalities including supranuclear ophthalmoplegia, decreased deep tendon reflexes, sphincter disturbance, loss of vision, and pyramidal signs may be found.

Table 18.6 Trinucleotide CAG repeat expansion disorders associated with dementia

• Huntington's disease
• Spinocerebellar ataxias
• Dentatorubropallidoluysial atrophy (DRPLA)

In some patients dementia and chorea may be inherited in an autosomal dominant pattern and the clinical suspicion of HD not supported by gene testing. In these patients dentatorubropallidoluysial atrophy (DRPLA) is a possibility. This is a rare disorder with a broad phenotypic spectrum due to CAG expansion in a new gene and protein called atrophin-1 (Becher *et al.* 1997). Myoclonus, cerebellar, ataxia, epilepsy, chorea, psychiatric disturbance, and dementia may occur in adults. CT and MRI reveal cerebral atrophy; MRI might show high signal lesions in cerebral white matter, globus pallidus, thalamus, midbrain, and pons.

3.9 CADASIL

A rare familial cause of stroke and vascular dementia in adults with a mean age of onset 45 years is cerebral autosomal dominant arteriopathy subcortical infarcts and leukoencephalopathy (CADASIL) (Ruchoux and Maurage 1997). The acronym describes the essential features of the condition. Dementia is common and may be associated with strokes, migraine with aura, and mood disturbances. The dementia may be dominated by a frontal lobe syndrome and cognitive decline occurs in a stepwise decline. Pseudobulbar palsy, gait disturbance, pyramidal signs and sphincter disturbance may be observed. CT shows white matter and basal ganglia lesions; MRI is more sensitive and high signal T2-weighted images are found in the white matter of the cerebral hemispheres, basal ganglia, and pons. Mutations in the *Notch 3* gene on chromosome 19 are the cause. These patients do not have vascular risk factors. This disorder is characterized by the deposition of granular osmiophilic material (GOM) detectable by electron microscopy in proximity to vascular smooth muscle cells in skin, muscle, peripheral nerve, and brain. Their presence in peripheral tissues may help to establish the diagnosis along with DNA testing if available.

3.10 Miscellaneous disorders

Disorders such as arteriosclerotic encephalopathy, alcohol-related dementia, Wernicke-Korsakoff psychosis, and communicating hydrocephalus are causes of dementia in young adults. Diagnosis of these entities requires a detailed history and imaging investigations. Psychiatric disorders like pseudodementia of depression occur and psychiatric assessment is essential. In pseudodementia of depression the dementing illness may start abruptly and is associated with symptoms of a depressive syndrome. Evidence of dementia may be mild and the patient may often report 'I don't know' to questions asked in a cognitive assessment.

Subacute sclerosing panencephalitis may masquerade as an aggressive dementing illness, and mimic a prion disease. Patients with demyelinating diseases like multiple sclerosis might also develop dementia. Multiple sclerosis, sarcoid, and syphilis are discussed in Chapter 17.

Dementia may occur in the context of alcoholism, narcotic addition, and heavy metal exposure. Organic toxins may also be implicated.

Dementia may be found in the presence of an endocrine disorder and vitamin deficiency — it is important to recognize that in such conditions the dementia is reversible if detected early. Hypothyroidism, B12 deficiency, thiamine deficiency, nicotinic acid deficiency, adrenal insufficiency, Cushing's syndrome, hypo- and hyperparathyroidism, and chronic hypoxaemia may be associated with cognitive decline. Clinical features should be sought which would raise the suspicion of these disorders like subacute combined degeneration of the cord in pernicious anaemia, and the features of Cushing's syndrome. Appropriate laboratory testing should be done in those cases where vitamin deficiency and an endocrine disorder are suspected.

4 Management

The approach to the care of patients with early onset dementia is probably best performed in a multidisciplinary team. The team should be lead by a neurologist, preferably with special expertise in behavioural neurology, neurogenetics, and neuropathology. In the team should be a psychiatrist, neuropsychologist, speech therapist, occupational therapist, and social worker. The neurologist must search for a potentially treatable cause and determine with as much certainty as possible the diagnosis using the investigations outlined above (Table 18.7).

Regular and long-term follow-up of our patients is thought essential to provide ongoing clinical and moral support for patient, carers, and family. This is imperative such that confirmation of the diagnosis with time may be made and evidence of progression can be monitored.

Confidence between the neurologist, management team, the patient, and carers must be such that the patient and family may be counselled on the importance of a post-mortem study to confirm the diagnosis and to contribute to research and understanding of their conditions.

Dementia in young adults represents particular diagnostic and management challenges, these patients and their families require a special approach. The key to this is a multidisciplinary team of caring and dedicated individuals. The complexity and cost of the care of young people with dementia is disproportional to their number.

5 Key points

1   Alzheimer's disease, frontotemporal dementia, progressive language disorders due to lobar atrophy remain the most common causes.

Table 18.7 Summary of key investigations in early onset dementia

Bloods:	FBC	ESR	U&E	LFT	BSL	Ca	B12/RBC folate	TFTs	ANF
Imaging:		CT		SPECT	MRI				
Neurophysiology:	EEG								
CSF:		14-3-3 protein may help in CJD							

Biochemical and DNA testing in special circumstances:	
Familial AD:	Presenilin and APP mutations
Familial prion disease:	Prion gene mutations
Familial frontal lobe atrophy:	Tau gene mutations
Huntington's disease SCA DRPLA:	CAG repeat testing
Wilson's disease:	Ceruloplasmin copper urinary copper Slit lamp exam for Kayser–Fleischer rings
Lysosomal storage disorders:	Blood film for vacuolated lymphocytes Enzymes in WBC serum fibroblasts tears Nerve conduction tests: metachromatic leukodystrophy Nerve biopsy: metachromatic leukodystrophy Skin and skeletal muscle: neuronal ceroid lipofuscinosis
Peroxisomal disorders:	VLCFA in plasma cultured fibroblasts
Mitochondrial disorders:	Skeletal muscle biopsy Mitochondrial DNA mutations
CADASIL:	*Notch 3* mutations

2   A detailed history is essential to help distinguish frontotemporal atrophy from Alzheimer's disease and language disorders due to lobar atrophy.

3   Look for behavioural phenomena suggestive of a frontal lobe syndrome.

4   Look for examination evidence that indicates disease outside of CNS that might suggest a rare metabolic or genetic cause.

5   Special investigations including biochemical and DNA testing may help to elucidate the diagnosis.

6   Management requires a caring multidisciplinary team committed to long-term management of this complex group of patients.

Acknowledgements

The author thanks the NH and MRC of Australia for their support.

References

Akil, M., Schwartz, J. A., Dutchak, D., Yuzbasiyan-Gurkan, V., and Brewer, G. J. (1991). The psychiatric presentations of Wilson's disease. *J. Neuropsychiatry Clin. Neurosci.*, **3**, 377–82.

Andreason, N., Vanmechelen, E., Vandevoorde, A., *et al.* (1998). Cerebrospinal fluid tau protein as a biochemical marker for Alzheimer's disease: A community based follow-up study. *J. Neurol. Neurosurg. Psychiatry*, **3**, 298–305.

Bauman, N., Masson, M., Carreau, V., *et al.* (1991). Adult forms of metachromatic leukodystrophy: Clinical and biochemical approach. *Dev. Neurosci.*, **13**, 211–15.

Becher, M. W., Rubinsztein, D. C., Leggo, J., *et al.* (1997). Dentatorubral and pallidoluysian atrophy (DRPLA). Clinical and neuropathological findings in genetically confirmed North American and European pedigrees. *Mov. Disorders*, **12**, 519–30.

Berkovic, S. F., Carpenter, S., Andermann, F., *et al.* (1988). Kufs' Disease: A critical reappraisal. *Brain*, **111**, 27–62.

Bosch, E. P. and Hart, M. N. (1978). Late adult onset metachromatic leukodystrophy. *Arch. Neurol.*, **35**, 475–7.

Brown, P. (1992). The phenotypic expression of different mutations in transmissible human spongiform encephalopathy. *Rev. Neurol. (Paris)*, **148**, 317–27.

Bull, P. C., Thomas, G. R., Rommens, J. M., *et al.* (1993). Wilson disease gene is a putative copper transporting P-type ATPase similar to the Menkes gene. *Nat. Genet.*, **5**, 327–37.

Burch, M., Fensom, A. H., Jackson, M., *et al.* (1986). Multiple sulphatase deficiency presenting at birth. *Clin. Genet.*, **30**, 409–15.

Cannizzaro, L. A., Chen, Y. Q., Rafi, M. A., and Wenger, D. A. (1994). Regional mapping of the human galactocerebrosidase gene (GALC). to 14q 31 by *in situ* hybridization. *Cytogenet. Cell Genet.*, **66**, 244–5.

Carstea, E. D., Morris, J. A., Coleman, K. G., *et al.* (1997). Niemann-Pick C1 disease gene: Homology to mediators of cholesterol homeostasis. *Science*, **277**, 228–31.

Ceuterick-de Groote, C. and Martin, J.-J. (1998). Extracerebral biopsy in lysosomal and peroxisomal disorders. Ultrastruchtural findings. *Brain Pathol.*, **8**, 121–32.

Dahl, N., Hillborg, P. O., and Olofsson, A. (1993). Gaucher disease (Norrbottnian type-II) – Probable founders identified by genealogical and molecular studies. *Hum. Genet.*, **92**, 513–15.

David, G., Abbas, N., Stevanin, G., *et al.* (1997). Cloning of the SCA7 gene reveals a highly unstalbe CAG repeat expansion. *Nat. Genet.*, **17**, 65–70.

Dening, T. R. and Berrios, G. E. (1989). Wilson's disease: Psychiatric symptoms in 195 cases. *Arch. Gen. Psychiatry*, **46**, 1126–34.

Erikson, A., Groth, C. G., Mansson, J. E., *et al.* (1990). Clinical and biochemical outcome of marrow transplantation for Gaucher disease of the Norrbottnian type. *Acta Paediatr. Scand.*, **79**, 680–5.

Galjaard, H., Willemsen, R., Hodgeveen, A. T., *et al.* (1987). Molecular heterogeneity in human beta-galactosidase and neuraminidase deficiency. *Enzyme*, **38**, 132–43.

Gambetti, P., Parchi, P., Petersen, R. B., Chen, S. G., and Lugaresi, E. (1995). Fatal familial insomnia and familial Creutzfeldt-Jakob disease: Clinical, pathological and molecular features. *Brain Pathol.*, **5**, 43–51.

Gelot, A., Maurage, C. A., Rodriguez, D., Perrier-Pallison, D., Larmande, P., and Ruchoux, M. M. (1998). *In vivo* diagnosis of Kufs' disease by extracerebral biopsies. *Acta Neuropathol.*, **96**, 102–8.

Geschwind, D. H., Perlman, S., Figueroa, C. P., Treiman, L. J., and Pulst, S. M. (1997). The prevalence and wide clinical spectrum of the spinocerebellar ataxia type 2 trinucleotide repeat in patients with autosomal dominant cerebellar ataxia. *Am. J. Hum. Genet.*, **60**, 842–50.

Ghetti, B., Dlouhy, S. R., Giaccone, G., Bugiani, O., Frangione, B., Farlow, M. R., *et al.* (1995). Gerstmann-Sträussler-Scheinker disease and the Indiana kindred. *Brain Pathol.*, **5**, 61–75.

Giannakopoulos, P., Hof, P. R., Savioz, A., Guimon, J., Antonarakis, S. E., and Bouras, C. (1996). Early-onset dementias: Clinical, neuropathological and genetic characteristics. *Acta Neuropathol.*, **91**, 451–65.

Gieselmann, V., Fluharty, A. L., Tonnesen, T., and von Figura, K. (1991). Mutations in the arylsulfatase A pseudodeficiency allele causing metachromatic leukodystrophy. *Am. J. Hum. Genet.*, **49**, 470–13.

Gieselmann, V., Zlotogora, J., Harris, A., *et al.* (1994). Molecular genetics of metachromatic leukodystrophy. *Hum. Mutat.*, **4**, 233–42.

Goebel, H. H. and Sharp, J. D. (1998). The neuronal ceroid-lipofuscinoses. Recent advances. *Brain Pathol.*, **8**, 151–62.

Graeber, M. B. and Muller, U. (1998). Recent development in the molecular genetics of mitochondrial disorders. *J. Neurol. Sci.*, **153**, 251–63.

Guerra, W. F., Verity, A., Fluharty, A. L., *et al.* (1990). Multiple sulphatase deficiency. Clinical, neuropathological, ultrastructural and biochemical studies. *J. Neuropathol. Exp. Neurol.*, **49**, 406–23.

Hock, C., Golombowski, S., Mullerspahn, F., *et al.* (1998). Cerebrospinal fluid levels of amyloid precursor protein and amyloid beta-peptide in Alzheimer's disease and major depression-inverse correlation with demential severity. *Eur. Neurol.*, **2**, 111–18.

Hodges, J. R., Patterson, K., Oxbury, S., and Funnell, E. (1992). Semantic dementia. Progressive fluent aphasia with temporal lobe atrophy. *Brain*, **115**, 1783–806.

Hsich, G., Kenney, K., Gibbs, C. J., Lee, K. H., and Harrington, M. G. (1996). The 14.3.3 brain protein in cerebrospinal fluid as a marker transmissible spongiform encephalopathies. *N. Engl. J. Med.*, **335**, 924–30.

Hurowitz, G. I., Silver, J. M., Brin, M. F., *et al.* (1993). Neuropsychiatric aspects of adult-onset Tay-Sachs disease: Two case reports with several new findings. *J. Neuropsychiatry Clin. Neurosci.*, **5**, 30–6.

Hutton, M., Lendon, C. L., Rizzu, P., *et al.* (1998). Association of missense and S^1-splice-site mutations in Tau with the inherited dementia FTDP-17. *Nature*, **393**, 702–5.

Kalimo, H., Lundberg, P. O., and Olsson, Y. (1979). Familial subacute necrotizing encephalomyelopathy of the adult form (adult Leigh syndrome). *Ann. Neurol.*, **6**, 200–6.

King, J. O. (1975). Progressive myoclonic epilepsy due to Gaucher's disease in an adult. *J. Neurol. Neurosurg. Psychiatry*, **38**, 849–54.

Kolodny, E. H., Raghavan, S., and Krivit, W. (1991). Late-onset Krabbe disease (globoid cell leukodystrophy): Clinical and biochemical features of 15 cases. *Dev. Neurosci.*, **13**, 232–9.

Kolter, T. and Sandhoff, K. (1998). Recent advances in the biochemistry of sphingolipidoses. *Brain Pathol.*, **8**, 79–100.

Kraus-Ruppert, R., Wildbolz, A., Matthieu, J. M., and Herschkowitz, N. (1972). The late form of metachromatic leukodystrophy I. A histochemical and neurochemical study. *J. Neurol. Sci.*, **17**, 373–81.

Krivit, W., Lockman, L. A., Watkins, P. A., Hirsch, J., and Shapiro, E. G. (1995). The future for treatment by bone marrow transplantation for adrenoleukodystrophy, metachromatic leukodystrophy, globoid cell leukodystrophy and Hurler syndrome. *J. Inherit. Metab. Disorders*, **18**, 398–412.

Lake, B. (1997). Lysosomal and peroxisomal disorders. In *Greenfield's neuropathology*, 6th edn (ed. D. I. Graham and P. L. Lantos), pp. 657–753. London: Arnold.

Long, R. G., Lake, B. D., Pettit, J. E., *et al.* (1977). Adult Niemann-Pick disease: Its relationship to the syndrome of the sea-blue histiocyte. *Am. J. Med.*, **62**, 627–35.

Lund and Manchester Groups, The (1994). Clinical and neuropathological criteria for frontotemporal dementia. *J. Neurol. Neurosurg. Psychiatry*, **57**, 416–18.

Lyon, G., Hagberg, B., Evrard, P., *et al.* (1991). Symptomatology of late onset Krabbe's leukodystrophy. The European experience. *Dev. Neurosci.*, **13**, 240–4.

Macfaul, R., Cavanagh, N., Lake, B. D., *et al.* (1982). Metachromatic leukodystrophy: Review of 38 cases. *Arch. Dis. Child.*, **57**, 168–75.

Majamaa, K., Moilanen, J. S., Uimonen, S., *et al.* (1998). Epidemiology of A3243G, the mutation for mitochondrial encephalomyopathy lactic acidosis, and stroke-like episodes: Prevalence of the mutation in an adult population. *Am. J. Hum. Genet.*, **63**, 447–54.

Martin, J.-J., Libert, J., and Ceuterick, C. (1987). Ultrastructure of brain and retina in Kufs' disease (adult type ceroid-lipofuscinosis). *Clin. Neuropathol.*, **6**, 231–5.

Medalia, A., Isaacs-Glaberman, K., and Scheinberg, I. H. (1988). Neuropsychological impairment in Wilson's disease. *Arch. Neurol.*, **45**, 502–4.

Miller, J. D., McCluer, R., and Kanfer, J. N. (1973). Gaucher's disease: Neurologic disorder in adult siblings. *Ann. Int. Med.*, **78**, 883–7.

Miyatake, T., Atsumi, T., Obayashi, T., *et al.* (1979). Adult type neuronal storage disease with neuraminidase deficiency. *Ann. Neurol.*, **6**, 232–44.

Mochizuki, H., Kamakura, K., Masaki, T., *et al.* (1997). Atypical MRI features of Wilson's disease: High signal in globus pallidus on T1-weighted images. *Neuroradiology*, **39**, 171–4.

Moser, H. W. (1997). Adrenoleukodystrophy: Phenotype, genetics, pathogenesis and therapy. *Brain*, **120**, 1485–508.

Mosser, J., Lutz, Y., Stoeckel, M. E., *et al.* (1994). The gene responsible for adrenoleukodystrophy encodes a peroxisomal membrane protein. *Hum. Mol. Genet.*, **3**, 264–71.

Nance, M. A. (1997). Clinical aspects of CAG repeat diseases. *Brain Pathol.*, **7**, 881–900.

Navon, R., Argov, Z., and Frisch, A. (1986). Hexosaminidase A deficiency in adults. *Am. J. Med. Genet.*, **24**, 179–96.

Navon, R. (1991). Molecular and clinical heterogeneity of adult Gm2 gangliosidosis. *Dev. Neurosci.*, **13**, 295–8.

Neary, D., Snowden, J. S., Northen, B., and Gouldine, P. (1988). Dementia of frontal lobe type. *J. Neurol. Neurosurg. Psychiatry*, **51**, 353–61.

Neary, D., Snowden, J. S., Gustafson, L., Passant, U., Stuss, D., Black, S., *et al.* (1998). Frontotemporal lobar degeneration: a consensus on clinical diagnostic criteria. *Neurology*, **51**, 1546–54.

Nebes, V. L. and Schmidt, M. C. (1994). Human lysosomal alpha-mannosidase: Isolation and nucleotide sequence of the full-length cDNA. *Biochem. Biophys. Res. Commun.*, **200**, 239–45.

Neville, B. G., Lake, B. D., Stephens, R., and Sanders, M. D. (1973). A neurovisceral storage disease with vertical supranuclear ophthalmoplegia, and its relationship to Niemann-Pick disease. A report of nine patients. *Brain*, **96**, 97–120.

Ockerman, P. A. (1967). A generalized storage disorder resembling Hurler's syndrome. *Lancet*, **ii**, 239–41.

Odone, A. and Odone, M. (1989). Lorenzo's oil. A new treatment for adrenoleukodystrophy. *J. Pediatr. Neurosci.*, **5**, 55–61.

Otto, M., Wiltfang, J., Schütz, E., *et al.* (1998). Diagnosis of Creutzfeldt–Jakob disease by measurement of S100 protein in serum: Prospective case-control study. *Br. Med. J.*, **316**, 577–82.

Panegyres, P. K., Goldswain, P., and Kakulas, B. A. (1989). Adult-onset adrenoleukodystrophy manifesting as dementia. *Am. J. Med.*, **87**, 481–3.

Patrick, A. D. (1965). A deficiency of glucocerebrosidase in Gaucher's disease. *Biochem. J.*, **97**, 17c–18c.

Powers, J. M. and Moser, H. W. (1998). Peroxisomal disorders: Genotype, phenotype, major neuropathologic lesions, and pathogenesis. *Brain Pathol.*, **8**, 101–20.

Rahman, S., Blok, R. B., Dahl, H. H., *et al.* (1996). Leigh syndrome: Clinical features and biochemical and DNA abnormalities. *Ann. Neurol.*, **39**, 343–51.

Richardson, E. P. and Masters, C. L. (1995). The nosology of Creutzfeldt-Jakob disease and conditions related to the accumulation of PrP[CJD] in the nervous system. *Brain Pathol.*, **5**, 33–41.

Rosselli, M., Lorenzana, P., Rosselli, A., and Vergara, I. (1987). Wilson's disease, a reversible dementia: Case report. *J. Clin. Exp. Neuropsychol.*, **9**, 399–406.

Ruchoux, M.-M. and Maurage, C.-A. (1997). CADASIL: Cerebral autosomal dominant arteriopathy with subcortical infarcts and leukoencephalopathy. *J. Neuropathol. Exp. Neurol.*, **56**, 947–64.

Schnabel, D., Schroder, M., and Sandhoff, K. (1991). Mutation in the sphingolipid activator protein 2 in a patient with a variant of Gaucher disease. *FEBS Lett.*, **284**, 57–9.

Silvestri, G., Ciafaloni, E., Santorelli, F. M., *et al.* (1993). Clinical features associated with the A→G transition at nucleotide 8344 of mtDNA ('MERRF mutation'). *Neurology*, **43**, 1200–6.

Snowden, J. S., Neary, D., Mann, D. M. A., Goulding, P. J., and Testa, H. J. (1992). Progressive language disorder due to lobar atrophy. *Ann. Neurol.*, **31**, 174–83.

Soffer, D. and Horoupian, D. S. (1979). Rosenthal fibers formation in the central nervous system. Its relation to Alexander's disease. *Acta Neuropathol.*, **47**, 81–4.

Starosta-Rubinstein, S., Young, A. B., Kluin, K., *et al.* (1987). Clinical assessment of 31 patients with Wilson's disease. Correlations with structural changes on magnetic resonance imaging. *Arch. Neurol.*, **44**, 365–70.

Suzuki, K., Parker, C. C., Pentchev, P. C., Katz, D., Ghetti, B., D'Agostino, A. N., *et al.* (1995). Neurofibrillary tangles in Niemann-Pick disease type C. *Acta Neuropathol.*, **89**, 227–38.

Tanaka, A., Hirabayashi, M., Ishii, M., *et al.* (1987). Complementation studies with clinical and biochemical characterizations of a new variant of multiple sulphatase deficiency. *J. Inherit. Metab. Disorders*, **10**, 103–10.

Vanier, M. T., Wenger, D. A., Comly, M. E., *et al.* (1998). Niemann-Pick disease group C: Clinical variability and diagnosis based on defective cholesterol esterification. A collaborative study on 70 patients. *Clin. Genet.*, **33**, 331–48.

Vanier, M. T. and Suzuki, K. (1998). Recent advances in elucidating Niemann-Pick C disease. *Brain Pathol.*, **8**, 163–74.

Vazquez-Memije, M. E., Shanske, S., Santorelli, F. M., *et al.* (1996). Comparative biochemical studies in fibroblasts from patients with different forms of Leigh syndrome. *J. Inherit. Metab. Disorders*, **19**, 43–50.

Waltz, G., Harik, S. I., and Kaufman, B. (1987). Adult metachromatic leukodystrophy. Value of computed tomographic scanning and magnetic resonance imaging of the brain. *Arch. Neurol.*, **44**, 225–7.

Winkelman, M. D., Banker, B. Q., Victor, M., and Moser, H. W. (1983). Noninfantile neuronopathic Gaucher's disease: A clinico-pathologic study. *Neurology*, **33**, 994–1008.

World Federation of Neurology: Research Committee Research Group on Huntington's Chorea. (1989). Ethical issues policy statement on Huntington's disease molecular genetics predictive test. *J. Neurol. Sci.*, **94**, 327–31.

Zevin, S., Abrahamov, A., Hadas Helpern, I., *et al.* (1993). Adult-type Gaucher disease in children: Genetics, clincial features and enzyme replacement therapy. *Q. J. Med.*, **86**, 565–73.

Zimran, A., Elstein, D., Kannai, R., *et al.* (1994). Low-dose enzyme replacement therapy for Gaucher's disease: Effects of age, sex, genotype and clinical features on response to treatment. *Am. J. Med.*, **97**, 3–13.

19 Drug interventions in dementia

Shibley Rahman, Barbara J. Sahakian, Carol A. Gregory

1 Introduction

There is now considerable optimism in the treatment of the presenile dementias. However, with this optimism has been the growing realization that therapeutic strategies in dementia should have very specific aims — to delay the progress of the disorder that is causing a progressive decline, to treat a range of emergent cognitive deficits, to ameliorate associated behavioural and affective disturbances, thereby reducing the consequences of functional disability and improving quality of life, and to address fully the needs of the caregiver. Whilst it remains the case that affective and behavioural symptoms of dementia, such as depression, difficult behaviour, and agitation, also often respond to interventions which are non-pharmacological in nature — e.g. trying to avoid circumstances which trigger behavioural outbursts, developing proper care environments, and teaching behavioural management to family members and nurses, — these 'symptoms often respond to therapeutic strategies aimed primarily at cognitive symptomatology.

Cognitive impairments in dementia may be the defining and perhaps the most easily measurable aspects of disease. However, behavioural disturbances and personality change are common, and may cause immense distress to the patients and their carers (such as family and friends or care staff if in residential or nursing accommodation). Behavioural changes such as physical aggression, shouting, and incontinence are a source of considerable burden to carers and may directly lead to admission to long-term care. Until relatively recently, behavioural changes in dementia were poorly characterized and a neglected area of research. These behaviours may be related to the development of psychiatric symptoms, but in some patients develop independently (Lyketsos *et al.* 1999). The clinician ideally needs to be aware of the possible beneficial effects of drugs upon both cognitive and behavioural symptomatology in dementia, and also, of course, be aware of the potential side-effects and drug interactions.

This book specifically addresses the subject of early onset dementia. However, little, if any, specific work on the pharmacological management of patients with early onset dementia exists. Research has more commonly been directed at dementia as a whole without reference to any particular diagnostic group. More recently, efforts have been directed at specific diagnostic categories such as dementia of the Alzheimer type (DAT) or the vascular dementias (VaD), where older patients predominate. The main focus of the first half of this chapter will be the current strategies for intervention in dementia of the Alzheimer type, with a review of how these strategies have been developed, and prospects for future intervention. We also consider briefly other important causes of dementia in this age group: frontotemporal dementia, multi-infarct dementia, and dementia with Lewy bodies. The management of Huntington's disease is discussed in Chapter 15 and of other rarer causes of dementia in Chapters 17 and 18. The second half of the chapter considers the profile, assessment, and treatment of common psychiatric symptoms of dementia with a critical evaluation of the precise rationale behind treatment.

2 Management of cognitive symptomatology in dementia of the Alzheimer type

Currently, the cholinesterase inhibitors represent the main drugs for the symptomatic treatment of dementia of the Alzheimer type (review, Lawrence and Sahakian 1998). The first to reach the market (in the USA and France) was tacrine, but its use was unfortunately limited by significant hepatotoxicity. Since then, donepezil has been successfully launched in the USA and in most countries of Western Europe. Rivastigmine and galanthamine have also been recently approved in Europe. The cholinesterase inhibitors therefore represent a major advance in the treatment of this condition. With the opportunity of early intervention using drug therapies, an early clinical, or ideally preclinical, diagnosis is clearly crucial. Early detection of neuropsychological deficits and differential diagnosis are both essential for therapeutic strategies to have the best chance of efficacy in improving symptoms and preventing further decline. Whilst sophisticated neuro-imaging is important, specialized neuropsychology is likely to become of increasing importance to reveal cognitive impairment before the disturbances reach a clinical level of dementia, particularly since laboratory investigations have generally not as yet yielded any reliable markers and to monitor therapeutic responses. Overall, a proper understanding of the spectrum of cognitive deficits and symptoms of disease provides the ideal approach for the therapeutic interventions in the senile dementias.

2.1 The pathology of DAT: implications for therapeutic strategies

Recently, there has been massive interest in the development of cholinesterase inhibitors for intervention in mild-to-moderate DAT. This interest ultimately arose from the observation from *post mortem* as well as biopsy studies that the earliest and most consistent biochemical abnormalities in the brains of DAT victims are found in the basal forebrain cholinergic system (e.g. Bowen *et al.* 1992). The major forebrain cholinergic pathways project from neurons in the nucleus basalis of Meynert, medial septum, and diagonal band of Broca to neocortex, amygdala, and hippocampus. Experimental lesions of the nucleus basalis in rats result in elevated cerebrospinal fluid APP secretion. DAT is associated with the loss of large pyramidal neurons in the cerebral cortex and depletion of several cholinergic, monoaminergic, and peptidergic markers (see Chapter 10). Given the range of abnormalities, repletion of a single neuro-transmitter may not reasonably be expected to produce complete clinical improvement particularly as the disease progresses. However, it is now well accepted that the cholinergic neurotransmitter system shows the largest deficits compared to other neurotransmitters. There may be interplay between the cholinergic neurotransmitter systems and other chemicals in the central nervous system; for example, presynaptic nicotinic receptors appear to control the release of excitatory amino acids in the hippocampus and the spinal cord. The nicotinic modulation of release of catecholamine and peptidic neurotransmitters has also been previously documented.

A key development in our understanding of DAT has been the development of the 'cholinergic hypothesis of geriatric dysfunction' (Drachman and Sahakian 1979; Bartus *et al.* 1982) which has generated much interest in the functions of central cholinergic systems and the neuro-pathological substrates underlying DAT. The synaptic loss, neuronal atrophy, and degeneration of cholinergic nuclei in the basal forebrain may be associated with reduced cholinergic activity in the hippocampus and a cortical loss of choline acetyltransferase, an enzyme that produces acetylcholine in the neurons (review, Perry 1986). Central cholinergic pathways have been found to have an important role in attentional function, as well as the processing and storage of information and memory. Perry *et al.* (1978) had previously demonstrated that the amount of cholinergic abnormalities correlated with mental state scores obtained from patients with DAT shortly before their death. Furthermore, systemic administration of the muscarinic acetylcholine receptor antagonist scopolamine to normal volunteers was found to reproduce many of the deficits in attention, visuospatial functions, and language seen in DAT (Drachman and Sahakian 1979). Importantly, cholinergic deficiency has been linked to a number of behavioural manifestations of DAT (Cummings and Kaufer 1996), and this shall be discussed later in this chapter. Certainly the cholinergic deficit hypothesis continues to fuel the studies of mechanisms of actions of systemically administered cholinergic drugs in patients with DAT.

As these pathological changes are known to be associated with evidence of inflammatory changes (e.g. Aisen and Davis 1994) and free radical formation due to oxidative metabolism, the development of anti-inflammatory and antioxidant agents has also been of considerable contemporary interest. A primary inflammatory process or an inflammatory reaction to deposition of abnormal proteins can cause neuronal damage; the roles of immune factors produced by vated astrocytes and microglia and the production of inflammatory factors such as interleukins and complement factors are also current areas of investigation into the pathobiology of DAT. It is acknowledged now that a much more ambitious strategy will be to attempt to retard, halt, or prevent disease progression. Nonetheless, even with the development of such agents, such drugs may not be able to improve existing symptoms, hence retaining the need for drugs such as cholinesterase inhibitors. Ultimately, through beneficial effects upon cognition and behavioural symptoms, it is hoped that cholinesterase inhibitors may improve substantially the quality of life for both patients and caregivers, delay institutionalization, and alleviate the financial burden of disease upon society.

Furthermore, in the overall development of rational therapeutic strategies, several practical issues inevitably arise from the fact that DAT is a heterogeneous disorder. The various subgroups include early versus late onset, familial versus sporadic disease, and rapid versus slow progression (see Petersen 1998, for review). Indeed, as is now being found to be the case for many neurodegenerative conditions, DAT may encompass a number of different clinical profiles, such as a Lewy body variant of DAT, and DAT in the presence of extrapyramidal symptoms and monoclonus (Petersen 1998). Not surprisingly, therefore, there is a corresponding heterogeneity in response to therapy, for example cholinesterase inhibitors, and it is a vital area of research to identify those patients who are most likely to respond to therapy. For example, a recent study suggested that after three months of therapy, gender was the only significant influence on the number of responders to anticholinesterase therapy (MacGowan et al. 1998). Whilst ApoE genotype did not modify response to therapy in the short-term, there were indications that it might affect response over the longer-term (up to 12 months) (MacGowan et al. 1998). It is likely that since attentional deficits show improvements following acute treatment with nicotine or treatments with tacrine (Sahakian and Coull 1993; Sahakian et al. 1989; Jones et al. 1992) that the baseline neuropsychological profile might help to predict those patients who show a beneficial response to cholinesterase inhibitors.

A plethora of drugs have so far been subjected to intense clinical investigation, some of which have been successful and are described below. In the field of DAT, pivotal clinical trials traditionally involve patients with 'probable DAT', defined by the Work Group on the Diagnosis of Alzheimer's disease established by the National Institute of Neurological and Communicative Disorders and Stroke and the Alzheimer's Disease and Related Disorders Association (McKhann et al. 1984). This standardization of diagnosis, whilst perhaps having helped to reduce some of the heterogeneity described above in dementia of the Alzheimer type, may have potentially limited the application of the results to a much large group of 'possibles' with variations in onset, presentation, or clinical course, or with associated conditions such as cerebrovascular disease (review, Gauthier 1998). Arguably, another major limitation of the trials thus far has been the failure to assess specific domains of cognitive function adequately. This has become particularly apparent, for example, in the assessment of attentional function which is not fully possible using many standard tools such as the ADAS-*cog*. Therefore, the observation that cholinesterase inhibitors such as tacrine or cholinergic agonists may improve attention in patients with mild DAT should not be overlooked, and indeed may be difficult to demonstrate quantitatively to a high standard using certain neuropsychological tools. The importance of this has become apparent when considering analogous work in the animal literature which involve AMPA-induced lesions of the nucleus basalis region. These specific lesions are used to investigate that the cholinergic hypothesis produces specific deficits in responding accurately in tests of visual attentional performance, which are reversed dose-dependently by treatment with systemic physostygmine or nicotine (review, Robbins *et al.* 1997). This clearly has important ramifications for our understanding of the cholinergic hypothesis and its application to the cognitive and neuropsychiatric aspects of DAT.

2.1.1 Pharmacoeconomics of cholinesterase inhibitors

An important consideration concerning cholinesterase inhibitors inevitably is their cost. At present, there is *a priori* no definite way to predict whether a patient with DAT will benefit from the drug, so it is clearly important for patients and carers to discuss possible benefits, risks, and costs, before deciding whether or not the drug should be tried. There is a pragmatic limit to treatment based upon the therapeutic indications for cholinesterase inhibitors (i.e. clinical progression to severe dementia). It should be acknowledged that the function of other central neurotransmitter pathways becomes compromised later on in the natural history of DAT and therefore, arguably, drugs that selectively target the cholinergic system may not have an underlying rationale in advanced disease. A complete analysis of cost-effectiveness would inevitably need to include the potential improvement in the quality of life for patients and carers, and in particular the environmental setting of the care. It is generally recognized that patients with DAT usually deteriorate to an end-stage requiring full nursing care. Although elderly patients may frequently die of other causes before dementia becomes severe, death is often from bronchopneumonia. The most widely quoted estimates of average survival are between five and eight years. The length of survival is highly variable, but recent data indicate that it is strongly associated with dementia severity as assessed using the MMSE. The mean survival from symptom onset was found to be 9.3 years. Results from various studies have implied is that it is actually important to consider the *relative* cost of putting a person on medication and keeping people at home, compared to the cost of being in a nursing home or in institutional care. Furthermore, maintaining improvements in the patients may make it possible for the carers to look after them for longer and this may cause them to stay out of a nursing home or institutional care. A final important consideration is that the role of cholinesterase inhibitors, in combination with other therapeutic strategies (e.g. antioxidants and anti-inflammatory agents), has yet to be properly evaluated.

2.2 The range of cholinesterase inhibitors

At the time of writing of this chapter, a number of experimental drugs are currently in different stages of development, and some cholinesterase inhibitors had licenses for the treatment of mild-to-moderate dementia of the Alzheimer type:

(a) Donepezil (both in the UK and the USA).

(b) Tacrine (in the USA only).

(c) Rivastigmine (in the UK and USA).

(d) Galanthamine (approved in the UK, and granted — at the time of writing — an approvable letter in the USA).

Other cholinesterase inhibitors are being considered for approval. In considering these drugs, direct comparisons are difficult because of differences in study design which include trial length, and patient inclusion criteria.

Furthermore, it is known that there are important subtle differences in the precise pharmacological properties of the cholinesterase inhibitors (review, Nordberg and Svensson 1998). In mammals, only a single gene encodes acetylcholinesterase (AChE), with its multiple forms arising from alternative mRNA, the function of the enzyme being to break down acetylcholine, as well as to have a number of useful neurotrophic and synaptogenic effects (see Chapter 10). Because the alternatively spliced forms of the enzyme have sequence identity in the domains affecting catalysis and inhibition, distinctions between cholinesterase inhibitors arise from differences in reaction mechanisms with the enzyme and from their pharmacokinetic properties (see review, Taylor 1998).

There are important subtle differences in the precise pharmacological properties of the cholinesterase inhibitors (review, Nordberg and Svensson 1998). For example, the mechanism of action of donepezil is similar to that of tacrine, in that it is a 'mixed type' reversible inhibitor, inhibiting acetylcholinesterase via both non-competitive mechanisms — by blockade of the deacetylation process — and ACh competitive mechanisms. Galanthamine is also a reversible inhibitor of ACh. However, the carbamates (such as rivastigmine) are pseudoirreversible cholinesterase inhibitors, in that they become cleaved by the enzyme resulting in a covalent modification of the enzyme. The term 'pseudoirreversible' reflects the effect of such compounds as intermediate between the reversible and irreversible inhibitors. Other key differences exist between the different drugs. For example, the elimination half-life is considerably longer for donepezil in comparison to other cholinesterase inhibitors, allowing a once-daily dosing (in comparison to tacrine which is administered four times daily and rivastigmine which is administered twice daily). Also, tacrine and donepezil are metabolized via the cytochrome P_{450} (cyt P_{450}) liver enzymes, whereas rivastigmine appears not to be.

Clinically, there are a number of important considerations with regards to practical use of cholinesterase inhibitors, which are summarized in Table 19.1. Ideally, cholinesterase inhibitors should show a minimal profile of adverse effects. The main common adverse effects will be discussed in relation to each cholinesterase inhibitor in turn. However, certain general points are worth noting. Because of their pharmacological action, cholinesterase inhibitors may have vagotonic effects on heart rate (e.g. bradycardia). The potential for this action may be particularly important to patients with 'sick sinus' syndrome or other supraventricular conduction abnormalities, such as sinoatrial or atrioventricular block. Patients at increased risk for developing ulcers, e.g. those with a history of ulcer disease or those receiving concurrent non-steroidal anti-inflammatory drugs, should be monitored for symptoms. Cholinesterase inhibitors may also theoretically cause bladder outflow obstruction.

2.3 The efficacy of cholinesterase inhibitors

There is likely to be fast progress in the next decades in the development of successful pharmacological therapies for mild-to-moderate DAT. It is important to note concerning the methodology of the majority of these trials to date are that patients are screened carefully, and in certain cases, individuals with important medical or neuropsychiatric comorbid symptoms, or more advanced disease are excluded from medical study.

Table 19.1 Profile of an ideal AChE inhibitor

1	It should be well tolerated within the clinically effective dosage range.
2	It should have minimal unwanted central or peripheral cholinergic effects (such as nausea, vomiting, headache, diarrhoea, dizziness, reduced appetite, abdominal pain).
3	It should display no organ toxicity (e.g. abnormal ECG, elevated liver enzyme levels).
4	It should be suitable for patients with concurrent illnesses (and who are also receiving long-term drug therapy). This is particularly important in the elderly population.
5	It should have minimal drug–drug interactions. This is particularly important in the elderly population.
6	The pharmacokinetics and duration of action should be consistent with a simple treatment regimen (with preferably oral administration once or twice a day).
7	Positive effects should ideally persist for years during treatment, and when therapy is stopped, there should not be any withdrawal effects such as an exaggerated cognitive deterioration.

2.3.1 Donepezil hydrochloride

Donepezil is a piperidine-based derivative that has been developed specifically for the symptomatic treatment of mild-to-moderate DAT. Donepezil may slow the rate of cognitive and noncognitive deterioration in about 40% of patients with DAT. Donepezil significantly is a highly selective, potent, reversible inhibitor of acetylcholinesterase according to *in vitro* data, being over 1000 times more potent an inhibitor of acetylcholinesterase than of butyrylcholinesterase, an enzyme found predominantly outside the central nervous system.

A number of trials of donepezil have been published in full examining the potential therapeutic benefit of donepezil and its safety (e.g. Rogers and Friedhoff 1996; Rogers *et al.* 2000). It should be noted that the designs of the trials would have been improved had the subjective clinical rating scales been complemented with objective neuropsychological tests which assessed a wide range of neuropsychological cognitive processes. A recent systematic review of donepezil demonstrates a significant improvement of 2.6 points on the ADAS-cog scale and an odds ratio of 2.4 for clinical global impression for the lower dose of 5 mg/day for a treatment duration of 12–24 weeks (Cochrane Collaboration: Birks and Melzer 1998). This review found no evidence of improvement with donepezil on a patient related quality of life scale, but lack of insight and decreased memory may make the use of ratings problematic in patients with DAT.

The most common adverse effects (incidence > 5% and twice the frequency of placebo) were diarrhoea, muscle cramps, fatigue, nausea, vomiting, and insomnia. In most cases, the adverse effects are mild, usually lasting from one to three weeks and reducing with continued use of the drug. As the clinical experience with donepezil is presently limited, the prescribing physician should be aware of the possibility of new, as yet unknown, interactions with donepezil. Donepezil hydrochloride and/or any of its metabolites does not inhibit the metabolism of theophylline, warfarin, cimetidine, or digoxin in humans. The metabolism of donepezil hydrochloride is not affected by concurrent administration of digoxin or cimetidine.

An important consideration regarding donepezil (as well as the other cholinesterase inhibitors) is that there is currently no information available that may help to predict which patients may benefit most. Studies are required to identify responders from non-responders, on the basis of objective neuropsychological tests. Prognostic variables that may also prove to be important include apolipoprotein ε2 genotype, presence of Lewy body pathology, and the risk of vascular dementia.

2.3.2 Tacrine hydrochloride (THA)

Tacrine, a first generation drug, produces non-specific reversible inhibition by forming an ionic bond at the anionic subsite (Silman *et al.* 1994). Tacrine has been shown to increase presynaptic ACh release through blocking slow K^+ channels, and is also thought to increase postsynaptic monoaminergic stimulation by blocking noradrenaline and serotonin uptake. These latter characteristics occur at concentrations higher than those required to achieve acetylcholinesterase inhibition, and therefore probably may not contribute to the drug's clinical effects. Tacrine has been shown to be successful in alleviating some aspects of the cognitive symptomatology in DAT as measured by improvements in subjective clinical rating scales, with manageable side-effects. For example, Farlow *et al.* (1992) demonstrated that after 12 weeks of treatment with tacrine in a double-blind, placebo-controlled, parallel group study, dose-related improvements were seen on the ADAS-cog as well as the CGIC. In contrast, a recent meta-analysis (Qizilbash *et al.* 1998) suggested that there was no convincing evidence as yet that tacrine was a useful treatment for DAT. It should however be noted that the authors of the meta-analysis conceded that only a few trials presented data in a format suitable for pooling.

Tacrine may have beneficial cognitive effects, in both acute and chronic dosage. For example, the acute effects of tacrine upon cognition in a group of patients meeting criteria for probable DAT have been assessed using objective computerized tests of learning, memory, and attention from the Cambridge Neuropsychological Test Automated Battery (CANTAB) (Sahakian and Coull 1993). Statistically significant beneficial effects of THA were found on the five choice reaction time task where significant improvements were seen in both speed and accuracy of performance. The pattern of results with CANTAB were supported by an improvement on the 'concentration/distractibility' subscore of the Rosen Alzheimer's Disease non-cognitive scale. It is important to note that the findings with tacrine parallel those with acute nicotine, described later in this chapter. In other words, there are beneficial effects on attentional function in patients with DAT, but these do not rule out a role for ascending cholinergic neurons in learning and memory: these functions may be subserved by other structures such as the hippocampus which also receives a substantial cholinergic innervation.

Interestingly, it is important to note that studies with tacrine have provided important clues into some of the factors determining response to cholinesterase inhibition therapy in patients with DAT. Riekkinen *et al.* (1998) recently described that 'responders' perform better than the 'non-responders' in tests measuring memory and frontal functions. The responders had less severe hippocampal atrophy and less prefrontal blood flow defect, and had a lower frequency of the apolipoprotein ε4 allele than the 'non-responders'. These results arguably suggested that severe dysfunction of hippocampus and prefrontal regions blocked the stimulatory effect of tetrahydroaminoacridine on short-term memory performance.

Because of the potential elevation of liver transaminases, correct dosing of tacrine and monitoring of liver function tests is mandatory. The wider significance of this is that both clinicians and researchers need, ideally, to identify those patients who are most likely to respond to such therapy for whom the benefits may outweigh the risk of adverse effects. Tacrine should therefore be prescribed with care in patients with current evidence or history of abnormal liver function indicated by significant abnormalities in serum transaminases, bilirubin, and γGT levels. The use of tacrine in patients without a prior history of liver disease is commonly associated with serum aminotransferase elevations, some to levels ordinarily considered to indicate clinically significant hepatic injury. Tacrine may also cause bladder outflow obstruction; and, also because of its cholinomimetic action, it should be prescribed with care to patients with a history of asthma. The most common adverse effects associated are elevated transaminases, ataxia, and also (in a dose-dependent manner) nausea and/or vomiting, diarrhoea, dyspepsia, myalgia, and anorexia. Tacrine is primarily eliminated by hepatic metabolism via cyt P_{450} drug metabolizing enzymes. Drug–drug interactions may occur when tacrine is given concurrently with agents such as theophylline and cimetidine. Because of its mechanism of action, tacrine also has the potential to interfere with the activity of anticholinergic medications (including amitriptyline, to a lesser extent other tricyclic antidepressants, and some neuroleptic agents). A synergistic effect is expected when tacrine is given concurrently with succinylcholine, cholinesterase inhibitors, or cholinergic agonists such as bethanecol.

2.3.3 Rivastigmine

Rivastigmine is long-acting reversible acetylcholinesterase inhibitor that is indicated as an oral treatment for patients with mild-to-moderately severe DAT. It is selective for the cortex and hippocampus areas of the brain (rather than the pons, medulla, or cerebellum). The efficacy of rivastigmine has been examined in a number of trials (review, Spencer and Noble 1998). Individual and pooled results from these trials indicate that rivastigmine 6–12 mg/day usually produces cognitive, global, and functional changes that indicate significantly less deterioration than observed in patients on placebo.

In humans, the duration of acetylcholinesterase inhibition is found to be sustained for approximately 10 hours (although the plasma half-life is short), and no neuromuscular effects were noted in preclinical studies. With brain-selectivity, therapeutic doses of rivastigmine had no effect on cardiac, respiratory, hepatic, or renal systems. Therefore, therapy can be considered safe for patients with concomitant medical illnesses. Rivastigmine is rapidly and extensively metabolized to a product that is eliminated renally. Given that rivastigmine is not metabolized via the cyt P_{450} system and exhibits relatively low protein-binding (approximately 40%), very few drug–drug interactions are to be theoretically expected. These pharmacokinetic properties are especially important in the elderly population, as multiple medications are often prescribed for numerous medical conditions. The adverse effects were those usually expected (predominantly gastrointestinal), and were usually of short duration and responsive to dosage reduction.

2.3.4 Galanthamine

Galanthamine is a tertiary alkaloid originally isolated from bulbs of snowdrop and narcissus. It has a dual action in both acting as a selective acetylcholinesterase inhibitor and in appearing to stimulate nicotinic acetylcholine receptors. Galanthamine attenuates drug- and lesion-induced cognitive deficits in animal models of learning and memory (review, Fulton and Benfield 1996). Furthermore, preliminary results in patients with DAT have reported galanthamine to be associated with a reduction in cognitive deterioration on some neuropsychiatric rating scales. Nausea and vomiting are the most commonly reported adverse effects; liver toxicity has not been reported to date. A recent six month double-blind trial (Raskind *et al.* 2000) has shown that galanthamine is effective and safe, and at six months significantly improved cognition and global function as measured by the ADAS-*cog* and the CIBIC-plus. Cognitive and daily function were maintained for 12 months at the 24 mg/day dose.

2.4 Other cholinesterase inhibitors in development

Therefore, it can be seen that the cholinesterase inhibitors currently available have considerable potential for the treatment of the dementia of the Alzheimer type. A summary of these compounds is given in Table 19.2. Promisingly, there are a number of other cholinesterase inhibitors in development, one of which is outlined below.

Table 19.2 Summary of the main features of currently available cholinesterase inhibitors

Cholinesterase inhibitor	Description
Donepezil	'Mixed-type' reversible inhibitor of acetylcholinesterase. Beneficial effects on cognition and behaviour. Most common adverse effects include dyspepsia, nausea, vomiting, diarrhoea, and facial flushing; less commonly, dizziness and headache. Donepezil does not inhibit the metabolism of theophylline, warfarin, cimetidine, or digoxin in humans.
Tacrine	Non-specific reversible inhibitor of acetylcholinesterase. Beneficial effects on cognition and behaviour. Adverse effects as donepezil, but also include elevated transaminases. There are possible interactions with theophylline and cimetidine.
Rivastigmine	Pseudoirreversible non-competitive carbamate acetylcholinesterase inhibitor. Beneficial effects on cognition and behaviour. Adverse effects as donepezil. No major drug–drug interactions.
Galanthamine	Reversible cholinesterase inhibitor and also stimulates nicotinic receptors. Beneficial effects on cognition and behaviour. Main adverse effects are nausea and vomiting.

2.4.1 Metrifonate

Metrifonate was first introduced as an insecticide in the 1950s, and has been used clinically as an anthelmintic for the treatment of schistosomiasis for more than three decades. Metrifonate is a pro-drug with a short life, but its metabolite forms a stable complex with AChE. The result is a consistent, long-lasting inhibition of AChE in the CNS. As with other cholinesterase inhibitors, mild-to-moderate dose-dependent cholinergic effects (typically nausea, vomiting, abdominal discomfort, diarrhoea, weakness, and leg cramps) have been most commonly associated with metrifonate. A key study by Cummings *et al.* (1998) evaluated critically the efficacy and safety of metrifonate in patients diagnosed with mild-to-moderate DAT in the form of a prospective 30 week multi-centre, double-blind, randomized parallel group dose-finding study. Metrifonate was found to improve cognitive function as assessed by the ADAS-*Cog* and enhance global function, as assessed using CIBIC-Plus. The drug was well tolerated; side-effects were predominantly gastrointestinal in nature, and no hepatic toxicity was observed. However, at the time of writing of the chapter, there was concern that a small yet significant proportion of patients on metrifonate had required respiratory support, hence necessitating a proper review of its safety and efficacy.

2.5 Cholinergic agonists — nicotine

There is evidence for a significant loss of nicotinic receptors in the cortex and the parahippocampal gyrus in DAT, as measured both at *post mortem* and through functional imaging studies. Jones *et al.* (1992) reported the effects of acute subcutaneous nicotine on attention, information processing and short-term memory in patients with DAT. Nicotine was found to improve significantly sustained visual attention, reaction time, and perception, with no effect on visual short-term memory. Clearly, the optimization of attentional processes may have substantial benefits for patients with DAT.

2.6 Other strategies in dementia of the Alzheimer type

The possible role of anti-inflammatory agents in the neurodegenerative process in DAT was suggested by evidence such as the discovery of an unexpectedly low prevalence of DAT amongst patients with rheumatoid arthritis. Case-control, cross-sectional, and longitudinal studies have found an inverse relation between the risk for DAT and non-steroidal anti-inflammatory drug (NSAID) use. In a recent trial of indomethacin for mild-to-moderate DAT (Rogers *et al.* 1993), at a dose of 100–150 mg/day indomethacin was found to improve cognitive function. However, about 20% of patients developed adverse effects, primarily gastrointestinal disturbance.

Experimental studies have demonstrated that loss of oestrogen predisposes to cognitive decline and neuronal degeneration. Human studies suggest that oestrogen hormone replacement therapy may prevent, delay, or reduce the symptoms of DAT. In a case-control study (Henderson *et al.* 1994), treatment with HRT at the time of enrolment was found to be significantly less common in women meeting criteria for DAT than control subjects. Furthermore, the patients with DAT using HRT performed significantly better on the MMSE. Obvious confounding factors include retrospective analysis, detailed information about dosage, and a previous history of HRT. Further information is clearly necessary.

Oxidative stress is believed to be a critical factor in normal ageing and neurodegenerative diseases such as Parkinson's disease and amyotrophic lateral sclerosis. The neuropathology of DAT may involve oxidative stress and the accumulation of free radicals, leading to raised intracellular calcium, excessive lipid peroxidation, and neuronal degeneration in the brain (Porta 1988). Selegiline, a monoamine oxidase (MAO) inhibitor, acts as an antioxidant since it inhibits oxidative deamination thereby reducing neuronal damage. It also increases levels of catecholamines, and adrenergic stimulation may improve the cognitive deficits associated with dementia of the Alzheimer type. Alpha-tocopherol may have beneficial effects in patients with DAT, as it is a lipid soluble vitamin that interrupts the chain reaction that damages cells. Sano *et al.* (1997) recently reported findings implying that selegiline and alpha-tocopherol could delay functional deterioration, particularly as reflected by the need for institutionalization. Another important recent area of research have utilized extracts of the leaf of the *Gingko biloba* tree which have actually been used in traditional Chinese medicine for thousands of years. Beneficial efficacy of this extract is still yet to be convincingly demonstrated.

2.7 Effects of drugs used to treat primarily psychiatric and behavioural problems on cognitive function

One area of concern — and one that will require continued research — relates to the potential effect of antipsychotics on cognitive function, about which conflicting reports currently exist in the literature (e.g. Barnes *et al.* 1982; Rosen 1979). In an out-patient study by Devanand *et al.* (1989), haloperidol was compared to placebo in nine people with DAT complicated by psychotic phenomena and disruptive problem behaviours. In this cross-over design study, haloperidol was significantly superior to placebo for target symptoms. However, deteriorated cognitive function and extrapyramidal effects limited improvement in the quality of life. In a subsequent paper by Devanand *et al.* (1998), moderate-to-severe extrapyramidal side-effects occurred in a significant minority of patients who were prescribed 2–3 mg haloperidol per day. Whilst the MMSE did not reveal a deterioration in cognitive function, the authors noted that this finding did not preclude deterioration in cognitive function from having occurred which was not detected by the MMSE. Clouding this issue is the fact that research suggests that psychosis, hallucinations, and aggressive behaviours have been associated with a more rapid decline in cognitive function (Burns and Jacoby 1990*b*; Rosen and Zubenko

1991; Levy *et al.* 1996). However, McShane *et al.* (1997) point out that there has been little research which adequately controls for the possibility that the decline in patients with these phenomena may be due to treatment with antipsychotics, and also noted use of antipsychotic drugs was associated with an increased rate of cognitive decline in dementia. This association was independent of the degree of dementia and also the behavioural symptoms for which the antipsychotic medications may have been prescribed.

2.8 Future strategies for dementia of the Alzheimer type

Future strategies for intervention in DAT are likely to be facilitated by the development of *in vivo* animal models. Animal models of dysfunction should hopefully enhance our understanding of the underlying substrates and mechanisms, and clarify a relationship between brain and behaviour, and should also help us to assess the effects of a number of different treatments. Such models may provide the opportunity for examination of cholinesterase inhibitors, as well as neurotrophic factor administration (such as NGF), and transplantation of cholinergic-enriched fetal grafts. Animal models may in addition provide complete novel approaches to therapy. For instance, point mutations in the presenilin 1 gene, a cause of familial DAT, result in a selective increase in the production of β-amyloid$_{1-42}$ by proteolytic processing of the amyloid precursor protein. In PS1 deficient mouse embryos, γ-secretase is unable to cleave APP, causing carboxyl-terminal fragments of APP to accumulate, indicating that PS1 inhibition may be a rationale target for anti-amyloidogenic therapy in DAT. Gene therapy also provides a tool for topographically restricted and selective delivery of therapeutic genes and their products to affected areas of brain.

2.9 Other forms of presenile dementias

Apart from DAT, there are a number of important other causes of presenile dementias, including vascular dementia, frontotemporal dementias, and dementia with Lewy bodies.

2.9.1 Vascular dementias

This is a term for dementias which are directly associated with cerebrovascular disease. Multi-infarct dementia is traditionally considered to be the second most common dementia in Europe and the US, and accounts for 15–30% of all cases of dementia (Konno *et al.* 1997). It is the most common kind of vascular dementia, and is more common in men and in people with a high risk of cardiovascular problems. The onset is usually relatively acute and the progression is stepwise, as minor infarcts cause damage to the cortex. Progressive damage leads to a decline in mental abilities, with the site and extent of infarcts determining cognitive effects. Risk factors need to be considered, and include older age, male gender, hypertension, hyperlipidaemia, diabetes mellitus, atrial fibrillation, congestive heart failure, carotid bruit, cigarette smoking, and alcohol abuse. It is important to acknowledge the risk factors may also contribute to the risk of DAT. The preliminary finding from the Syst-Eur trial that treatment of isolated systolic hypertension reduced the incidence of dementia by 50% emphasized the importance of vascular risk factors as possible targets for prevention. Hypertension should be treated with appropriate anti-hypertensives. Also, any coexisting conditions that predispose to emboli formation (e.g. cardiac arrhythmias, valvular disease) should be treated appropriately. Daily low-dose enterically-coated aspirin is indicated because of its antithrombotic effects. Anticoagulants should only be considered only where there is an identified source of cerebral emboli and when the risk of falls and intracerebral haemorrhage does not counterindicate their use. Ticlodipine may be warranted in patients who are unresponsive to aspirin or who cannot tolerate that drug.

Chronic progressive subcortical encephalopathy or *leucoariosis* (Binswanger's disease) is another slowly evolving type of dementia. Symptoms include lethargy and slowness, emotional lability, and unsteadiness of gait. The patients are often hypertensive and there is patchy or diffuse loss of the periventricular cerebral white matter evident on CT scan or MRI. Risk factors, including hypertension, amyloid angiopathy, cerebral autosomal dominant arteriopathy with subcortical infarcts and leukoencephalopathy (CADASIL) amongst others should be as far as possible considered in the management of the disease, using also similar strategies as in multi-infarct dementia.

2.9.2 Frontotemporal dementias

There are currently no pharmacological treatments for frontotemporal dementias (FTD) in routine usage. However, recent reports of an improvement in executive function in patients with fvFTD following increased noradrenergic activity produced by the α_2 antagonist idazoxan (IDZ) (Coull *et al.* 1996) suggest a promising approach to the development of new treatments for this type of dementia. IDZ was found to produce dose-dependent improvements in three patients with the frontal variant of FTD (where the prefrontal cortex is predominantly affected), particularly on tests of planning, sustained attention, verbal fluency, and episodic memory. It is now known that IDZ is an agonist at 5-HT_{1A} autoreceptors modulating serotonin synthesis in the rat brain *in vivo*, causing overall a reduction in the synthesis of serotonin in the cerebral cortex. This may be of some relevance in relation to the reports from Sparks and Markesbery (1991) of decreased serotonin receptor binding in the frontal lobes, temporal lobes, and hypothalamus in autopsy-proven FTD cases and the study by Francis *et al.* (1993) also finding reduced serotonin receptors. There is therefore a decent scientific rationale that many of the cognitive and behavioural symptoms (including disinhibition, depressive symptoms, carbohydrate craving, and compulsions) may also respond to serotonergic agents. This possibility is discussed in more detail later in this chapter.

2.9.3 Dementia with Lewy bodies

In dementia with Lewy bodies (DLB), neocortical choline acetyltransferase levels tend to be consistently low (see Chapter 9), and hence the potential utility of therapeutic trials of cholinesterase inhibitors should be seriously considered. In relation to this, it is noteworthy that two patients with DLB have recently reported with extremely low cholinergic activity who were found to respond to tacrine. Most recently, it has been observed that patients with DLB may respond to the newer cholinesterase inhibitor donepezil (Kaufer *et al.* 1998). More research is needed to examine this further. It is important to note that dopamine receptor blockers should be avoided because of possible shortened survival and neuroleptic sensitivity syndrome in patients. As described in the chapter by Perry and colleagues, this neuroleptic sensitivity may be a consequence partly of the low level of dopamine D_2 receptors with increased susceptibility to D_2 antagonistic neuroleptic drugs.

3 The pharmacological management of psychiatric symptoms and behavioural disturbance in dementia

Certain psychiatric symptoms have been linked to carer burden, and may even play a part in determining the need for placement in residential settings (Rabins *et al.* 1982). Clinicians involved in the care of patients with dementia are frequently asked whether any treatment will help when mood symptoms, psychotic phenomena, or behavioural disturbance develop. Effective treatment of such complications, whether pharmacologically, with psychological interventions or manipulation of the environment, would hopefully improve the quality of the patients and carers' life, and perhaps delay the need for institutional care which has significant cost implications.

There are several questions that the clinician caring for patients with dementia needs to consider:

(a) How common are psychiatric symptoms and behavioural disturbance in dementia?

(b) What is the evidence for treating them?

(c) When should these problems be treated?

(d) When should treatment be stopped?

This part of the chapter will examine the nature of psychiatric symptoms and behavioural changes in dementia, as well as their clinical assessment. We will consider the prevalence of mood symptoms, psychotic phenomena, and behavioural disturbance, and the data supporting the pharmacological treatment of these problems. Also, we intend to review the literature to date that may help inform decisions on when to withdraw treatment.

3.1 The nature of psychiatric symptomatology in dementia

Patients with dementia may develop a variety of psychiatric symptoms and syndromes, for example, depression and anxiety, and more rarely mania, delusions, and hallucinations. In addition, patients may demonstrate marked behavioural disturbance, e.g. aggression, wandering, and shouting. In some patients, these changes may be linked. It is sometimes hard to compare the prevalence of such complications because study characteristics can vary considerably, e.g. variation in the diagnostic groups studied, the severity and stage of dementia, the stringency of criteria for inclusion in the study, and whether standardized assessment instruments were used. The characteristics of the population under study can also differ, e.g. community sample versus hospital inpatients (see later). However, despite these methodological differences, it seems clear that psychiatric symptoms and behavioural change are common in patients with dementia. The term 'non-cognitive symptoms' has been used to cover the psychiatric symptoms and behavioural changes seen in dementia as opposed to the more 'cognitive' or 'neurological' changes in the domains of memory, attention, language, and visuospatial ability. This distinction does not sit easily with all clinicians, but many 'non-cognitive' symptoms are driven by cognitive deficits, for example delusions of misidentification being secondary to cognitive deficits in face processing.

3.2 The clinical assessment of psychiatric symptomatology in dementia

The onset of psychiatric symptoms or behavioural disturbance in dementia requires careful assessment in order that interventions and treatments can be carefully planned. The quality of the history available from the patient or their carer will determine how much needs to be performed in the way of investigation. In general, the areas to consider are: health changes in the patient, alterations in the environment including changes in the care or routine of the patient, psychological factors, and the natural history of the underlying condition. Abrupt onset of behavioural problems or psychiatric symptoms should alert one to the possibility of a superimposed physical problem. Common problems are those of the elderly in general (see Table 19.3) and include infections, constipation, metabolic abnormalities, undiagnosed pain, or confusion secondary to

Table 19.3 Common psychiatric symptoms in dementia

Ballpark figures vary considerably across studies	
Depressive symptoms	Very common (> 50%)
Depressive syndrome	Common (up to 20%)
Mania	Uncommon (< few %)
Delusions — particularly of theft	Common (up to one-third)
Misidentification syndromes	Common (up to one-third)
Hallucinations — usually visual	Common (up to 15%)

medication. Problems such as failing hearing aids or lost glasses may have a substantial impact on the ability of an impaired patient to make sense of their immediate environment. Environmental factors may also play a role in affecting patients. For example, illness or stress in a carer may result in less skilled handling, or changes in routine such as changes in care staff or starting at a day centre, may in turn lead to changes in behaviour. Psychological factors also need to be considered; the patient's own awareness of loss of practical skills or deterioration in intellectual skills, as well as interpersonal difficulties with families, friends, or staff may underpin the development of mood related symptoms or behavioural change.

A more thorough assessment of psychiatric symptomatology or behavioural change is sometimes required, and it may be particularly useful to have a measurement against which to assess the efficacy of any given intervention for which a number of instruments are available, some of which are specific (e.g. the Cornell Scale for Assessment of Depression in Dementia), others better designed to capture a wider range of problems, e.g. MOUSEPAD (Allen *et al.* 1996), the Behave-AD scale (Reisberg *et al.* 1987), the Alzheimer's Disease Assessment Scale (Rosen *et al.* 1984), the Present Behavioural Examination (Hope and Fairburn 1992), and the Neuropsychiatric Inventory (Cummings *et al.* 1994).

3.3 The nature of mood symptoms in dementia

Depression occurs frequently in patients with dementia although the exact prevalence and nature remains uncertain. Assessment and diagnosis of depression in the elderly, with or without dementia, is not always easy. Medical problems may mimic the biological/vegetative symptoms of depression and masked presentations, for example, marked somatic symptoms, may occur. Many of the assessment schedules designed for the assessment of depression rely on information provided by the patient or are even self-rated. Deficits in concentration, memory, or judgement may therefore confound the use of such instruments. The difficulty of diagnosing depression in a significantly cognitively impaired individual, because of a poor history, etc., means that a high level of awareness must be maintained, together with an understanding that behavioural disturbance may be the presenting problem when a superadded depression occurs (Lyketsos *et al.* 1999). In some cases where there is clinical doubt a trial of antidepressants may be worth pursuing.

Wragg and Jeste (1989) and Burns (1991) highlight the considerable variation in the rates of psychiatric phenomena between different studies and discuss possible reasons for this variation (even when standard diagnostic criteria are applied), with rates varying between 0–87%, and a depressive disorder between 0–86%, with most figures being in the range of 40–50% and 10–20% respectively. Elevated mood, or mania, in DAT, on the other hand, is found much less frequently. Ranges of 3–17%, for example, have been found (Burns 1991), and in the study by Burns and Jacoby (1990c), only one patient out of 110 reported feelings of elation. Comparisons of the rates of affective symptoms in DAT with other diagnostic groups have also been undertaken. Sultzer *et al.* (1993) reported that blunted affect, depressed mood, low motivation, emotional withdrawal, anxiety, and somatic concerns were more common in vascular dementia than in DAT. Patients with fvFTD may present with an amotivational state or with disinhibition, perhaps suggestive of a depressive disorder or a manic state respectively, in up to a third of patients (Gustafson 1987). Reports of significant or enduring mood change are, however, much less common (Gregory and Hodges 1996).

3.4 The pharmacological treatment of depression

The rationale for the drug treatment of depression in the context of dementia is based on rather limited data. Clinicians treat on the empirical basis that experiencing significant depressive symptoms is distressing, and that depressed mood may worsen cognitive or functional abilities. In more advanced cases of dementia, depression may lead to behavioural disturbance which is lessened by antidepressant therapy.

It is useful to consider whether any of these clinical decisions are based on current evidence. Only a small number of placebo-controlled trials have been performed and these are reviewed by Kumar *et al.* (1998). The studies are, on the whole, limited by low sample sizes, the inclusion of mixed or poorly characterized dementia syndromes, a lack of randomization, or the use of rather uncommon psychotropic agents. Reifler *et al.* (1989) studied patients with DAT with and without depression. Depressed patients were randomized to receive either placebo or treatment with imipramine in double-blind conditions. Doses of imipramine were, on average, approximately 80 mg. Depressive symptoms improved considerably and equally in both medication and placebo groups. However, there was some evidence to suggest that, rather than experiencing an improvement in cognitive function as depressive symptoms resolved, drug treatment may have had a detrimental effect on cognitive function possibly through anticholinergic mechanisms. The authors attributed the improvement in symptoms in the depressed patients treated with placebo to the involvement of the nurse coordinator and the study doctor. There were no significant differences in side-effects reported between the active and placebo groups, suggesting that at these doses imiprimine was well tolerated. In a six week double-blind trial to assess the effect of citalopram in the treatment of depression in a mixed group of patients with depression and dementia, or somatic disorders (Nyth and Gottfries 1990), depression (both depressive symptoms and the subgroup with DSM-IIIR major depression) and cognitive function improved more in the citalopram-treated group.

The data on which to base decisions about *which* antidepressant to use is even more limited, with only one study to date comparing two antidepressants in this group of patients. Katona *et al.* (1998) compared imiprimine and paroxetine in an eight week double-blind study investigating the efficacy of these two agents. Both treatment groups improved significantly. Treatment-emergent adverse effects were equally high in both groups, but there were trends to suggest that paroxetine was better tolerated in terms of anticholinergic effects than imiprimine. However, given the finding from the study by Reifler *et al.* (1989) of no significant differences between imiprimine and placebo, the lack of control group in the study by Katona *et al.* (1998) may prevent strict differentiation between active treatment and placebo response.

Arguably, until further research is available in this particular area, it is sensible to be guided by general principles of prescribing in the elderly. Specific serotonin reuptake inhibitors (SSRIs) are, on the whole, well-tolerated in the elderly, require single dosing, and avoid the theoretical risk of deteriorating cognitive ability in many domains and the potential for delirium through additional anticholinergic mechanisms. Side-effects tend to be predominantly gastrointestinal (nausea and vomiting), agitation, akathisia, and the development of parkinsonian syndrome. The SSRIs have varying effects on the cytochrome P_{450}, and hence require attention as regards concomitant prescription of other medication. Tricyclic antidepressants, particularly the older agents, whilst generally effective may be less well tolerated in the elderly due to potential adverse effects, such as dizziness, postural hypotension, falls, and cardiac arrhythmias. MAO inhibitors may lead to postural hypotension and a risk of falls; dietary and drug restrictions are likely to be the most problematic areas in cognitively impaired individuals unless closely supervised. Many clinicians in the UK use trazodone which appears to be, on the whole, a well tolerated and helpfully sedative (at night) drug, and relatively safe with respect to the cardiovascular system. Some of the newer antidepressants such as nefazadone, venlafaxine, and mirtazepine, may have theoretical advantages in this group of patients, but there are no available data as yet.

Although, as stated earlier in this chapter, mania or elevated mood are much less common complications of dementia, clinicians will occasionally encounter such patients. Judgements about when to treat and what to treat with need to be based on sound general principles of the treatment of mania, as unfortunately there is no data to assist clinical decisions specifically for patients with dementia.

In summary, the limited data, in keeping with clinical experience, suggest that antidepressant medication should be considered in patients with depression and dementia and that patients will benefit from treatment. The choice of drug has not been fully addressed by researchers, and physicians should use their clinical experience of prescribing in the elderly (with or without cognitive impairment) to guide their treatment decisions. The issue of whether cognitive function is altered beneficially or indeed detrimentally in the face of antidepressant treatment warrants further study. Data are not available on the course of depression in dementia, hence decisions as to when to cease therapy should be supported by the usual principles of regular reassessment of mood state, development of side-effects, and the progression of underlying dementia. In addition, it is useful to note that the study by Reifler *et al.* (1989) highlighted a substantial placebo response in depressed patients with dementia, and this may have important implications for the role of non-pharmacological psychosocial interventions.

Finally, an important final point is that successful pharmacological intervention is obviously dependent upon accurate diagnosis. Levy *et al.* (1998) found that across different dementia diagnostic groups apathy did not correlate with depression, lending support to the idea that apathy is a specific neuropsychiatric syndrome distinct from depression. Correctly distinguishing these two syndromes has therapeutic implications, as apathy may potentially be amenable to interventions affecting dopaminergic neurotransmission.

3.5 Psychotic symptoms — delusions, hallucinations, and misidentification syndromes

Most readers of this book will be familiar with the terms *delusions* and *hallucinations*, delusions being the presence of firmly held false beliefs which are not open to reason or argument and which are outside the generally accepted norms for the individual's cultural group, while hallucinations are perceptions in the absence of any external stimulus. A number of studies provide useful information about the prevalence of delusions in dementia. In a review of 30 studies by Wragg and Jeste (1989), the reported frequency of delusions in patients with DAT ranged from 10–73%, with most results clustered between 30–38% of patients (see also Burns and Jacoby 1990a; Ballard *et al.* 1995). In a case-controlled study, Cummings *et al.* (1987) compared the frequency of persecutory delusions in DAT and MID. Delusions occurred in 30% of patients with DAT compared to 40% of patients with MID; however, the authors pointed out that the patients with DAT were more cognitively impaired, and hypothesized that this may have contributed to the disparity. A large study by Cohen *et al.* (1993), including patients with DAT and MID found that there was no significant difference in the prevalence of delusions across the two groups. Misidentification syndromes also seem to occur commonly and this has been borne out by the study of Burns and Jacoby (1990*c*). They examined reports of additional people in the house (a variant of the 'phantom boarder syndrome'), misidentification of mirror image, misidentification of the television (as taking place in reality), and misidentification of people. In total, 30% of patients had demonstrated these phenomena.

The reported frequency of hallucinations also varies considerably. The analysis of Wragg and Jeste (1989) of patients with DAT reported the range to be 21–49%, with visual hallucinations occurring more frequently than auditory hallucinations. Whilst there were higher rates of hallucinations were found in hospitalized patients, it was not possible to exclude a diagnosis of superimposed delirium on the basis of the data available to them. Ballard *et al.* (1995) found that the prevalence of hallucinations ranged between 17–34% in all dementia, with visual hallucinations reported in the region of 10–15% of patients. The frequency of auditory hallucinations varied greatly (see also Burns and Jacoby 1990*b*). The study by Cohen *et al.* (1993) of patients with DAT and MID reported no significant difference in the prevalence of hallucinations across the two groups (12% and 16% respectively). Overall the prevailing view seems to be that psychotic symptoms across these two diagnostic groups do not vary significantly.

3.6 Psychotic symptoms in early onset dementia

Few studies have specifically looked at psychotic symptoms in patients with early onset dementia, and which suggest that the symptoms are common in younger patients too. Most studies are unfortunately flawed by a lack of standardized instruments and operational criteria, but figures range from 18–42% across dementia groups (Ballard *et al.* 1995). In a study of younger patients with mild or very mild DAT by Rubin *et al.* (1993), five out of 17 patients had delusions and three had hallucinations; however the numbers involved in this study were relatively small. Gustafson and Risberg (1992) compared the frequency of delusions and hallucinations in three groups of patients including many with early onset dementia; the groups were — early onset DAT (mean age, 57), fvFTD (mean age, 55), and DAT in older patients (mean age, 76). Hallucinations and delusions were reported in approximately a quarter of the two younger groups and about half of the older DAT patients. Delusions were more common in VaD (60%) compared to DAT (38%). Patients with FTD had surprisingly high rates of delusions (63%) and half of the patients with DLB experienced delusions. Hallucinations were present in 28% of DAT patients, and 56% of patients with VaD. Unfortunately, psychotic symptoms cause distress in 30% of cases and represent a significant problem for both patients and carers (e.g. Reisberg *et al.* 1987).

3.7 Treatment of psychotic symptoms

Antipsychotics are widely used in the treatment of psychotic symptoms functional psychiatric disorders such as schizophrenia and so it is not surprising therefore to find them used in patients with psychotic symptoms in the presence of organic brain disease. The use of antipsychotic medication in the treatment of 'non-cognitive' symptoms is widespread, but the evidence for their use certainly necessitates review. Although there are many case reports and open label studies there remain relatively few placebo controlled trials (reviews, see Raskind 1998; Lanctot *et al.* 1998). Substantial placebo effects have been shown to occur even in markedly cognitively impaired individuals; therefore, placebo controlled studies remain the gold standard in this important area of research. Studies vary in the choice of criteria for diagnosis, the assessment of the target symptoms, and the population under consideration (for example, outpatient versus inpatient groups).

A study by Petrie *et al.* (1982) of 61 patients, the majority of whom had either DAT or MID, found that global improvements were found in one-third of patients who were randomly assigned to active antipsychotic (loxapine or haloperidol) versus 9% who responded to placebo, with hostility, hallucinations, or unco-operativity responding best. However, rates of adverse events in both the placebo and drug groups were high. Barnes *et al.* (1982) compared loxapine, thioridazine, and placebo and found that the effects of antipsychotics were modest at best. Reisberg *et al.* (1987) found that over half of their patient group with DAT responded to thioridazine, which is commonly used to treat either psychotic phenomena or behavioural disturbance usually agitation. However, high rates of adverse effects (over 50%) and extrapyramidal effects (17%) occurred. A single-blind study of nine patients with DAT treated with haloperiod in doses of 1–5 mg daily demonstrated improvements in behavioural ratings, but significant treatment-emergent extrapyramidal symptoms were found to occur particularly at higher doses (Devanand *et al.* 1989).

A meta-analysis of controlled trials of antipsychotic treatment in dementia (Schneider and Sobin. 1991) examined the clinical efficacy of a wide range of antipsychotics and concluded that the effects of antipsychotics were modest, with 18% of patients with agitated behavioural symptoms (usually agitation, unco-operativeness, and hallucinations) benefiting from treatment with these agents. The meta-analysis also concluded that no one antipsychotic was particularly superior to another. It was noteworthy that the dose of antipsychotic agent was not correlated with the magnitude of benefit. The authors did highlight that a substantial number of older patients with dementia may receive antipsychotics unnecessarily, either because they would have responded to those factors associated with placebo or because they continue to receive antipsychotic medication even though there has been no obvious benefit. Adverse effects were common, but specific rates were not given. A more recent meta-analysis (Lanctot *et al.* 1998) re-examined the literature to assess both the efficacy and safety of antipsychotics in dementia. The therapeutic effect of the antipsychotics was 26%, i.e. similar to the findings of the Schneider *et al.* (1990) study. No differences were identified between different antipsychotics (regardless of potency) in terms of their efficacy, side-effects, or drop-out rate. Doses of antipsychotic were on the whole low, and more than 80% of patients were prescribed less than half of the standard daily dosage, but treatment-emergent side-effects were significantly greater than in the placebo group. The review stated that the current literature could not assist over the issue of optimal dosage; dosage should be individualized.

The question of optimal dosing in the treatment of disruptive behaviours and psychosis has been examined recently by Devanand *et al.* (1998). The authors of this study assessed in a six week random assignment double-blind placebo-controlled trial doses of haloperidol 2–3 mg/day (as a standard dose) versus haloperidol, 0.5–0.75 mg/day (low dose) or placebo in patients with DAT. The dose of 2–3 mg of haloperidol was chosen to be towards the high end of doses used clinically but below the dose of 5 mg/day which has been shown to result in severe extrapyramidal signs (Devanand *et al.* 1989). The lower (0.5–1.0 mg) dose was considered to be a dosing regime that clinicians frequently prescribe. Analysis of the results showed that low dose haloperidol was indistinguishable from placebo for all efficacy and adverse effect measures. Both psychosis and disruptive behaviours (aggression and agitation) improved on the standard dose haloperidol, but a subgroup of patients (20%) did develop moderate to severe extrapyramidal signs. On the basis of this study, the authors recommended a starting dose of 1 mg haloperidol adjusted according to the clinical response and the development of adverse effects.

The above studies highlight the high levels of adverse effects that elderly patients with dementia sadly suffer when exposed to antipsychotics. In addition to extrapyramidal side-effects, postural hypotension and falls are common problems. Other adverse effects of medication, e.g. sedation or delirium, may also exacerbate any behavioural disturbance. Tardive dyskinesia is of particular concern, the risk being about 30% for elderly patients with significant exposure. Being female, elderly, and having dementia are generally regarded as risk factors for the development of tardive dyskinesia (Jeste *et al.* 1995). A recent large prospective study (Woerner *et al.* 1998) found cumulative rates of 25%, 34%, and 53% after one, two, and three years of treatment, and interestingly found that patients with multi-infarct dementia had higher rates than patients with DAT.

Accurate clinical diagnosis is increasingly important since there is considerable evidence that patients with DLB are particularly susceptible to adverse consequences of antipsychotic medication. McKeith *et al.* (1992) reported that 29% of patients with DAT versus 81% of patients with DLB developed neuroleptic sensitivity, defined as a development or worsening of extrapyramidal features or acute and severe physical deterioration, in response to antipsychotic medication. In 54% of cases of DLB and 7% of DAT patients, this was judged to precipitate terminal decline. In contrast, the pathological study by McShane *et al.* (1997) did not find that those patients exposed to antipsychotics, found to have DLB at *post mortem*, had a more rapid rate of decline than patients with other non-DLB of dementia.

Another major problem in clinical practice when trying antipsychotic treatment for distressing psychotic symptoms or behavioural disturbance is to establish the patient on a dose which is helpful clinically but which does not produce unacceptable adverse effects. The new atypical antipsychotics such as clozapine, risperidone, olanzepine, and quietiapine offer theoretical advantages, but to date there have been a few case reports only of their overall efficacy (e.g. Kumar 1997). An open-label study of risperidone (with potent antagonism at 5-HT$_2$ receptors and relatively weak antagonism at D2 receptors) suggested promising effects on a number of target symptoms in behaviourally disturbed institutionalized elderly with dementia when used at doses of 0.5–1.0 mg daily (Goldberg and Goldberg 1996). Risperidone has also been assessed in a large number of hospitalized psychogeriatric patients with mixed diagnoses of which 53% had dementia with psychosis or behavioural disturbance. Risperidone was found to be reasonably well tolerated if initiated at a low dose (0.5 mg daily) and titrated slowly (Zarate *et al.* 1997). There are also encouraging reports of the successful treatment of patients with DLB dementia with either risperidone (Lee *et al.* 1994) or clozapine (Chacko *et al.* 1993), but also, unfortunately, reports that newer agents such as risperidone may cause some degree of neuroleptic sensitivity (Ballard *et al.* 1998; McKeith *et al.* 1995).

In summary, it seems that the balance of evidence is certainly in favour of cautious prescribing of antipsychotics for psychotic symptoms or disruptive behaviours (generally agitation, suspiciousness, unco-operativeness). Doses are substantially smaller than those used in the elderly with psychiatric disorders, and the likelihood of response is more modest with significant rates of adverse effects. In view of this, dosing should be 'low and slow', with consideration to using one of the atypical agents. Although data suggests that there are no significant differences between the efficacy of standard antipsychotics, most clinicians would perhaps feel that switching to a different agent would be an appropriate strategy if faced with a lack of efficacy or development of adverse effects. The use of anticholinergics for antipsychotic treatment-emergent side-effects is not recommended (APA 1997).

3.8 Behavioural changes in dementia

The importance of behavioural changes in dementia is easy to underestimate. Burns and Jacoby (1990*d*) reported a number of behavioural abnormalities in patients with DAT, including aggression (20%), wandering (19%), binge-eating (10%), and hyperorality (6%). These behavioural deficits were related to the severity of dementia. In a study of physical aggression in patients with dementia, 79 of 541 people exhibited physically aggressive behaviour in the two weeks prior to the study (Lyketsos *et al.* 1999). Aggression was closely associated with moderate or severe depression, male sex, and greater impairment of activities of daily living even after adjustment for delusions and hallucinations and cognitive impairment. Hope *et al.* (1997) recently examined a group of patients with DAT or VaD who were still living in the community and identified three behavioural syndromes, implying different underlying neuropathologies:

(a) An overactivity syndrome.

(b) Aggressive behaviour.

(c) Psychosis.

These syndrome clusters appeared to be robust as they persisted over a period of longitudinal follow-up. Interestingly, in this study, depression segregated as a separate factor from behavioural syndromes.

Although commonly prescribed, the data supporting the use of a wide range of non-antipsychotic therapies is generally based on small numbers of case reports or open label studies (for reviews, see Kumar *et al.* 1998).

Trazadone, a serotonergic antidepressant, has been found to be useful in the treatment of agitation in dementia in a number of case reports and series (Aisen *et al.* 1993; Lebert *et al.* 1994). Initial doses are in the region of 25–50 mg twice a day (Zayas and Grossberg 1996). Dose-limiting adverse effects are most often those of sedation and postural hypotension. In the only placebo-controlled study in ten patients with DAT, trazadone (at maximal doses of 50 mg three times a day) produced small but significant effects compared to placebo or buspirone (Lawlor *et al.* 1994). Some patients were not able to tolerate 150 mg/day because of sedation.

Carbamazepine has been assessed in a number of studies including case reports, case series, open label trials, and a few controlled trials. Two placebo-controlled studies have shown encouraging results (Tariot *et al.* 1996; Cooney and Mortimer 1996) with one study showing a 70% response rate on carbamazepine versus 17% response rate with placebo (Tariot *et al.* 1996). Doses were in the range of 200–600 mg carbamazepine daily, with serum levels in the range of 17–38 μmol/ml. The potential of the drug to induce leucopaenia and altering liver function needs to be considered.

Sodium valproate has also been used, but to date is based on case series and open trials only (APA 1997). Doses suggested range between 500–2500 mg daily (Mellow *et al.* 1993; Sandborn *et al.* 1995). In the largest prospective study to date 16 patients with total daily doses of 700–2500 mg per day had significantly reduced scores on the Behave-AD. However, half of the patients did not show improvement, the reasons for which remain uncertain. Doses commenced at 125 mg twice a day with slow titration. Response occurred over two to four weeks.

Benzodiazepines have also been used in the treatment of behavioural disturbance in dementia. A small number of double-blind trials have compared benzodiazepines (diazepam or oxazepam) to antipsychotics, although the studies are limited by poorly defined diagnoses and target symptoms. Both benzodiazepine and antipsychotic groups improved significantly, but with a greater improvement in the antipsychotic group (Kirven and Montero 1973).

Cholinergic enhancers. The efficacy of cholinesterase inhibitors for the treatment of the cognitive aspects of DAT was evaluated earlier, and their potential for treating psychiatric symptoms and behavioural disturbance also deserves proper attention. Cummings and Back (1998) have outlined the utility of a cholinergic hypothesis of DAT in understanding the range of neuropsychiatric symptoms seen in DAT and the productive application of cholinomimetic therapy to ameliorate the behavioural disturbances accompanying DAT.

Selective serotonin reuptake inhibitors. The cognitive effects of drugs in frontal variant fronto-temporal dementias was discussed earlier in this chapter. As mentioned earlier, post-mortem studies provide some, albeit limited evidence, that abnormalities in serotonergic receptor numbers may contribute to the cognitive and behavioural presentation of patients with fvFTD relatively early in the course of disease (also see Chapter 9). A recent study by Swartz *et al.* (1997) demonstrated benefits in at least half of the patients; however, the study was uncontrolled and unblinded in design and used three different SSRIs. It is evident that more studies have to be done in this area to examine objectively the effects of serotonin-boosting compounds upon behavioural symptoms, and to consider in particular whether a specific pattern of presenting clinical symptoms may predict a response to therapy. A theoretically driven approach which makes use of the considerable literature of serotonin on diverse aspects of behaviour, such as impulsivity, depression, aggressive behaviour, or carbohydrate craving, is obviously likely to become particularly fruitful in the immediate future. This approach has also considerable relevance to DAT, where there is growing realization that a combination of disturbances in cholinergic and serotonergic function may play also a role in the cognitive impairment in DAT, with serotonergic dysfunction potentially responsible for a significant portion of the behavioural aspects seen later in disease (e.g. impulsive behaviour). In the future, advances in neuroimaging for example with PET shall be able to examine the direct involvement of 5-HT neurons in the cognitive and behavioural features of disease.

Buspirone, a 5-HT$_{1A}$ agonist, has been subjected to a small number of studies. For example, Cantillon *et al.* (1996) found that buspirone at 15 mg/day compared favourably with haloperidol 1.5 mg, both producing significant improvement but with greater reduction in anxiety in the buspirone group.

3.9 The natural history of psychiatric symptoms and the withdrawal of treatment

It is therefore clear that a number of psychiatric symptoms occur commonly in dementia, and are amenable to pharmacological intervention. Knowledge of the natural history of behavioural disturbance and psychiatric symptoms in patients with dementia should, theoretically, be helpful in making rational decisions about the cessation of treatment. However, longitudinal studies are scarce. Levy *et al.* (1996) in a large sample of patients with DAT found that psychiatric symptoms frequently reoccurred during a one year follow-up period. Hope *et al.* (1999) who assessed prospectively 100 patients with dementia found that behavioural and psychiatric changes occurred over a wide range of cognitive impairment and that some behavioural deficits, once they had emerged, tended to persist until death, e.g. verbal aggression, aggressive resistance, physical aggression, and hypophagia. Other changes occurred as discrete episodes. The authors suggested that predicting the likely duration of a specific episode of behavioural change may be helpful in deciding when to stop treatment and suggested eight-monthly review and withdrawal of medication. Whatever the exact timing of reviews of medication, attempts at reduction should occur in order to reduce the development of adverse effects, as symptoms may diminish with the course of time and the progression of the underlying dementing process.

There are a few studies which examine antipsychotic withdrawal in patients with dementia. For example, Bridges-Parlet *et al.* (1997) found that withdrawing institutionalized dementia patients from neuroleptics for an extended period of time was successful in most but not all patients. Because of concerns related to injudicious prescribing of antipsychotics to patients in nursing homes, in the US since 1987, nursing homes have been highly regulated with the enactment of the Omnibus Budget Reconciliation Act (review, Sunderland 1996). This act requires that doctors document the diagnostic indication for the use of antipsychotics and reassess to justify the continued use of such agents. The main criterion for prescribing of antipsychotics in dementia is that the behaviour must be harmful to the patient — including behaviour that prevents staff from caring for the patient — or that the behaviour causes a reduction in the functional abilities of the patient. A second requirement is that the behaviour must be characterized both qualitatively and quantitatively, allowing the effects of prescribed medication to be objectively assessed.

4 Conclusion

This chapter has examined the options for treatment of the symptoms of dementia. The success of this treatment depends upon a sophisticated neuropsychological approach to the early detection and differential diagnosis of dementia, and this has shown to be essential for treatments to have the best possible chance of success. Using neuropsychology as well as other scientific tools clearly provides considerable insight into the nature of disease, and may be in addition extremely informative about normal brain mechanisms of cognition. Understanding the cognitive symptomatology of different dementias provides a precise and rational strategy for the development of novel pharmacological treatments which target specific neurochemical abnormalities. A cognitive psychopharmacological approach therefore offers justified optimism for the millennium for the development of the treatment of these distressing disorders, leading to improvement in patients' symptoms and the quality of life both for them and their carers. In this chapter, we have also identified the common psychiatric symptoms in dementia, including depression and psychotic symptoms, and outlined the principal arguments underlying the initiation, maintenance, and cessation of treatment. Objective assessment of the effects of any intervention with a patient — whether pharmacological, psychological, or environmental — is clearly good practice. Further research into the pharmacological management of specific changes in the context of well characterized dementia will help to allow clinicians to make informed decisions.

5 Key points

1   Cholinesterase inhibitors have been found to produce beneficial effects on both cognitive and behavioural symptoms of dementia of the Alzheimer type.
2   Cholinesterase inhibitors may also be useful in dementia of Lewy body type. In this condition, neuroleptics should be avoided.
3   Examination of risk factors is the mainstay of prevention and management of vascular dementias.
4   There are no routine pharmacological treatments for frontotemporal dementia. Interventions to boost noradrenergic or serotonergic function are likely to be of use in the future.
5   Psychiatric symptoms (depression, delusions particularly of theft, hallucinations, and misidentification syndromes) occur commonly in dementia.
6   Before assuming development of psychiatric symptoms represent progression of the underlying dementing process through assessment to exclude superadded medical problems and to address any changes in environmental/social factors should take place.
7   Psychiatric symptoms are worth treating if they cause distress or behavioural disturbance.
8   Depression has been shown to be effectively treated by antidepressants including tricyclics and SSRIs. There is little data as yet regarding other newer agents, but they may too have theoretical benefits.
9   Psychotic symptoms can be helped by antipsychotics. Data does not suggest obvious superiority of any particular agent. Guiding principles of starting low and increasingly slowly as a proportion are very susceptible to extrapyramidal side-effects.

10 On balance the data suggest that neuroleptics should be avoided where possible in patients with presumed diffuse Lewy body dementia. The very limited data suggests that very new atypicals may not be problem free, although theoretically safer.

11 Some forms of behavioural disturbance, e.g. agitation, may be helped by antipsychotics or other medications including carbamazepine, sodium valproate, benzodiazepines, and cholinergic enhancers.

12 It is important to review the continuing need for any psychotropics prescribed in this group of patients.

Acknowledgements

The work of S. R. is funded by a MRC Research Studentship. The research of B. J. S. is funded by an MRC LINK grant (G9705363). This work was completed within the MRC Co-operative group in Brain, Behaviour, and Neuropsychiatry.

References

Aisen, P. S. and Davis, K. L. (1994). Inflammatory mechanisms in Alzheimer's disease: implications for therapy. *Am. J. Psychiatry*, **151**, 1105–13.

Aisen, P. S., Johannessen, J. D., and Marin, D. B. (1993). Trazadone for behavioural disturbance in Alzheimer's disease. *Am. J. Geriatr. Psychiatry*, **1**, 349–50.

Allen, N. H. P., Gordon, S., Hope, T., and Burns, A. (1996). Manchester and Oxford University scale for the psychopathological assessment of dementia. *Br. J. Psychiatry*, **169**, 293–307.

American Psychiatric Association (APA). (1997). Practice guidelines for the treatment of patients with Alzheimer's disease and other dementias of late life. *Am. J. Psychiatry*, **154**, 1–39.

Ballard, C., Bannister, C., Graham, C., Oyebode, F., and Wilcock, G. (1995). Associations of psychotic symptoms in dementia sufferers. *Br. J. Psychiatry*, **167**, 537–40.

Ballard, C., Grace, J., McKeith, I., and Holmes, C. (1998). Neuroleptic sensitivity in dementia with Lewy bodies and Alzheimer's disease. *Lancet*, **351**, 1032–3.

Barnes, R., Veith, R., Okimoto, J., Raskind, M., and Gumbrecht, G. (1982). Efficacy of antipsychotic medication in behaviourally disturbed patients. *Am. J. Psychiatry*, **139**, 1170–4.

Bartus, R. T., Dean, R. L. I., Beer, B., and Lippa, A. S. (1982). The cholinergic hypothesis of geriatric memory dysfunction. *Science*, **217**, 408–17.

Birks, J. S. and Melzer, D. (1998). The efficacy of donepezil for mild and moderate Alzheimer's disease. In *Cochrane collaboration*. Cochrane Library. Issue 4. Oxford: Update Software.

Bowen, D. M., Francis, P. T., Pangalos, M. N., Stephens, P. H., and Procter, A. W. (1992). Treatment strategies for Alzheimer's disease. *Lancet*, **339**, 132–3.

Bridges-Parlet, S., Knopman, D., and Steffes, S. (1997). Withdrawal of neuroleptic medications from institutionalized dementia patients: results of a double-blind baseline-treatment-controlled pilot study. *J. Geriatr. Psychiatry Neurol.*, **10**, 119–26.

Burns, A. and Jacoby, R. (1990*a*). Psychiatric phenomena in Alzheimer's disease I. Disorders of thought content. *Br. J. Psychiatry*, **157**, 72–6.

Burns, A. and Jacoby, R. (1990*b*). Psychiatric phenomena in Alzheimer's disease II. Disorders of perception. *Br. J. Psychiatry*, **157**, 76–81.

Burns, A. and Jacoby, R. (1990*c*). Psychiatric phenomena in Alzheimer's disease III. Disorders of mood. *Br. J. Psychiatry*, **157**, 81–6.

Burns, A. and Jacoby, R. (1990*d*). Psychiatric phenomena in Alzheimer's disease IV. Disorders of behaviour. *Br. J. Psychiatry*, **157**, 86–94.

Burns, A. (1991). Affective symptoms in Alzheimer's disease. *Int. J. Geriatr. Psychiatry*, **6**, 371–6.

Cantillon, M., Brunswick, R., *et al.* (1996). Buspirone vs haloperidol: a double-blind trial for agitation in a nursing home population with Alzheimer's disease. *Am. J. Geriatr. Soc.*, **4**, 263–7.

Chacko, R., Hurley, R., and Jancovic, J. (1993). Clozapine use in diffuse Lewy body dementia. *J. Neuropsychiatry Clin. Neurosci.*, **5**, 206–98.

Cohen, D., Eisdorfer, C., Gorelick, P., Paveza, G., Luchins, D. J., Freels, S., *et al.* (1993). Psychopathology associated with Alzheimer's disease and related disorders. *J. Gerontol.*, **48**, M255–60.

Cooney, C. and Mortimer, A. (1996). Carbamazepine use in aggressive behaviour associated with senile dementia. *Int. J. Geriatr. Psychiatry*, **11**, 901–5.

Coull, J. T., Sahakian, B. J., and Hodges, J. R. (1996). The alpha(2) antagonist idazoxan remediates certain attentional and executive dysfunction in patients with dementia of frontal type. *Psychopharmacology (Berl)*, **123**, 239–49.

Cummings, J. L. and Back, C. (1998). The cholinergic hypothesis of neuropsychiatric symptoms in Alzheimer's disease. *Am. J. Geriatr. Psychiatry*, **6**, S64–78.

Cummings, J. L., Cyrus, P. A., Bieber, F., Mas, J., Orazem, J., and Gulanski. B. (1998). Metrifonate treatment of the cognitive deficits of Alzheimer's disease. Metrifonate Study Group. *Neurology*, **50**, 1214–21. Published erratum appeared in *Neurology*, 1998, **51**, 332.

Cummings, J. L. and Kaufer, D. (1996). Neuropsychiatric aspects of Alzheimer's disease: the cholinergic hypothesis revisited. *Neurology*, **47**, 876–83.

Cummings, J. L., Mega, M., and Gray, K. (1994). The neuropsychiatric inventory: comprehensive assessment of psychopathology in dementia. *Neurology*, **44**, 2308–14.

Cummings, J., Miller, B., Hill, M. A., and Neshkes, R. (1987). Neuropsychiatric aspects of multi-infarct dementia and dementia of Alzheimer type. *Arch. Neurol.*, **44**, 389–93.

Devanand, D. P., Marder, K., Michaels, K. S., Sackheim, H. A., Bell, K., Sullivan, M. A., *et al.* (1998). A randomized, placebo-controlled dose-comparison trial of haloperidol for psychosis and disruptive behaviours in Alzheimer's disease. *Am. J. Psychiatry*, **155**, 1512–20.

Devanand, D. P., Sackheim, H., and Brown, R. P. (1989). A pilot study of haloperidol treatment of psychosis and behavioural disturbance in Alzheimer's disease. *Arch. Neurol.*, **46**, 854–7.

Drachman, D. A. and Sahakian, B. J. (1979). The effects of cholinergic agents on human learning and memory. In *Nutrition and brain*, Vol. 5 (ed. A. Barbeau, J. H. Growden, and R. J. Wurtman), pp. 351–66. New York, Raven Press.

Farlow, M., Gracon, S. I., Hershey, L. A., Lewis, K. W., Sadowsky, C. H., and Dolan-Ureno, J. (1992). A controlled trial of tacrine in Alzheimer's disease: The Tacrine Study Group. *J. Am. Med. Assoc.*, **268**, 2523–9.

Francis, P. T., Holmes, C., Webster, M. T., Stratmann, G. C., Procter, A. W., and Bowen, D. M. (1993). Preliminary neurochemical findings in non-Alzheimer dementia due to lobar atrophy. *Dementia*, **4**, 172–7.

Fulton, B. and Benfield, P. (1996). Galanthamine. [Review.] *Drugs Aging*, **9**, 60–5; discussion 66–7.

Gauthier, S. (1998). Clinical trials and Therapy. [Review.] *Curr. Opin. Neurol.*, **11**, 435–8.

Goldberg, R. J. and Goldberg, J. (1996). Anti-psychotics for dementia related behavioural disturbances in elderly institutionalised patients. *Clin. Geriatr.*, **4**, 58–68.

Gregory, C. A. and Hodges, J. R. (1996). Dementia of frontal type: use of consensus criteria and prevalence of psychiatric symptoms. *Neuropsychiatry Neuropsychol. Behav. Neurol.*, **9**, 145–53.

Gustafson, L. (1987). Frontal lobe degeneration of non-Alzheimer's type II: Clinical picture and differential diagnosis. *Arch. Geronotol. Geriatr.*, **6**, 209–23.

Gustafson, L. and Risberg, J. (1992). Deceptions and delusions in Alzheimer's disease and frontal lobe dementia. Delusions and hallucinations in old age (ed. C. Katona and R. Levy), pp. 216–27. London; Gaskell.

Henderson, V. W., Paganini-Hill, A., Emanuel, C. K., Dunn, M. E., and Buckwalter, J. G. (1994). Estrogen replacement therapy in the treatment of the cognitive decline and neurodegeneration associated with Alzheimer's disease. *Neurobiol. Aging*, **15**, S195–7.

Hope, T., Keene, J., Fairburn, C. G., McShane, R., and Jacoby, R. (1997). Behavioural changes in dementia 2: Are there behavioural syndromes? *Int. J. Geriatr. Psychiatry*, **12**, 1074–8.

Hope, T., Keene, J., Fairburn, C. G., McShane, R., and Jacoby, R. (1999). The natural history of behavioural changes and psychiatric symptoms in Alzheimer's disease. *Br. J. Psychiatry*, **174**, 39–44.

Jeste, D. V., Caliguiri, M. P., Paulsen, J. S., Heaton, R. K., Lacro, J. P., Harris, M., *et al.* (1995). Risk of tardive dyskinesia in older patients: a prospective longitudinal study of 266 out-patients. *Arch. Gen. Psychiatry*, **52**, 756–65.

Jones, G. M. M., Sahakian, B. J., Levy, R., Warburton, D. M., and Gray, J. A. (1992). The effects of acute subcutaneous nicotine on attention, information processing and short-term memory in Alzheimer's disease. *Psychopharmacology*, **108**, 485–94.

Katona, C. L., Hunter, B. N., and Bray, J. (1998). A double-blind comparison of the efficacy and safety of paroxetine and imprimine in the treatment of depression with dementia. *Int. J. Geriatr. Psychiatry*, **13**, 102–8.

Kaufer, D. I., Catt, K. E., Lopez, O. L., and DeKosky, S. T. (1998). Dementia with Lewy bodies: response of delirium-like features to donepezil. *Neurology*, **51**, 1512.

Kirven, L. E. and Montero, E. F. (1973). Comparison of thioridazine and diazepam in the control of non-psychotic symptoms associated with senility: a double-blind study. *J. Am. Geriatr. Soc.*, **21**, 546–51.

Konno, S., Meyer, J. S., Terayama, Y., Margishvili, G. M., and Mortel, K. F. (1997). Classification, diagnosis and treatment of vascular dementia. *Drugs Aging*, **5**, 361–73.

Kumar, V. (1997). Use of atypical antipsychotic agents in geriatric patients; a review. *Int. J. Geriatr. Psychopharmacol.*, **1**, 15–23.

Kumar, V., Durai, N. B., and Jobe, T. (1998). Pharmacologic management of Alzheimer's disease. *Clin. Geriatr. Med.*, **14**, 129–46.

Lanctot, K. L., Best, T. S., Mittmann, N., Liu, B. A., Oh, P. I., Einarson, T. R., *et al.* (1998). Efficacy and safety of neuroleptics in behavioural disorders associated with dementia. *J. Clin. Psychiatry*, **59**, 550–61.

Lawlor, B. A., Radcliffe, J., and Molchan, S. E. (1994). A pilot placebo-controlled study of trazadone and buspirone in Alzheimer's disease. *Int. J. Geriatr. Psychiatry*, **9**, 55–9.

Lawrence, A. D. and Sahakian, B. J. (1998). The cognitive psychopharmacology of Alzheimer's disease: focus on cholinergic systems. *Neurochem. Res.*, **23**, 787–94.

Lebert, F., Pasquier, F., and Petit, H. (1994). Behavioural effects of trazadone in Alzheimer's disease. *J. Clin. Psychiatry*, **55**, 536–8.

Lee, H., Cooney, J. M., and Lawlor, B. A. (1994). The use of risperidone, an atpyical neuroleptic in Lewy body disease. *Int. J. Geriatr. Psychiatry*, **9**, 415–17.

Levy, M., Cummings, J. L., Fairbanks, L. A., Bravi, D., Calvani, M., and Carta, A. (1996). Longitudinal assessment of symptoms in depression, agitation and psychosis in 181 patients with Alzheimer's disease. *Am. J. Psychiatry*, **153**, 1438–43.

Levy, M. L., Cummings, J. L., Fairbanks, L. A., Masterman, D., Miller, B. L., Craig, A. H., *et al.* (1998). Apathy is not depression. *J. Neuropsychiatry Clin. Neurosci.*, **10**, 314–19.

Lyketsos, C. G., Steele, C., Galik, E., Rosenblatt, A., Steinberg, M., Warren, A., *et al.* (1999). Physical aggression in dementia patients and its relationship to depression. *Am. J. Psychiatry*, **156**, 66–71.

MacGowan, S. H., Wilcock, G. K., and Scott, M. (1998). Effect of gender and apolipoprotein E genotype on response to anticholinesterase therapy in Alzheimer's disease. *Int. J. Geriatr. Psychiatry*, **13**, 625–30.

McKeith, I. G., Ballard, C., and Harrison, R. W. S. (1995). Neuroleptic sensitivity to risperidone in Lewy Body dementia *Lancet*, **346**, 699.

McKeith, I. G., Fairbairn, A., Perry, R., Thompson, P., and Perry, E. (1992). Neuroleptic sensitivity in patients with senile dementia of the Lewy body type. *Br. Med. J.*, **305**, 673–8.

McKhann, G., Drachman, D., Folstein, M., Katzman, R., Price, D., and Stadlan, E. (1984). Clinical diagnosis of Alzheimer's disease: report of the NINCDS-ADRDA Work Group under the auspices of Department of Health and Human Services Task Force on Alzheimer's disease. *Neurology*, **34**, 939–44.

McShane, R., Keene, J., Gedling, K., Fairburn, C., Jacoby, R., and Hope, T. (1997). Do neuroleptic drugs hasten cognitive decline in dementia? Prospective study with necroscopy follow-up. *Br. Med. J.*, **314**, 266–70.

Mellow, A. M., Solano-Lopez, C., and Davis, S. (1993). Sodium valproate in the treatment of behavioural disturbance in dementia. *J. Geriatr. Psychiatry Neurol.*, **6**, 205–9.

Nordberg, A. and Svensson, A. L. (1998). Cholinesterase inhibitors in the treatment of Alzheimer's disease: a comparison of tolerability and pharmacology. *Drug Saf.*, **19**, 465–80.

Nyth, A. L. and Gottfries, C. G. (1990). The clinical efficacy of citalopram in the treatment of emotional disturbances in dementia disorders. *Br. J. Psychiatry*, **157**, 894–901.

Perry, E. K. (1986). The cholinergic hypothesis – ten years on. [Review]. *Br. Med. Bull.*, **42**, 63–9.

Perry, E. K., Tomlinson, B. E., Blessed, G., Bergman, K., Gibson, P. H., and Perry, R. H. (1978). Correlation of cholinergic abnormalities with senile plaques and mental test scores in senile dementia. *Br. Med. J.*, **2**, 1457–9.

Petersen, R. C. (1998). Clinical subtypes of Alzheimer's disease. *Dement. Geriatr. Cogn. Disord.*, **9**, 16–24.

Petrie, W. M., Ban, T. A., and Berney, S. (1982). A placebo and standard controlled clinical investigation. *J. Clin. Psychopharmacol.*, **2**, 122–6.

Qizilbash, N., Whitehead, A., Higgins, J., Wilcock, G., Schneider, L., and Farlow, M. (1998). Cholinesterase inhibition for Alzheimer disease: a meta-analysis of the tacrine trials. Dementia Trialists' Collaboration. *J. Am. Med. Assoc.*, **280**, 1777–82.

Rabins, P., Mace, M., and Lucas, M. (1982). The impact of dementia on the family. *J. Am. Med. Assoc.*, **248**, 333–5.

Raskind, M. A. (1998). Psychopharmacology of non-cognitive abnormal behaviours in Alzheimer's disease. *J. Clin. Psychiatry*, **59**, 28–32.

Raskind, M. A., Peskind, E. R., Wessel, T., and Yuan, W. (2000). Galanthamine in AD: A 6-month, randomised, placebo-controlled trial with a 6-month extension. *Neurology*, **54**, 2261–8.

Reifler, B. V., Teri, L., Raskind, M., Veith, R., Barnes, R., White, E., *et al.* (1989). Double-blind trial of imiprimine in Alzheimer's disease patients with and without depression. *Am. J. Psychiatry*, **146**, 45–9.

Reisberg, B., Borenstein, J., Salob, S. P., Ferris, S. H., Franssen, E., and Georgotsas, A. (1987). Behavioural symptoms in Alzheimer's disease: phenomenology and treatment. *J. Clin. Psychiatry*, **48**, 9–15.

Riekkinen, M., Soininen, H., Riekkinen, P. Sr., Kuikka, J., Laakso, M., Helkala, E. L., *et al.* (1998). Tetrahydroaminoacridine improves the recency effect in Alzheimer's disease. *Neuroscience*, **83**, 471–9.

Robbins, T. W., McAlonan, G., Muir, J. L., and Everitt, B. J. (1997). Cognitive enhancers in theory and practice: studies of the cholinergic hypothesis of cognitive deficits in Alzheimer's disease. [Review.] *Behav. Brain Res.*, **83**, 15–23.

Rogers, S. L., Doody, R. S., Pratt, R. D., and Ieni, J. R. (2000). Long-term efficacy and safety of donepezil in the treatment of Alzheimer's disease: final analysis of a US multi-centre open label study. *Eur. Neuropsychopharmacol.*, **10**, 195–203.

Rogers, S. L. and Friedhoff, L. T. (1996). The efficacy and safety of donepezil in patients with DAT. Results of a US multicentre randomised, double-blind, placebo-controlled trial. The DSG. *Dementia*, **7**, 293–303.

Rogers, J., Kirby, L. C., Hempelman, S. R., Berry, D. L., McGeer, P. L., Kaszniak, A. W., *et al.* (1993). Clinical trial of indomethacin for Alzheimer's disease. *Neurology*, **43**, 1609–11.

Rosen, J. H. (1979). Double-blind comparison of haloperidol and thioridazine in geriatric outpatients. *J. Clin. Psychiatry*, **40**, 17–20.

Rosen, W., Mohs, R., and Davis, K. (1984). A new rating scale for Alzheimer's disease. *Am. J. Psychiatry*, **141**, 1356–64.

Rosen, J. and Zubenko, G. S. (1991). Emergence of psychosis and depression: the longitudinal assessment of Alzheimer's disease. *Biol. Psychiatry*, **29**, 224–32.

Rubin, E. H., Kinscherf, D. A., and Morris, J. C. (1993). Psychopathology in younger versus older persons with very mild and mild dementia of the Alzheimer type. *Am. J. Psychiatry*, **150**, 637–9.

Sahakian, B. J. and Coull, J. T. (1993). Tetrahydroaminoacridine (THA) in Alzheimer's disease: an assessment of attentional and mnemonic function using CANTAB. *Acta Neurol. Scand. Suppl.*, **149**, 29–35.

Sahakian, B., Jones, G., Levy, R., Gray, J., and Warburton, D. (1989). The effects of nicotine on attention, information processing, and short-term memory in patients with dementia of the Alzheimer type. *Br. J. Psychiatry*, **154**, 797–800.

Sandborn, W. D., Bendfeldt, F., and Hamdy, R. (1995). Valproic acid for physically aggressive behavior in geriatric patients. *Am. J. Geriatr. Psychiatry*, **3**, 239–42.

Sano, M., Ernesto, C., Thomas, R. G., Klauber, M. R., Schafer, K., Grundman, M., *et al.* (1997). A controlled trial of selegiline, alpha-tocopherol, or both as treatment for Alzheimer's disease. *N. Eng. J. Med.*, **336**, 1216–22.

Schneider, L. S., Pollock, V. E., and Lyness, S. A. (1990). A meta-analysis of controlled trials of neuroleptic treatment in dementia. *J. Geriatr. Soc.*, **38**, 553–63.

Schneider, L. S. and Sobin, P. B. (1991). Non-neuroleptic medications in the management of agitation in Alzheimer's disease and other dementia: a selective review. *Int. J. Geriatr. Psychiatry*, **6**, 691–708.

Silman, I., Harel, M., Eichler, J., *et al.* (1994). Structure-function relationships in the binding of reversible inhibitors in the active-site gorge of acetylcholinesterase. In *Alzheimer disease: therapeutic strategies* (ed. R. Becker and E. Giacobini), pp. 88–92. Birkhauser: Boston.

Sparks, D. L. and Markesbery, W. R. (1991). Altered serotonergic and cholinergic synaptic markers in Pick's disease. *Arch. Neurol.*, **48**, 796–9.

Spencer, C. M. and Noble, S. (1998). Rivastigmine: a review of its use in Alzheimer's disease. [Review.] *Drugs Aging*, **13**, 391–411.

Sultzer, D. L., Levin, H. S., Mahler, M. E., High, W. M., and Cummings, J. L. (1993). A comparison of psychiatric symptoms in vascular dementia and Alzheimer's disease. *Am. J. Psychiatry*, **150**, 1806–12.

Sunderland, T. (1996). Treatment of the elderly suffering from psychosis in dementia. *J. Clin. Psychiatry*, **57**, 53–6.

Swartz, R., Miller, B. L., Lesser, I. M., and Darby, A. L. (1997). Frontotemporal dementia: treatment response to serotonin selective reuptake inhibitors. *J. Clin. Psychiatry*, **58**, 212–16.

Tariot, P. N., Erb, R., and Leibovici, A. (1996). Carbamazepine in the treatment of agitation in nursing home patients with dementia: a preliminary study. *J. Am. Geriatr. Soc.*, **42**, 1160–6.

Taylor, P. (1998). Development of acetylcholinesterase inhibitors in the therapy of Alzheimer's disease. [Review.] *Neurology*, **51**, S30–35.

Woerner, M. G., Alvir, J. M., Saltz, M. D., Lieberman, J. A., and Kane, J. M. (1998). Prospective study of tardive dyskinesia in the elderly; rates and risk factors. *Am. J. Psychiatry*, **155**, 1521–7.

Wragg, R. E. and Jeste, D. V. (1989). Overview of depression and psychosis in Alzheimer's disease. *Am. J. Psychiatry*, **146**, 577–87.

Zarate, C. A. Jr., Baldessarini, R. J., Siegel, A. J., Nakamura, A., McDonald, J., Muir Hutschison, L. A., *et al.* (1997). Risperidone in the elderly: a pharmacoepidemiologic study. *J. Clin. Psychiatry*, **58**, 311–17.

Zayas, E. M. and Grossberg, G. T. (1996). Treating the agitated Alzheimer patient. *J. Clin. Psychiatry*, **57**, 46–51.

20 Practical issues in the management of early onset dementia

Carol A. Gregory and Sinclair Lough

1 Introduction

This chapter covers a number of practical issues encountered in the management of patients with dementia. The first section considers issues in the management of challenging behaviour. The second examines the advice patients and their families often require regarding driving, legal, and financial matters.

As a dementing illness progresses disruptive or challenging behaviours often emerge. It is well established that behavioural disturbances are common in dementia (Hope 1992). Often it is repeated exposure to a sufferer's challenging behaviours that leads the carer to initiate contact with the medical services (Silver and Yudofsky 1987). Coping on a daily basis with challenging behaviours is a major cause of carer stress (Gilleard *et al.* 1984). Whilst many carers, both informal and formal, can manage the physical or labour-intensive chores of their role, attempting to deal with disruptive behaviour often leads to extreme strain and intolerance and this can result in the institutionalization of the sufferer (Pearlin *et al.* 1990). A major challenge for clinical services involved in dementia care is therefore the management of challenging behaviour.

Patients of all ages with dementia, and their families, need advice regarding driving, managing their finances, and making wills, and benefits they may be entitled to. Whereas driving and legal issues are similar regardless of age, the financial support system for younger patients who are no longer able to work is different from that of older retired patients and these differences will be outlined below. Two important points need to be made, first that these issues are reported on from an English perspective and may of course be different in other countries and secondly, although providing an overview, specialist advice from the DVLA (for driving licence issues), Social Services (for benefits), or solicitors (regarding wills etc.) may be necessary or helpful in individual cases.

2 Management of challenging behaviour

Over the past couple of decades the major approach to the management of challenging behaviour in dementia in the UK has been underpinned by two major tenets:-

(a) That the behaviour is learned.

(b) That it is often the expression of an unmet need.

Much is therefore drawn from learning theory and in particular the principles of operant conditioning (Skinner 1953). In clinical practice most of the referrals to psychological services are for very difficult behaviours expressed within a residential/nursing setting by elderly people with very limited communication skills and in the moderate-to-severe stages of dementia. However it can be argued that the management approach outlined below can be applied to younger sufferers, in the earlier stages of a dementia, who are living at home.

Common challenging behaviours include rejection of care or control, withdrawal or apathy, stereotyped and repetitive behaviours, excessive demands, socially inappropriate behaviours, dangerous behaviours such as self-neglect or wandering, and hostile or aggressive behaviours (Wattis and Martin 1986). The definition of exactly what constitutes a 'challenging behaviour' is not without its difficulties. Concern has been expressed (Hope and Patel 1993; Stokes 1996) over the use of vague, ambiguous, and unstructured descriptions of behaviour that exist in the literature and in clinical practice. These authors argue the need for clear, objective definitions of the observable characteristics of behaviour.

In clinical practice, the initial complaint or referral typically describes and labels the challenging behaviour. Obtaining an operational definition follows from assessment involving interview and observation. Following a precise description of the behaviour it is essential to examine the biological, social, environmental, and personal factors that may be acting as determinants of the behaviour (Stokes and Goudie 1990). Sometimes one factor predominates. For example, the onset of pain in a person with limited or non-existent communication may often result in an upsurge of shouting or screaming. However, more frequently, the challenging behaviour ensues from an interaction of many factors. Consider the case of an elderly man who has just moved into a residential home, which is staffed mostly by young, untrained women. He is suffering from a vascular dementia which has produced a severe deficit in short-term memory with accompanying deficits in primary perception and visuo-spatial organization. His comprehension and expressive language remain intact. He is an ex-headmaster, pre-morbidly of high intelligence with a reputation for having been a strict disciplinarian. Very soon after his placement in the home he becomes verbally aggressive towards care staff. On assessment it is apparent that the interaction of three key factors lie behind the behaviour. His presentation in the home is of a person who cannot find his way around and who cannot learn the names of staff (Biological factor). The untrained staff tar all residents with dementia with the brush of moderate-to-severe Alzheimer's disease. They treat this gentleman accordingly (Social factor) whilst failing to recognize his intact verbal intelligence (Biological factor). His background (Personal factor) predisposes him to react aggressively.

In order to develop a constructive management plan it is necessary to obtain details of the occurrences of the challenging behaviour, and in particular the surrounding circumstances, through measurement of the behaviour. Interviews with carers can be guided and supplemented with tools such as the Motivation Assessment Scale (Durand and Crimmins 1988) or the Functional Analysis Interview Form (O'Neil *et al.* 1990), which, although developed for use with the learning disabled, can be adapted for use with people with dementia. Observation of the challenging behaviour may be conducted either directly by the clinician or by asking staff to record incidents. If the behaviour is of high frequency then direct observation is preferred. This is also the case if it occurs only at particular times of the day, for example at meal times. Direct observation affords a much richer description of the behaviour and its circumstances than recording. Perrin (1996) provides an excellent and concise overview of the different observational methods. If the presentation of the behaviour is of low frequency and seemingly random in its occurrence then recording by carers is the method of choice. Table 20.1 is an example of a typical recording sheet.

Table 20.1 Example of a chart for recording challenging behaviour[a]

Behaviour recording chart			
Name:_____ Date of Birth:_____		Date:_____ Target Behaviour:_____ _____	
Setting:_____			
Date Time Place	**Antecedents**	**Behaviour**	**Consequences**
	* What was the person doing immediately before the behaviour? * Who was present? * What were they doing?	* What exactly did the person do? * For how long did did it last?	* What did the person do immediately after the behaviour? * Who else was present? * What did they do?

[a] The details of each occurrence of a target challenging behaviour is recorded in order to identify frequency, timing, situation, antecedents, and consequences.

The first two columns give an idea of the frequency of the behaviour and whether there is any temporal pattern. The third column allows assessment of whether it occurs in a particular location. The remaining three columns are designed to obtain a description of the behaviour itself and its surrounding circumstances. This then permits a functional analysis of the behaviour. This entails reaching some understanding of the relative contributions to the presentation of the behaviour of triggering events (Antecedents) and reinforcers (Consequences). Once this is reached, a hypothesis can be formed about the activation and maintenance of the behaviour, the unmet need it expresses, and an intervention can be implemented to modify the behaviour. If the behaviour is largely antecedent driven it is often relatively easy to modify or eliminate the triggering stimuli.

Case 1 provides a good example of this.

Case 1

Background

Mr A was a resident in a home for the elderly and was in the moderate-to-severe stages of Alzheimer's disease. He was referred following an incident during the night whereby he assaulted two members of staff in the corridor outside his room with a fire extinguisher.

On interviewing the staff it transpired the aggressive act had taken place when staff had confronted Mr A about urinating in a corner of the corridor. Subsequent recordings indicated that Mr A regularly urinated in the corridor during the night and was only ever aggressive within that context if prevented or interrupted by staff. The target behaviour to be modified was therefore urination in the corridor.

Functional analysis

Antecedent	Leaves bedroom
Behaviour	Urinates in corridor
Consequences	Urge to urinate met

Intervention

The key to eliminating the behaviour lay in understanding why Mr A left his room when he had the urge to urinate, particularly as it contained an en suite toilet. Examination of his room indicated that when Mr A rose from his bed to approach the toilet the door directly in front of him was the exit door to the corridor. The door to the toilet was at a 45 degree angle to this off to the right. The hypothesis was that Mr A was not spotting the toilet door. It was recommended that the toilet door should be left ajar with the light on and that a sign saying 'Toilet' with an indicating arrow should be attached to the exit door. This was done and the behaviour ceased.

Mr A is an example where a simple modification of an environmental factor antecedent to a behaviour can lead to its elimination. Sometimes recordings indicate that there are no obvious antecedents or consequences associated with the behaviour. In these circumstances the antecedent may be internal and biochemically associated with the pathological processes of dementia. In such cases a pharmacological intervention is often indicated. However when it is thought that the behaviour, for example screaming, is a form of self-stimulation, it may be reduced by providing other forms of stimulation.

Observations and recordings of challenging behaviour often reveal that it is the consequences of the behaviour that are maintaining its presentation. Operant conditioning theory indicates that the behaviour is rewarding in that it satisfies a need and therefore has a reinforcing outcome. Full accounts of this theory and its applications in behaviour modification are contained in Bandura (1970) and Blackman (1973). Martin and Pear (1988) gives a practical description and Perrin (1996) provides a concise account with good case examples.

In brief, there are two types of reinforcement: positive and negative. Positive reinforcement increases the likelihood of a behaviour occurring. Common examples are social contact and material/consumable gain. Need for social contact is often the genesis for challenging behaviour in badly run nursing homes. Positive reinforcement can also consist of the removal of a noxious stimulus. For example, consider a wheelchair bound male resident in a home who is hypersensitive to sound. Every time he is wheeled into the day room he starts shouting and banging his fists. In order not to disturb the other residents he is removed from the room and the behaviour ceases. The day room contains a television set which is set at a high volume. His behaviour serves to remove him from a noxious stimulus.

In contrast to positive, negative reinforcement decreases the frequency of a behaviour. It consists of the presentation of an aversive stimulus, for example physical punishment or reprimand, or the removal of positive reinforcement, for example 'time out' or denial of material/consumable objects. As a method of intervention it is ethically questionable and is of dubious therapeutic efficacy. It is also clearly open to abuse unintentionally or otherwise.

Case 2 provides a typical example of how two different forms of positive reinforcement interact in a care setting to maintain challenging behaviour.

Case 2

Background

Mrs D was a resident in a nursing home. She was suffering from a vascular dementia in a mild-to-moderate form. She was referred for high frequency calling out at night. Baseline recording on one night showed 27 episodes. Mrs D acknowledged her behaviour, but could not give an explanation for it. Interviews with the staff indicated that they responded very quickly to her calls.

Functional analysis

Antecedent	Mrs D wakes up
Behaviour	She calls out
Consequences	She gains immediate social contact

Mrs D's calling out is therefore being rewarded with rapid positive reinforcement. However another chain of positive reinforcement is also operating:-

Antecedent	Staff hear calls and worry about other residents waking
Behaviour	They respond as quickly as possible to prevent others waking
Consequences	Mrs D immediately quietens

Staff are therefore rewarded for responding as quickly as possible to Mrs D. A vicious circle of dual positive reinforcement had been constructed which had served to escalate the frequency of the challenging behaviour .

Intervention

Further observation by staff showed that Mrs D was awake for most of the night. A programme was set up to keep her active and awake during the day (this was only very minimally successful) and a behavioural programme was instigated at night. Clearly social contact had a calming effect on Mrs D. The idea was to initially give her social contact at a higher frequency than her calling out and then to progressively fade this out.

Within a week her calling out had fallen off markedly and from at first holding her hand every 15 minutes, staff were only looking into her room every half hour.

The above account serves to outline the bare bones of the behavioural approach to the management of challenging behaviour. In clinical practice most cases are more complex than the above two and the need for a multidisciplinary assessment cannot be stressed enough as a means to tease out the various factors at work behind the behaviour.

In the broader context, over the course of the past decade dementia management in general is moving from a largely biomedically focused model of care towards an approach with its roots in social psychology. The person-centred approach advocated by Kitwood and his colleagues (Kitwood 1997; Kitwood and Bredin 1992) has, at its procedural heart, rigorous behavioural observation. However, this is within the context of emphasizing the importance of viewing challenging behaviour more as a response to a 'malignant' social or psychological environment, rather than as an inevitable product of incremental brain pathology. Stokes (1996) has made a start at providing an integrative framework for the management of challenging behaviour within the person-centred approach.

Much can be taken from the behavioural approach and applied to the management of challenging behaviour in early onset dementia. However it works at its best with persons with moderate-to-severe cognitive decline within a residential setting. There are limitations to its applicability to a younger person living at home in the early stages of a dementia. This is especially the case in sufferers with a non-cognitive presentation.

The most likely challenging behaviours exhibited by a younger person in the early stages of AD are repetitive questioning and importuning behaviour. This results directly from the initial loss of short-term memory (STM) and is often an indirect result of associated anxiety. The task here for the clinician is to reduce the behaviour by constructing a 'safe' psychological environment for the sufferer through memory and anxiety management. Wilson and Moffat (1992) give a broad overview of memory management and many of the techniques can be applied to circumvent or alleviate difficulties encountered in the early stages of dementia. Clare and Wilson (1997) have produced a self-help manual which carers and sufferers can use to ease many of the problems caused by memory impairment. Many of the techniques of anxiety management (Clark 1989) are readily applicable in the early stages of AD.

The relatively high prevalence of FTD in younger dementia sufferers suggests that the management of any challenging behaviour associated with this dementia will be a major focus within early onset dementia care. Over the past decade several studies have documented the characteristics of the early stages of FTD and contrasted them with those of AD. Whilst AD sufferers present with deficits in memory, language, and construction, those with FTD show deterioration in personality, social behaviour, and executive functioning (Cummings and Benson 1992). Whilst some doubts exist regarding how easy it is to distinguish neuropsychological characteristics between the two patient groups (Pachana *et al.* 1996), there seems to be a consensus within the literature that FTD patients are more likely to present with behavioural or psychiatric disturbance rather than with the cognitive decline associated with Alzheimer's disease (Gregory and Hodges 1996).

Sometimes the behavioural disturbance can be quite severe. Miller *et al.* (1997) described a group of 22 FTD patients of whom almost one-half exhibited aggressive and antisocial behaviours such as physical assault, theft, offensive language, and public urination and masturbation. In contrast only one of 22 AD patients described exhibited such behaviour.

Table 20.2 Types of challenging behaviour often seen in frontotemporal dementia

Perseveration
Distractability
Disinhibition
Apathy
Utilization behaviour
Obsessionality

Miller *et al.* (1997) argue that the aberrant behaviours found in their FTD patients are a result of regional alterations in brain function which predisposes them to conduct themselves in a completely alien way to lifelong behaviour patterns. This is in contrast to challenging behaviour in Alzheimer's disease where, as discussed above, the behaviour is more likely to be multi-factorial in origin. Even one of the most vociferous advocates of social causes of behaviour in dementia acknowledges the direct link between challenging behaviour and frontal pathology (Kitwood 1997).

The quality of the challenging behaviour often present in FTD is different to AD. It rarely presents as a learned communication of unmet need. Instead the behaviour appears to be the result of release from, or loss of, executive control. It is often accompanied by a loss of insight (Gregory and Hodges 1996) and empathy (Eslinger 1998). Those living with the sufferer often fail to appreciate the implications of loss of insight. They often perceive the behaviour as deliberate and, when reasoning fails, think the sufferer to be callous. In addition to straining the carer/sufferer interpersonal relationship, the carer loses a sense of control over the situation. A start can be made by instilling a sense of control through educating the carer about the nature of FTD. This is necessary prior to commencement of any intervention. Types of challenging behaviour commonly found in FTD are listed in Table 20.2.

A major task for the clinician in the management of early onset dementia is therefore likely to be the reduction or elimination of challenging behaviour in FTD sufferers. A theoretical framework within which to undertake this task can incorporate learning theory, but must venture beyond it into the realms of neurorehabilitation (Eslinger *et al.* 1996), cognitive neuropsychology (Morris 1996), and cognitive therapy (Beck 1976). Within this lies the prospect of exploiting the patient's relatively intact memory and manipulating deficits for therapeutic gain. Case 3 illustrates an intervention which combines learning theory with positive use of behavioural deficit.

Case 3

Background

Mrs E lived at home with her husband. Her mobility was limited due to multiple sclerosis. She constantly complained about a pain in her left hand. Repeated demands were made on her husband to medicate and call in the medical services. No physical cause for the pain was discovered. Observations of her behaviour at home indicated there was a large anxiety component associated with her calling out and that there was a perseverative aspect to it.

Functional analysis

Antecedent	Anxiety through perception of pain
Behaviour	Calling on husband to attend
Consequences	Attention by husband relieves anxiety

Intervention

Mr E's ability to cope with his wife became so severely strained that she was admitted to the local psychiatric hospital. It was noted on the ward that Mrs E was highly distractable. An intervention was constructed whereby as soon as she began to call out she was given a magazine and engaged in conversation about it. Mrs E then continued to read the magazine until distracted by something else. She was discharged home with the recommendation to her husband that he should use distraction to halt his wife's calling out.

Case 3 demonstrates exploitation of distractability in managing behavioural disturbance. It is one of the most often recommended methods for tackling perseverative behaviour. Anecdotes abound about sufferers being distracted to a jigsaw which they then spend hours perseveratively completing.

Utilization behaviour or the environmental dependency syndrome (Lhermitte 1986) could also be exploited in the management of challenging behaviour. This syndrome is characterized by an excessive dependence upon environmental cues to the extent that the patient appears to lose personal autonomy. The therapeutic implication is that antisocial behaviour could be switched off by restructuring the environment. It could be argued that Case 3 became almost clinically obsessed with the perceived pain and obsessive compulsive disorder is described in FTD (Tonkonogy *et al.* 1994). Case 4 demonstrates the use of cognitive behaviour therapy (Salkovskis and Kirk 1989) in the elimination of a challenging behaviour which was the result of obsessional thinking about contamination and harm.

Case 4

Background

Mr B was a man in his fifties who had been diagnosed with FTD some three years prior to referral. Before this diagnosis he had been thought to have been suffering from OCD.

He was referred because his wife's ability to cope with him at home was at breaking point. He was systematically destroying the large bungalow in which they lived. He refused to go out of the house and he was rude and offensive to family and visitors.

Discussion with Mrs B revealed that in the previous two weeks he had attempted to demolish a ceiling and had stripped the kitchen walls of tiles. He had also ordered his daughter and family to leave the house during an evening meal. He had a history of some years of ordering objects in the environment and of compulsive cleanliness. Mr B speech was rambling and occasionally anomic. He claimed his memory was often vague, but he could give an account of his recent behaviour. He stated that he had attempted to demolish the ceiling after observing a crack in it. He knew his grandchildren were visiting imminently and he became concerned that the ceiling might collapse on them. He therefore attempted to remove it. Concern over potential harm to the grandchildren featured in his other behaviour. He had noticed a blemish on a kitchen tile and became concerned that the tiles might be contaminated and that the children might be harmed. During the evening meal, he had vague, non-specific anxieties about impending harm to the children if they remained in the house. The only way to alleviate this fear was for the children to leave.

Functional analysis

A functional analysis of the incident with the kitchen tiles is:-

Antecedent	Notices blemish which elicits anxiety about contamination
Behaviour	Immediate removal of contaminated objects
Consequences	Reduction in anxiety

In other words Mr B had learned to reduce anxiety by compulsive behaviour.

Intervention

Mr B presented as quite an anxious person in general , therefore he was taught anxiety management in the form of relaxation. However an intervention was needed to target the link between the antecedent and the behaviour. This took the form of thought stopping (Salkovskis and Kirk 1989). This technique consists of using a startle response to break a chain of thought. Mr B was instructed to wear an elastic band on his wrist. When he noticed a potentially harmful or contaminating stimulus he was told to pull and release the band rapidly and then to go immediately to the kitchen and turn on the radio. This intervention was successful in eliminating his destructive behaviour and reduced his cleaning and ordering.

The thought stopping technique was also applied to his social behaviour. He used the band whenever he felt he was about to make some offensive remark. There was only partial success with the technique in this instance. It could be speculated that this was because the mechanism behind the behaviour was more disinhibition rather than obsessionality and therefore lacked the intervening stage of cognition which thought stopping targets.

Difficulties with social self-regulation in FTD occur along a continuum ranging from apathy to disinhibition. The latter involves decreased or absent appreciation for interpersonal boundaries and difficulty in inhibiting impulsive responses in social contexts. Case 5 illustrates a cognitive behavioural intervention for disinhibition.

Case 5

Background

Mr C was a man in his late fifties with a recent diagnosis of FTD. His wife had been unable to cope with his sexual disinhibition towards her and other women. Consequently at the time of referral Mr C was living in a residential home. His disinhibited behaviour continued in the home and was directed at all female staff, residents, and visitors. Mr C was both verbally and physically sexually disinhibited. This was causing great concern and the staff were perplexed because Mr C would always remember his behaviour later and apologize for it. Since there was perceived to be a deliberate element to the behaviour Mr C was increasingly alienated and isolated.

At interview Mr C acknowledged his challenging behaviour. He could describe recent incidents and was extremely remorseful. He did not want to engage in such behaviour and stated that it gave him no gratification.

Functional analysis

Mr C's challenging behaviour did not fit fully into the ABC framework since the consequences appeared irrelevant to the maintenance of the behaviour. There seemed to be a direct link between the antecedent and the behaviour:-

Antecedent   Sight or close proximity of a female
Behaviour   Physical and verbal sexual behaviour

Intervention

The key to intervention lay in breaking the link between antecedent and behaviour. The sexual behaviour was unregulated internally and directly released in a reflex fashion. An attempt was made to devise a system of external regulation.

In anxiety management the use of self-control statements is commonplace (Clark 1989). In extreme cases, where in some situations the anxiety can become so overwhelming that the person forgets the self-control statements, flashcards with written statements are used. Mr C was asked to generate statements which he might use to control sexual behaviour. These were the written out on cards. Mr C was asked to carry one with him at all times and two were strategically placed in his room. All female staff were issued with cards and a programme was set up whereby staff were requested to increase their visual and proximal contact with Mr C. He was asked to refer to a card the moment he caught sight of a female and staff were asked to present a card to him at arm's length.

There was an immediate and dramatic reduction in the challenging behaviour.

Cases 3, 4, and 5 were seen in routine clinical practice by one of the authors (S. L.), and in the absence of hard data are anecdotal. Few clearly documented interventions exist. There is a need for good case studies to advance our knowledge about how to intervene and manage challenging behaviour in FTD. In this regard much can be learned from the neurorehabilitation literature. For example, Yuen (1997) describes a training programme for a man with a 20 year history of frontal pathology who was verbally and physically aggressive. Underlying this behaviour were deficits in interpersonal skills, the primary one being negative verbal expression towards others. The intervention consisted of a positive talk programme with a therapist using modelling and role-playing techniques. This was incorporated into a programme of social skills training. After four weeks the patient was able to make positive statements whenever he was given prompts and a generalized improvement in social behaviour followed. This is a good example of how achieving an understanding of the deficits that influence a patient's behaviour can lead to the design of an appropriate treatment plan.

Whilst the concept of rehabilitation seems contrary to the process of dementia, it can be argued that much can be learned from it and applied to the management of the types of challenging behaviours seen in FTD. Certainly theoretical frameworks are emerging with the potential for guiding the search for effective assessment and management methods.

Clinical experience suggests that perhaps the most concerning challenging behaviour to carers is antisocial behaviour. Eslinger *et al.* (1995) propose a model of social processes mediated by the frontal lobes within which the antisocial behaviours associated with FTD may be better understood. Central to the operation if this model is the concept of a social executor.

Figure 20.1 presents a model for analysing antisocial behaviour associated with FTD which is directly adapted from Eslinger *et al.*'s (1995) model for social behaviour following acquired injury to the frontal lobes. These authors argue that the frontal lobes operate as an executor of a complex functional system from which social behaviour emerges. When the frontal lobes are intact personality and social behaviour systems function in an organized and unique pattern for each person. However in a pathological state personality and social behaviour can become unregulated, disorganized, and fragmented resulting in behaviour that is inappropriate to the emotional state of the individual and the social context.

Eslinger *et al.*'s model of social executors includes processes that facilitate or obstruct the initiation and maintenance of meaningful and effective interpersonal relationships. The social

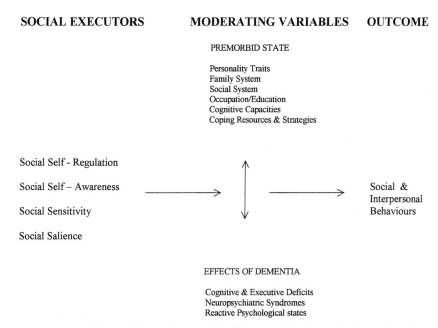

Figure 20.1 Summary of a model specifying several of the variables that underlie social and interpersonal impairments after cerebral damage. Adapted from Eslinger *et al.* (1995)

executors mediate how emotional and reactive states are expressed within the context of the individual's needs, goals, and social knowledge. Figure 20.1 indicates that the precise manner in which an impairment in this system is presented is moderated by the pre-morbid characteristics of the individual and the specific effects of the dementia.

The model includes four specific aspects of social and interpersonal behaviour.

Social self-regulation refers to the ability to manage the initiation, rate, intensity, and duration of social interaction. Problems with social self-regulation range from social withdrawal, through reduced appreciation of interpersonal boundaries, to difficulty in inhibiting impulses in social settings. The disinhibition described above in Case 5 is an example of dysfunctional social self-regulation.

Social self-awareness refers to having knowledge and insight about one's self in social situations. This involves the ability to accurately perceive one's own emotional state, to manage one's emotions, and to recognize the effect of one's behaviour on others. Deficits in social self-awareness lead to under or over estimations of the impact of social and emotional behaviour upon others.

Social sensitivity is the ability to take another person's point of view and to understand another's emotional state. Carers of FTD patients often describe the sufferer as showing a loss of empathy as indicated by insensitivity and self-centred behaviour. Eslinger *et al.* argue that this social executor closely resembles the construct of empathy.

Social salience is a composite of the cognitive, autonomic, and visceral processes that regulate somatic and emotional states. A deficit in this executor can result in reduced autonomic responsiveness to the social environment (Damasio *et al.* 1991) and an inability to share the emotional experiences of others. Eslinger *et al.* argue that a flattening of social salience will lead to all interpersonal and social stimuli having similar emotional values, thus preventing stimuli being assigned degrees of meaningfulness or social relevance. A result of this is the inability to learn from positive or negative social events.

Through applying Eslinger *et al.*'s model to the antisocial behaviour often found with FTD patients a much finer level of behavioural description can be obtained through detailed assessment of emotional processing and social cognition. This in turn should lead to innovative and more effective methods of management. Eslinger *et al.* (1995) provide example of the sorts of intervention strategies might be employed when deficits exist in particular social executors and suggest that these often need to be embedded within a more general psychotherapeutic program for interpersonal problems. With some interventions success will be determined by the degree of integrity of memory and cognition.

Suggested interventions in social self-regulation involve implementing external cueing systems and verbal mediation. For the disinhibited patient external cues are necessary to help inhibit behaviour, as was seen in the example of Case 5. In more apathetic or withdrawn patients a programme of time limited and focused periods of social exchange with interpersonal cueing is recommended.

Individual psychotherapy is advocated for reduced social awareness. This could then progress to carefully tailored group work in, for example, a day hospital setting.

Cognitive-behavioural techniques may have a role to play in the amelioration of reduced social sensitivity. Exercises in alternative thinking and problem solving could help the patient to begin to consider other perspectives in social encounters and help to bring about a challenge to any inaccurate perceptions of others. Role-playing activities could also be effective.

Eslinger *et al.* state that interventions for deficits in social salience are limited. They suggest encouraging the use of cognitive processes to make associations between emotion and social encounters as a means to guide interpersonal behaviour. Major developments are occurring in the study of the relationship between cognition and emotion (Teasdale and Barnard 1993; Power and

Dalgleish 1999) and these may help to guide management strategies for this executor. It is encouraging that Bender and Wainwright (1998) are applying Teasdale and Barnard's (1993) Interactive Cognitive Subsystems approach to the study of the role of emotion in the dementing process.

In order to capitalize on the neurorehabilitation framework and intervene successfully, new methods of assessment are necessary. These are emerging from studies that examine links between particular deficits in social behaviour and areas of pathology within the frontal lobe (e.g. Hornak *et al.* 1996; Stone *et al.* 1998). Hornak *et al.* (1996) describe a patient who could be said to be suffering from a deficit in social sensitivity. They developed procedures which finely dissected this, revealing that the patient had a severe impairment in identifying vocal emotion, but an intact ability to recognize facial expression. On the basis of this, strategies were devised to facilitate communication within the family.

Stone *et al.* (1998) describe procedures which can distinguish between deficits in emotional processing and impairments in social reasoning. These have been applied to FTD patients with a view to eventually developing new assessment tools (Gregory *et al.* in press). Studies such as these are a rich source of ideas for the clinician in the attempt to accurately describe the precise target behaviour and devise an appropriate intervention.

In the practical management of early onset dementia a major challenge for clinical services is the design and implementation of effective and ethically sound interventions for challenging behaviour. Much can be gained from the traditional, behavioural approach and its integration (Stokes 1996) into the person-centred approach (Kitwood 1997). However there are limitations in applying management strategies based solely on learning theory to sufferers of FTD, who represent a significant proportion of early onset sufferers (see Chapter 2) and who may present with disturbing antisocial behaviour within a family environment. It is necessary to venture beyond this and incorporate constructs and procedures from the fields of neurorehabilitation, cognitive neuropsychology and cognitive therapy.

3 Dementia and driving

Driving is a sophisticated skill requiring interacting cognitive, motor, and sensory functions; these include attention, memory, visuospatial skills, judgement and planning, motor co-ordination, good visual acuity, and ability to make and carry out rapid decisions. Healthy people undergo changes in some of these domains later in life, with studies showing reductions in dynamic visual acuity, reaction times, and divided attention (Ponds *et al.* 1988). It has also been shown that the healthy elderly do not necessarily recognize age related deficits in sensory abilities which are relevant to driving (Holland and Rabbitt 1991). Elderly drivers are involved in more accidents per distance travelled than middle-aged drivers, with accident rates resembling those of 15–25 year olds (OECD 1985; Evans 1988). Additionally drivers over the age of 65 are progressively more likely to be involved in fatal motor accidents than those aged 30–60 (Evans 1988). Research has shown that up to 70% of crashes are due primarily to human error (Treat 1980), and therefore as O'Neill *et al.* (1992) state it is paradoxical that in many European countries vehicles are routinely tested as they age, while their drivers are not.

3.1 Driving licence law in the UK

In the UK driving licences for private vehicles are issued until the age of 70 years and thereafter renewal occurs three-yearly by self-certification. At renewal the onus is on the individual to report both active relevant medical conditions and those that may become relevant with the passage of time. If, at any other time, the licence holder becomes aware that he or she is suffering from a disability he must inform the Driver and Vehicle Licensing Authority — DVLA (Medical Aspects of Fitness to Drive). If a licence is refused or revoked on medical grounds there is a right of appeal to a Magistrate Court in England or to a Sheriffs Court in Scotland.

Currently the guidelines published in 'Medical Aspects of Fitness to Drive' state that in general a patient able to attend to day-to-day needs, retaining adequate insight and judgement, and not disorientated in time or place may be fit to drive. In such cases a licence may be issued on a yearly basis with reassessment on each renewal. In doubtful cases assessment at a mobility centre may be required, and where serious doubt exists a medical adviser at the DVLA may require a test to be taken. This, on the face of it, seems straightforward, but in practice driving issues are often fraught with concerns for the patient, their families and friends, and clinicians.

Notification of a diagnosis of dementia to the DVLA may often be considerably more problematic than these guidelines suggest. For example, not all patients with early or even moderate dementia will necessarily have had a formal diagnosis of dementia made, nor need they be in contact with the medical services. Because of this, and because in many cases an individual may have limited insight into deficits in cognitive or functional abilities, self-declaration of a diagnosis of dementia or its associated problems may not be made. Driving issues in patients with frontal variant frontotemporal dementia, with its insidious onset, may be particularly problematic given the presenting features which often include impulsivity and poor judgement and planning, coupled with lack of insight (Gregory and Hodges 1996). Additionally younger patients with dementia may, in theory, pose more of a risk, being more likely to be involved in the transportation of family and often driving greater mileages.

What is known about the risks that patients with dementia pose when driving? While it is clear that individuals with advanced dementia undoubtedly have impaired driving skills, the relationship between driving skills and mild or moderate degrees of dementia or less common forms of dementia, such as the lobar atrophies, needs to be clarified. There are a number of retrospective studies that suggest that patients with dementia have higher rates of driving accidents. For example, O'Neill et al. (1992) studied a group of patients fulfilling DSM-IIIR criteria for dementia attending a memory disorders clinic and found that nearly 1/5 of patients with documented dementia continued to drive and that impaired driving ability had been noticed in two-thirds of these. Families reported great difficulty persuading patients to stop driving and had to invoke outside help in two-thirds. Nearly 50% of the patients studied became occasionally or regularly lost and 43% were involved in crashes before they ceased to drive. In a case-controlled study, Friedland et al. (1988) found that individuals with Alzheimer's disease were five times more likely to be involved in a motor vehicle accident than healthy age-matched controls and that 58% of the AD patients stopped driving only after an accident. In contrast, a study by Trobe et al. (1996), found that the crash rates of 99 patients with Alzheimer's disease was not significantly different compared to age- and sex-matched controls, although of course crash index remains a crude outcome.

It has been suggested that cognitive screening measures may be able to predict driving ability and identify individuals at risk, and as a consequence various neuropsychological measures have been studied in relation to driving. One of the most common screening tests for dementia used in clinical practice is the Mini-Mental State Examination (Folstein et al. 1975). On the whole research suggests that this is not a useful tool in predicting driving skills. O'Neill et al. (1992), found no correlation between the MMSE or a visuospatial task in a group of patients with impaired versus non-impaired driving skills, while in the same study there was a significant correlation between Activities of Daily Living and driving skills. Similarly, in a study by Fitten et al. (1995), the MMSE in isolation was unhelpful in distinguishing between those patients with dementia judged to have preserved driving ability, and those with diminished driving ability. However, in this same study, a combination of a task of memory search (Sternberg Memory Search), visual tracking, and the Mini-Mental State Examination, were found to account for two-thirds of the variance in driving score. In contrast a study by Fox *et al.* (1997) did identify the MMSE as a significant predictor of an on-the-road evaluation of driving skills. Other studies have examined more specific aspects of cognitive function such as attentional processing, for example aspects of visual attention (Duchek *et al.* 1998). In this study of individuals with very mild or mild dementia and healthy controls, visual search performance was predictive of performance in an on-the-road driving assessment over and above simple dementia severity. Carr *et al.* (1998) developed a two minute traffic sign test that successfully identified 74% of patients who had mild-to-moderate Alzheimer's disease, but misclassified 10% of patients as normal, although the authors did not look at whether failure on the traffic sign test was related to poor driving performance.

At face value a driving test would appear to offer a practical solution to this complex situation. However there are few prospective studies which have assessed on-the-road driving ability in dementia, and none which have looked at on-the-road driving skills of more unusual forms of dementing disorders. Fitten *et al.* (1995) found that patients with mild AD performed significantly worse on a road test than either a group of healthy control subjects or diabetic controls. Specifically the AD patients made more errors, for example driving into a road saying do not enter, particularly in the more complex part of the test. In a study by Hunt *et al.* (1997), 3% of healthy controls failed an on-the-road test, compared to 19% of a *very* mild AD group and 41% of a mild AD group. This also means of course, that 81% of very mild AD patients and 59% of mild AD patients *passed* the test. This suggests that there is a relationship between a diagnosis of dementia and its severity and impaired driving abilities as judged by these more 'real-life tests'. However the relationship is likely to be a complex one and does not help in determining at what point an individual becomes sufficiently impaired to cease driving.

Even on-the-road tests are not without their detractors. As Dobbs *et al.* (1998) state in their review, studies that have assessed driving performance have generally reported their findings in terms of pass or fail and have used small groups of patients, usually without control groups, thus making it difficult to judge whether errors made reflect a decline in competence related to the dementia, or are commonly made errors amongst experienced healthy elderly drivers. These workers emphasize that the conventional criteria used for licensing new drivers may well be inappropriate for license removal in experienced drivers.

It is important that researchers continue to address the important issue of driving and dementia and much work needs to be done. Many general and specific questions need to be answered. For instance, what level of risk should society accept in our elderly drivers with dementia, what is our cut-off to be? For any given individual, what factors should be taken into account and what weight should they be given; for example how should reports of safe driving from family member or the availability of a 'co-pilot' influence the decision about ability to drive? Can we improve on tests of general intellectual function or specific psychometric tests or aspects of processing to predict driving ability? Are on-the-road tests the best form of assessment? Do we know enough about driving performance in the healthy elderly to understand errors made during on-the-road tests in patients with dementia?

3.2 Practical management of driving issues

In practice, once a diagnosis of dementia is made and an assessment of the severity has taken place and discussed with the patient, the issue of driving should be discussed including views on the individuals driving ability from family members. The physician should remind the patient of his/her legal obligation to inform the DVLA. Families are often very concerned and may be helpful and supportive in encouraging the patient to give up their driving, but as the study by O'Neill *et al.* (1992) shows in a significant number of cases the patient may resist advice. Where the patient and family are not prepared to inform the DVLA, and the medical adviser is concerned that there will be serious consequences if the individual continues to drive, informing the DVLA directly of his or her concerns would be in 'accordance with the guidelines on professional confidence laid down by the General Medical Council' (Medical Aspects of Fitness to Drive). The Physician can point out to the patient that it is then DVLA medical adviser who makes a decision. In reality there is a circularity to this as the medical adviser may well ask for further information and a view from the referring clinician. DVLA assessment is becoming more sophisticated with moves towards reassessment of driving skills and regular review in some cases. In cases where a patient is unable to inform the DVLA due to the severity of the dementia, the medical adviser is advised to phone the DVLA without delay. In cases, where a licence has been revoked, and the patient is continuing to drive it may even be necessary to inform the police. In these difficult circumstances many practitioners may wish to discuss such decisions with colleagues, or a medical defence organization.

In some states in the USA, for example California, there is a mandate requiring the physician to submit a confidential report to the County Health Department when an individual is diagnosed as having a dementing disorder. This information is then forwarded to the Department of Motor Vehicles (DMV) which is authorized to take action against the driving privileges of any individual who is unable to safely operate a motor vehicle. The DMV has determined that only those people with mild dementia may continue to drive, and if a medical evaluation reports this to be the case the individual is asked to attend a re-examination with the DMV, consisting of both a written test on driving rules and an interview which concentrates on short-term and long-term memory of events. After a good performance in these areas a driving test is taken. Success in these areas generally means that the licence is not revoked but that restrictions are placed upon it, such as no freeway or night driving, and a limit placed upon the mileage that can be undertaken in a single journey. Regular review involving the same process is then undertaken six monthly or annually (California Department of Motor Vehicle 1993).

O'Neill *et al.* (1992) argue persuasively for a graded and flexible approach to the issue of driving in dementia, stating that an all or nothing scenario is limiting and stigmatizing to those in the early stages of the disease. This is likely to become increasingly important as more patients are diagnosed at an earlier stage of their illness.

Finally on a practical note, one study has shown that if an individual drives less than 4000 miles per year, the cost of taxis and public transport may well cost less than running and using a car (MCAP/AA working group).

4 Financial matters

Many families in this country, especially where financial affairs are simple, continue to manage the patient's affairs informally. However formal arrangements are important, in order to safeguard both the interests of the individual and the family. The particular type of legal arrangement will depend on whether the individual has capacity when legal arrangements are sought. If the patient has capacity (as defined below) to make decisions and issue instructions, then he/she may set up a power of attorney or an enduring power of attorney. For those patients who no longer have capacity, application to the Court of Protection is the appropriate way forward.

4.1 Capacity

Capacity is a legal question and ultimately it is the role of the court to decide whether an individual has capacity (BMA and Law Society 1995). However decisions about capacity, which do not ever reach court, are made on a regular basis by professionals who come into contact with patients with dementia, i.e. clinicians, solicitors, and social workers. It is a basic premise that all individuals are regarded as being competent and thus having capacity until proved otherwise. An individual is assumed to have capacity if there is an:

- ability to comprehend the information
- ability to retain and believe the information
- ability to form and express an opinion

Individuals who have capacity may decide to appoint another individual to manage his or her affairs by setting up a power of attorney or an enduring power of attorney. If an individual no longer has capacity through mental disorder and is no longer capable of managing their affairs then someone must apply on behalf of the patient to the Court of Protection in order that a receiver may be appointed to manage the affairs of that individual.

4.2 Enduring power of attorney

A power of attorney is a means whereby one person (the donor) gives legal authority to another person (the attorney) to manage his affairs. A power of attorney may be given to manage the individual's (donor's) affairs generally or may be limited to a specific task or tasks. There are two types of power of attorney. An ordinary power of attorney is automatically revoked by law if the donor loses his or her mental capacity. This tends to be used in situations where a capable adult is travelling or living abroad and wishes to have someone to temporarily manage their home affairs. This has little value when managing the affairs of dementia patients. An enduring power of attorney enables an individual to decide who should look after their affairs if/after they become mentally incapable. This Act came into existence in 1986, subsequently over 15 000 EPAs have been registered with the public trust office (BMA and Law Society 1995). The attorney must register the enduring power when the individual is no longer capable. Notice of intended registration of the enduring power registration must take place in a prescribed manner defined in the Act. This lays out the requirements of who must be informed, in what order, and by what means. Information regarding this is available from the Public Trust Office (see Appendix). The degree of capacity to create an enduring power of attorney has been tested legally with elements as outlined above.

Although the donor need not have the capacity to do the things which the attorney will do on their behalf they should understand that the attorney will be able to assume complete authority over the patient's affairs, and that the attorney will be able to do anything with the donors property that the donor might have done. Additionally, to have capacity to set up a power of attorney, the donor needs to understand that the power will continue if the donor should become mentally incapable and that if mentally incapable the power will be irrevocable without confirmation by the court of protection. The capacity to revoke an enduring power is said to require the same degree of understanding as that required to set it up. The enduring power does not take into account capacity to manage personal affairs or to make medical decisions, areas of considerable importance in patients with dementia. Recent recommendations have been made by the Law Commission that these areas be included in a new form of enduring power.

4.3 Court of Protection

The Court of Protection is an office of the Supreme Court and is described in the Mental Health Act 1983. Its judicial functions are carried out by judges nominated by the Lord Chancellor. It exists to protect the property and affairs of persons who through mental disorder are incapable of managing their own affairs. As stated above for an individual to become subject to a Court of Protection, it is necessary for the patient to be both suffering from a mental disorder and incapable of managing their own affairs. In these circumstances the Court of Protection nominates a receiver (e.g. family member, solicitor, etc.).The public trust office is responsible for the overall running of the patient's affairs alongside the receiver.

4.4 Testamentary capacity

The capacity to make a will is known as testamentary capacity and in English law requires that at the time of making a will the testator understands:
- the nature of the act (making a will) and its effects
- the extent of the property which is being left
- who might justifiably make claims upon that property

Important riders to this are that the testator (will-maker) is not under undue pressure from any other individual to make a particular will, and that no mental disorder exists which would interfere with the above requirements. After a will is made, subsequent illness or mental decline does not invalidate that will, for example a will made by a middle-aged adult would not be invalidated twenty years later even if the individual had developed a dementia. It is the persons capacity at the time of making the will that is important. Similar criteria also apply to the act of revoking a will.

4.5 Welfare benefits

Carers of people with dementia will require advice regarding welfare benefits that they may be entitled to. General advice regarding this may be obtained from the Citizens Advice Bureau, the Alzheimer's Disease Society, or from professionals with specialist knowledge, such as a social worker. This section of the chapter is not intended to be comprehensive, the benefits system is both complex and changes fairly frequently. However it is important that any clinician involved with dementia patients is at least aware of the kinds of benefits that are available and where to advise the individual to go in order to seek further information.

Benefits are broadly divided into those provided for the person with dementia and those available to the carer. Additionally, benefits may differ depending on whether the patient is under or over 65 years. Entitlement to benefits will also differ depending on whether National Insurance contributions have been paid, the amount of weekly income or savings, or on the practical effects of disability.

4.6 Attendance allowance and disability living allowances

These two benefits are determined by the effects of the disability and can be claimed by people who need help with personal care, or supervision to avoid danger, and are not determined by whether the person with dementia lives independently or with family. Individuals entitled to these benefits claiming before the age of 65 will receive disability living allowance which has a

Table 20.3 Levels of care for attendance allowances

	Attendance allowance
Lowest level	In need of help with personal care for some of the day.
Lower rate	In need of frequent help with personal care or supervision during the day or night.
Higher rate	In need of frequent help with personal care or continual supervision to avoid danger during the day and either help with personal care or supervision for a prolonged period or several times during the night.

component for care and for mobility, while those over the age of 65 receive attendance allowance. There are variable rates for both of these allowances depending on the degree of physical need the patient has. As an example a guide to the level of need which determines the rate of benefit when applying for attendance allowance, is shown in Table 20.3.

4.7 Invalid care allowance

This benefit is paid to carers who spend more than 35 hours per week looking after someone who is receiving either the attendance allowance at the higher or lower rates (but not the lowest) or the middle or higher rates of the disability living allowance. Carers have to be below the age of 65 when they first apply.

In summary, patients with dementia and their families may encounter a range of difficulties and problems which require expert advice. Of particular concern are issues related to behavioural disturbance and uncertainties related to driving skills. Although there is some data available to assist clinicians' advice in these areas, much work needs to be done. Younger patients and those with more unusual dementias such as FTD have particularly challenging problems, making multidisciplinary assessment an essential procedure.

5 Key points

1 Challenging behaviour is a major cause of carer stress and is an important issue for clinical services involved in dementia care.

2 Established procedures for the psychological management of challenging behaviour exist based on learning theory and the concept of unmet need.

3 These methods were developed for older people in the moderate/severe stages of Alzheimer's disease. Their applicability to younger persons, particularly those suffering from frontotemporal dementia is limited.

4 Appropriate management of challenging behaviour in early onset dementia needs a framework which includes constructs from learning theory, cognitive neuropsychology, and neurorehabilitation.

5 Although advanced dementia is undoubtedly associated with diminished driving abilities there is a more complex relationship between driving skills and more mild levels of dementia. Likely to become an increasingly important issue as patients are diagnosed earlier.

6 The Driving and Vehicle licensing authority requires that relevant medical conditions or those that may become relevant with time are reported to the DVLA.

7   Where there is a diagnosis of mild dementia the DVLA may allow retention of driving license following further reports or assessment at a mobility centre.

8   The best means of identifying those patients with dementia who have impaired driving skills has not been established.

Appendix

Public Trust Office, Protection Division, Stewart House, 24 Kingsway, London WC2B 6JX, UK.
Alzheimer's Disease Society, Gordon House, 10 Greencoat Place, London SW1P 1PH, UK.
info@alzheimers.org.uk

References

Bandura, A. (1970). *Principles of behaviour modification*. Holt Rinehart Winston.

Beck, A. (1976). *Cognitive therapy and the emotional disorders*. International Universities Press.

Bender, M. P. and Wainwright, A. (1998). Dementia: Reversing out of the dead end. *PSIGE Newsletter*, **66**, 22–4.

Blackman, D. (1973). *Operant conditioning: an experimental analysis of behaviour*. Methuen.

BMA and The Law Society. (1995). *Assessment of mental capacity: Guidance for doctors and lawyers*. British Medical Association.

California Department of Motor Vehicles. (1993). *DMVI's Policies for evaluating persons reported with dementia*. Published by Department of Motor Vehicles.

Carr, D. B., LaBarge, E., Dunnigan, K., and Storandt, M. (1998). Differentiating drivers with dementia of the Alzheimer's type from healthy older persons with a traffic sign naming test. *Journal of Gerontology*, **53**, 135–9.

Clare, L. and Wilson, B. A. (1997). *Coping with memory problems: a guide. People with memory impairments and their relatives and friends*. Thames Valley Test Company.

Clark, D. (1989). Anxiety states: Panic and generalised anxiety. In *Cognitive behaviour therapy for psychiatric problems. A practical guide* (ed. K. Hawton, P. M. Salkovskis, J. Kirk, and D. M. Clark). Oxford Medical Publications.

Cummings, J. L. and Benson, D. F. (1992). *Dementia: a clinical approach*. Butterworth–Heinemann.

Damasio, A. R., Tranel, D., and Damasio, H. C. (1991). Somatic markers and the guidance of behaviour: Theory and preliminary testing. In *Frontal lobe function and dysfunction* (ed. H. S. Levin, H. M. Eisenberg, and A. L. Benton), pp. 217–29. Oxford University Press.

Dobbs, A. R., Heller, R. B., and Schoplocher, D. (1998). A comparative approach to identify unsafe older drivers. *Journal of Accident Analysis and Previews*, **30**, 363–70.

Driver and Vehicle Licensing Agency. (1996). *Medical aspects of fitness to drive*. DVLA.

Duchek, J. M., Hunt, L., Ball, K., Buckles, V., and Morris, J. C. (1998). Attention and driving performance in Alzheimer's disease. *Journal of Gerontology*, **53**, 130–41.

Durand, V. M. and Crimmins, D. B. (1988). Identifying the variables maintaining self-injurious behaviour. *Journal of Autism and Developmental disorders*, **18**, 99–117.

Eslinger, P. J. (1998). Neurological and neuropsychological bases of empathy. *European Neurology*, **39**, 193–9.

Eslinger, P. J., Grattan, L. M., and Geder, L. (1995). Impact of frontal lobe lesions on rehabilitation and recovery from acute brain injury. *NeuroRehabilitation*, **5**, 161–82.

Eslinger, P. J., Grattan, L. M., and Geder, L. (1996). Neurologic and neuropsychologic aspects of frontal lobe impairments in postconcussive syndrome. In *Head injury and postconcussive syndrome* (ed. M. Rizzo and D. Tranel), pp. 415–40. Churchill Livingstone.

Evans, L. (1988). Older driver involvement in fatal and severe traffic crashes. *Journal of Gerontology*, **43**, 186–93.

Fitten, L. J., Perryman, K. M., Wilkinson, C. J., Little, R. J., Burns, M. M., Pachana, N., *et al.* (1995). Alzheimer and vascular dementias and driving: A prospective road and laboratory study. *Journal of the American Medical Association*, **273**, 1360–5.

Folstein, M. F., Folstein, S. E., and McHugh, P. R. (1975). Mini-Mental state: A practical method for grading the cognitive state of patients for the clinician. *Journal of Psychiatric Research*, **12**, 189–98.

Fox, G. K., Bowden, S. C., Bashford, G. M., and Smith, D. S. (1997). Alzheimer's disease and driving: Prediction and assessment of driving performance. *Journal of the American Geriatric Society*, **45**, 949–53.

Friedland, R. P., Koss, E., Kumar, A., Gaine, S., Meltzer, D., Haxby, J. V., *et al.* (1988). Motor vehicle crashes in dementia of the Alzheimer type. *Annals of Neurology*, **24**, 782–6.

Gregory, C. A. and Hodges, J. R. (1996). Dementia of Frontal Type: Use of consensus criteria and prevalence of psychiatric symptoms. *Neuropsychiatry, Neuropsychology and Behavioural Neurology*, **9**, 145–53.

Gregory, C. A., Lough, S., Stone, V. E., Baron-Cohen, S. and Hodges, J. R., (in press). Is theory of mind disproportionately impaired in patients with frontal variant fronto-temporal dementia: theoretical and practical implications. *Brain*.

Gilleard, C. J., Belford, H., Gilleard, E., Whittick, J. E., and Gledhill, A. (1984). Emotional distress among the supporters of the elderly mentally infirm. *British Journal of Psychiatry*, **145**, 172–7.

Holland, C. A. and Rabbitt, P. M. A. (1991). Peoples awareness of age related sensory and cognitive deficits and the implications for road safety. *Journal of Applied Cognitive Psychology*, **5**, 464–479.

Hope, R. A. (1992). Behaviour and personality change in dementia. In *Dementia and normal ageing* (ed. F. A. Huppert, C. Brayne, and D. W. O'Conner). Cambridge University Press.

Hope, P. A. and Pattel, V. (1993). Assessment of behavioural phenomena in dementia. In *Ageing and dementia: a methodological approach* (ed. A. Burns), pp. 221–36. Edward Arnold.

Hornak, J., Rolls, E. T., and Wade, D. (1996). Face and voice expression identification in patients with emotional and behavioural changes following ventral frontal lobe damage. *Neuropsychologia*, **34**, 247–61.

Hunt, L., Carr, D., Duchek, J. M., Grant, E., Buckles, V., and Morris, J. C. (1997). Reliability of the Washington University road test: A performance based assessment for drivers with dementia of the Alzheimer type. *Archives of Neurology*, **57**, 702–12.

Kitwood, T. (1997). *Dementia reconsidered*. Open University Press.

Kitwood, T. and Bredin, K. (1992). Towards a theory of dementia care: personhood and well-being. *Ageing and Society*, **12**, 269–87.

Lhermitte, F. (1986). Human autonomy and the frontal lobes. Part II: Patient behaviour in complex and social situations: The 'environmental dependency syndrome'. *Annals of Neurology*, **19**, 335–43.

Martin, G. and Pear, J. (1988). *Behaviour modification: what it is and how to do it*. Prentice–Hall.

MCAP/AA working group. (1990). *Helping the older driver*. The Medical Commission on Accident Prevention and the Automobile Association.

Miller, B. L., Darby, A., Benson, F., Cummings, J. L., and Miller, M. H. (1997). Aggressive, socially disruptive and anti-social behaviour associated with fronto-temporal dementia. *British Journal of Psychiatry*, **170**, 150–4.

Morris, R. G. (1996). *The cognitive neuropsychology of Alzheimer's disease*. Oxford University Press.

O'Neill, D. O., Neubauer, K., Boyle, M., and Gerrard, J. (1992). Dementia and driving. *Journal of the Royal Society of Medicine*, **85**, 199–202.

O'Neill, R. E., Horner, R. H., Albin, R. W., Storey, K., and Sprague, J. R. (1990). *Functional analysis of problem behaviour: a practical assessment guide*. Sycamore Publishing Company.

Organisation for economic co-operation and development. (1985). Traffic safety of elderly road users. OECD, Paris.

Pachana, N. A., Boone, K. B., Miller, B. L., Cummings, J. L., and Berman, N. (1996). Comparison of neuropsychological functioning in Alzheimer's disease and frontotemporal dementia. *Journal of the International Neuropsychological Society*, **2**, 505–10.

Pearlin, L. I., Mullan, J. T., Semple, S. J., and Skaff, M. M. (1990). Caregiving and the stress process: an overview of concepts and their measures. *Gerontologist*, **30**, 583–94.

Perrin, T. (1996). *Problem behaviour and the care of elderly people*. Winslow Press.

Ponds, R. W., Brouwer, W. H., and van Woeffelaar, P. C. (1988). Age differences in divided attention in a simulated driving task. *Journal of Gerontology*, **43**, 151–6.

Power, M. J. and Dalgleish, T. (1999). Two routes to emotion: Some implications of multi-level theories of emotion for therapeutic practice. *Behaviuoral and Cognitive Psychotherapy*, **27**, 129–41.

Salkovskis, P. M. and Kirk, J. (1989). Obsessional disorders. In *Cognitive behaviour therapy for psychiatric problems. A practical guide* (ed. K. Hawton, P. M. Salkovskis, J. Kirk, and D. M. Clark). Oxford Medical Publications.

Silver, J. M. and Yudofsky, S. C. (1987). Documentation of aggression in assessment of the violent patient. *Psychiatric Annals*, **17**, 375–84.

Skinner, B. F. (1953). *Science and human behaviour*. Macmillan.

Stokes, G. (1996). Challenging behaviour in dementia: A psychological approach. In *Handbook of clinical psychology of ageing* (ed. R. T. Woods). John Wiley and Sons.

Stone, V. E., Baron-Cohen, S., and Knight, R. T. (1998). Frontal lobe contributions to theory of mind. *Neuropsychologia*, **34**, 247–61.

Teasdale, J. and Barnard, P. (1993). *Affect, cognition and change*. Erlbaum.

Tonkonogy, J. M., Smith, T. W., and Barreira, P. J. (1994). Obsessive-compulsive disorders in Pick's disease. *Journal of Neuropsychiatry and Clinical Neurosciences*, **6**, 176–80.

Treat, J. R. (1980). A study of precrash factors involved in traffic accidents. *HSRI Research Review*, **10**, 1–35.

Trobe, J. D., Waller, P. F., Cook-Flannagan, C. A., Teshima, S. M., and Bieliauskas, L. A. (1996). Crashes and violations among drivers with Alzheimer's disease. *Archives of Neurology*, **53**, 411–16.

Wattis, J. and Martin, C. (1986). *Practical psychiatry of old age*. Chapman and Hall.

Wilson, B. A. and Moffat, N. (1992). *Clinical management of memory problems*. Chapman and Hall.

Yuen, H. K. (1997). Positive talk training in an adult with traumatic brain injury. *The American Journal of Occupational Therapy*, **51**, 780–3.

Index

Note: References to figures are indicated by 'f' and references to tables are indicated by 't' when they fall on a page not covered by the text reference. Plates are indicated by bold font.